OTHER PMIC TITLES OF INTEREST

CODING AND REIMBURSEMENT TITLES

Collections Made Easy!
CPT & HCPCS Coding Made Easy!
CPT Coding Guides by Medical Specialty
CPT Plus! Coders Choice®
DRG Plus!
E/M Coding Made Easy!
Getting Paid for What You Do
HCPCS Coders Choice®,
Health Insurance Carrier Directory
HIPAA Compliance Manual
ICD-9-CM, Coders Choice®,
ICD-9-CM Coding for Physicians' Offices
ICD-9-CM Coding Made Easy!
ICD-9-CM, Home Health Edition
Medical Fees in the United States
Medicare Compliance Manual
Medicare Rules & Regulations
Physicians Fee Guide
Reimbursement Manual for the Medical Office

PRACTICE MANAGEMENT TITLES

Accounts Receivable Management for the Medical Practice
Achieving Profitability With a Medical Office System
Encyclopedia of Practice and Financial Management
Managed Care Organizations
Managing Medical Office Personnel
Marketing Strategies for Physicians
Medical Marketing Handbook
Medical Office Policy Manual
Medical Practice Forms
Medical Practice Handbook
Medical Staff Privileges
Negotiating Managed Care Contracts
Patient Satisfaction
Performance Standards for the Laboratory
Professional and Practice Development
Promoting Your Medical Practice
Starting in Medical Practice
Working With Insurance and Managed Care Plans

Dictionary of Coding and Billing Terminology

PMIC

ISBN 978-1-57066-525-7

Practice Management Information Corporation

4727 Wilshire Boulevard Los
Angeles, California 90010
http://www.pmiconline.com

Printed in the China

FOREWORD

The *Dictionary of Coding and Billing Terminology* is a comprehensive reference designed for medical coders, billing professionals, HIPAA compliance staff, and third party payers.

The reference includes definitions of coding, billing, compliance, procedural and diagnostic words, terms, phrases, acronyms, eponyms and abbreviations. The reference includes:

- Introduction to medical terminology prefixes and suffixes and root words.
- Full-color anatomical illustrations
- Definitions of surgical, diagnostic and medical services and procedures from the CPT® coding system
- Definitions of illnesses, injuries, signs, symptoms and conditions from the ICD-9-CM coding system
- Definition of equipment and supplies from the HCPCS coding system
- Definitions of CMS and HIPAA common terms

As experienced coders know, and beginning coders quickly learn, in-depth knowledge of medical terminology is essential to the coding process. While there are numerous medical dictionaries available, these references do not specifically address the needs of medical coders and billers. As a result, coders frequently have to research terminology, coding, and compliance definitions from different resources.

The Dictionary of Coding and Billing Terminology provides definitions to the most common coding, compliance, coverage, reimbursement and terminology words, terms and phrases encountered by medical coding and billing personnel. The reference includes definitions for over 7,500 words, terms, phrases, abbreviations, acronyms and eponyms.

James B. Davis, Publisher

DISCLAIMER

This publication is designed to offer definitions of medical words, terms, phrases, acronyms, eponyms and abbreviations covering the coding and billing of medical services, supplies and procedures using the CPT, HCPCS, MS-DRG, CDT and ICD-9-CM coding systems, and selected definitions of Medicare and HIPAA terms. The information presented is based on a thorough review of the CPT, HCPCS, MS-DRG, CDT and ICD-9-CM coding systems, information obtained from official U.S. government resources, and the experience and interpretations of the editors. Though all of the information has been carefully researched and checked for accuracy and completeness, neither the editor nor the publisher accept any responsibility or liability with regard to errors, omissions, misuse or misinterpretation.

CONTENTS

INTRODUCTION

Coding based on medical terminology is the *language* of medical billing and reimbursement. Fluency in this language is required for all medical personnel involved in the processes of billing for medical services, chart abstracting, coding, medical transcription, and reimbursement management.

If the medical practice insurance billing staff is not fluent in this language, the practice will not receive the reimbursement it deserves and audit liability will increase. If hospital coders and patient accounting personnel are not fluent in this language, the hospital will not be paid properly and likewise may find itself with higher audit liability. If health insurance company claims processing personnel are not fluent in this language, claims processing errors may be made which result in improper denial or low payment of claims, or improper payment or overpayment of claims.

Medical nomenclature is an evolving language. New words, phrases, acronyms, eponyms, and abbreviations appear frequently as diseases and illnesses are discovered or understood more clearly, new diagnostic and operative procedures are developed, and new technology is implemented. While the fundamentals of the nomenclature are easy after the basics have been mastered, the constant additions requires regular review and updates of medical terminology resources.

WHAT IS MEDICAL CODING?

Medical coding refers to any set of codes used to encode data elements, such as tables of terms, medical concepts, medical diagnostic codes, or medical procedure codes. This includes both the codes and their descriptions.

Medical coding provides universal definition and recognition of diagnoses, procedures and level of care that allows sharing of information among physicians, hospitals, other health care providers and health insurance companies.

Coding is important not only as a method of transmitting information about what medical services were provided and why they were done, but also because it is the basis for reimbursement for these services, as well as a method of measuring appropriateness and quality of care. Coding errors, defined as documentation errors in which a treatment is miscoded or the codes used to describe procedures do not match those used to identify the diagnosis, cost health care providers billions of dollars annually.

But medical coding is also the process of translating words and phrases that describe medical procedures and diagnoses into numeric or alpha-numeric codes that are recorded in computer systems and on health insurance claim forms.

When the code is selected and posted, the code by itself defines the medical procedure, supply or diagnosis.

But we humans do not converse in codes. So in order to code properly, we must learn and understand human anatomy, physiology, and medical terminology as well as understanding the words, terms and phrases of the various medical coding systems. Add to that the numerous administrative and management words, terms and phrases that must be understood to review and comply with HIPAA regulations, Medicare policies and procedures, and health insurance company rules, and the importance and complexity of medical coding becomes more apparent.

CODING SYSTEMS

The purpose of this dictionary is to provide definitions for the most common words, terms and phrases encountered during the process of reviewing medical documentation and selecting codes for procedures, diagnoses, and supplies. There are no medical codes (other than examples) included in this dictionary, but a brief introduction of the various coding systems and other resources will be helpful for beginning coders.

Current Procedural Terminology (CPT)

The CPT coding system is a listing of over 8,000 codes and descriptions used to report medical services and procedures performed by physicians and other medical professionals. The purpose of the CPT coding system is to provide a uniform language that accurately describes medical, surgical, and diagnostic services and to provide an effective means for reliable nationwide communication among physicians, hospitals, and health insurance companies.

CPT codes and terminology serve a variety of important functions in the field of medical nomenclature for the reporting of physician procedures and services under government and private health insurance programs. CPT is also used for administrative management purposes such as claims processing and for the development of guidelines for medical care review.

International Classification of Diseases, 9th Revision, Clinical Modification (ICD-9-CM)

ICD-9-CM is a statistical classification system that arranges diseases and injuries into groups according to established criteria. There are over 23,000 codes in the ICD-9-CM coding system. Most ICD-9-CM codes are numeric and consist of three, four or five numbers and a description. The codes are revised approximately every 10 years by the World Health Organization and annual updates are published by Center for Medicare and Medicaid Services (CMS).

Volume 1 of ICD-9-CM, also known as the Tabular List, lists diagnosis codes and descriptions. Volume 3 of ICD-9-CM, also known as Procedures: Tabular List lists procedure codes and descriptions used by hospitals.

Healthcare Common Procedure Coding System (HCPCS)

HCPCS is a two-level coding system incorporating CPT codes as Level I and nationally mandated codes designated as HCPCS Level II. There are over 5,600 codes in the HCPCS Level II coding system. HCPCS codes must be used when billing Medicare carriers and, in some states, Medicaid carriers. Some private health insurance companies allow or mandate the use of HCPCS codes, mostly those processing Medicare claims.

The HCPCS Level II codes are used to bill Medicare for ambulance services, durable medical equipment, orthotics, prosthetics, supplies, materials, and injections. HCPCS Level II may also include codes for certain procedures and services that are not defined in the current edition of the CPT coding system.

Medicare Severity Diagnosis Related Group (MS-DRG)

MS-DRG is a classification system developed for the Medicare program as part of the prospective payment system for inpatient services. Until Fiscal Year 2008, these were known as DRGs. Each MS-DRG category is based on patient characteristics such as age and sex, plus the final diagnoses and any medical procedures performed during the hospital stay.

The MS-DRG classification is determined by a "grouper" program based on diagnoses and procedures coded in ICD-9-CM, and on patient age, sex, length of stay, and other factors. The MS-DRG assigned to the hospital stay determines the amount of money paid to the hospital by Medicare, regardless of the actual charges that the hospital may have incurred.

MS-DRG codes are defined by the Centers for Medicare and Medicaid (CMS) for adult Medicare billing. For other patient categories and payers, such as Medicaid, CHAMPUS, commercial payers for neonatal claims, and worker's compensation, modified groups and additional DRG codes are used.

Current Dental Terminology (CDT)

CDT is a listing of codes and descriptions used to report dental services performed by dentists, oral surgeons and ancillary professionals. The purpose of the CDT coding system is to provide a uniform language that accurately describes dental services and to provide an effective means for reliable nationwide communication among dentists and health insurance companies.

CDT codes and terminology serve a variety of important functions in the field of medical nomenclature for the reporting of dental procedures and services under government and private health insurance programs. CDT is also used for administrative management purposes such as claims processing and for the development of guidelines for medical care review.

Health Insurance Portability and Accountability Act (HIPAA)

The acronym HIPAA stands for the Health Insurance Portability & Accountability Act of 1996, Public Law 104-191, which amends the Internal Revenue Service Code of 1986. The Act is also known as the Kennedy-Kassebaum Act.

The HIPAA legislation includes a section, Administrative Simplification, requiring standardized electronic data interchange, and protection of confidentiality and security of health data through setting and enforcing standards. HIPAA calls for standardization of electronic patient health, administrative and financial data; unique health identifiers for individuals, employers, health plans and health care providers; security standards protecting the confidentiality and integrity of "individually identifiable health information," past, present or future.

All Health Care organizations are impacted by HIPAA. This includes all health care providers, even solo-physician offices, health plans, employers, public health authorities, life insurers, clearinghouses, billing agencies, information systems vendors, service organizations, and universities.

Medicare and Administrative Terminology

In addition to medical words, terms and phrases there are numerous other words, terms and phrases used in the medical field. Many of these other words are used to describe insurance coverage and policies, Medicare rules and regulations, and other non-clinical items.

Medical Acronyms, Eponyms And Abbreviations

Medical words, terms and phrases, as well as hand-written physician's orders can be long and cumbersome. As a result, thousands of medical acronyms, abbreviations and eponyms are in widespread use in the medical community.

An acronym is a word formed by the initial letters of a phrase or title. For example, the phrase "coronary artery bypass graft" is commonly represented by the acronym CABG.

An eponym is a procedure, disease, process, or device derived from the name of a person. For example, the phrase "Doppler ultrasound", is named after Christian Andreas Doppler, an Austrian physicist and mathematician, born november 29, 1803, Salzburg; died March 17, 1853, Venice. The Doppler-effect made possible the ultrasonic registration of the flow in blood vessels, because ultrasonic sound is reflected from red moving red blood corpuscles.

An abbreviation is simply a shortened form or phonetic representation of a word or phrase. Examples of abbreviations include "appy" for appendectomy, "hx" for history, and "subq" for subcutaneous.

Acronyms and abbreviations were originally designed to 1) reduce the amount of writing by doctors when writing orders or making medical record entries, 2) facilitate the abstracting of medical records, particularly for tests and medications, and 3) to simplify and standardize the communication process among medical personnel.

However, in addition to simplifying the communication process, there is also the potential for confusion and incorrect interpretation of acronyms and abbreviations. For example the acronym AMA can mean " "Advanced maternal age," "Against medical advice," "Anti-mitochondrial antibody," or "American Medical Association." Obviously the context in which an acronym is used is critical to proper understanding of what the acronym is supposed to mean. The medical specialty, clinical status, diagnosis, location, along with administrative and legal policies and procedures must be taken into consideration.

WORD ROOTS

Medical terminology is a vocabulary for accurately describing the human body and associated components, conditions, processes and process in a scientific manner. The systematic approach to medical word building and comprehension is based on word roots combined with prefixes and/or suffixes.

The word root is a term derived from a source language such as Greek or Latin and usually describes a body part, but may also describe bodily concepts, color, quantity, position or description. For example, the English word heart is represented in medical terminology by the Greek word root cardi(o)- or the Latin word root cordi-.

This section contains lists of different root classification (e.g. body components, quantity, description, etc.). Each list is alphabetized by English meanings, with the corresponding Greek and Latin roots given.

ROOTS OF BODILY CONCEPTS

BODILY CONCEPT	GREEK ROOT	LATIN ROOT
Digestion	-pepsia	-
Disease	-pathy	-
Eating	-phagia	-

ROOTS OF BODY PARTS AND COMPONENTS
(Internal Anatomy, External Anatomy, Body Fluids, Body Substances)

BODY PART/COMPONENT	GREEK ROOT	LATIN ROOT
abdomen	lapar(o)-	abdomin-
aorta	aort(o)-	aort(o)-
arm	brachi(o)-	-
armpit	-	axill-
artery	arteri(o)-	-
back	-	dors-
big toe	-	allic-
bladder	cyst(o)-	vesic(o)-
blood	hemat- (hem-)	sangui-, sanguine-
blood clot	thromb(o)-	-
blood vessel	angi(o)-	vascul-, vas-
body	somat-, som-	corpor-
bone	oste(o)-	ossi-
bone marrow, marrow	myel(o)-	medull-
brain	encephal(o)-	cerebr(o)-
breast	mast(o)-	mamm(o)-
chest	steth(o)-	-

BODY PART/COMPONENT	GREEK ROOT	LATIN ROOT
cheek	-	bucc-
ear	ot(o)-	aur-
eggs, ova	oo-	ov-
eye	ophthalm(o)-	ocul(o)-
eyelid	blephar(o)-	cili-; palpebr-
face	-	faci(o)-
fallopian tubes	salping(o)-	-
fat, fatty tissue	lip(o)-	adip-
finger	dactyl(o)-	digit-
forehead	-	front(o)-
gallbladder	cholecyst(o)-	fell-
genitals, sexually undifferentiated	gon(o)-, phall(o)-	-
gland	aden(o)-	-
glans *penis* or *clitoridis*	balan(o)-	-
gums	-	gingiv-
hair	trich(o)-	capill-
hand	cheir(o)-, chir(o)-	manu-
head	cephal(o)-	capit(o)-
heart	cardi(o)-	cordi-
hip, hip-joint	-	cox-
horn	cerat(o)-	cornu-
intestine	enter(o)-	-
jaw	gnath(o)-	-
kidney	nephr(o)-	ren-
knee	gon-	genu-
lip	cheil(o)-, chil(o)-	labi(o)-
liver	hepat(o)- (hepatic-)	jecor-
loins, pubic region	episi(o)-	pudend-
lungs	pneumon-	pulmon(i)- (pulmo-)
marrow, bone marrow	myel(o)-	medull-
mind	psych-	ment-
mouth	stomat(o)-	or-
muscle	my(o)-	-
nail	onych(o)-	ungui-
navel	omphal(o)-	umbilic-
neck	trachel(o)-	cervic-
nerve; nervous system	neur(o)-	nerv-
nipple, teat	thele-	papill-, mammill-
nose	rhin(o)-	nas-
ovary	oophor(o)-	ovari(o)-

BODY PART/COMPONENT	GREEK ROOT	LATIN ROOT
pelvis	pyel(o)-	pelv(i)-
penis	pe(o)-	-
pupil (of the eye)	cor-, corc-, coro-	-
rib	pleur(o)-	cost(o)-
rib cage	thorac(i)-, thorac(o)-	-
shoulder	om(o)-	humer(o)-
sinus	-	sinus-
skin	dermat(o)- (derm-)	cut-, cuticul-
skull	crani(o)-	-
stomach	gastr(o)-	ventr(o)-
testis	orchi(o)-, orchid(o)-	-
throat (upper throat cavity)	pharyng(o)-	-
throat (lower throat cavity/voice box])	laryng(o)-	-
thumb	-	pollic-
tooth	odont(o)-	dent(i)-
tongue	gloss-, glott-	lingu(a)-
toe	dactyl(o)-	digit-
tumour	cel-, onc(o)-	tum-
ureter	ureter(o)-	ureter(o)-
urethra	urethr(o)-, urethr(a)-	urethr(o)-, urethr(a)-
urine, urinary System	ur(o)-	urin(o)-
uterine tubes	sarping(o)-	sarping(o)-
uterus	hyster(o)-, metr(o)-	uter(o)-
vagina	colp(o)-	vagin-
vein	phleb(o)-	ven-
vulva	episi(o)-	vulv-
womb	hyster(o)-, metr(o)-	uter(o)-
wrist	carp(o)-	carp(o)-

ROOTS OF COLOR

COLOR	GREEK ROOT	LATIN ROOT
black	melano-	nigr-
blue	cyano-	-
gray, grey	polio-	-
green	chlor(o)-	vir-
purple	porphyr(o)-	purpur-, purpureo-
red	erythr(o)-, rhod(o)-	rub-, rubr-
red-yellow	cirrh(o)-	-
white	leuc-, leuk-	alb-

COLOR	GREEK ROOT	LATIN ROOT
yellow	xanth(o)-	flav-

ROOTS OF DESCRIPTION

DESCRIPTION	GREEK ROOT	LATIN ROOT
bad, incorrect	cac(o)-, dys-	mal(e)-
bent, crooked	ankyl(o)-	prav(i)-
big	mega-, megal(o)-	magn(i)-
biggest	megist-	maxim-
broad, wide	eury-	lat(i)-
cold	cry(o)-	frig-
dead	necr(o)-	mort-
equal	is(o)-	equ(i)-
false	pseud(o)-	fals(i)-
female, feminine	thely-	-
flat	platy-	plan(i)-
good, well	eu-	ben(e)-, bon(i)-
great	mega-, megal(o)-	magn(i)-
hard	scler(o)-	dur(i)-
heavy	bar(o)-	grav(i)-
hollow	coel(o)-	cav-
huge	megal(o)-	magn(i)-
incorrect, bad	cac(o)-, dys-	mal(e)-
large; extremely large	mega-	magn(i)-
largest	megist-	maxim-
long	macr(o)-	long(i)-
male, masculine	arseno-	vir-
narrow	sten(o)-	angust(i)-
new	neo-	nov(i)-
normal, correct; straight	orth(o)-	rect-
old	paleo-	veter-
sharp	oxy-	ac-
short	brachy-	brev(i)-
small	micr(o)-	parv(i)- (rare)
smallest	-	minim-
slow	brady-	tard(i)-
fast	tachy-	celer-
soft	malac(o)-	moll(i)-
straight, normal, correct	orth(o)-	rect(i)-
thick	pachy-	crass(i)-

DESCRIPTION	GREEK ROOT	LATIN ROOT
varied, various	poikilo-	vari-
well, good	eu-	ben(e)-
wide, broad	eury-	lat(i)-

ROOTS OF POSITION

DESCRIPTION	GREEK ROOT	LATIN ROOT
around	peri-	circum-
left	-	sinistr-
middle	mes(o)-	medi-
right	dexi(o)-	dextr(o)-
surrounding	peri-	circum-

ROOTS OF QUANTITY

DESCRIPTION	GREEK ROOT	LATIN ROOT
double	diplo-	dupli-
equal	iso-	equi-
few	oligo-	pauci-
half	hemi-	semi-
many, much	poly-	multi-
twice	dis-	bis-

PREFIXES & SUFFIXES

As stated in the previous section on Word Roots, the systematic approach to medical word building and comprehension is based on word roots combined with prefixes and/or suffixes. The **word root** is a term derived from a source language such as Greek or Latin and usually describes a body part. Using the previous example, the English word heart is represented in medical terminology by the Greek word root cardi(o)- or the Latin word root cordi-.

Most medical terms involve the combination of a prefix, combined with a word root and a suffix. The **prefix** can be added in front of the term to modify the word root by giving additional information about the location of an organ, the number of parts, or time involved. Continuing with the Greed word root cardi(o)- we can add a prefix, such as peri-, meaning something with a position 'surrounding' or 'around' another, to create the medical term pericardium, which is defined as a thin membranous covering of the outer surfaces of the heart.

Suffixes are attached to the end of a word root to add meaning such as condition, disease process, or procedure. In the process of creating medical terminology, certain rules of language apply. To create the complete word pericardium, the final step is to add the suffix –ium, meaning structure, tissue.

Following is an alphabetical list of common medical prefixes and suffixes, along with their meanings, origin, and an English example.

PREFIX/SUFFIX	MEANING	EXAMPLE(S)
a-, an-	Denotes an absence of	apathy, analgia
ab-	away from	abduction
abdomin(o)-	Of or relating to the Abdomen	abdomen
-ac	pertaining to	cardiac
acanth(o)-	thorn or spine	acanthocyte
acous(io)-	Of or relating to hearing	acoustic
acr(o)-	extremity, topmost	acromegaly
-acusis	hearing	presbycusis
-ad	toward, in thc dircction of	dorsad
ad-	increase, adherence, motion toward, very	adduction
aden(o)-, aden(i)-	Of or relating to a gland	adenology
adip(o)-	Of or relating to fat or fatty tissue	adipocyte
adren(o)-	Of or relating to adrenal glands	adrenal artery
aer(o)-	air, gas	aerosinusitis

PREFIX/SUFFIX	MEANING	EXAMPLE(S)
-al	pertaining to	abdominal
alb-	Denoting a white or pale color	albino
alge(si)-	pain	analgesic
-algia	pain	myalgia
alg(i)o-	pain	myalgia
allo-	Denoting something as different, or as an addition	alloantigen, allopathy
ambi-	Denoting something as positioned on both sides; Describing both of two	ambidextrous
amnio-	Pertaining to the membraneous fetal sac (amnion)	amniocentesis
an-	not, without	analgesia
an(o)	anus	
andr(o)-	pertaining to a man	andrology, android
angi(o)-	blood vessel	angiogram
aniso-	Describing something as unequal	anisotropic
ankyl(o)-, ancyl(o)-	Denoting something as crooked or bent	ankylosis
ante-	Describing something as positioned in front of another thing	antepartum
anti-	Describing something as 'against' or 'opposed to' another	antibody, antipsychotic
apo-	separated from, derived from	apoptosis
arteri(o)-	Of or pertaining to an artery	artery, arteriole
arthr(o)-	Of or pertaining to the joints, limbs	arthritis
articul(o)-	joint	articulation
-ary	pertaining to	bilary tract
-ase	enzyme	lactase
-asthenia	weakness	myasthenia gravis
-ation	process	

PREFIX/SUFFIX	MEANING	EXAMPLE(S)
aur(i)-	Of or pertaining to the ear	aural
aut(o)-	sclf	autoimmunc
axill-	Of or pertaining to the armpit [uncommon as a prefix]	axilla
balano-	Of the glans penis or glans clitoridis	balanitis
bi-	twice, double	
bio-	life	biology
blast(o)-	germ or bud	blastomere
blephar(o)-	Of or pertaining to the eyelid	blepharoplast
brachi(o)-	Of or relating to the arm	brachium
brachy-	Indicating 'short' or less commonly 'little'	brachycephalic
brady-	Indicating 'slow'	bradycardia
bronch(i)-	bronchus	bronchiolitis obliterans
bucc(o)-	Of or pertaining to the cheek	buccolabial
burs(o)-	bursa	bursitis
capill-	Of or pertaining to hair	capillus
capit-	Pertaining to the head (as a whole)	capitation
carcin(o)-	cancer	carcinoma
cardi(o)-	Of or pertaining to the heart	cardiology
carp(o)-	Of or pertaining to the wrist.	carpopedal
cata-	down	cataract
-cele	pouching, hernia	hydrocele
-centesis	surgical puncture for aspiration	amniocentesis
cephal(o)-	Of or pertaining to the head (as a whole)	cephalalgy
cerat(o)-	Of or pertaining to the cornu; a horn	ceratoid
cerebell(o)-	Of or pertaining to the cerebellum	cerebellum
cerebr(o)-	Of or pertaining to the brain	cerebrology

PREFIX/SUFFIX	MEANING	EXAMPLE(S)
cervic-	Of or pertaining to the neck, the cervix	cervicodorsal
chem(o)-	chemistry, drug	chemotherapy
chir(o)-, cheir(o)-	Of or pertaining to the hand	chiropractor
chlor(o)-	Denoting a green color	chlorophyll
chol(e)-	Of or pertaining to bile	cholaemia
cholecyst(o)-	Of or pertaining to the gallbladder	cholecystectomy
chondr(i)o-	cartilage, gristle, granule, granular	chondrocalcinosis
chrom(ato)-	color	hemachromatosis
-cidal, -cide	killing, destroying	
cili-	Of or pertaining to the cilia, the eyelashes; eyelids	ciliary
circum-	Denoting something as 'around' another	circumcision
cis-	on this side	
clast	break	
co-	with, together, in association	
col-, colo-, colono-	colon	colonoscopy
colp(o)-	Of or pertaining to the vagina	colposcopy
com-	with, together	
contra	against	contraindicate
cor-	with, together	
cor-, core-, coro-	Of or pertaining to eye's pupil	corectomy
cordi-	Of or pertaining to the heart [uncommon as a prefix]	commotio cordis
cornu-	Applied to processes and parts of the body describing them likened or similar to horns	
cost(o)-	Of or pertaining to the ribs	costochondral
cox-	Of or relating to the hip,	coxopodite

PREFIX/SUFFIX	MEANING	EXAMPLE(S)
	haunch, or hip-joint	
crani(o)-	Belonging or relating to the cranium	craniology
-crine	to secrete	endocrine
cry(o)-	cold	cryoablation
cutane-	skin	subcutaneous
cyan(o)-	Denotes a blue color	cyanopsia
cycl-	circle, cycle	cylic somatostatin
cyph(o)-	Denotes something as bent [uncommon as a prefix]	cyphosis
cyst(o)-, cyst(i)-	Of or pertaining to the urinary bladder	cystotomy
cyt(o)-	cell	cytokine
-cyte	cell	leukocyte
dacryo-	tear	
dactyl(o)-	Of or pertaining to a finger, toe	dactylology
de-	away from, cessation	
dent-	Of or pertaining to teeth	dentist
dermat(o)-, derm(o)-	Of or pertaining to the skin	dermatology
-desis	binding	arthrodesis
dextr(o)-	right, on the right side	dextrocardia
di-	two	
di-	apart, separation	
dia-	(same as Greek meaning)	diacetyl
dif-	apart, separation	
digit-	Of or pertaining to the finger [rare as a root]	digit
dis-	separation, taking apart	dissection
dors(o)-, dors(i)-	Of or pertaining to the back	dorsal, dorsocephalad
duodeno-	duodenum, twelve: upper part of the small intestine (twelve inches long on average), connects to the stomach	duodenal atresia
dynam(o)-	force, energy, power	dynamometry

PREFIX/SUFFIX	MEANING	EXAMPLE(S)
-dynia	pain	
dys-	bad, difficult	dysphagia, dysphasia
-eal	pertaining to	
ec-	out, away	
ect(o)-	outer, outside	ectopic pregnancy
-ectasis	expansion, dilation	bronchiectasis
-ectomy	Denotes a surgical operation or removal of a body part	mastectomy
-emesis	vomiting condition	hematemesis
-emia	blood condition	anemia
encephal(o)-	Of or pertaining to the brain. Also see Cerebro.	encephalogram
endo-	Denotes something as 'inside' or 'within'	endocrinology, endospore
enter(o)-	Of or pertaining to the intestine	gastroenterology
epi-	[Same as Greek meaning: on, upon]	epistaxis, epicardium, episclera, epidural
episi(o)-	Of or pertaining to the pubic region, the loins	episiotomy
erythr(o)-	Denotes a red color	erythrocyte
-esophageal, -esophago	gullet	
esthesio-	sensation	
eu-	true, good, well, new	eukaryote
ex-	out of, away from	
exo-	Denotes something as 'outside' another	exoskeleton
extra-	outside	extracorporeal
faci(o)-	Of or pertaining to the face	facioplegic
fibr(o)	fiber	fibroblast
filli-	fine, hair like	
-form, -iform	Used to form adjectives indicating 'having the form of'	cuneiform
front-	Of or pertaining to the forehead	frontonasal
galact(o)-	milk	galactorrhea
gastr(o)-	Of or pertaining to the	gastric bypass

PREFIX/SUFFIX	MEANING	EXAMPLE(S)
	stomach	
-gen	(1) Denotes the sense 'born in, from' (2) Denotes the sense 'of a certain kind'	(1) endogen; (2) heterogenous
-genic	Formative	cardiogenic shock
genu-	Of or pertaining to the knee	genu valgum
gingiv-	Of or pertaining to the gums	gingivitis
glauc(o)-	Denoting a grey, bluish-grey color	glaucoma
gloss(o)-, glott(o)-	Of or pertaining to the tongue	glossology
gluco-	glucose	glucocorticoid
glyco-	sugar	glycolysis
gnath(o)-	Of or pertaining to the jaw	gnathodynamometer
gon(o)-	seed, semen; also, reproductive	gonorrhea
-gram	record or picture	angiogram
-graph	record or picture	electrocardiograph
-graphy	process of recording	angiography
gyn(ec)o-	woman	gynecomastia
halluc-	to wander in mind	hallucinosis
hemat-, (hem-)	Of or pertaining to blood	hematology, older form haematology
hema or hemo-	blood	hematological malignancy
hemi-	one-half	cerebral hemisphere
hepat- (hepatic-)	Of or pertaining to the liver	hepatology
heter(o)-	Denotes something as 'the other' (of two), as an addition, or different	heterogeneous
hidr(o)-	sweat	hyperhidrosis
hist(o)-, histio-	tissue	histology
home(o)-	similar	homeopathy
hom(o)-	Denotes something as	homosexuality

PREFIX/SUFFIX	MEANING	EXAMPLE(S)
	'the same' as another or common	
humer(o)-	Of or pertaining to the shoulder (or [rarely] the upper arm)	humerus
hydr(o)-	water	hydrophobe
hyper-	Denotes something as 'extreme' or 'beyond normal'	hypertension
hyp(o)-	Denotes something as 'below normal'	hypovolemia,
hyster(o)-	Of or pertaining to the womb, the uterus	hysterectomy
-i-asis	condition	mydriasis
iatr(o)-	Of or pertaining to medicine, or a physician [uncommon as a prefix; common as as suffix, see -iatry]	iatrochemistry
-iatry	Denotes a field in medicine of a certain body component	podiatry, psychiatry
-ic	pertaining to	hepatic artery
-icle	small	ovarian follicle
-ics	organized knowledge, treatment	
idio-	self, one's own	idiopathic
ileo-	ileum	ileocecal valve
infra-	below	infrahyoid muscles
inter-	between, among	interarticular ligament
intra-	within	intracranial hemorrhage
irid(o)-	iris	iridectomy
ischio-	Of or pertaining to the ischium, the hip-joint	ischiorrhogic
-ism	condition, disease	dwarfism
-ismus	spasm, contraction	
iso-	Denoting something as being 'equal'	isotonic

PREFIX/SUFFIX	MEANING	EXAMPLE(S)
-ist	one who specializes in	pathologist
-ite	the nature of, resembling	hermaphrodite
-itis	inflammation	tonsillitis
-ium	structure, tissue	pericardium
isch-	Restriction	ischemia
karyo-	nucleus	eukaryote
kerat(o)-	cornea (eye or skin)	keratoscope
kin(e)-, kin(o), kinesi(o)-	movement	kinesthesia
koil(o)-	hollow	koilocyte
kyph(o)-	humped	kyphoscoliosis
labi(o)-	Of or pertaining to the lip	labiodental
lacrim(o)-	tear	lacrimal canaliculi
lact(i)-, lact(o)	milk	lactation
lapar(o)-	Of or pertaining to the abdomen-wall, flank	laparotomy
laryng(o)-	Of or pertaining to the larynx, the lower throat cavity where the voice box is	larynx
latero-	lateral	lateral pectoral nerve
lei(o)-	smooth	leiomyoma
-lepsis, -lepsy	attack, seizure	epilepsy, narcolepsy
lept(o)-	light, slender	
leuc(o)-, leuk(o)-	Denoting a white color	leukocyte
lingu(a)-, lingu(o)-	Of or pertaining to the tongue	linguistics
lip(o)-	fat	liposuction
lith(o)-	stone, calculus	lithotripsy
log(o)-	speech	
-logist	Denotes someone who studies a certain field: _____-logy	oncologist, pathologist
-logy	Denotes the academic study or practice of a certain field	hematology, urology
lymph(o)-	lymph	lymphedema
lys(o)-, -lytic	dissolution	lysosome

PREFIX/SUFFIX	MEANING	EXAMPLE(S)
-lysis	Destruction	paralysis
macr(o)-	large, long	macrophage
-malacia	softening	osteomalacia
mamm(o)-	Of or pertaining to the breast	mammogram
mammill(o)-	Of or pertaining to the nipple	
manu-	Of or pertaining to the hand	manufacture
mast(o)-	Of or pertaining to the breast	mastectomy
meg(a)-, megal(o)-, megaly	enlargement	splenomegaly
melan(o)-	Denoting a black color	melanin
mening(o)-	membrane	meningitis
mero-	part	merocrine, meroblastic
mes(o)-	middle	mesoderm
meta-	after, behind	metacarpus
-meter	measurement	sphygmomanometer
-metry	process of measuring	optometry
metr(o)-	Pertaining to conditions or instruments of the uterus	metrorrhagia
micro-	denoting something as small, or relating to smallness	microscope
mon(o)-	single	infectious mononucleosis
morph(o)-	form, shape	morphology
muscul(o)-	muscle	musculoskeletal system
my(o)-	Of or relating to muscle	myoblast
myc(o)-	fungus	onychomycosis
myel(o)-	Of or relating to bone marrow	myeloblast
myring(o)-	eardrum	myringotomy
myx(o)-	mucus	myxoma
narc(o)-	numb, sleep	narcolepsy
nas(o)-	Of or pertaining to the nose	nasal
necr(o)-	death	necrotizing fasciitis

PREFIX/SUFFIX	MEANING	EXAMPLE(S)
neo-	new	neoplasm
nephr(o)-	Of or pertaining to the kidney	nephrology
nerv-	Of or pertaining to nerves and the nervous system [Uncommon as a root: neuro- mostly always used]	nerve
neur(i)-, neur(o)-	Of or pertaining to nerves and the nervous system	neurofibromatosis
normo-	normal	normocapnia
ocul(o)-	Of or pertaining to the eye	oculist
odont(o)-	Of or pertaining to teeth	orthodontist
odyn(o)-	pain	stomatodynia
-oid	resemblance to	sarcoidosis
ole	small or little	
olig(o)-	Denoting something as 'having little, having few'	oligotrophy
om(o)-	Of or pertaining to the shoulder	omoplate
-oma (singular), -omata (plural)	tumor	sarcoma, teratoma
omphal(o)-	Of or pertaining to the navel, the umbilicus	omphalotomy
onco-	tumor, bulk, volume	oncology
onych(o)-	Of or pertaining to the nail (of a finger or toe)	onychophagy
oo-	Of or pertaining to the an egg, a woman's egg, the ovum	oogenesis
oophor(o)-	Of or pertaining to the woman's ovary	oophorectomy
ophthalm(o)-	Of or pertaining to the eye	ophthalmology
optic(o)-	Of or relating to chemical properties of the eye	opticochemical
or(o)-	Of or pertaining to the	oral

PREFIX/SUFFIX	MEANING	EXAMPLE(S)
	mouth	
orchi(o)-, orchido-	testis	orchiectomy, orchidectomy
orth(o)-	Denoting something as straight or correct	orthodontist
-osis	a condition, disease or increase	harlequin type ichthyosis
osseo-	bony	
ossi-	bone	peripheral ossifying fibroma
ost(e)-, oste(o)-	bone	osteoporosis
ot(o)-	Of or pertaining to the ear	otopathy
-ous	pertaining to	
ovari(o)-	Of or pertaining to the ovaries	ovariectomy
ovo-, ovi-, ov-	Of or pertaining to the eggs, the ovum	ovogenesis
oxo-	addition of oxygen	
oxy-	sharp, acid, acute, oxygen	
pachy-	thick	pachyderma
palpebr-	Of or pertaining to the eyelid [uncommon as a root]	palpebra
pan-, pant(o)-	Denoting something as 'complete' or containing 'everything'	panophobia, panopticon
papill-	Of or pertaining to the nipple (of the chest/breast)	papillitis
papul(o)-	Indicates papulosity, a small elevation or swelling in the skin, a pimple, swelling	papulation
para-	alongside of, abnormal	
-paresis	slight paralysis	hemiparesis
path(o)-	disease	pathology
-pathy	Denotes (with a negative sense) a disease, or disorder	sociopathy, neuropathy

PREFIX/SUFFIX	MEANING	EXAMPLE(S)
ped-, -ped-, -pes	Of or pertaining to the foot; -footed	pedoscope
pelv(i)-, pelv(o)-	hip bone	pelvis
-penia	deficiency	osteopenia
peo-	Of or pertaining to the penis	peotomy
-pepsia	Denotes something relating to digestion, or the digestive tract.	dyspepsia
per-	through	
peri-	Denoting something with a position 'surrounding' or 'around' another	periodontal
-pexy	fixation	nephropexy
phaco-	lens-shaped	
-phage, -phagia	Forms terms denoting conditions relating to eating or ingestion	sarcophagia
-phago-	eating, devouring	phagocyte
phagist-:	Forms nouns that denote a person who 'feeds on' the first element or part of the word	lotophagis
-phagy	Forms nouns that denotes 'feeding on' the first element or part of the word	anthropophagy
phallo-	phallus	aphallia
pharmaco-	drug, medication	pharmacology
pharyng(o)-	Of or pertaining to the pharynx, the upper throat cavity	pharyngitis, pharyngoscopy
-phil(ia)	attraction for	hemophilia
phleb(o)-	Of or pertaining to the (blood) veins, a vein	phlebography, phlebotomy
phob(o)-	exaggerated fear, sensitivity	arachnophobia

PREFIX/SUFFIX	MEANING	EXAMPLE(S)
phon(o)-	sound	
phos-	Of or pertaining to light or its chemical properties, now historic and used rarely. See the common root phot(o)- below.	phosphene
phot(o)-	Of or pertaining to light	photopathy
phren(i)-, phren(o)-, phrenico	diaphragm	phrenic nerve
-plasia	formation, development	achondroplasia
-plasty	surgical repair, reconstruction	rhinoplasty
-plegia	paralysis	paraplegia
pleur(o)-, pleur(a)	Of or pertaining to the ribs	pleurogenous
-plexy	stroke or seizure	cataplexy
pneum(o)-	Of or pertaining to the lungs	pneumonocyte, pneumonia
pneumat(o)-	air, lung	
pod-, -pod-, -pus	Of or pertaining to the foot, -footed	podiatry
-poiesis	production	hematopoiesis
polio-	Denoting a grey color	poliomyelitis
poly-	Denotes a 'plurality' of something	polymyositis
por(o)-	pore, porous	
porphyr(o)-	Denotes a purple color	porphyroblast
post-	Denotes something as 'after' or 'behind' another	postoperation, postmortem
pre-	Denotes something as 'before' another (in [physical] position or time)	prematurity
presby(o)-	old age	presbyopia
prim-	Denotes something as 'first' or 'most-important'	primary
pro-	Denotes something as 'before' another (in [physical] position or time)	procephalic
proct(o)-	anus, rectum	proctology

PREFIX/SUFFIX	MEANING	EXAMPLE(S)
prot(o)-	Denotes something as 'first' or 'most-important'	protoneuron
pseudo-	Denotes something false or fake	
psych(e)-, psych(o)	Of or pertaining to the mind	psychology, psychiatry
-ptosis	falling, downward placement, prolapse	apoptosis
-ptysis	(a spitting), spitting	hemoptysis
pulmon-, pulmo-	Of or relating to the lungs.	pulmonary
pyel(o)-	pelvis	pyelonephritis
pyo-	pus	pyometra
pyro-	fever	antipyretic
quadr(i)-	four	quadriceps
radio-	radiation	radiology
re-	again, backward	
rect(o)-	rectum	rectum
ren(o)-	Of or pertaining to the kidney	renal
reticul(o)-	net	reticulocyte
retro-	backward, behind	retroverted
rhabd(o)-	rod shaped, striated	
rhachi(o)-	spine	
rhin(o)-	Of or pertaining to the nose	rhinoceros, rhinoplasty
rhod(o)-	Denoting a rose-red color	rhodophyte
-rrhage	burst forth	hemorrhage
-rrhagia	rapid flow of blood	
-rrhaphy	surgical suturing	glossorrhaphy
-rrhea	flowing, discharge	galactorrhea
-rrhexis	rupture	
rubr(o)-	Of or pertaining to the red nucleus of the brain	rubrospinal
salping(o)-	Of or pertaining to the fallopian tubes	salpingectomy
sangui-, sanguine-	Of or pertaining to blood	sanguine
sarco-	muscular, fleshlike	sarcoma
schist(o)-	split, cleft	
schiz(o)-	Denoting something	schizophrenia

PREFIX/SUFFIX	MEANING	EXAMPLE(S)
	'split' or 'double-sided'	
scler(o)-	hardness	atherosclerosis
scoli(o)-	twisted	scoliosis
-scope	instrument for viewing	stethoscope
-scopy	use of instrument for viewing	endoscopy
semi-	one-half, partly	
sial(o)-	saliva, salivary gland	sialagogue
sigmoid(o)-	sigmoid, sigmoid colon	sigmoidoscopy
sinistr(o)-	left, left side	
sinus-	Of or pertaining to the sinus	sinusitis
-sis	condition of	osteoperosis
sito-	food, grain	
somat(o)-, somatico-	body, bodily	somatotropin
spasmo-	spasm	
sperma-, spermo-, spermato-	semen, spermatozoa	spermatogenesis
splanchn(i)-, splanchn(o)-	viscera	splanchnicectomy
splen(o)-	spleen	splenectomy
spondyl(o)-	Of or pertaining to the spine, the vertebra	spondylitis
squamos(o)-	Denoting something as 'full of scales' or 'scaly'	squama
-stasis	stop, stand	homeostatis
-staxis	dripping, trickling	epistaxis
sten(o)-	Denoting something as 'narrow in shape' or pertaining to narrow-ness	stenography
steth(o)-	Of or pertaining to the upper chest, chest, the area above the breast and under the neck	stethoscope
stheno-	strength, force, power	
stom(a)	mouth	stomatognathic system
stomat(o)-	Of or pertaining to the mouth	stomatogastric
-stomy	creation of an opening	colostomy
sub-	beneath	subcutaneous tissue

PREFIX/SUFFIX	MEANING	EXAMPLE(S)
super-	in excess, above, superior	superior vena cava
supra-	above, excessive	supraorbital vein
sy(l)-, sym-, syn-, sys-	Indicates similarity, likeness, or being together; Assimilates before some consonants: before l to syl-, s o sys-, before a labial to sym-.	synalgia, synesthesia, syssarcosis
tachy-	Denoting something as fast, irregularly fast	tachycardia
-tension, -tensive	blood pressure	hypertension
thel(e)-, thel(o)-	Of or pertaining to a nipple [uncommon as a prefix]	theleplasty
thely-	Denoting something as 'relating to a woman, feminine'	thelygenous
therm(o)-	heat	
thorac(i)-, thorac(o)-, thoracico-	Of or pertaining to the upper chest, chest; the area above the breast and under the neck	thorax
thromb(o)-	Of or relating to a blood clot, clotting of blood	thrombus, thrombocytopenia
thyr(o)-	thyroid	thyroidectomy
-tic	pertaining to	
toco-	childbirth	
-tome	cutting instrument	
-tomy	cutting operation	cystotomy
tono-	tone, tension, pressure	tonometry
-tony	tension	
top(o)-	place, topical	
tox(i)-, tox(o)-, toxico-	toxin, poison	toxoplasmosis
trache(o)-	trachea	tracheotomy
trachel(o)-	Of or pertaining to the neck	
trans-	Denoting something as moving or situated 'across' or 'through'	transfusion
trich(i)-, trichia, trich(o)-	Of or pertaining to hair, hair-like structure	trichotomy

PREFIX/SUFFIX	MEANING	EXAMPLE(S)
-tripsy	crushing	lithotripsy
-trophy	nourishment, development	
tympan(o)-	eardrum	tympanostomy
-ula, -ule	small	nodule
ultra-	beyond, excessive	
umbilic-	Of or pertaining to the navel, the umbilicus	umbilical
ungui-	Of or pertaining to the nail, a claw	unguiform, ungual
un(i)-	one	unilateral hearing loss
ur(o)-	Of or pertaining to urine, the urinary system; (specifically) pertaining to the physiological chemistry of urine	urology
uri(c)-, urico-	uric acid	
urin-	Of or pertaining to urine, the urinary system	uriniferous

CONVENTIONS

MAIN ENTRIES

All main entries appear in boldface type.

SUBENTRIES

Some main entries include subentries. The subentries are indented under the main term in bold, italicized type. For example:

anemia: Condition in which the number of red blood cells or hemoglobin (oxygen carrying substance in blood) are inadequate.

anemia, aplastic: Serious disease characterized by decreased bone marrow production of all blood cells.

MULTIPLE ENTRIES

Words, terms or acronyms that have more than one meaning are presented as sequentially numbered entries. For example:

cordectomy: 1) Surgical removal of a vocal cord. 2) Surgical removal of part of the spinal cord.

ACRONYMS

Acronyms are presented without periods. Most acronyms include only a definition of the acronym, while some include a more complete definition of the concept represented by the acronym. Example:

CVS: Chorionic Villi Sampling

EPONYMS

Eponyms are presented in both possessive and non-possessive forms. Examples:

Ramstedt operation: A surgical procedure on the pylorus in order to relax a stenotic or closed-by-spasm sphincter. *Synonym*: pyloromyotomy.

Raynaud's phenomenon: Circulation system disorder affecting fingers and toes. A complication of an underlying disease or emotional disturbance.

ABBREVIATIONS

Abbreviations are (mostly) presented in lower case as they are most usually encountered in medical records and physician orders. Examples:

pre-op: Preoperative

prn: As needed.

SYNONYMS:

Some entries include a listing of synonyms for the main term. These entries are identified by the term *Synonym:* in italics following the definition. Example:

pulmonary sequestration: A condition where a piece of tissue that develops into lung tissue is not attached to the pulmonary blood supply and does not communicate with the other lung tissue. *Synonym*: cystic lung lesion.

ANATOMICAL ILLUSTRATIONS

The full-color anatomical illustrations following this section provide visual reinforcement of human anatomy and physiology.

ILLUSTRATIONS

There are illustrations throughout the content that help to illustrate words, terms, concepts and medical procedures.

ANATOMICAL ILLUSTRATIONS

A fundamental knowledge and understanding of basic human anatomy and physiology is a prerequisite for accurate coding. While a comprehensive treatment of anatomy and physiology is beyond the scope of this text, the large scale, full color anatomical illustrations on the following pages are designed to facilitate the understanding of basic anatomy by providing a visual reference to the various organ systems.

Male Figure
(Anterior View)

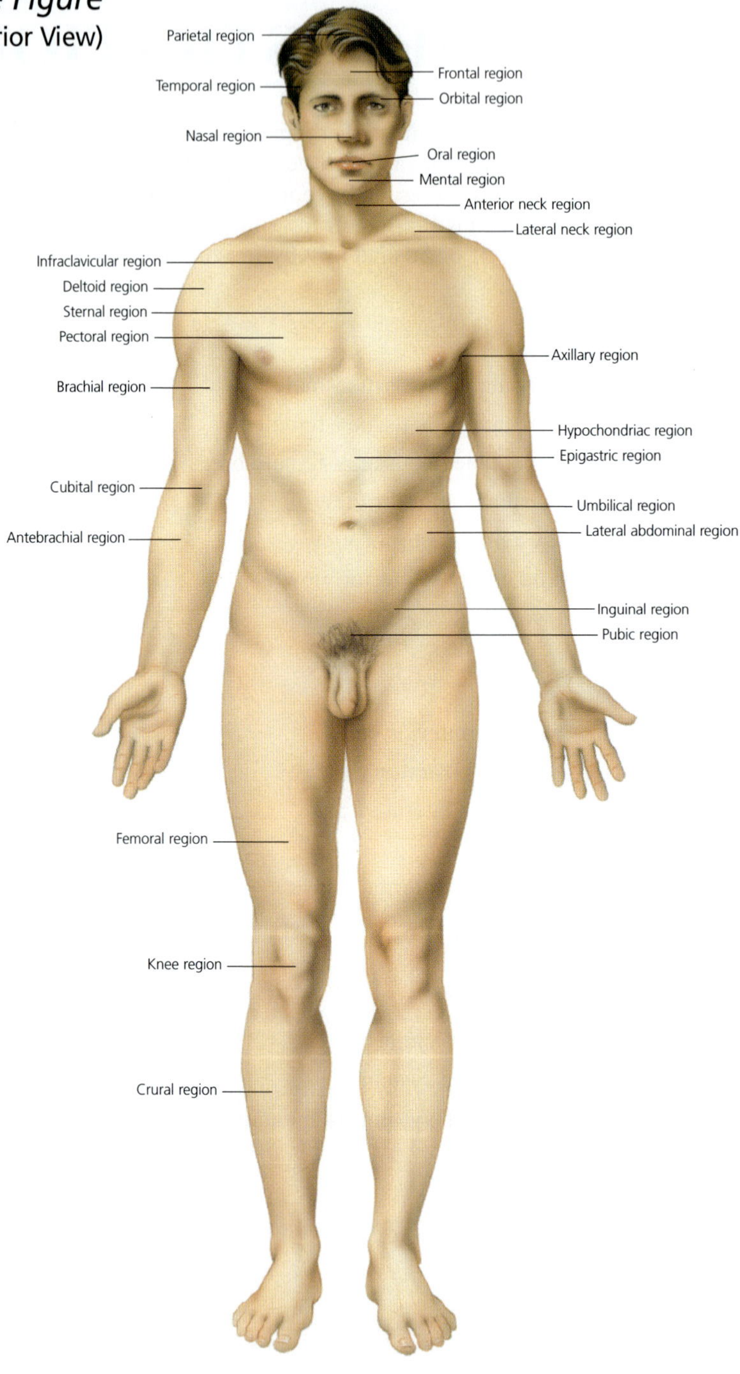

Female Figure
(Anterior View)

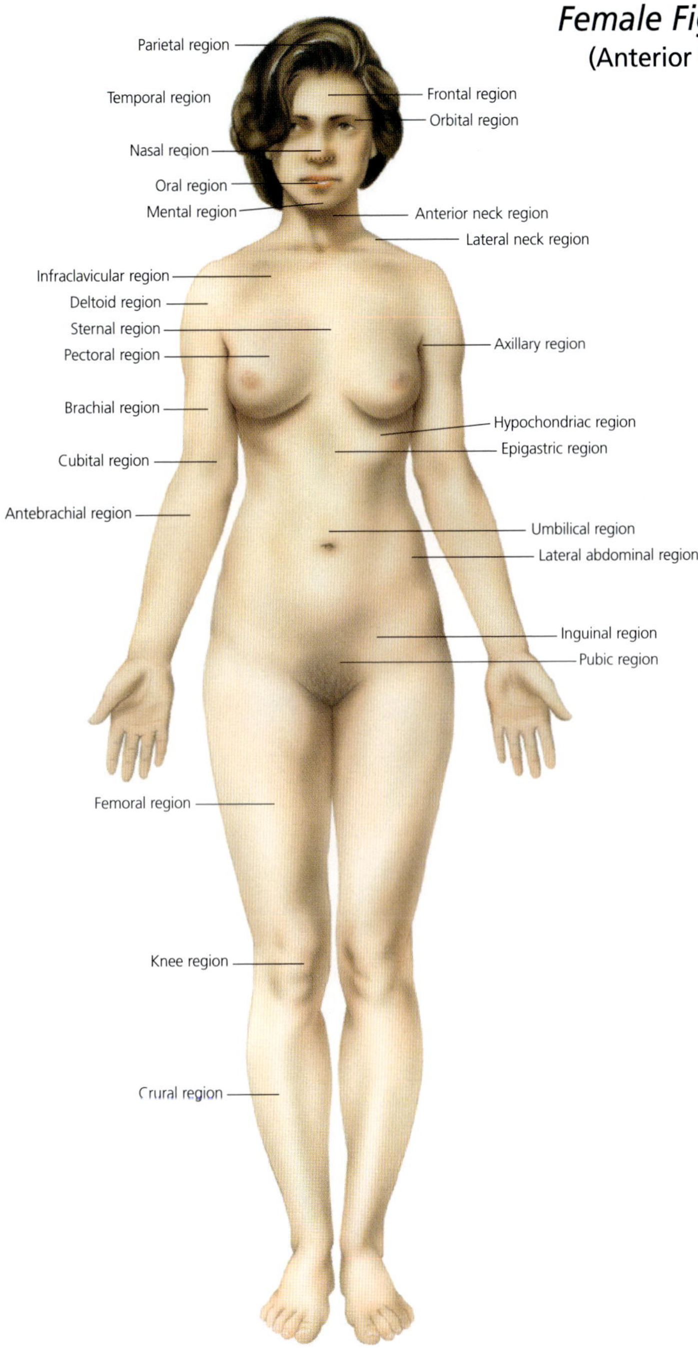

Female Breast

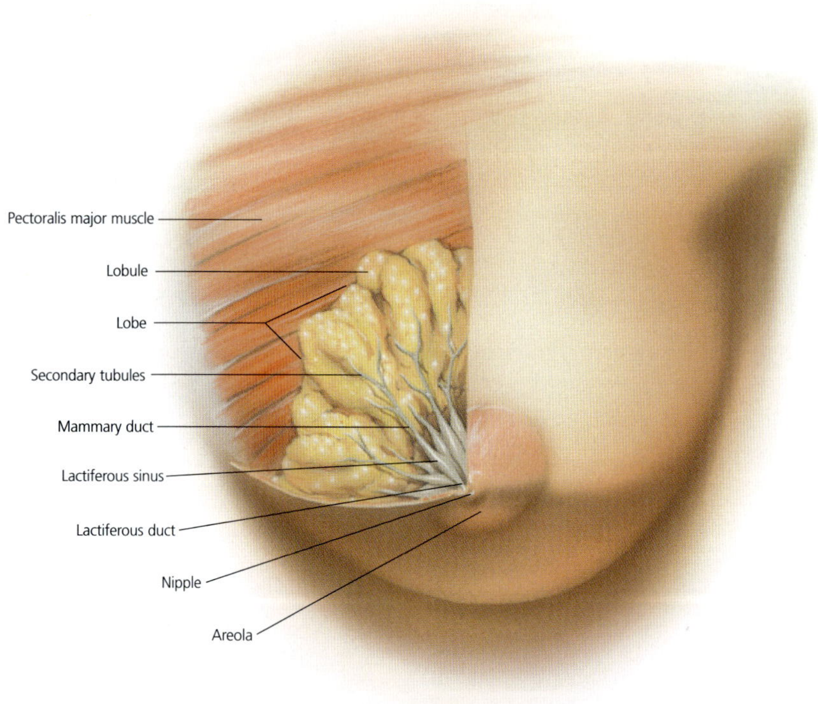

Muscular System
(Anterior View)

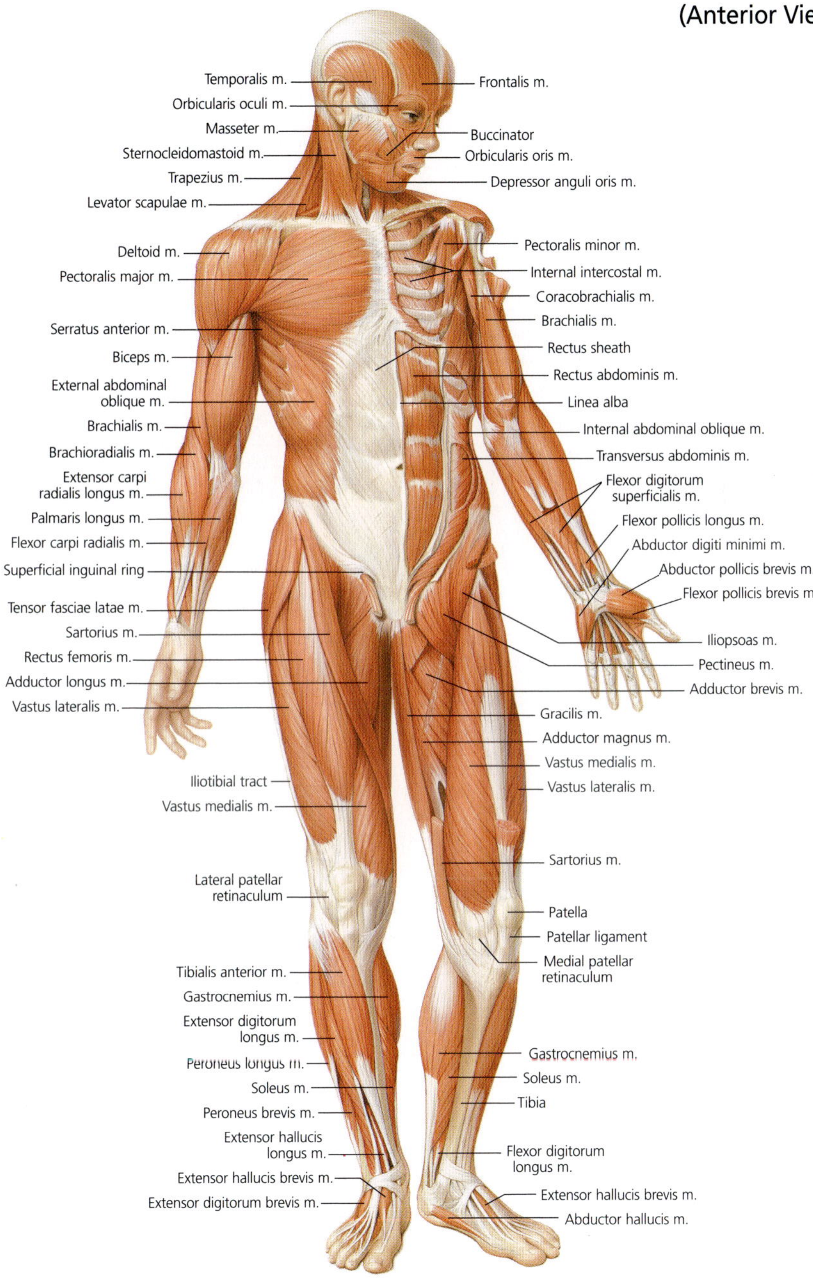

Muscular System

(Posterior View)

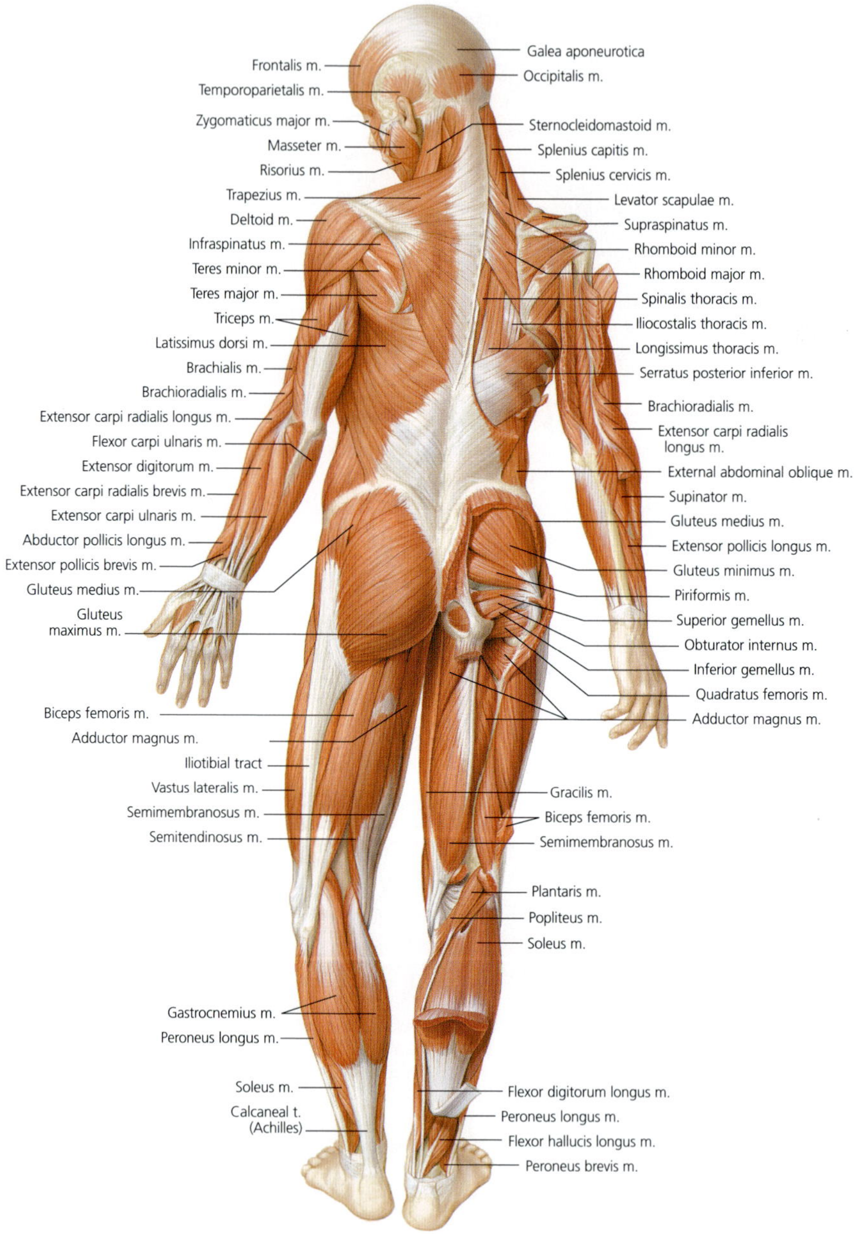

Shoulder and Elbow

(Anterior View)

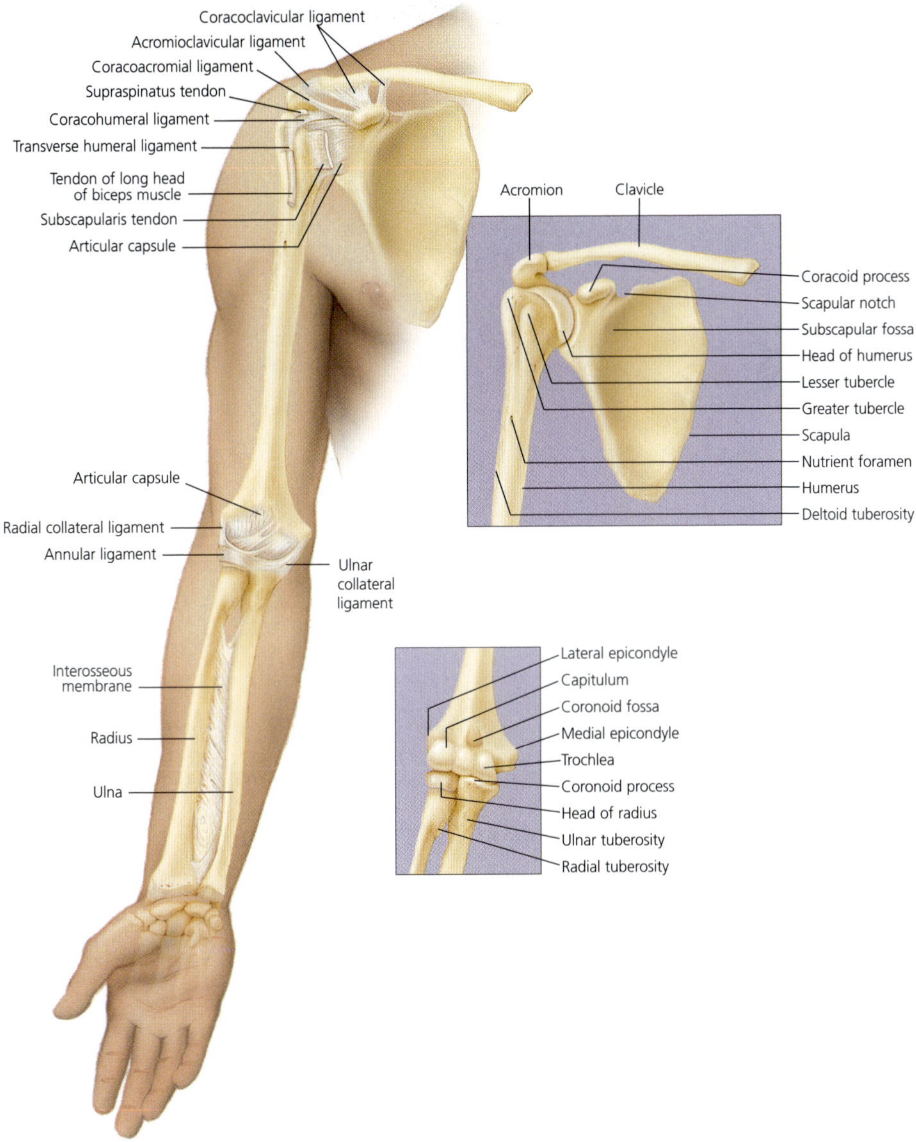

Hand and Wrist

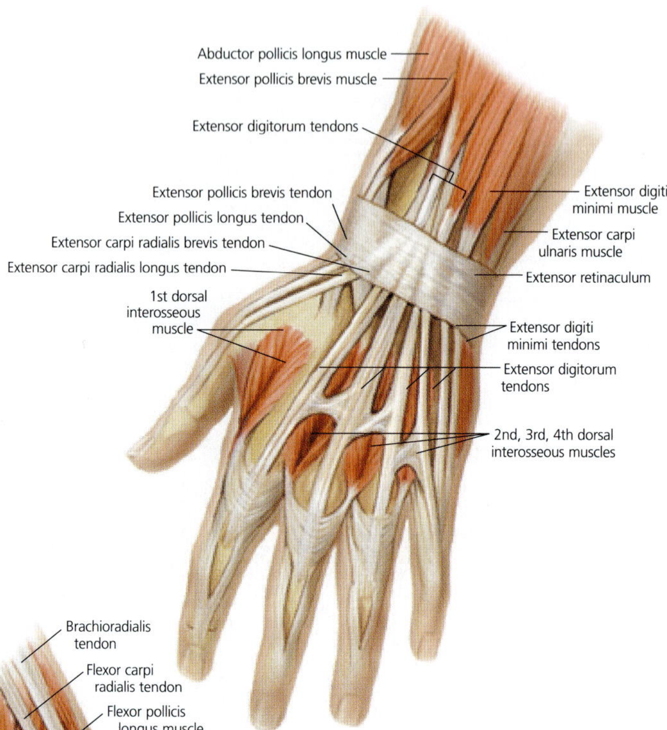

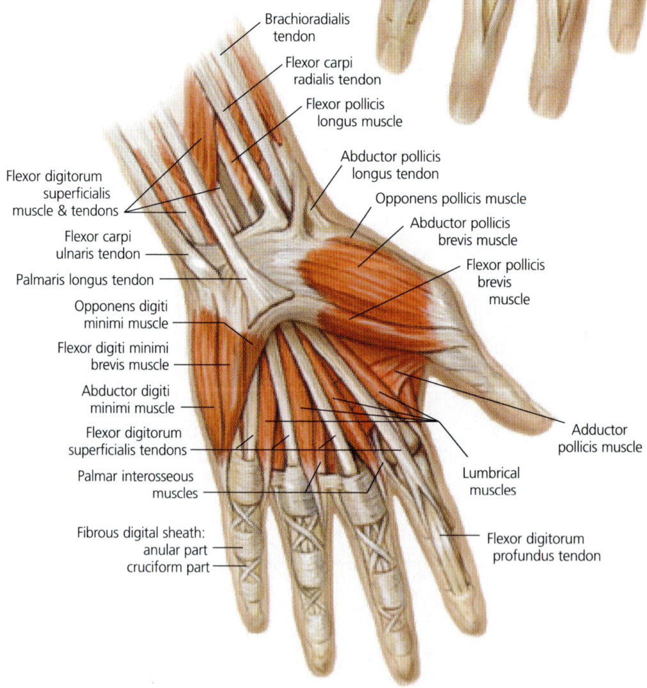

Hip and Knee

(Anterior View)

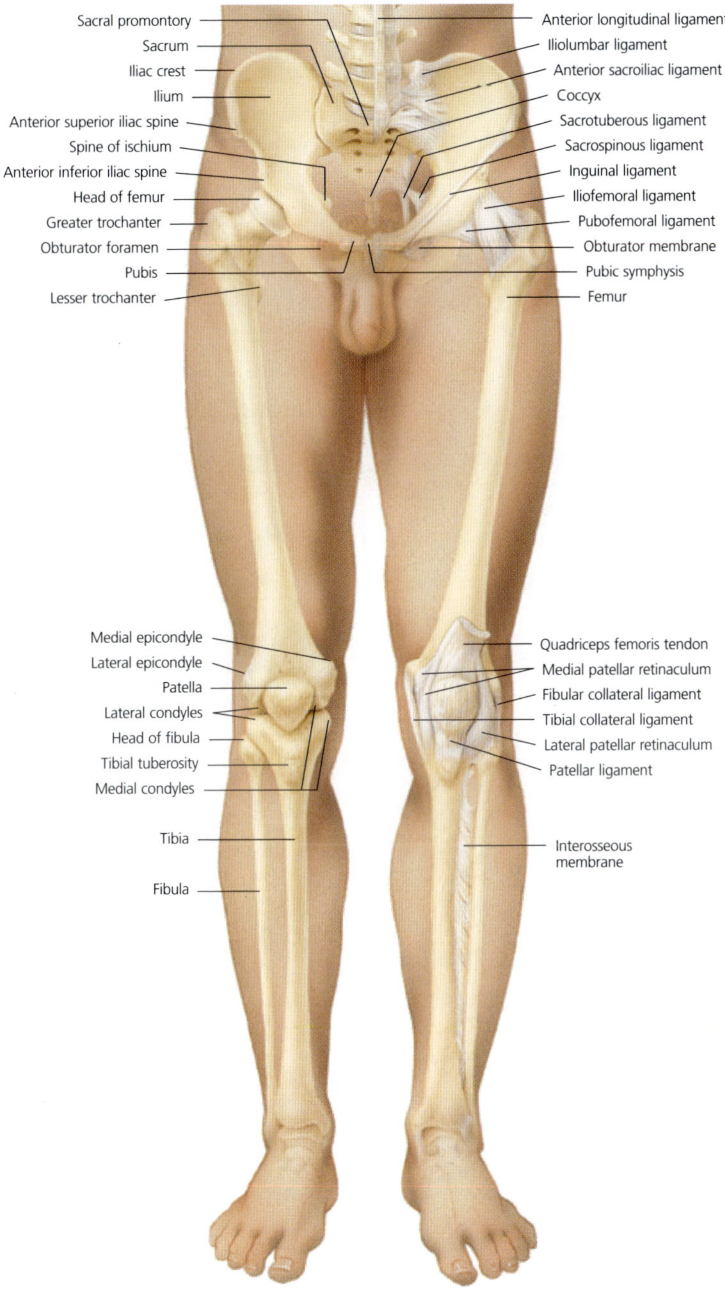

Foot and Ankle

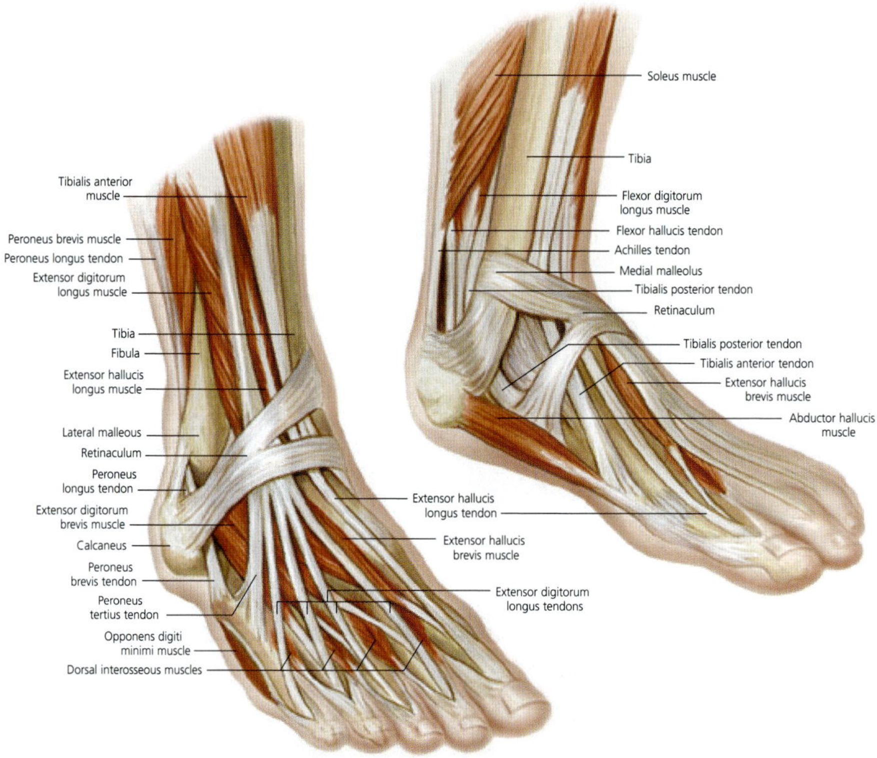

Skeletal System
(Anterior View)

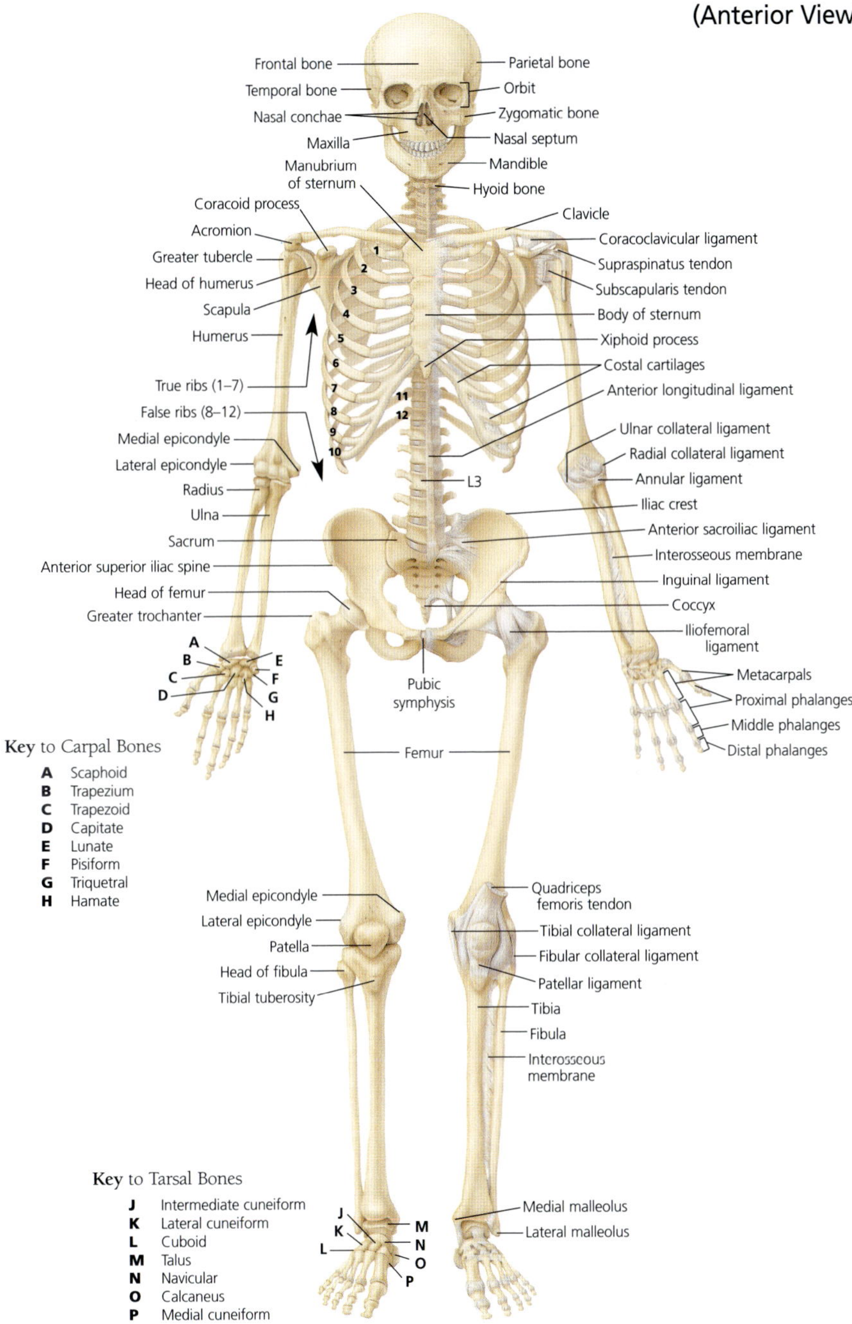

Skeletal System
(Posterior View)

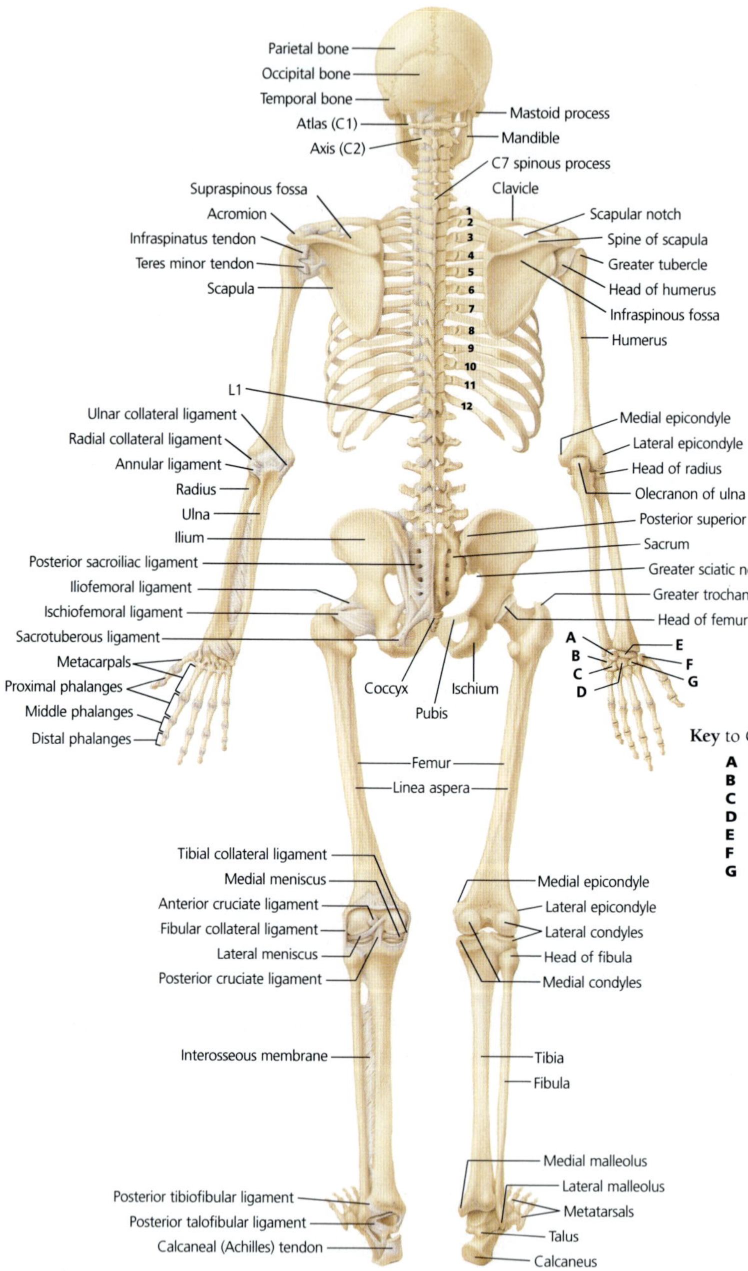

Key to Carpal Bones

A Lunate
B Triquetral
C Hamate
D Capitate
E Scaphoid
F Trapezium
G Trapezoid

Vertebral Column
(Lateral View)

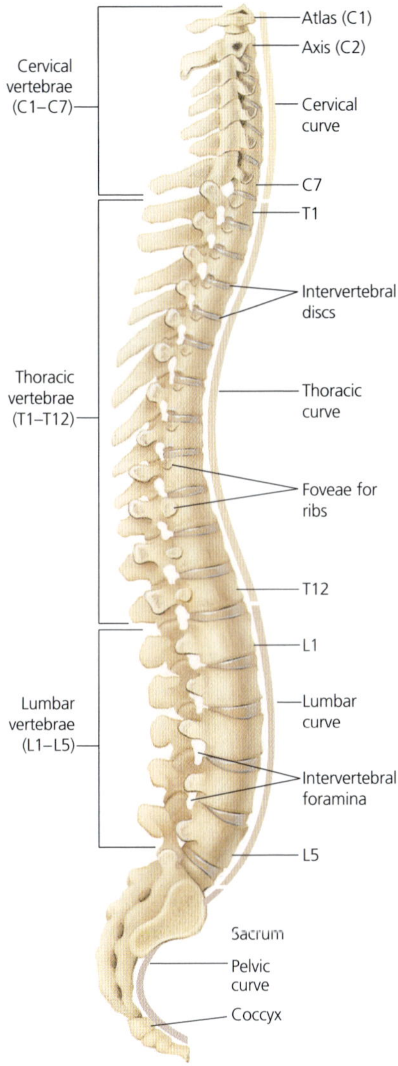

Respiratory System

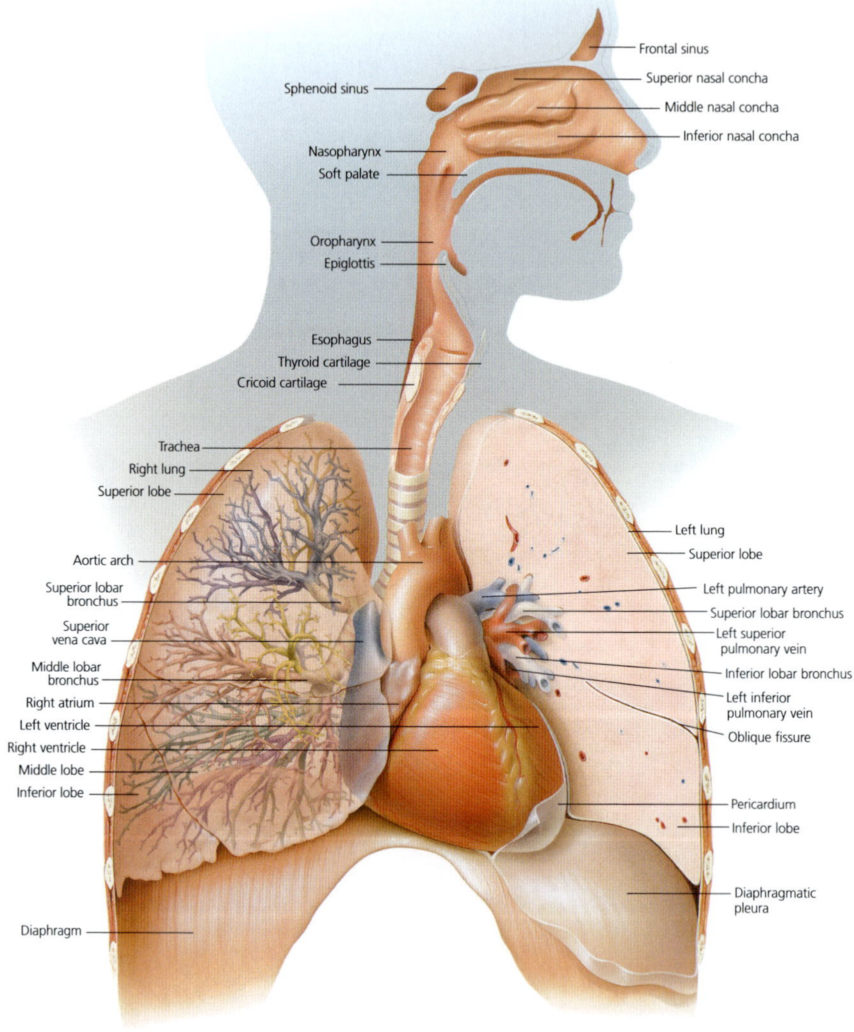

Heart
(External View)

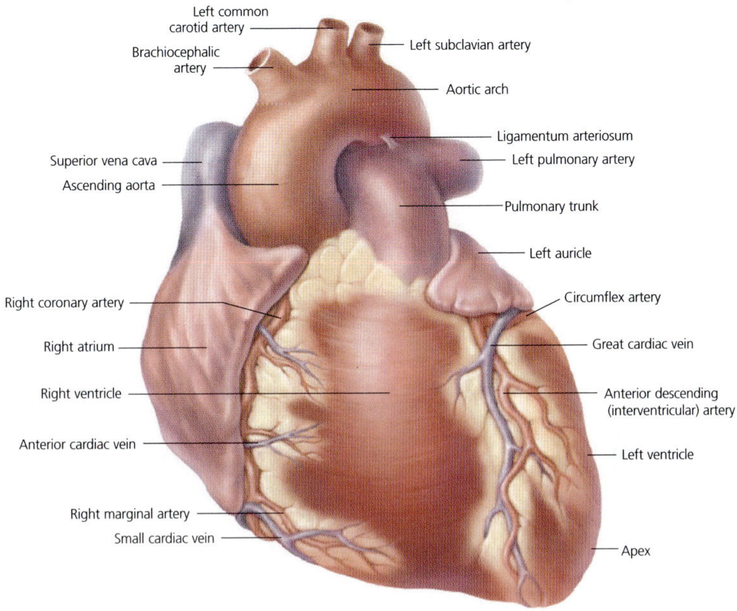

Heart
(Internal View)

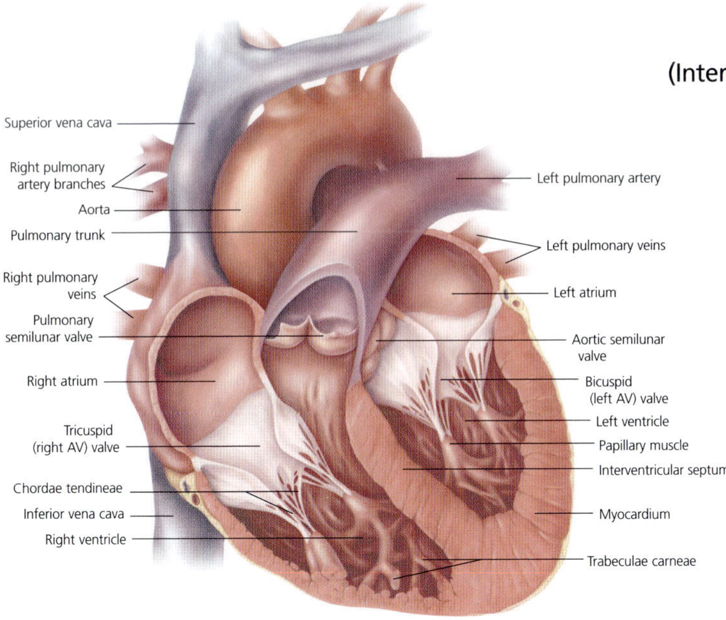

Vascular System

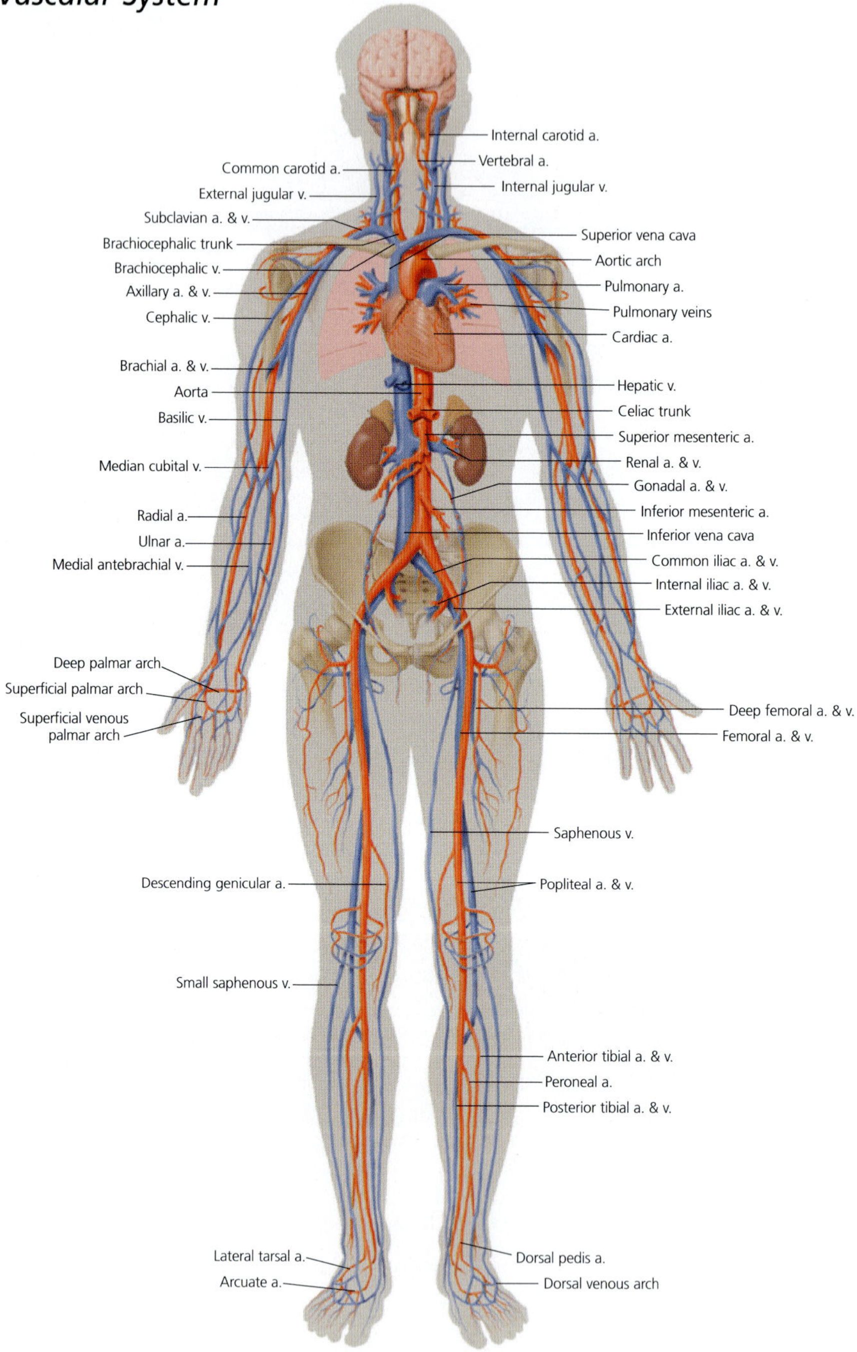

Digestive System

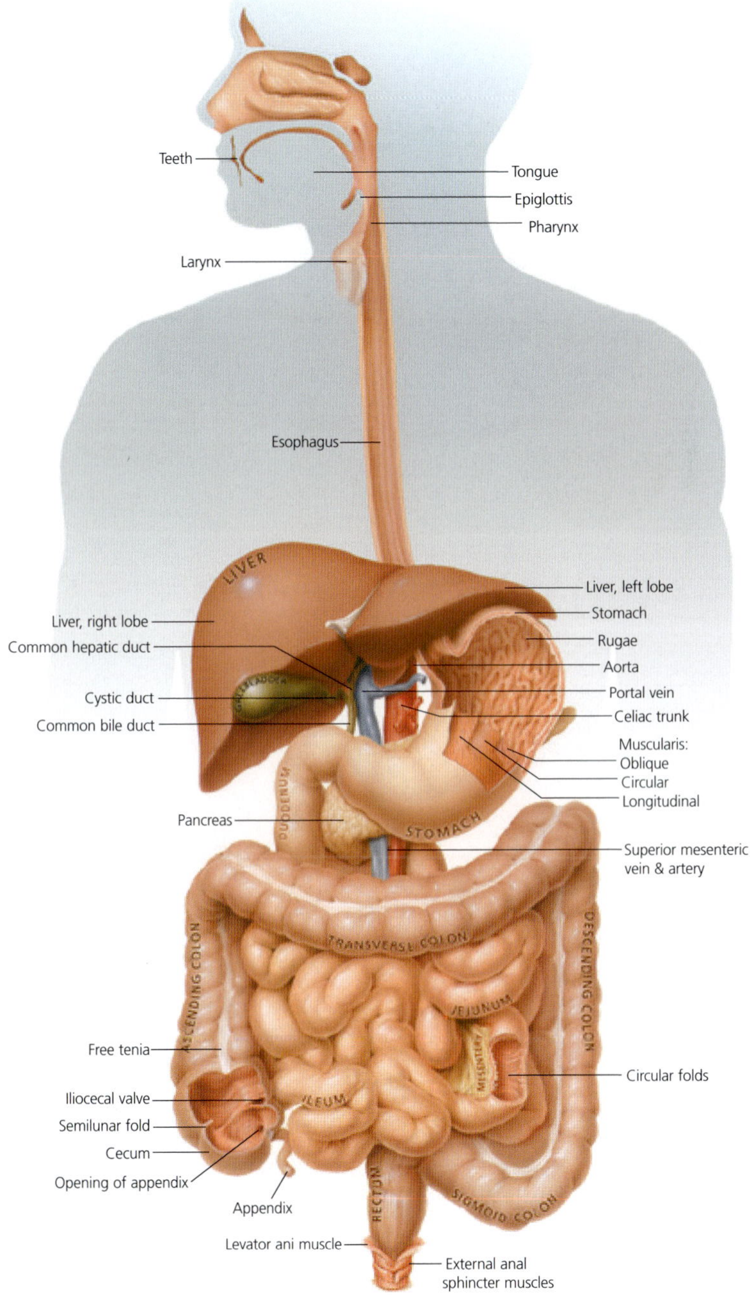

Urinary System

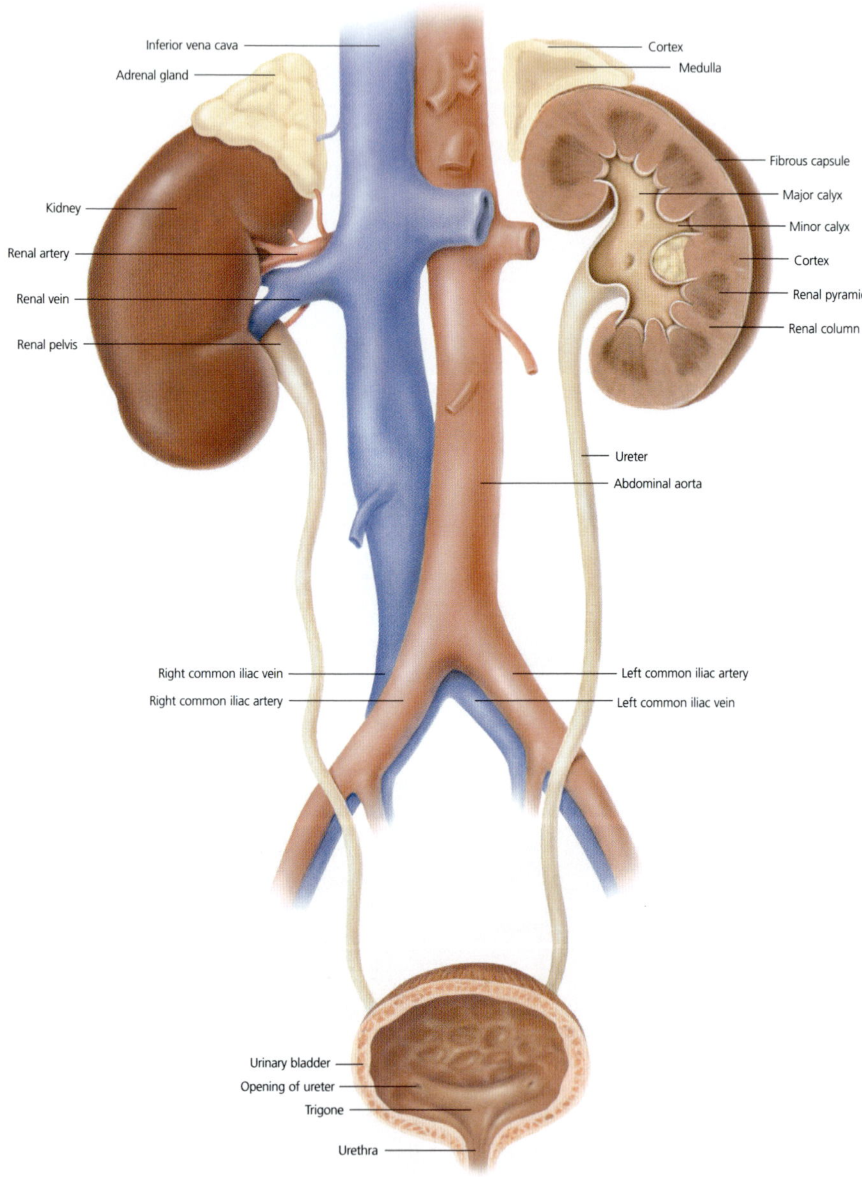

Male Reproductive System

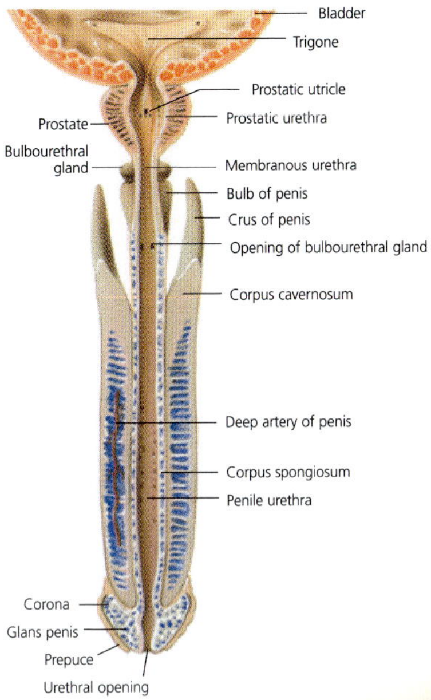

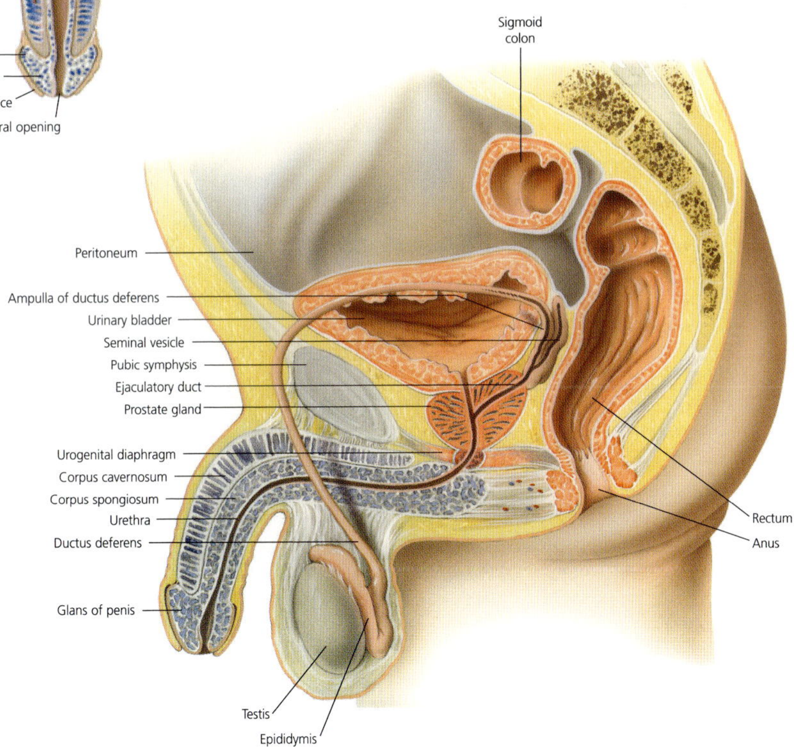

Female Reproductive System

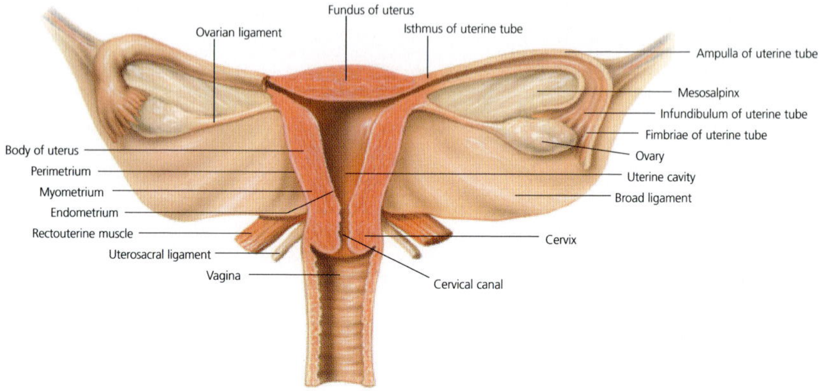

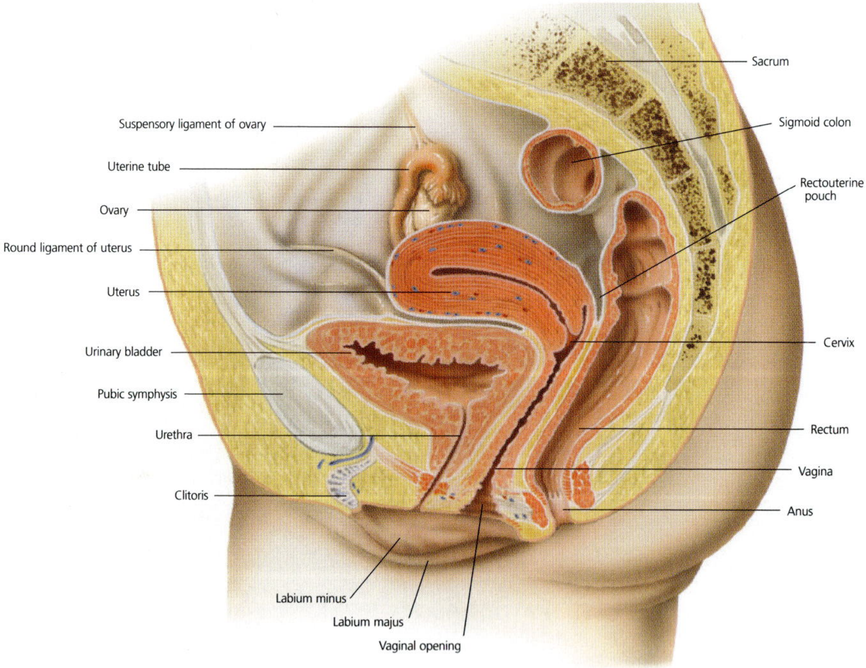

Female Reproductive System: Pregnancy

Lateral View)

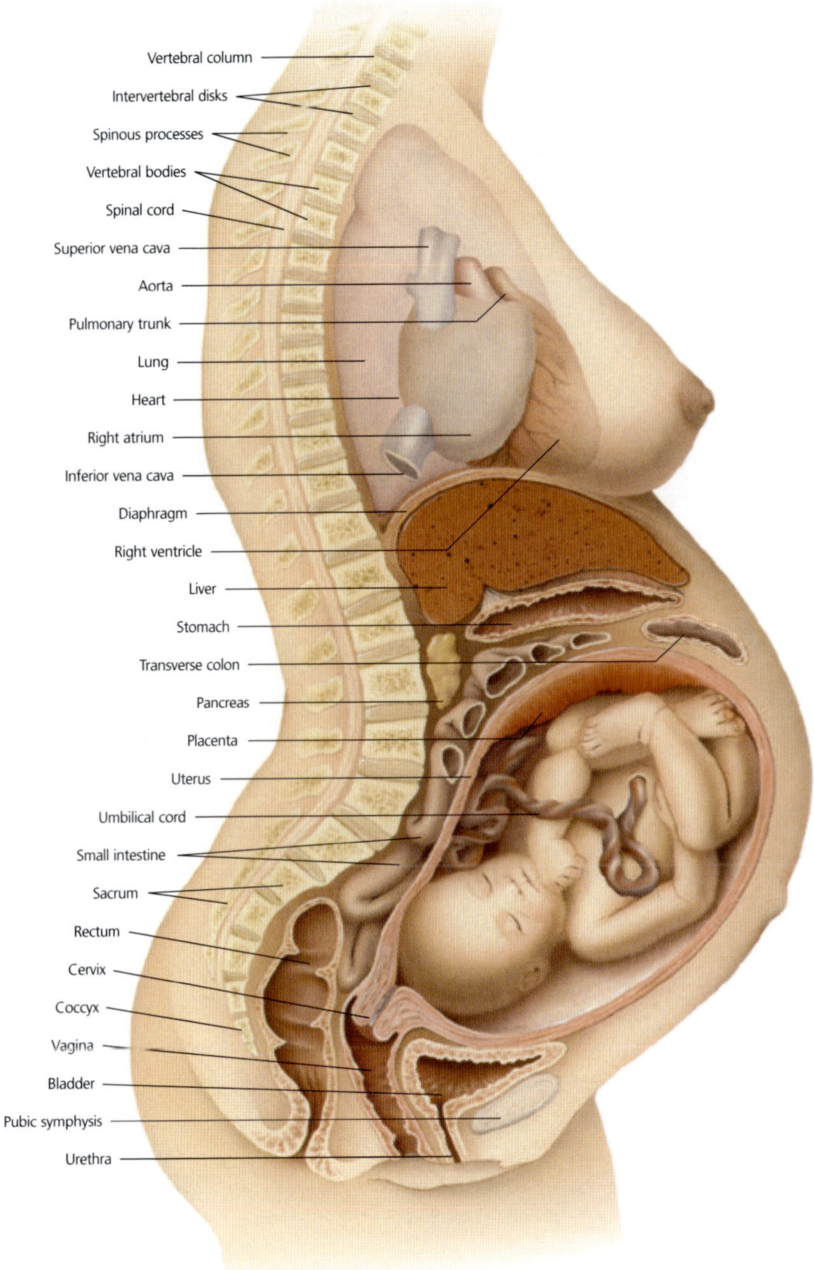

Brain
(Base View)

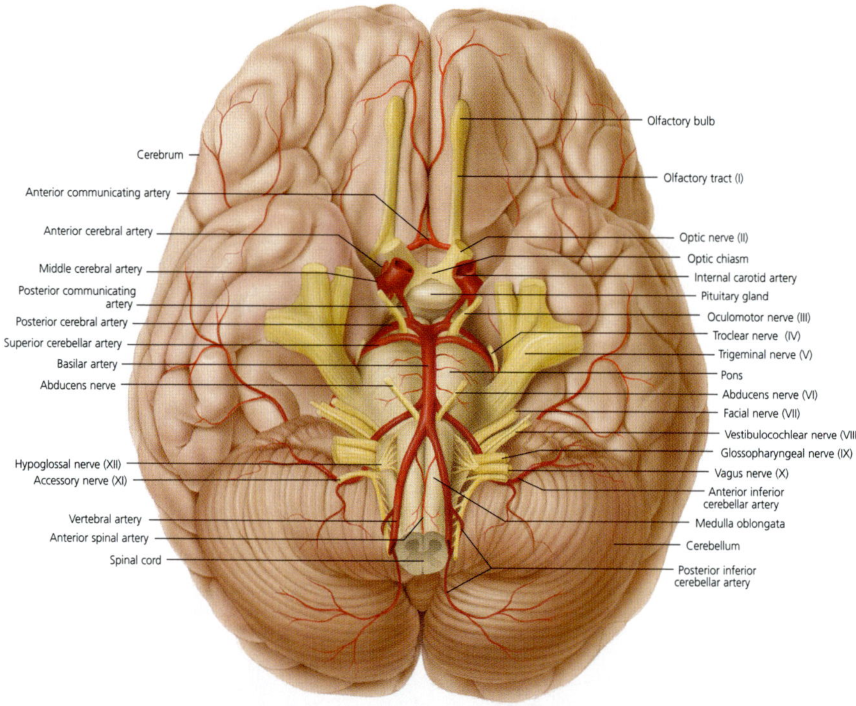

Nervous System

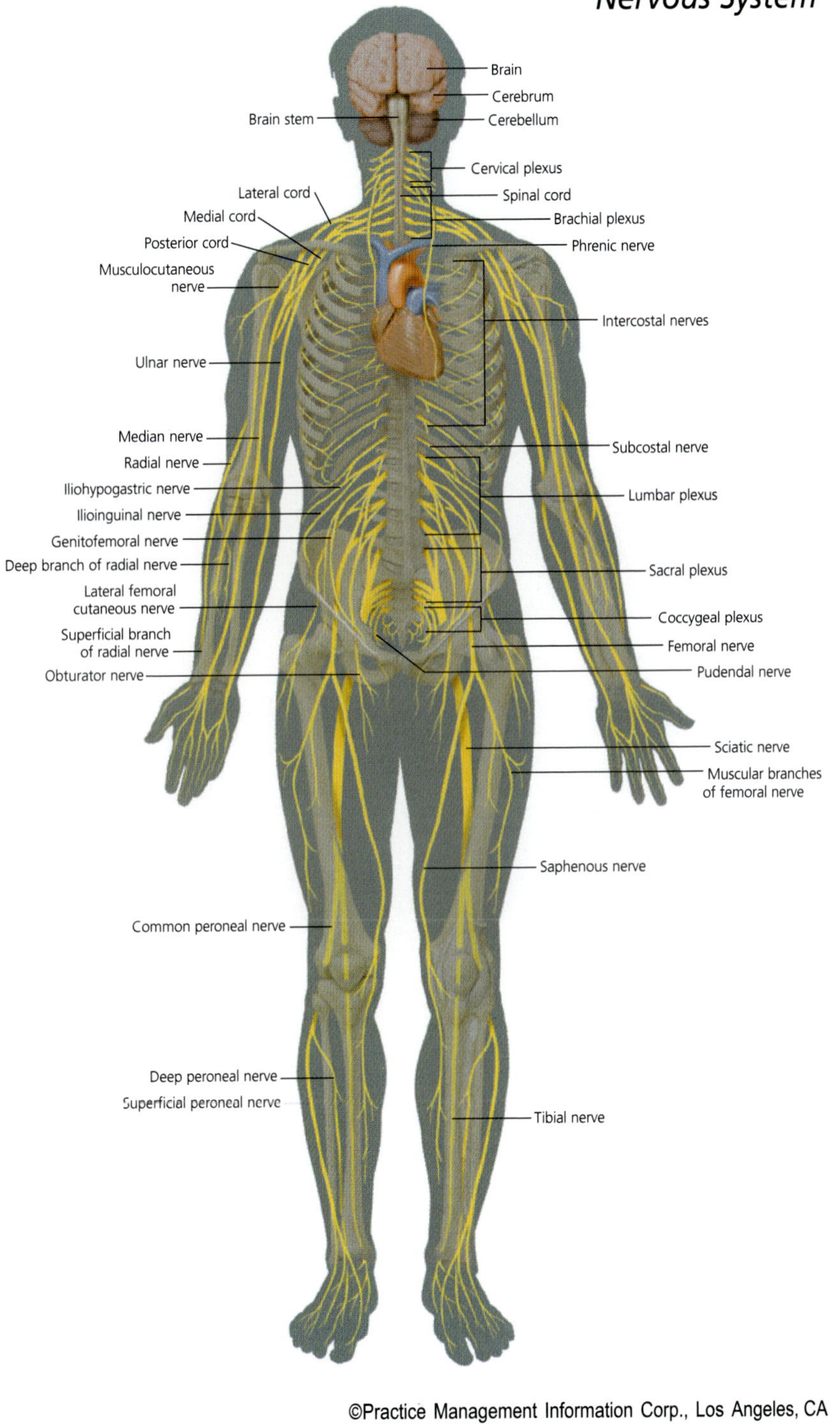

Right Eye
(Horizontal Section)

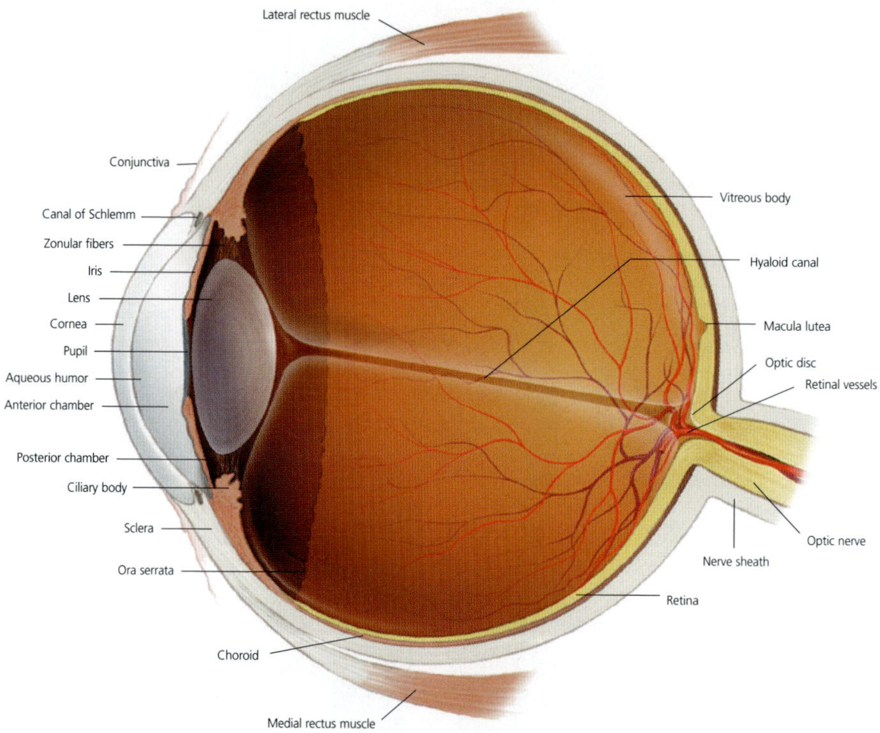

The Ear

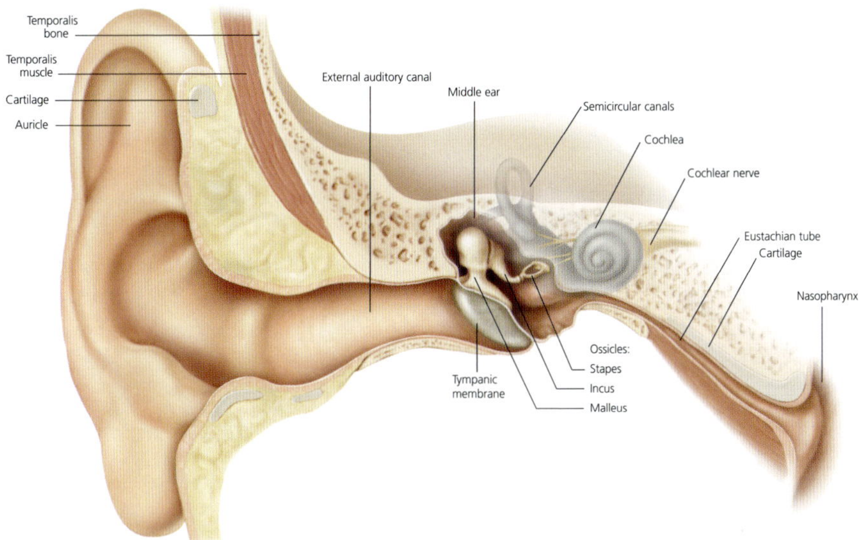
Temporalis
bone
Temporalis
muscle
Cartilage
Auricle
External auditory canal
Middle ear
Semicircular canals
Cochlea
Cochlear nerve
Eustachian tube
Cartilage
Nasopharynx
Tympanic
membrane
Ossicles:
Stapes
Incus
Malleus

A

A & H Accident And Health Insurance.

a-, an- Denotes an absence of.

A/G Ratio Albumin and globulin are the primary constituents of the protein found in blood. An abnormal ratio is seen when levels of albumin or globulin are elevated or decreased. Abnormal ratios are seen in various disorders, include-ing kidney and liver diseases. *Synonym:* albumin or globulin ration.

A/R Accounts Receivable.

AAA Abdominal Aortic Aneurysm.

AAAI American Academy of Allergy and Immunology.

AAC Antibiotic-Associated Colitis.

AAFA Asthma And Allergy Foundation of America.

AAFP American Academy of Family Physicians.

AAGP American Academy of General Practice.

AAHP American Association of Health Plans.

AAMA American Association of Medical Assistants.

AAME Acetylargenine Methyl Ester.

AAMS Acute Aseptic Meningitis Syndrome.

AAN American Academy of Neurology.

AANS American Academy of Neurological Surgery • American Association of Neurological Surgeons.

AAO American Academy of Ophthalmology.

AAOG American Association of Obstetricians and Gynecologists.

AAOS American Academy of Orthopaedic Surgeons.

AAP American Academy of Pediatrics.

AAPA American Academy of Physician Assistants.

AAPC American Association of Professional Coders • Annual Average Per Capita.

AAPCC Average annual per capita cost.

Aaron's sign Pain in the epigastric or precordial region in appendicitis.

Aarskog syndrome Faciogenital dysphasia.

AAU Acute Anterior Uveitis.

AAV Adeno-Associated Virus.

ab abortion.

ab- Away from.

Abadie's sign Spasm of the levator palpebrae superioris in thyro-toxicosis.

Abbe's operation Using a triangular portion of the lower lip to repair a defect in the upper lip.

Abbott's method Treatment of scoliosis by pulling the spine into the proper position and then applying a plaster cast to hold in place.

abd abdomen, abdominal.

Abderhalden-Kauffman-Lignac syndrome Renal rickets with systinosis.

abdomen The part of the body between the pelvis and the thorax.

abdomin(o)- of or relating to the abdomen.

abdominal of or referring to the abdomen.

abdominal aorta The largest artery in the abdominal cavity. As part of the aorta, it is a direct continuation of descending aorta (of the thorax).

abdominal cavity A cavity within the abdomen, the space between the abdominal wall and the spine.

abdominal pain Sensation of discomfort, distress, or agony in the abdominal region.

abdominal reflex The quadrants of the abdomen are stroked towards the midline above, parallel to and below the umbilicus. In corticospinal tract lesions, the reflex contraction of the abdominal muscles is lost on the side ipsilateral (same side) as the lesion.

abdominal wall The abdominal wall represents the boundaries of the abdominal cavity. The abdominal wall is split into the posterior (back), lateral (sides) and anterior (front) walls.

abdominohysterectomy hysterectomy through an abdominal incision.

abdominopelvic amputation Amputation of a lower limb through the sacroiliac joint.

abdominoperineal resection A surgery in which the anus, rectum, and sigmoid colon are removed. It is used to treat cancer located very low in the rectum or in the anus, close to the sphincter muscles.

abdominoplasty A cosmetic surgery procedure used to make the abdomen more firm. The surgery involves the removal of excess skin and fat from the middle and lower abdomen in order to tighten the muscle and fascia of the abdominal wall. *Synonym:* tummy tuck.

abducens nerve A small motor nerve supplying the lateral rectus muscle of the eye.

abduction A motion that pulls a structure or part away from the midline of the body (or, in the case of fingers and toes, spreading the digits apart, away from the centerline of the hand or foot). Abduction of the wrist is called radial deviation. Raising the arms laterally, to the sides, is an example of abduction.

abductor muscle Any muscle used to pull a body part away from the midline of the body.

ABE Acute Bacterial Endocarditis.

Abernethy's fascia Fascia iliaca.

ABG Arterial blood Gases.

ablation The removal or destruction of a body part or tissue or its function. Ablation may be performed by surgery, hormones, or drugs.

ABN Advance Beneficiary Notice.

abnormal Not normal; not typical or usual or regular or conforming to a norm.

abnormality An abnormal physical condition resulting from defective genes or developmental deficiencies.

ABO blood group The method of classifying human blood on the basis of the inherited properties of red blood cells. People may have type a, type b, type o, or type ab blood.

abortifacient agents Chemical substances that interrupt pregnancy after implantation.

abortion The termination of a pregnancy by the removal or expulsion from the uterus of a fetus or embryo, resulting in or caused by its death. An abortion can occur spontaneously due to complications during pregnancy or can be induced.

ABP Arterial blood Pressure.

ABR Auditory brain-stem response.

Abraham's sign A percussive sound heard over the lung with early tuberculosis.

Abrams' heart reflex Contraction of the myocardium when the precordial region is irritated.

abrasion A surgical procedure that involves the controlled wearing away of the upper layers of the skin with sandpaper or other mechanical means.

Abrikossov's tumor Granular cell tumor. Achard's syndrome Arachnodactyly associated with a receding mandible and joint laxity in the hands and feet.

abruptio placenta Separation of the placenta from the uterus during the last trimester of pregnancy.

ABS Acute Brain Syndrome • American Board of Surgery.

abscess A collection of pus (dead neutrophils) that has accumulated in a cavity formed by the tissue on the basis of an infectious process or other foreign materials. It is a defensive reaction of the tissue to prevent the spread of infectious materials to other parts of the body.

absence Refers to the lack of an organ, body part, or chemical substance.

absence seizure A seizure that takes the form of a staring spell. The person suddenly seems to be absent. An absence seizure involves a brief loss of awareness, which can be accompanied by blinking or mouth twitching.

absolute blood cell count Measurement of the total number of the white blood cell subtypes (neutrophils, lymphocytes, monocytes, eosinophils, and basophils) based on the percentage of each blood cell type and the total white blood cell (WBC) count. Abnormal absolute counts are seen in severe infections and blood disorders.

absorptiometry A diagnostic technique for measuring bone mineral density in which an image of bone is produced from computerized analysis of absorption rates of photons directed in a focused beam at a body part.

abstract The collection of information from the medical record via hard copy or electronic instrument.

abuse A range of the following improper behaviors or billing practices including, but not limited to; billing for a non-covered service; misusing codes on the claim (i.e., the way the service is coded on the claim does not comply with national or local coding guidelines or is not billed as rendered); or inappropriately allocating costs on a cost report.

abuse (personal) When another person does something on purpose that causes you mental or physical harm or pain.

abutment A tooth or implant used to support a prosthesis; the natural teeth (or implanted teeth) that hold a fixed or removable bridge in place.

AC Actual Charge.

-ac Pertaining to.

academic medical centers Medical complexes consisting of medical school, hospitals, clinics, libraries, administrative facilities, etc.

acanthosis An abnormal but benign thickening of the prickle-cell layer of the skin (as in psoriasis).

acariasis Infestation with arthropod parasites of the order acarina including the ticks and mites.

ACC American College of Cardiology.

access A patient's ability to obtain medical care. The ease of access is determined by components such as the availability to the patient, availability of insurance, the location of health care facilities, transportation, hours of operation, affordability and cost of care.

access authorization HIPAA information use policies or procedures that establish the rules for granting and/or restricting access to a user, terminal, transaction, program, or process.

access control HIPAA methods of restricting access to resources, allowing only privileged entities access. Types of access control include, among others, mandatory access control, discretionary access control, time-of-day, classification, and subject-object separation.

access controls HIPAA protection of sensitive communications transmissions over open or private networks so that it cannot be easily intercepted and interpreted by parties other than the intended recipient.

access establishment HIPAA security policies, and the rules established therein, that determine an entity's initial right of access to a terminal, transaction, program, or process.

access level A level associated with an individual who may be accessing information (for example, a clearance level) or with the information which may be accessed (for example, a classification level).

access modification The security policies, and the rules established therein, that determine types of, and reasons for, modification to an entity's established right of access to a terminal, transaction, program, or process.

accessory nerve A nerve that controls specific muscles of the neck.

accident and health insurance Health insurance under which benefits are payable in case of disease, accidental injury or accidental death.

accommodation The process by which the eye changes optical power to maintain a clear image on an object as its distance changes.

accountability The property that ensures that the actions of an entity can be traced uniquely to that entity.

ACCP American College of Chest Physicians.

Accountable Health Plans (AHP) : Under the Managed Care Act, providers and insurance companies would be encouraged (through tax incentives) to form AHPs, similar to HMOs, PPOs, and other group practices. Accountable health plans would compete on thc basis of offering high-quality, low-cost care and would offer insurance and health care as a single product. They would be responsible for looking after the total health of members and reporting medical outcomes in accordance with Federal guidelines.

accreditation An evaluative process in which a health care organization undergoes an examination of its operating procedures to determine whether the procedures meet designated criteria as defined by the accrediting body, and to ensure that the organization meets a specified level of quality.

accreditation for deeming Some states use the findings of private accreditation organizations, in part or in whole, to supplement or substitute for state oversight of some quality related standards. This is referred to as deemed compliance with a standard.

accreditation for participation State requirement that plans must be accredited to participate in the Medicaid managed care program.

Accredited Means that a facility or health care organization has met certain quality standards. These standards are set by private, nationally recognized groups that check on the quality of care at health care facilities and organizations. Organizations that accredit Medicare managed care plans include the national committee for quality assurance, the joint commission on accreditation of health care organizations, and the american accreditation health care commission or URAC.

accrete The addition of new enrollee to a health plan, usually used in reference to Medicare.

accumulation period Timeframe within a policy period in which deductible and out-of-pocket amounts are calculated. For most health insurance policies, the accumulation period is a calendar year.

ACE Angiotensin-Converting Enzyme.

ACE inhibitor A group of pharmaceuticals that are used primarily in treatment of hyper-tension and congestive heart failure.

acellular Not made up of or divided into cells.

ACEP American College of Emergency Physicians.

acetabular Refers to the acetabulum.

acetabuloplasty Plastic repair involving repair or enlargement of the cavity of the acetabulum to restore its normal state.

acetabulum The cup-shaped cavity at the base of the hipbone into which the ball-shaped head of the femur fits.

acetonuria Excessive amounts of ketone bodies in the urine as in diabetes mellitus or starvation.

ACF Accessory Clinical Findings.

ACF Ambulatory Care Facility.

ACG Ambulatory Care Group.

ACG Angiocardiogram, Angiocardiography.

ACH Acetylcholine.

ACH Adrenal Cortical (adreocortical) Hormone.

achalasia A condition of the esophagus that disrupts normal swallowing.

Achard's syndrome Arachnodactyly associated with a receding mandible and joint laxity in the hands and feet.

Achard-thiers syndrome Women with diabetes and aspects of both adrenogenital syndrome and Cushing syndrome including masculinization and menstrual disorders.

Achilles tendon The large tendon connecting the heel bone to the calf muscle of the leg.

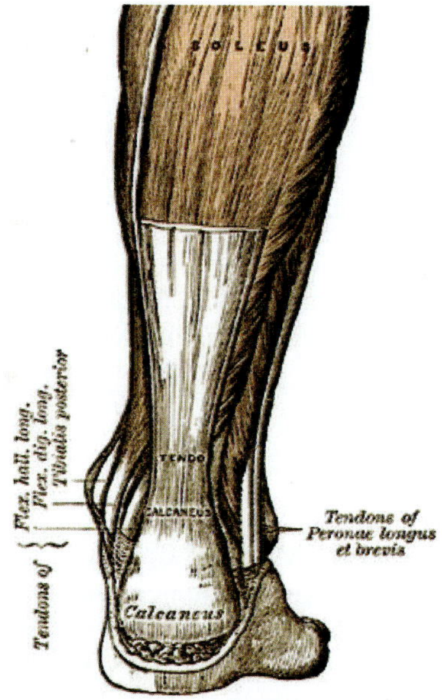

Achilles' tendon

achlorhydria An abnormal deficiency or absence of free hydrochloric acid in the gastric juice; often associated with severe anemias and cancer of the stomach.

achromatopsia An hereditary disorder of sight due to a lack of cone vision - that type of vision provided by the cone photoreceptors in the retina.

acid elution test Air-dried blood smears are fixed in 80 per cent methanol and immersed in a pH 3.3 buffer; all hemoglobins are eluted except fetal hemoglobin, which is seen in red cells after staining.

acid perfusion test A method to reproduce symptoms of heartburn. It is usually done with other tests to measure esophageal function. *Synonym:* bernstein test.

acid reflux disease A condition in which the esophagus becomes irritated or inflamed because of acid backing up from the stomach.

acid-base imbalance An imbalance that occurs when body retains too much acid or too much base.

acidified serum test Incubation of red cells in acidified serum; after centrifugation, the supernatant is examined by colorimetry for hemolysis, which indicates paroxysmal nocturnal hemoglobinuria.

acidosis Excessive acidity of body fluids due to accumulation of acids as may happen in diabetes or kidney disease.

acidosis, metabolic Too much acid in the body due to loss of base.

acidosis, respiratory Too much acid in the body due to accumulation of excess carbon dioxide.

Ackerman tumor Verrucous carcinoma of the larynx.

ACL Anterior Cruciate Ligament.

ACLS Advance Cardiac Life Support.

acne A skin condition characterized by the excessive production of oil from the sebaceous glands in which the hair follicles become blocked.

ACOG American College of Obstetricians and Gynecologists.

ACOMS American College of Oral and Maxillofacial Surgeons.

ACOS American College of Osteopathic Surgeons.

Acosta disease Hypoxic disease caused by high elevation.

acous(o)- of or relating to hearing.

acoustic Pertaining to the sense of hearing, the organs of hearing, or the science of sounds.

acoustic reflex test Measurement of the acoustic reflex threshold; used to differentiate between conductive and sensorineural deafness and to diagnose acoustic neuroma.

acoustic nerve A nerve in the inner ear that sends sound information to the brain.

acoustic neuroma A non-cancerous tumor that develops on the nerve that connects the ear to the brain.

acoustic reflex test Measurement of the acoustic reflex threshold; used to differentiate between conductive and sensorineural deafness and to diagnose acoustic neuroma.

acoustic reflex testing Brief, involuntary closure of the eyes due to stimulation of the acoustic nerve by a sudden sound.

ACPS Acrocephalopolysyndactyly.

acquired deformity A deformity acquired after birth from injury or disease.

acquired hypothyroidism acquired glandular disorder resulting from insufficient production of thyroid hormones.

Acquired Immune Deficiency Syndrome (AIDS) Major failure of body's immune system. It decreases body's ability to fight infection and suppress multiplication of abnormal cells, such as cancer cells. Caused by a sexually transmitted virus, contaminated blood or via the placenta to a fetus of an infected mother.

ACR American College of Radiology.

acr(o)- Extremity or topmost.

acrocephalosyndactyly Congenital disorder characterized by malformations of the skull, face, hands and feet.

acromegaly Condition characterized by a gradual, marked enlargement of the bones of the face, jaw and extremities. Caused by overproduction of growth hormone by pituitary gland.

acromial of or referring to the acromion.

acromial process The outermost point of the spine of the shoulder blade.

acromioclavicular joint A joint at the top of the shoulder. It is the junction between the acromion (part of the scapula that forms the highest point of the shoulder) and the clavicle.

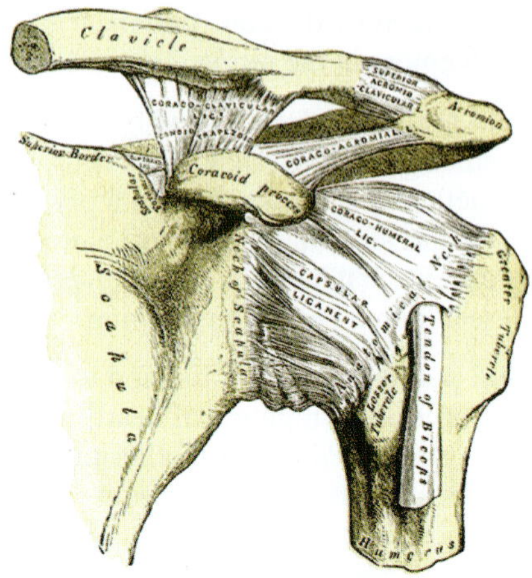

acromioclavicular joint

.acromion The outermost point of the spine of the shoulder blade.

acromionectomy Partial or total surgical excision of the acromion.

acromioplasty a arthroscopic surgical procedure of the acromion. Generally, it implies removal of a small piece of the surface of the bone (acromion) that is in contact with a tendon causing, by friction, damage to the latter tissue.

ACTD Actinomycin D.

ACTH Adrenocorticotropic hormone. A hormone produced by the pituitary gland. It stimulates adrenal glands to secrete the hormones they produce, including cortisone and cortisol.

ACTH deficiency A condition in which too little ACTH is produced by the pituitary gland; often the result of a pituitary tumor. Symptoms include weakness, fatigue and gastrointestinal disturbances.

actigraphy The use of a small instrument called an actigraph worn on the wrist or ankle to measure body movement. It creates a pattern based on activity that is useful in assessing sleep-wake cycles across many consecutive days and nights. It is useful for assessing advanced and delayed sleep phase disorders.

actinic keratosis A premalignant condition of thick, scaly, or crusty patches of skin.

actinomyces A genus of anaerobic, gram-positive bacteria that may cause disease in humans. The bacteria are normally present in the mouth and throat. Disease activity is normally limited to periodontal disease.

aActinomycosis Infection primarily caused by the bacterium actinomyces Israeli. Infection most often occurs in the face and neck region and is characterized by the presence of a slowly enlarging, hard, red lump.

actinotherapy The treatment of disease (especially cancer) by exposure to a radioactive substance.

activated partial thromboplastin time A blood test that measures the length of time (in seconds) that it takes for clotting to occur when certain substances are added to the liquid portion of blood in a test tube. It is used to detect clotting factor deficiencies and to monitor heparin's effectiveness.

activities of daily living Routine activities that people tend do everyday without needing assistance. There are six basic ADLs eating, bathing, dressing, toileting, transferring (walking) and continence. An individual's ability to perform ADLs is important for determining what typc of long-tcrm care (e.g. Nursing-home care or home care) and coverage the individual needs (i.e. Medicare, Medicaid or long-term care insurance).

actual charge The amount a physician or other provider actually bills a patient for a particular medical service, procedure or supply in a specific instance. The actual charge may differ from the usual, customary, prevailing, and/or reasonable charge.

actuarial cost of **coverage** The expected dollar value of a health plan's benefits. The method of determining this value may be based entirely on a plan's provisions, or may adjust for the geographic location and demo-graphic characteristics of enrollees, the actual health care utilization level by plan participants, or the type of plan under which the benefits are provided.

actuarial rates One half of the expected monthly cost of the SMI program for each aged enrollee (for the aged actuarial rate) and one half of the expected monthly cost for each disabled enrollee (for the disabled actuarial rate) for the duration the rate is in effect.

actuarial soundness A measure of the adequacy of Hospital Insurance (HI) and Supplementary Medical Insurance (SMI) financing as determined by the difference between trust fund assets and liabilities for specified periods.

actuarial status A measure of the adequacy of the financing as determined by the difference between assets and liabilities at the end of the periods for which financing was established.

acuity Clearness, as in visual acuity. The most common measure of visual acuity is the Snellen acuity chart.

acupuncture Refers to the insertion of thin needles through the skin at specific points on the body to control pain and other symptoms. It is a type of complementary and alternative medicine.

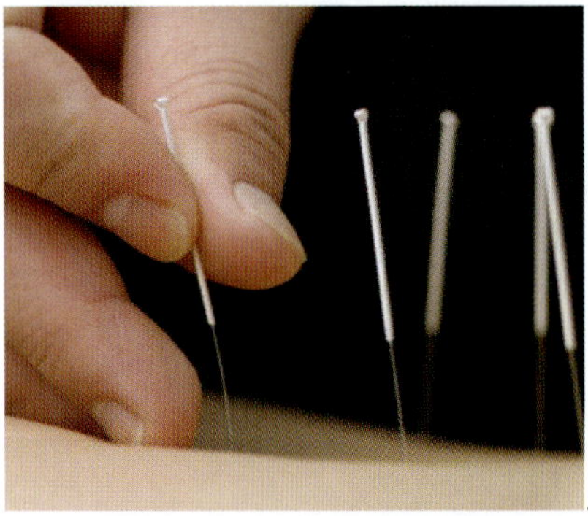

Application of acupuncture needles

-acusis Hearing.

acute of abrupt onset, in reference to a disease. Acute often also connotes an illness that is of short duration, rapidly progressive, and in need of urgent care.

acute care Hospital care given to patients who generally require a stay of up to seven days and that focuses on a physical or mental condition requiring immediate intervention and constant medical attention, equipment and personnel.

acute coronary syndrome A classification encompassing clinical presentations ranging from unstable angina through non, sometimes also including Q wave infarction.

acute hemolytic transfusion reaction Acute hemolytic transfusion reaction can cause serious, potentially fatal consequences. HTRs are most often caused by ABO blood type incompatibility between the blood product needed by the patient and red blood cells given the patient during transfusion.

acute intermittent porphyria Disease of porphyrin metabolism. Symptoms include recurrent attacks of abdominal pain, gastrointestinal symptoms, neurological disturbances and an excess of porphobilinogen in the urine.

acute pulmonary edema Set of dramatic, life-threatening symptoms, including extreme shortness of breath, rapid breath-ing, anxiety, cough, bluish lips and nails, and sweating. Usually caused by congestive heart failure. *See* Congestive heart failure.

acute respiratory distress syndrome Fulminant pulmonary interstitial and alveolar edema, which usually develops within a few days after the initiating trauma, thought to result from alveolar injury that has led to increased capillary permeability.

acute retinal necrosis syndrome Necrotizing retinitis with uveitis and other retinal pathology, severe loss of vision, and often retinal detachment; of viral etiology.

ACVD Acute Cardiovascular Disease.

-ad Toward, in the direction of.

ad- Increase, adherence, motion toward, very.

ad lib Freely, as desired (ad libitum).

ADA American Dental Association.

Adair Dighton's syndrome Osteogenesis imperfecta.

adamantinoma A slow growing cancerous bone tumor that is most often found in the shin bone (tibia) or the jaw bone (mandible). Occasionally, these tumors are found in the forearm, hands or feet. It is a rare tumor, occurring primarily in males between the ages of 10-30, usually after skeletal maturity is reached.

Adams Stokes syndrome Episodic cardiac arrest and syncope due to failure of normal and escape pacemakers, with or without ventricular fibrillation; the principal manifestation of severe heart attack.

ADAS Alzheimer's Disease Assessment Scale.

ADD Attention deficit disorder.

addenda Official updates to ICD-9-CM published continuously since 1986 that become effective on October 1st of each year.

Addison's disease Condition caused by inactive or underactive adrenal glands. Symptoms include weakness, low blood pressure, behavior changes, abdominal pain, diarrhea, appetite loss and brown skin. *Synonym:* hypoadreno-corticism, hypoadrenalism.

add-on codes Many surgical procedures are performed secondary to primary surgical procedures. These procedures are classified as additional or supplemental proce-dures and are designated as add-on codes in the cpt coding system. Add-on cpt codes are identified.

adduction A motion that pulls a structure or part towards the midline of the body, or towards the midline of a limb. Dropping the arms to the sides, or bringing the knees together, are examples of adduction. In the case of the fingers or toes, adduction is closing the digits together. Adduction of the wrist is called ulnar deviation.

adductor A muscle that moves a body part (e.g. an arm or leg) towards the midline of the body.

aden(o)-, aden(i)- of or relating to a gland.

adenocarcinoma Any of a large group of cancerous tumors of a gland or gland tissue.

adenoidectomy Surgical removal of the adenoids.

adenoiditis Inflammation of the adenoid tissue.

adenoids A mass of lymphoid tissue situated at the very back of the nose, in the roof of the nasopharynx, where the nose blends into the mouth.

adenoma Benign tumor of glandular cells. May cause excess hormone secretion by the affected gland.

adenomatosis An abnormal condition in which hyperplasia or tumor development affects two or more glands, usually the thyroid, adrenals, or pituitary.

adenopathy A glandular disease or enlargement of glandular tissue (especially of the lymph glands).

adenovirus A group of viruses that cause respiratory tract and eye infections.

adequacy The extent to which a network offers the appropriate types and numbers of providers in the appropriate geographic distribution according to the needs of the plan's members.

ADG Ambulatory Diagnostic Group.

ADH A test that measures the amount of antidiuretic hormone (ADH) in blood. ADH is found in the body, and it may be given as a medication.

ADHD Attention-deficit or hyperactivity disorder.

adhesiolysis A surgical procedure used to remove scar tissue formed as a result of prior surgery or infections involving reproductive tact, urinary tract or vaginal canal causing severe pain.

adhesions Small strands of fibrous tissue that cause organs in the abdomen and pelvis to cling together abnormally, creating a risk of intestinal obstruction.

Adie's syndrome Tonic pupil associated with absence or diminution of certain tendon reflexes.

adip(o)- of or relating to fat or fatty tissue.

adipose tissue Specialized connective tissue that functions as the major storage site for fat in the form of triglycerides. *Synonym:* fatty tissue.

adjudication The process of deciding whether to pay, pend, or reject a claim based upon the information submitted, the eligibility of the recipients, and the available benefits.

adjusted average per capita cost An estimate of the average per capita cost incurred by Medicare per beneficiary in the fee-for-service system, adjusted by county for age, sex, and program entitlement.

adjusted community rating A rating method under which a health plan or MCO divides its members into classes or groups based on demographic factors such as geography, family composition, and age, and then charges all members of a class or group the same premium. The plan cannot consider the experience of a class, group, or tier in developing premium rates. *Synonym:* modified community rating, community rating by class.

adjusted historical payment basis The average historical payment in aspecific locality for a specific service.

Adjusted Payment Rate (APR) The Medicare capitated payment to risk-contract HMOs. For a given plan, the APR is determined by adjusted county-level AAPCCs to reflect the relative risks of the plan's enrollees.

adjustment A chiropractic term which describes the skilled application of force to a joint or motion segment to improve intersegmental motion, decrease localized muscle tension, and restore normal motion and position.

adjustment disorder A classification of mental disorder that is a psychological response from an identifiable stressor or group of stressors that causes significant emotional or behavioral symptoms that does not meet criteria for more specific disorders.

ADL Activities of Daily Living.

administrative code sets Code sets that characterize a general business situation, rather than a medical condition or service. Under HIPAA, these are sometimes referred to as non-clinical or non-medical code sets.

administrative costs Costs related to activities such as utilization review, marketing, medical under-writing, commissions, premium collection, claims processing, insurer profit, quality assurance, and risk management for purposes of insurance.

administrative data Information that is collected, processed, and stored in automated information systems. Administrative data include enrollment or eligibility information, claims information, and managed care encounters. The claims and encounters may be for hospital and other facility services, professional services, prescription drug services, laboratory services, or other services.

administrative procedures to guard data integrity, confidentiality and availability Under HIPAA, documented, formal practices to manage (1) the selection and execution of security measures to protect data, and (2) the conduct of personnel in relation to the protection of data.

administrative simplification Title II, Subtitle F, of HIPAA which authorizes HHS to (1) adopt standards for transactions and code sets that are used to exchange health data; (2) adopt standard identifiers for health plans, health care providers, employers, and individuals for use on standard transactions; and (3) adopt standards to protect the security and privacy of personally identifiable health information.

admission date The date the patient was admitted for inpatient care, outpatient service, or start of care. For an admission notice for hospice care, enter the effective date of election of hospice benefits.

admitting physician The physician responsible for admitting a patient to a hospital or other inpatient health facility.

admitting privileges The right granted to a physician to admit patients to a particular hospital.

adnexa Accessory or adjoining anatomical parts.

adren(o)- of or relating to adrenal glands.

adrenal Pertaining to one or both glands located adjacent to the kidneys. These glands secrete many hormones, including adrenalin, and play an important part in the body's endocrine system.

adrenal cortex Outer layer of the adrenal gland. Secretes various hormones including cortisone, estrogen, testosterone, cortisol, androgen, aldosterone and progesterone.

adrenal gland A gland located on each kidney that secretes hormones regulating metabolism, sexual function, water balance, and stress.

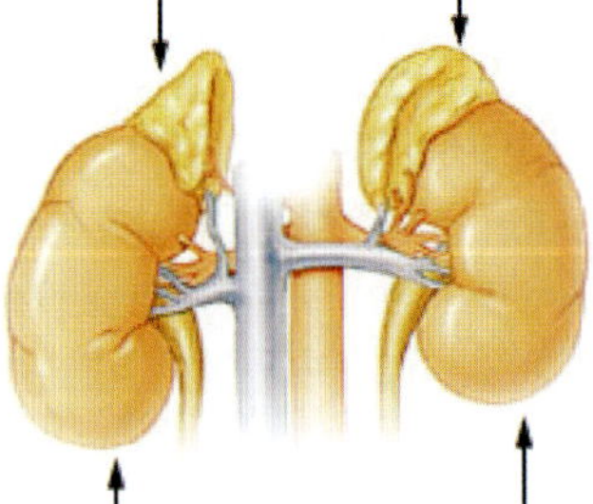

adrenal hyperplasia Abnormal increase in the number of normal cells in the adrenal gland(s).

adrenal medulla Middle part of the adrenal gland. Secretes epinephrine (adrenalin) and norepinephrine.

adrenal medulla tumors Tumors of the medulla, an inner layer of the adrenal gland, called pheochromocytomas. Tumors are rare and secrete norepinephrine and epinephrine. They are characterized by episodes of hypertension, headache, palpitations, sweating and apprehension. *Synonym:* pheochromocytoma.

adrenalectomy The surgical removal of one or both adrenal glands. *Synonym:* suprarenalectomy.

adrenaline Properly referred to as epinephrine, is a hormone and neurotransmitter that participates in the fight or flight response of the sympathetic nervous system.

adrenergic Activated by, characteristic of, or secreting epinephrine or related substances, particularly the sympathetic nerve fibers that liberate norepinephrine at a synapse when a nerve impulse passes.

adrenocortical hyperplasia Increase in the number of cells of the adrenal cortex. Adrenal cortex secretes cortisol, androgens and aldosterone. Increased production of any or all of these hormones may result in a variety of disorders, such as Cushing's syndrome and hypertension. *See* Cushing's syndrome; hypertension.

adrenocorticotropic hormone A hormone produced and secreted by the anterior pituitary gland often produced in response to biological stress. Its principal effects are increased production of androgens and cortisol from the adrenal cortex.

adrenocorticotropic hormone deficiency Insufficient ACTH is produced by the pituitary gland. *See* ACTH.

adrenogenital syndrome A group of disorders caused by adreno-cortical hyperplasia or malignant tumors, resulting in abnormal secretion of adrenocortical horm-ones and characterized by masculi-nization of women, feminization of men, or precocious sexual develop-ment in children.

adrenoleukodystrophy Disturbance in brain substance caused by abnormal function of the adrenal gland.

Adson's test one for thoracic outlet syndrome; with the patient in a sitting position, hands on thighs, the examiner palpates both radial pulses as the patient rapidly fills the lungs by deep inhalation and, holding breath, hyperextends the neck, turning the head toward the affected side. If the radial pulse on that side is markedly or completely obliterated, the result is positive.

adult day care A program of social and health-related services provided during the day in a community group setting. The purpose of the program is to support frail or impaired elderly, or other disabled adults who can benefit from care in a group setting outside the home.

adult foster care An elderly person's placement with another family when independent living is no longer possible, but nursing care is not necessary.

adult living care facility To be used when billing services rendered at a residential care facility that houses beneficiaries who cannot live alone but who do not need around-the-clock skilled medical services. The facility services do not include a medical component.

Advance Beneficiary Notice (ABN) A report given to Medicare beneficiaries to let the patient know that Medicare is not likely to pay for certain services. The notice must be given to the patient before services are performed.

CMS has modified its form and given explicit instructions how the locater form should be completed. According to regulations, providers include physicians, institutions such as outpatient hospitals, practitioners and suppliers paid under Part B, and hospice providers and religious non-medical health care institutions (RNHCIs) paid exclusively under Part A.

The ABN form must be verbally reviewed with the beneficiary or their representative before they sign it. Once completed and the form is signed, a copy is given to the beneficiary or representative. In all cases, the notifier must retain the original notice on file. These forms are not required in emerg-ency or urgent care situations.

advance medical directive Written ahead of time, a health care advance directive is a written document that defines how a patient wants medical decisions to be made if the patient loses the ability to make decisions for themselves. A health care advance directive may include a Living Will and a Durable Power of Attorney for health care.

adverse Any response to a drug that is noxious and unintended and occurs with proper dosage.

adverse effect A harmful and undesired effect resulting from a medication or other intervention such as chemotherapy or surgery.

adverse event Any harm a patient suffers that is caused by factors other than the patient's underlying condition.

adverse selection Among applicants for a given group or individual health insurance program, the tendency for those with an impaired health status, or who are prone to higher-than-average utilization of benefits, to be enrolled in disproportionate numbers in lower deductible plans.

advocacy Any activity done to help a person or group to get something the person or group needs or wants.

AEG air encephalogram.

AEP Auditory evoked potential.

AER Acoustic Evoked Response.

aer(o)- air, gas.

aerobacter Any bacteria of a former genus (Aerobacter) normally found in the intestine now in either of two genera (Enterobacter or Klebsiella).

aerobic Depending on free oxygen or air; aerobic fermentation.

aerosol A cloud of solid or liquid particles in a gas.

AF Atrial fibrillation, atrial flutter.

AFB Acid-Fast Bacillus.

AFDC Aid to Families with Dependent Children.

affective disorder A category of mental health problems that includes a disturbance in mood, usually profound sadness or apathy, euphoria or irritability, such as the disorder depression. *Synonym:* mood disorder.

afferent loop syndrome Chronic partial obstruction of the proximal loop (duodenum and jejunum) after gastrojejunostomy, resulting in duodenal distention, pain, and nausea following ingestion of food.

affiliated provider A health care provider or facility that is paid by a health plan to give service to plan members.

aflatoxin A toxin produced by mold that can damage the liver and may lead to liver cancer.

AFMS Affective Family Member Syndrome.

AFO Ankle-Foot Orthosis (Splint).

AFP alpha-fetoprotein.

AFRD Acute Febrile Respiratory Disease.

aftercare The care or follow-up treatment needed by a patient who has recently undergone surgery, been involved in an accident or has experienced an illness requiring hospitalization.

after-cataract Secondary cataract. Remnants of an opaque lens remaining in the eye, or opacities forming, after extracapsular cataract removal.

AG Atrial gallop.

age or sex rating A method of structuring capitation payments based on enrollee or membership age and sex.

aged enrollee An individual aged 65 or over, who is enrolled in the SMI program.

agenesis The failure of an organ to develop during embryonic growth and development.

age/sex factor A measurement used in insurance underwriting. It represents the age and sex risk of medical costs of one population relative to another. For example, a group with an age/sex factor of 1.05 would be expected to incur medical costs 5% greater than the average.

Age/Sex Rates (ASR) Set of rates for a grouping based on age and sex categories used to calculate premiums. This type of premium structure is often preferred over single and family rating in small groups because it automatically adjusts to demographic changes in the group. *Synonym:* table rates.

Agency for Health Care Policy and Research (AHCPR) A Federal agency within the Public Health Service responsible for research on quality, appropriateness, effectiveness and cost of health care.

AGG Agammaglobulinemia.

agglutination The process by which suspended bacteria, cells, or other particles are caused to adhere and form into clumps.

agglutination test Cells containing antigens to a given antibody are mixed into the solution being tested for a particular antibody, with agglutination indicative of antibody presence.

AGL Acute Granulocytic Leukemia.

aglossia A developmental anomaly in which a portion or all of the tongue is absent.

agoraphobia anxiety disorder characterized by a fear of open, public places or of being in crowds. Agoraphobics often experience panic attacks in a place or situation from which escape may be difficult or embarrassing.

AGOS American Gynecological and Obstetrical Society.

AGPA American Group Practice Association.

agranulocytosis Agranulocytosis means a failure of the bone marrow to make enough white blood cells (neutrophils). Bone marrow is the soft tissue inside bones that helps form blood cells.

AGS Adrenogenital Syndrome.

AGTH Adrenoglomerulotropin.

AGTT Abnormal glucose tolerance test.

AHA Acquired Hemolytic Anemia, American Hospital Association.

ahaptoglobulinemia Without haptoglobin in the blood. Condition is often seen with hemolytic anemia, severe liver disease and infectious mononucleosis. *See* Anemia, hemolytic; infectious mononucleosis.

Aid to Families with Dependant Children (AFDC) A Federally supported, state-administered program established by the Social Security Act of 1935 that provides financial support for children under the age of 18 (and their caretakers) who have been deprived of parental support or care because of the parent's death, continued absence from the home, unemployment, or physical or mental illness.

AHD Arteriosclerotic Heart Disease • Atherosclerotic Heart Disease.

AHFS American Hospital Formulary Service.

AHIMA American Health Information Management Association.

AHIP Assisted Health Insurance Plan.

AHPB Adjusted Historical Payment Basis.

AICD Automatic Implantable Cardioverter Defibrillator.

AIDS Acquired Immune Deficiency Syndrome.

AIHD Acquired Immune Hemolytic Disease.

air abrasion, dental A technique using a pneumatic, high-pressure stream of aluminum oxide to remove dental enamel; dentin; and restorative materials from teeth.

airborne A term used to describe any particles or substances that float in the air.

airway The path air follows to get into and out of the lungs. The mouth and nose are the normal entry and exit ports.

AK above knee.

AKA 1) above-knee amputation, 2) also known as.

akinetic-rigid syndrome Muscular rigidity with varying degrees of slowness of movement; seen in parkinsonism and disorders of the basal ganglia.

-al Pertaining to.

alb- Denoting a white or pale color.

Albarran test A test for renal insufficiency.

Albee lumbar fusion Fusion of the spine using grafts across the spinous processes in spondylolisthesis.

Albee's operation An operation for ankylosis of the hip.

Albers-Schönberg disease An extremely rare inherited disorder whereby the bones harden, becoming denser. *Synonym:* Osteopetrosis, marble bone disease.

albinism An inherited disorder in which there is no pigmentation in skin, hair or eyes, due to the absence of melanin, the substance that gives skin its color.

Albrecht's bone Basiotic bone.

Albrights' syndrome Inherited hypoparathyroidism associated with skeletal defects; polyostotic fibrous dysplasia.

albumin Major blood protein. Monitors nutritional status, or sometimes kidney status in protein-losing kidney problems.

albumin, serum Albumin is the main protein in human blood and the key to the regulation of the osmotic pressure (the movement of water between the bloodstream and tissues) of blood. This test helps in determining if a patient may have liver disease or kidney disease, or if not enough protein is being absorbed by the body. Albumin is the protein of the highest concentration in plasma.

Alcock canal Tunnel enclosing pudendal vessels and nerves.

alcohol cardiomyopathy Disease of the myocardium (muscle layer) of the heart, due to chronic alcoholism. Results in enlargement of the heart. Heart muscle is weakened and cannot pump blood efficiently.

alcohol dependence syndrome The most severe stage of a group of drinking problems which begins with binge drinking and alcohol abuse. *Synonym:* alcoholism.

alcohol deterrents Substances interfering with the metabolism of ethyl alcohol, causing unpleasant side effects thought to discourage the drinking of alcoholic beverages. Alcohol deterrents are used in the treatment of alcoholism.

alcoholic A person who drinks alcohol to excess habitually.

alcoholic cirrhosis A chronic disease interfering with the normal functioning of the liver; caused by chronic alcoholism.

alcoholic polymyopathy Disease affecting several muscles simultaneously. Caused by alcoholism.

alcoholic psychosis A severe mental disorder in which contact with reality is lost or highly distorted; caused by alcoholism.

alcohol-induced mental disorders alcohol-induced psychological or behavioral pattern that occurs in an individual and is thought to cause distress or disability that is not expected as part of normal development or culture.

alcoholism Habitual intoxication; prolonged and excessive intake of alcoholic drinks leading to a breakdown in health and an addiction to alcohol such that abrupt deprivation leads to severe withdrawal symptoms.

aldosterone test Measures the level of aldosterone (a hormone made by the adrenal glands), in the blood. Aldosterone helps regulate sodium and potassium levels in the body. This helps control blood pressure and the balance of fluids and electrolytes in the blood.

aldosteronism, primary Overproduction of aldosterone, which is secreted by adrenal glands. Caused by adrenal hyperplasia (increase in number of adrenal cells) or a tumor of the adrenal gland (Conn's syndrome). Symptoms may include hypertension, muscle weakness or cramping, kidney disease and abnormal heart rhythm. *See* Adrenal hyperplasia; Conn's syndrome; hypertension.

ALE allowable limits of error.

alexia Word blindness (inability to perceive written words).

alg(i)o- Pain.

alge(si)- Pain.

-algia Pain.

algoneurodystrophy A chronic progressive disease characterized by severe pain, swelling and changes in the skin.

alimentary canal The pathway by which food enters the body and solid wastes are expelled. The alimentary canal includes the mouth, pharynx, esophagus, stomach, small intestine, large intestine, and anus.

alimentation Feeding, being fed; the provision of food and other necessities.

alkali denaturation test A spectrophotometric method for determining the concentration of fetal (F) hemoglobin.

alkaline phosphatase An enzyme made in the liver, bone, and the placenta and normally present in high concentrations in growing blood and in bile and in low concentrations in the blood. Alkaline phosphatase is released into the blood in increased amounts during liver cell injury and during such normal activities as bone growth and pregnancy. Abnormally low levels of alkaline phosphatase are present in a genetic condition and also in hypothyroidism. It is measured in a routine blood test.

alkaline phosphorus A material found in the blood related to liver and bone.

alkalosis Abnormally high alkalinity (low hydrogen-ion concentration) of the blood and other body tissues.

alkalosis, metabolic Abnormal condition in which body fluids are more alkaline than normal. Can result from loss of acid from prolonged vomiting or excess intake of bicarbonate.

alkalosis, respiratory Abdominal pain, diarrhea, appetite loss and brown skin. Abnormal condition when body fluids are more alkaline than normal. Caused by conditions that decrease the level of carbon dioxide in the blood, such as breathing too rapidly or congestive heart failure. *See* congestive heart failure.

alkali denaturation test A spectrophotometric method for determining the concentration of fetal (F) hemoglobin.

ALL Acute Lymphatic Leukemia.

All Patient Diagnosis Related Groups (APDRG) An enhancement of the original Diagnostic Related Groups, designed to apply to a population broader than that of Medicare beneficiaries, who are predom-inately older individuals. The APDRG set includes groupings for pediatric and maternity cases as well as of services for HIV-related conditions and other special cases.

all-payer system A plan to impose uniform prices on medical services, regardless of who's paying.

alleles Alternate forms or varieties of a gene. The alleles for a trait occupy the same locus or position on homologous chromosomes and thus govern the same trait. However, because they are different, their action may result in different expressions of that trait.

allergen Any substance that can cause an allergy.

allergen immunotherapy Allergen immunotherapy is the process by which increasing doses of an allergen (allergy-causing substance) are injected subcutaneously over time as a treatment to prevent allergic symptoms that usually occur on exposure to the allergen.

allergenic Relating to or having the effect of an allergen.

allergic rhinitis A group of symptoms similar to those of a cold such as runny nose and sore throat, caused by an allergic reaction to an allergen such as dust, plant pollens or animal dander.

allergy Allergy is a disorder (or improper reaction) of the immune system often also referred to as atopy. Allergic reactions occur to normally harmless environmental substances known as allergens.

allergy and immunology Refers to diagnostic services performed to determine a patient's sensitivity to specific substances, the treatment of patients with allergens by the administration or allergenic extracts, and/or medical conference services.

allied health General term referring to a variety of non-physician and non-nursing clinicians, practitioners, therapists, technologists and technicians working in the health field.

allied health personnel or allied health professional Specially trained and often licensed health workers other than physicians, dentists, optometrists, chiropractors, podiatrists, and nurses. The term is sometimes used synonymously with paramedical personal, all health workers who perform tasks that must otherwise be performed by a physician, or health workers who do not usually engage in independent practice.

allo- Denoting something as different, or as an addition.

alloantibody A type of antibody directed against substances recognized as foreign to the host. *See* alloimmunization.

allochiria tests Errors in identifying left from right assist in locating lesions near the angular gyrus.

allogeneic blood Blood from one person that matches that of another, usually from a volunteer blood donor. *Synonym:* homologous blood.

allogeneic stem cell transplant A procedure in which a person receives blood-forming stem cells from a genetically similar, but not identical, donor. This is often a sister or brother, but could be an unrelated donor.

allograft A transplant process wherein a tissue or organ is taken from one individual (donor) and placed into another (recipient). *Synonym:* homograft.

allograft valves Replacement valves recovered from the hearts of humans who have died (cadavers).

alloimmunization or alloantibody The process whereby antibodies are formed which are directed towards antigens from other people, including leukocytes. It is one of the most serious transfusion complications.

allopathic One of two schools of medicine that treats disease by inducing effects opposite to those produced by the disease. The other school of medicine is osteopathic.

alloplastic Refers to nonbiologic material such as metal, ceramic, and plastic.

allotransplantation A transplant in which transplanted cells, tissues, or organs are sourced from a genetically non-identical member of the same species. Most human tissue and organ transplants are allografts.

allowable costs Charges for services rendered or supplies furnished by a health care provider, which qualify as covered expenses for insurance purposes.

allowable charge Generic term referring to the maximum fee that a third party will use in determining reimbursement for a given service or supply. An allowable charge may not always be the same as the actual charge.

allowed amount The amount Medicare determines to be the maximum amount allowable for any given service. There is a 5% differential between the approved charges for services rendered by participating providers and the approved charges for services rendered by nonparticipating providers. The participating approved amount is 5% higher.

allowed charge (approved charge) Payment for a physician service under the customary, prevailing and reasonable system; includes the payment from Medicare and the beneficiary's coinsurance, but not any balance bill. *See* Balance Bill; Coinsurance; Customary, Prevailing and Reasonable.

alopecia The complete or partial loss of hair.

ALOS Average length of stay.

Alper's disease Progressive cerebral poliodystrophy.

alphabetic index The portion of the ICD-9-CM diagnosis coding system that lists definitions and codes in alphabetic order. *Synonym:* Volume 2.

alphabetic index to procedures The portion of the ICD-9-CM Volume 3 procedures that lists definitions of procedures in alphabetic order.

ALS Advanced Life Support.

Alternative Delivery and Financing Systems (ADFS) *See* alternative delivery system.

alternative delivery sites Substitute for traditional inpatient sites for care such as ambulatory care centers, surgicenters, home care, hospice care, or alternative delivery and financing systems such as health maintenance organizations (HMOs), or preferred provider arrangements.

Alternative Delivery System (ADS) An alternative to traditional inpatient care such as ambulatory care, home health care and same day surgery. Also used as an expression to describe all forms of health care delivery systems other than traditional fee-for-service indemnity health care.

alternative levels of care Alternatives to traditional acute impatient care, such as ambulatory care centers, surgicenters, home care, skilled nursing facilities, and hospices.

alternative medicine Refers to any healing practice that does not fall within the realm of conventional medicine. In practice, alternative medicine encompasses therapies with a historical or cultural, rather than a scientific, basis. Commonly cited examples include naturopathy, chiropractic, herbalism, traditional chinese medicine, unani, ayurveda, meditation, yoga, biofeedback, hypnosis, homeopathy, acupuncture, and diet-based therapies, in addition to a range of other practices.

alveolar Pertaining to the alveoli sac, the site of gas exchange in the lungs.

alveolar bone The jaw bone that anchors the roots of teeth.

alveolar edema Swelling of the smallest branches of the bronchial tubes (alveoli).

alveolectomy The excision of a portion of the alveolar process to aid in the removal of teeth, modification of the contour after.

alveolitis 1) inflammation in the socket of a tooth; sometimes occurs after a tooth is extracted and a blood clot fails to form 2) inflammation of the alveoli in the lungs caused by inhaling dust; with repeated exposure the condition may become chronic. *Synonym:* dry socket.

alveoloplasty Surgical shaping of the alveolar ridges in preparation for dentures or after the removal of several teeth.

alveolus Air sacs in the lungs where oxygen and carbon dioxide are exchanged.

Alzheimer's disease An irreversible, progressive brain disease that slowly destroys memory and thinking skills, and eventually even the ability to carry out the simplest tasks. In most people with AD, symptoms first appear after age 60.

AD is the most common cause of dementia among older people. Dementia is the loss of cognitive functioning thinking, remembering, and reasoning—to such an extent that it interferes with a person's daily life and activities. According to recent estimates, as many as 2.4 to 4.5 million Americans are living with AD.

AMA Against Medical Advice • American Medical Association.

amalgam A metal alloy, typically composed of mercury, silver, tin and copper, used in dental restorations.

ambi- Denoting something as positioned on both sides; describing both of two.

ambiguous genitalia External genitals that are not normal for the sex.

amblyopia Reduced vision in an eye that appears to be normal when examined with an ophthalmoscope (an instrument used to examine the interior of the eye). Sometimes associated with strabismus. May also be caused by certain toxins. *Synonym:* lazy eye.

ambulance A vehicle used to transport the sick or injured.

ambulance (air or water) An air or water vehicle specifically designed, equipped, and staffed for life saving and transporting the sick or injured.

ambulance (land) A land vehicle specifically designed, equipped, and staffed for life saving and transporting the sick or injured.

ambulatory Able to walk, i.e. mobility not relying on walker, crutch, cane, other physical object, or use of wheelchair.

ambulatory blood pressure monitoring The recording of a patient's blood pressure at regular intervals under normal living and working conditions.

ambulatory care Refers to all types of health services that do not require an overnight hospital stay.

ambulatory care facility A medical care center that provides a wide range of health care services, including preventive care, acute care, surgery, and outpatient care, in a centralized facility. *Synonym:* medical clinic.

Ambulatory Patient Group (APG) A payment system that pays a fixed price for certain types of outpatient procedures.

ambulatory payment class A payment type for outpatient PPS claims.

ambulatory setting An institutional health setting in which organized health services are provided on an outpatient basis, such as surgery center, clinic or other outpatient facility. Ambulatory care settings also may be mobile units of services, e.g., mobile mammography, MRI.

ambulatory surgical center (ASC) A freestanding facility, other than a physician's office, where surgical and diagnostic services are provided on an ambulatory basis.

ambulatory surgical procedures Surgery performed on an outpatient basis. It may be hospital-based or performed in an office or surgicenter.

ambulatory utilization management Review prior to service against established standards to determine the medical necessity and appropriateness of the care to be provided in an ambulatory setting. The selection of treatment plans subject to pre-service review may be based upon criteria such as proposed care that would require frequent visits, expensive therapy, an extended course of therapy, or costly technology. Concurrent review would be applied as appropriate.

AMD age-related macular degeneration.

AME Agreed Medical Examiner.

amebiasis An inflammation of the intestines caused by infection with Entamoeba histolytica (a type of amoeba) and characterized by frequent, loose stools flecked with blood and mucus.

amebic dysentery Inflammation of the intestines caused by Endamoeba histolytica; usually acquired by ingesting food or water contaminated with feces; characterized by severe diarrhea.

amenorrhea There are two categories of amenorrhea. In primary amenorrhea, menstruation has not begun in a young woman who has passed puberty and is at least 16 years old. Cause is usually unknown. In secondary amenorrhea, there is cessation of menstruation for at least 3 months in a woman who has previously menstruated. Causes include pregnancy, breast feeding, eating disorders, endocrine disorders, psychological disorders, menopause (usually 35 years of age or older), surgical removal of uterus or ovaries, or very strenuous athletic activities.

American Accreditation Health care Commission (AAHC/URAC) Formerly known as the Utilization Review Accreditation Commission, AAHC/URAC is an independent not-for-profit corporation which develops national standards for utilization review and managed care organizations.

American Association For Homecare An industry association for the home care industry, including home IV therapy, home medical services and manufacturers, and home health providers.

American Association of Blood Banks (AABB) The professional society for institutions and individuals involved in blood banking.

American College of Health care Executives (ACHE) An international professional society of nearly 30,000 health care executives. ACHE is known for its prestigious credentialing and educational programs. ACHE is also known for its journal and magazines as well as groundbreaking research and career development and public policy programs. ACHE'S publishing division is a major publisher of books and journals on all aspects of health services management in addition to textbooks for use in college and university courses. Through its efforts, ACHE works toward its goal of improving the health status of society by advancing health care management excellence.

American Dental Association (ADA) A professional organization for dentists. The ADA maintains a hardcopy dental claim form and the associated claim submission specifications, and also maintains the Current Dental Terminology (CDT) medical code set.

American Health Care Association (AHCA) A trade association representing nursing homes and long term care facilities in the United States.

American Health Information Management Association (AHIMA) An association of health information management professionals.

American Hospital Association (AHA) A health care industry association that represents the concerns of institutional providers. The AHA hosts the NUBC, which has a formal consultative role under HIPAA.

American Hospital Formulary Service (AHFS) Drug reference published annually by the American Society of Health-System Pharmacists (ASHP). AHFS references are evidence-based and peer-reviewed, compiled without the influence of manufacturers, insurers, regulators, or other interested parties.

American Medical Association (AMA) The national voluntary non-profit organization of professional medical personnel, composed of state and territorial medical societies and component county medical societies. The AMA conducts education and publication services to members, and sponsors research to improve medical knowledge. The AMA advocates for the medical profession and for public health.

American Medical Informatics Association (AMIA) A professional organization that promotes the development and use of medical informatics for patient care, teaching, research, and health care administration.

American National Standards Institute (AHSI) An organization that accredits various standards-setting committees, and monitors their compliance with the open rule-making process that they must follow to qualify for ANSI accreditation. HIPAA prescribes that the standards mandated under it be developed by ANSI-accredited bodies whenever practical.

Americans with Disabilities Act (ADA) A Federal law which prohibits employers of more than 25 employees from discriminating against any individual with a disability who can perform the essential functions, with or without accommodations, of the job that the individual holds or wants.

Ames test Test for carcinogens using strains of Salmonella typhinium that will mutate if carcinogens are present.

ametropia Any imperfection in refractive state of the eye. Examples would be hyperopia (farsighted, longsighted vision), myopia (nearsighted, shortsighted vision), or astigmatism (irregular cornea).

AMHT Automated multiphasic health testing.

AMI Acute Myocardial Infarction.

amine Organic chemical compound containing nitrogen.

amino acids A group of 20 different kinds of small molecules that link together in long chains to form proteins. Often referred to as the "building blocks" of proteins. The sequence of amino acids in a protein determines the structure and function of the protein.

AML Acute Myeloid Leukemia.

AMLOS Arithmetic Mean Length of Stay.

amnesia Loss of memory.

amnestic disorder A brain disorder marked by memory impairment. *Synonym:* amnesia.

amnio- Pertaining to the membranous fetal sac (amnion).

amnioinfusion A procedure whereby a solution such as normal saline or lactated ringer's solution is infused through a catheter into the uterus to alleviate cord compression and to help dilute meconium staining.

amniotic cavity The fluid-filled cavity that surrounds the developing embryo.

amount, duration and scope How a Medicaid benefit is defined and limited in a state's Medicaid plan. Each state defines these parameters, thus state Medicaid plans vary in what is actually covered.

ampulla The dilated portion of a canal or duct especially of the semicircular canals of the ear.

Ampulla of Vater Enlarged area where the pancreatic duct and common bile duct come together before entering the duodenum (section of small intestine).

amputation The removal of a body extremity by trauma or surgery. As a surgical measure, it is used to control pain or a disease process in the affected limb, such as malignancy or gangrene.

AMRS Automated Medical record system.

amygdalohippocampectomy A surgical procedure for the treatment of epilepsy.

amylase A pancreatic digestive enzyme. Elevated in pancreatitis, or with injury to the bowel.

amyloid Starchy substance.

amyloidosis Disease in which a waxy, starch like, translucent material accumulates in tissues and organs, impairing function. If kidneys are involved, kidney dialysis or a kidney transplant may be part of the treatment.

amyotrophic lateral sclerosis A progressive, fatal, neurodegenerative disease caused by the degeneration of motor neurons, the nerve cells in the central nervous system that control voluntary muscle movement. *Synonym:* Lou Gehrig's disease.

amyotrophy The progressive wasting of muscle tissues. Muscle pain is also a symptom.

an- Not, without.

an(o) anus.

anabolic steroid class of steroid hormones related to the hormone testosterone.

anaerobes Any organism that does not require oxygen for growth.

anal of or referring to the anus.

anal fissure A crack-like sore in the anal region. It is the most common reason for pain in this area.

anal fistula A channel that develops between the anus and the skin. Most fistulas are the result of an abscess that spreads to the skin.

anal sphincter Circular muscles that allow waste materials to pass through the anal opening.

anal tag Are shapeless lumps and flaps of skin or flesh found at the anal verge. Anal skin tags are an extremely common condition and are frequently associated with other anorectal problems. Anal skin tags are usually the result of a prior anorectal insult or injury.

analgesia Loss of sensation of pain that results from an interruption in the nervous system pathway between sense organ and brain.

analgesic Compounds capable of relieving pain without the loss of consciousness or without producing anesthesia.

analysis A psychology term for processes used to gain understanding of complex emotional or behavioral issues.

anaphylactic shock A sudden, severe, potentially life-threatening allergic reaction caused by food allergy, insect stings or medications. Symptoms can include hives, swelling, difficulty breathing, vomiting, diarrhea, cramping and a fall in blood pressure.

anaphylaxis Severe, life-threatening allergic response to medications or other allergy-causing substances.

anaplastic The histologic grade of a tumor. Anaplastic tumors are poorly differentiated, meaning that their cells look primitive and do not resemble normal cells.

anaspadias Urethral opening on the dorsum of the penis.

anastomosis To join together two hollow organs (viscus), usually to restore continuity after resection, or to bypass an unresectable disease process. Historically such proce-dures were performed with suture material, but increasingly mechanical staplers and biological glues are employed.

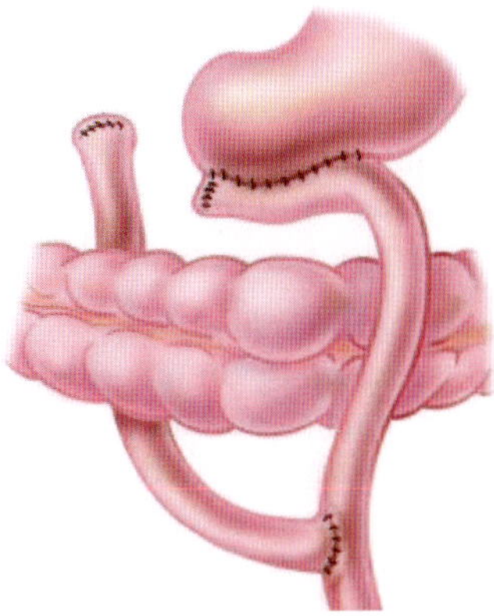

Roux-en-Y anastomosis.

anastomotic suturing The delicate sewing process of stitching the end of the bypass graft vessel to the artery.

anatomic pathology The diagnosis of disease based on the gross, microscopic, chemical, immunologic and molecular examination of organs, tissues, and whole bodies (autopsy).

anatrophic nephrolithotomy A surgical procedure for the removal of large renal calculi, specifically branched or staghorn calculi.

ancillary care A term used to describe additional services performed related to care, such as lab work, X-ray and anesthesia.

ancillary charge Also referred to as hospital "extras" or miscellaneous hospital charges. They are supplementary to a hospital's daily room and board charge. They include such items as charges for drugs, medicines and dressings; laboratory services; x-ray examinations; and use of the operating room.

ancillary services Auxiliary or supplemental services, such as diagnostic services, home health services, physical therapy, and occupational therapy, used to support diagnosis and treatment of a patient's condition.

ancylostoma Infestation by a species of hookworm.

ancylostomiasis A disease caused by hookworm infestation and marked by progressive anemia. *Synonym:* hookworm disease, tunnel disease.

Anders disease A disease accompanied by painful localised fatty swellings and by various nerve lesions. It is usually seen in women and may cause death from pulmonary complications.

Andersen disease Type IV glycogenosis.

Andersen's syndrome Cystic fibrosis of the pancreas, bronchiectasis and vitamin A deficiency.

Andrade's syndrome A hereditary form of amyloidosis characterized by predominantly neurological symptoms.

andrenogenital syndrome Endocrine disorder resulting from adrenocortical hyperplasia. Less than normal amounts of cortisol and greater than normal amounts of androgens are produced. This results in precocious puberty in boys and masculinization of the external genitals in girls. Usually a congenital disorder.

androgenic arrhenoblastoma Ovarian tumor in which cells resemble those in male testes; they secrete male sex hormone. Causes appearance of male secondary sex characteristics in a woman, such as a husky, deep-pitched voice, excessive body hair and enlarged clitoris.

andrenogenital syndrome An endocrine disorder resulting from adrenocortical hyperplasia. See Adrenal hyperplasia. Less than normal amounts of cortisol and greater than normal amounts of androgens are produced. This results in precocious puberty in boys and masculinization of the external genitals in girls. Usually a congenital disorder.

anemia Condition in which the number of red blood cells or hemoglobin (oxygen carrying substance in blood) are inadequate.

anemia, aplastic Serious disease characterized by decreased bone marrow production of all blood cells. Symptoms may include paleness, weakness, frequent infection, spontaneous bleeding from the nose, mouth, gums, vagina, rectum, brain and other sites, unexplained bruising, and ulcers in the mouth, throat or rectum. May be caused by disease in the bone marrow or destruction of the bone marrow by exposure to certain chemicals, anticancer drugs, immunosuppressive drugs or antibiotics. Cause is sometimes unknown. Curable if cause can be identified and treated successfully. If response to treatment is poor, complications of uncontrollable infections and bleeding may be fatal.

anemia, autoimmune hemolytic Anemia due to the breakdown of an individual's blood cells by his own serum. Exact cause is unknown and still under investigation. *See* Serum.

anemia, chronic hemolytic Anemia caused by an inherited disorder, such as hereditary spherocytosis, G-6-PD deficiency, sickle cell anemia or thalassemia. Currently no cure is known. *See* Anemia; hemolytic anemia; G-6-PD deficiency; sickle cell anemia; thalassemia.

anemia, diserythropoietic Any anemia caused by a disorder that diminishes the body's normal ability to produce red blood cells.

anemia, hemolytic Anemia due to the premature destruction of mature red blood cells. Bone marrow cannot produce red blood cells fast enough to compensate for those being destroyed.

anemia, hypochromic Any of a large group of anemias characterized by a decreased concentration of hemoglobin in red blood cells. *See* Red cell indices.

anemia, hypoplastic Anemia characterized by decreased bone marrow production of red blood cells.

anemia, idiopathic acquired hemolytic Anemia characterized by a shortened lifespan of red blood cells. Cause is unknown, but it is not hereditary.

anemia, iron deficiency Decreased number of circulating red blood cells or insufficient hemoglobin in the cells. Caused by inadequate supplies of iron.

anemia, macrocytic Blood disorder characterized by abnormal presence of large, fragile red blood cells. Mean corpuscular hemoglobin (MCH) and mean corpuscular volume (MCV) are increased. *See* Red cell indices. Often the result of folic acid and vitamin-B12 deficiency.

anemia, megaloblastic (folic acid deficiency) Anemia caused by folic acid deficiency. Often accompanied by iron deficiency anemia.

anemia, microcytic Any anemia characterized by abnormally small red blood cells, usually associated with chronic blood loss or nutritional anemia, such as iron deficiency anemia. *See* Anemia, iron deficiency; anemia, megaloblastic; red cell indices.

anemia, non-spherocytic hemolytic Inherited disorder of red blood cells in which shortened red cell survival is associated with membrane defects, unstable hemoglobins and intracellular defects.

anemia, pernicious Anemia caused by inadequate absorption of vitamin B12.

anemia, pyridoxine-responsive Decreased red blood cells in circulation, which increase to normal with pyridoxine treatment.

anemia, sickle cell Severe, incurable anemia that occurs in people who have an abnormal form of hemoglobin in their blood cells. It is an inherited disease.

anemia, sideroblastic A special type of anemia in which the bone marrow deposits iron prematurely into red blood cells. These cells do not transport oxygen to the body as efficiently as normal cells.

anencephalus The congenital absence of most of the brain and spinal cord.

anesthesia Anesthesia is a pharmacologically induced reversible state of amnesia, analgesia, loss of consciousness, loss of skeletal muscle reflexes and decreased stress response.

anesthesia by surgeon Regional or general anesthesia provided by the surgeon. Reported by adding the CPT modifier – 47 to the primary procedure code.

anesthesia physical status modifiers The physical status modifiers are consistent with the american society of anesthes-iologists ranking of patient physi-cal status, and distinguishing various levels of complexity of the anesthesia provided.

anesthesia recovery period The period of emergence from general anesthesia, where different elements of consciousness return at different rates.

anesthetics Agents that are capable of inducing a total or partial loss of sensation, especially tactile sensation and pain. They may act to induce general anesthesia, in which an unconscious state is achieved, or may act locally to induce numbness or lack of sensation.

aneuploidy Any variation in chromosome number that involves individual chromosomes and not entire sets of chromosomes. There may be fewer chromosomes, as in Turner's syndrome, or more chromosomes, as in Down's syndrome. *See* Turner's syndrome; Down's syndrome. Abnormal traits vary depending on which set of chromosomes is involved.

aneurysm Abnormal enlargement or ballooning of an artery. Caused by a weak artery wall.

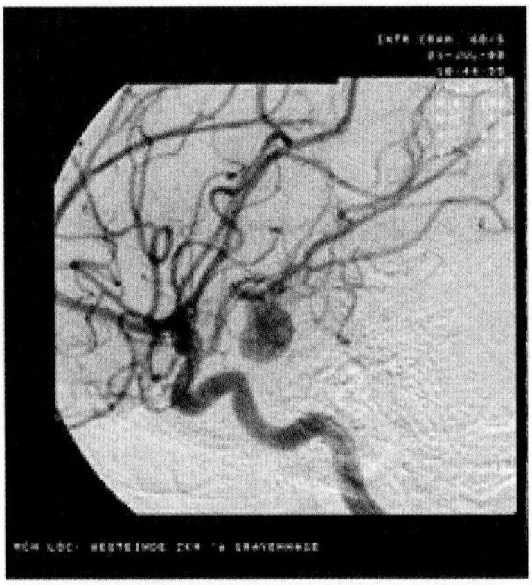

Angiography of an aneurism.
in a cerebral artery.

aneurysmal Relating to or affected by an aneurysm.

aneurysmectomy Surgical procedure performed to repair a weak area in the aorta.

ANG Angiogram • Angiography.

angiitis An inflammatory condition of the walls of blood or lymph vessels.

angina (angina pectoris) Chest pain or pressure usually beneath the sternum (breastbone). Caused by inadequate blood supply to the heart. Often brought on by exercise, emotional upset or heavy meals in someone who has heart disease.

angina pectoris Angina pectoris, commonly known as angina, is severe chest pain due to ischemia (a lack of blood and hence oxygen supply) of the heart muscle.

anginal of or related to the pain of angina pectoris.

angio Angiogram.

angiodysplasia Small blood vessel abnormalities.

angioedema Allergic disorder characterized by skin changes with raised areas, redness and itching.

angiography A medical imaging technique used to visualize the inside, or lumen, of blood vessels and organs of the body, with particular interest in the arteries, veins and the heart chambers. This is traditionally done by injecting a radio-opaque contrast agent into the blood vessel and imaging using x-ray based techniques such as fluoroscopy.

angiomas Benign tumor made up of blood vessels or lymph vessels. Most are congenital.

angiopathy Any disease of the blood vessels or lymph ducts.

angioplasty A procedure where a tiny balloon is inserted into the blocked coronary artery and inflated at the site of blockage.

Inflating the balloon reopens the vessel by pushing the plaque back against the walls of the artery.

angioscopy Endoscopic examination, therapy or surgery performed on the interior of blood vessels.

angiotensin Any of several vasoconstrictor substances (trade name Hypertension) that cause narrowing of blood vessels.

anhidrosis The reduced ability or inability to sweat.

anion gap Measure combining laboratory analysis of sodium, chloride and bicarbonate. A quick, noninvasive calculation.

aniridia A rare congenital condition characterized by the underdevelopment of the eye's iris. This usually occurs in both eyes.

anisakiasis Infestation by a species of parasitic nematodes.

aniseikonia A visual defect in which the shape and size of an ocular image differ in the two eyes.

aniso- Describing something as unequal.

anisocoria A condition characterized by an unequal size of the pupils.

anisocytosis Condition which is characterized by a considerable variation in the size of cells, especially red blood cells.

anisometropia A condition where the eyes have a significantly different refractive power from each other.

ankle The joint which connects the foot with the leg.

ankle jerk reflex The Achilles tendon is struck by the examiner to test the reflex reactions related to L5-S1.

ankyl(o)-, ancyl(o)- Denoting something as crooked or bent.

ankylosing spondylitis A long-term disease that causes inflammation of the joints between the spinal bones and the joints between the spine and the pelvis. It eventually causes the affected spinal bones to join together.

ankylosis A stiffness of a joint, the result of injury or disease.

anniversary The beginning of a benefit year for a subscriber group.

annual maximum benefit amount The maximum dollar amount set by an MCO that limits the total amount the plan must pay for all health care services provided to a subscriber in a year.

annuloplasty Surgical reconstruction of an incompetent cardiac valve.

annulus The outer ring of a vertebral disc.

anodontia A congenital condition in which all the teeth fail to develop.

anogenital Refers to the external genitalia and perineal area.

anogenital examination Examine the external genitalia and perineal area for injury, foreign materials, and other findings for suspected sexual molestation or assault.

anomaloscope An instrument used to test for color blindness.

anomaly A health problem or feature not normally present in a healthy individual, a deviation from the normal.

anoperineal Relating to the anus and surrounding perineum.

anophthalmia Congenital absence of eyes.

anophthalmos The congenital absence of one or both eyes.

anopia Absence of eyes.

anoplasty Reconstructive surgery on the anus.

anopsia A defect in the visual field. If the defect is only partial, then the portion of the field with the defect can be used to isolate a lesion.

anorectal Relating to the anus and the rectum.

anorectal abscess Abscess occurring in the rectum (last segment of the large intestine) and anus (opening of the rectum on the body surface). *See* Abscess.

anorexia Loss of appetite.

anorexia nervosa Syndrome in which the primary features include excessive fear of becoming overweight, body image disturbance, significant weight loss, refusal to maintain minimal normal weight, and amenorrhea. This disorder occurs most frequently in adolescent females.

anosognosia tests In cases of non-dominant side, frontal and parietal lobe lesions, the patient denies his paralysis of an affected side or limb.

anovulation Failure of ovaries to produce, mature or release eggs.

anoxia A condition in which tissues are severely or totally deprived of oxygen, severe hypoxia.

ANS Autonomic nervous system.

ANSI American National Standards Institute.

ante Before (ante).

ante- Describing something as positioned in front of another thing.

antenatal Refers to the period before birth. *Synonym:* prenatal.

antenatal screening Testing for diseases or conditions in a fetus or embryo before it is born.

antepartum Occurring or existing before birth.

antepartum care Refers to medical care provided during the period before birth. *Synonym:* prenatal period.

antepartum hemorrhage Bleeding before delivery.

anterior Front or forward portion. The front portion of the body. It is often used to indicate the position of one structure relative to another. *Synonym:* ventral.

anterior chamber The fluid-filled space inside the eye between the iris and the cornea's innermost surface, the endothelium. Aqueous humor is the fluid that fills the anterior chamber.

anterior horn cell disease Diseases characterized by a selective degeneration of the motor neurons of the spinal cord, brainstem, or motor cortex. Clinical subtypes are distinguished by the major site of degeneration.

anterior ocular segment The part of the eye anterior to the crystalline lens, including the cornea, anterior chamber, iris and ciliary body.

anterior segment The front third of the eye that includes the structures in front of the vitreous humor the cornea, iris, ciliary body, and lens.

anterior teeth The six upper or six lower front teeth.

anterograde Motion in the normal direction of flow. For example, passage of food from the mouth to the stomach.

anterolateral A combination of the words anterior and lateral, it means both in front of and to the side (both anterior and lateral).

anteroposterior Anterior to posterior; front-to-back.

anthrax An acute disease in humans and animals caused by the bacterium Bacillus anthracis which is highly lethal in some forms.

anti- Describing something as 'against' or 'opposed to' another.

anti-allergic and respiratory system agents A collective term for drugs used to treat allergic reactions as well as those drugs that produce an effect on the respiratory system.

anti-arrhythmia agents Agents used for the treatment or prevention of cardiac arrhythmias. They may affect the polarization-repolarization phase of the action potential, its excitability or refractoriness, or impulse conduction or membrane responsiveness within cardiac fibers.

antibiotic A drug that stops or slows the growth of bacteria.

anti-dyskinesia agents Drugs used in the treatment of movement disorders. Most of these act centrally on dopaminergic or cholinergic systems.

anti-inflammatory agents, anti-rheumatic agents, and inflammation mediators Both endogenous and exogenous substances used to counteract the inflammatory process or alleviate or prevent rheumatic diseases, and the compounds that mediate the inflammation process.

Anti-Kickback Statute A Federal law that prohibits the paying or receiving of remuneration in exchange for the referral of patients or businesses paid by a Federal health care program.

anti-obesity agents Agents that increase energy expenditure and weight loss by neural and chemical regulation. Beta-adrenergic agents and serotoninergic drugs have been experimentally used in patients with noninsulin dependent diabetes mellitus (NIDDM) to treat obesity.

antibiotic Any substance that can destroy or inhibit the growth of bacteria and similar micro-organisms.

antibiotic prophylaxis Antibiotics taken before a surgical or dental procedure to prevent infection of an abnormal or artificial heart valve called prophylactic antibiotics.

antibodies Proteins created in blood and body tissue by the immune system to neutralize or destroy sources of disease.

antibody-coated bacteria test, urinary Fluorescent antibody technique for visualizing antibody-bacteria complexes in urine. The presence or absence of antibody-coated bacteria in urine correlates with localization of urinary tract infection in the kidney or bladder, respectively.

anticoagulant management anti-coagulant services are intended to describe the outpatient management of warfarin therapy, including ordering, review and interpretation of international normalized ratio (INR) testing, communication with patient, and dosage adjustments as appropriate.

anticoagulant z A type of medication, commonly referred to as a blood thinner, that causes the blood to take a longer time to form a blood clot. Used to prevent the formation of blood clots or to treat blood clots. they may be given by injection, either into a vein or under the skin (e.g., heparin, low-molecular-weight heparin), or by mouth (warfarin). Learn More.

anticoagulants Medications that interfere with, or inhibit, blood from clotting are sometimes recommended for patients with atrial fibrillation or an artificial valve.

anticonvulsant A drug or treatment that prevents seizures or makes them less severe.

antidepressants Medications that treat depression, as well as other psychiatric disorders.

antidiuretic An agent or drug that, administered to an organism, helps control body water balance by reducing urination.

anti-DNA test An immunoassay that uses native double-stranded DNA as an antigen to detect and monitor increased serum levels of anti-DNA antibodies; used in the detection and management of systemic lupus erythematosus.

antiemetics Drugs used to prevent nausea or vomiting. Antiemetics act by a wide range of mechanisms. Some act on the medullary control centers (the vomiting center and the chemoreceptive trigger zone) while others affect the peripheral receptors.

antifungal A medication used to treat fungal infections such as athlete's foot, ringworm, candidiasis (thrush), serious systemic infections such as cryptococcal meningitis, and others.

antigen A substance on the surface of red blood cells that elicits an immune response when transfused into a patient who lacks that antigen.

antiglobulin test A test for non-agglutinating antibodies against red cells, using antihuman globulin antibody to agglutinate red cells coated with the nonagglutinating antibody. The direct antiglobulin test detects antibodies bound to circulating red cells in vivo. It is used in the evaluation of autoimmune and drug-induced hemolytic anemia and hemolytic disease of the newborn. The indirect antiglobulin test detects serum antibodies that bind to red cells in an in vitro incubation step. It is used in typing of erythrocyte antigens and in compatibility testing (cross-match).

antihistamines Drugs that combat the histamine released during an allergic reaction by blocking the action of the histamine on the tissue.

antihypertensive agents Drugs used in the treatment of acute or chronic hypertension regardless of pharmacological mechanism.

anti-lipemic of or pertaining to a regimen, diet, agent or drug that reduces the amount of fat or fat-like substances (lipids) in the blood.

antimetropia A condition in which one eye is myopic and the fellow eye is hyperopic.

antimicrobial A substance that kills or inhibits the growth of microorganisms such as bacteria, fungi, or protozoans, as well as destroying viruses.

antimycobacterial An antimycobacterial is a type of drug used to treat Mycobacteria infections.

antineoplastic and immunosuppressive agents Collective grouping for substances used to arrest the proliferation of malignant cells and those that suppress the immune response.

antinuclear antibody A substance that appears in the blood indicating presence of an autoimmune disease. *See* Autoimmune disease.

antiphospholipid antibody This antibody, which is directed against one's own tissues (autoantibody), is associated with an increased risk for forming blood clots and/or recurrent miscarriages.

antiphospholipid antibody syndrome This rare autoimmune disorder is characterized by recurrent blood clots and/or miscarriages in which there is an elevated antiphospholipid antibody level in the blood. APS may occur in those with lupus or related autoimmune diseases. It may also occur as a primary syndrome (Primary ABS) in otherwise healthy individuals.

antipruritics Agents, usually topical, that relieve itching (pruritus).

antipsychotic A group of psychoactive drugs commonly but not exclusively used to treat psychosis, which is typified by schizophrenia.

antipyretic Drugs that reduce body temperature in situations such as fever.

antirheumatics A category of otherwise unrelated drugs defined by their use in rheumatoid arthritis to slow down disease progression.

antiselection The tendency of people who have a greater-than-average likelihood of loss to seek health care coverage to a greater extent than individuals who have an average or less-than-average likelihood of loss. *Synonym:* adverse selection.

antiserum Human or animal serum containing antibodies that are specific for one or more antigens.

antisocial personality disorder A personality disorder whose essential feature is a pervasive pattern of disregard for, and violation of, the rights of others that begins in childhood or early adolescence and continues into adulthood.

antispasmodic A drug or an herb that suppresses spasms usually caused by smooth muscle contraction, especially in tubular organs. The effect is to prevent spasms of the stomach, intestine or urinary bladder.

antithrombin III A protein found in our bloodstream that controls our clotting mechanism and prevents excessive clotting. It functions as a naturally occurring mild blood thinner.

antithrombin III Deficiency a disorder that increases the risk for blood clots. It can be (a) acquired, or (b) inherited, or (c) based on a misinterpretation of lab tests (values can be temporarily low at the time of the acute clot or during heparin therapy).

antitrust laws Legislation designed to protect commerce from unlawful restraint of trade, price discrimination, price fixing, reduced competition, and monopolies. *See* also Sherman Antitrust Act, Clayton Act, and Federal Trade Commission Act.

antitussive agents Agents that suppress cough. They act centrally on the medullary cough center.

antiviral drug An agent that kills a virus or that suppresses its ability to replicate and, hence, inhibits its capability to multiply and reproduce.

antrostomy The operation of making an opening into an antrum for purposes of drainage.

antrotomy Incision through the wall of a cavity or chamber (antrum).

antrum A general term for a cavity or chamber which may have specific meaning in reference to certain organs or sites in the body.

ANUG Acronym for Acute Necrotizing Ulcerative Gingivitis, commonly known as trench mouth or Vincent's disease.

anuresis The absence of urine formation. *Synonym:* anuria.

anxiety A relatively permanent state of worry and nervousness occurring in a variety of mental disorders, usually accompanied by compulsive behavior or attacks of panic.

anxiety disorders Disorders in which anxiety (persistent feelings of apprehension, tension, or uneasiness) is the predominant disturbance.

anxiolytic A drug prescribed for the treatment of symptoms of anxiety.

any willing provider A physician, hospital, or other health care provider that agrees to accept the plan's terms and conditions related to payment and that meets other requirements for coverage.

any willing provider laws Legislation that requires health care plans to accept into their PPO and HMO networks any provider willing to agree to the network's terms and conditions.

AOA American Osteopathic Association.

AOD Arterial Occlusive Disease.

AODM Adult-Onset Diabetes Mellitus.

AOM Acute Otitis Media.

aorta The largest blood vessel in the body, originating from the left ventricle of the heart and bringing oxygenated blood to all parts of the body in the systemic circulation.

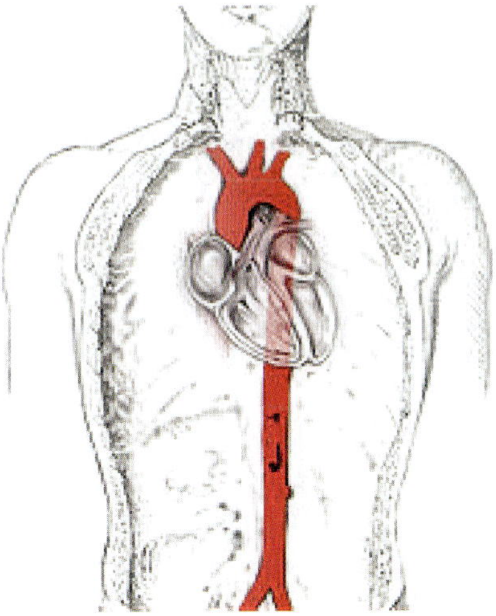

aortic Refers to the aorta.

aortic aneurysm A localized, abnormal and persistent dilation of a section of the aorta. This usually results from a weakness in the vessel wall. If severe enough, rupture of the aorta with severe hemorrhage a potential hazard.

aortic arch The superior left bend of the aorta between the ascending and descending portions.

aortic body One of several small clusters of chemoreceptors, baroreceptors, and supporting cells located along the aortic arch.

aortic dissection A tear in the wall of the aorta that causes blood to flow between the layers of the wall of the aorta and force the layers apart. Aortic dissection is a medical emergency and can quickly lead to death, even with optimal treatment. If the dissection tears the aorta completely open (through all three layers), massive and rapid blood loss occurs. Aortic dissections resulting in rupture have an 80% mortality rate, and 50% of patients die before they even reach the hospital.

aortic stenosis The obstruction of blood flow across the aortic valve.

aortic valve A semilunar valve between the left ventricle and the aorta; prevents blood from flowing from the aorta back into the heart.

aortic-valve stenosis Heart abnormality characterized by narrowing or stricture of the aortic valve due to a congenital malformation of the valve or fusing of segments of the valve, such as from rheumatic fever. This results in obstruction of blood flow out of the heart into the aorta; heart cannot pump effectively. Signs of the disease include intolerance for exercise, heart pain and heart murmur. Treatment usually includes surgery to repair the defective valve.

aortitis Inflammation of the aorta.

aorto of or referring to the aorta.

aortobifemoral bypass surgery Surgery to bypass diseased large blood vessels in the abdomen and groin.

aortocoronary Relating to the aorta and the coronary arteries.

aortofemoral The joining the abdominal aorta and the femoral arteries.

aortogram An image or set of images of the aorta made after the injection of a radiopaque substance.

aortography Examination of the aorta using x-rays following the injection of a radiopaque substance.

aortoiliac Refers to joining the abdominal aorta and the iliac arteries.

aortoiliac occlusive disease Complete or partial blocking of the lower part of the aorta as it enters the leg, at the level of the groin.

aortopexy a surgical procedure in which the aortic arch is fixated to the sternum.

aortoplasty Surgical repair of the aorta.

aortopulmonary window A rare heart defect in which there is a hole between the major blood vessel feeding the heart (the aorta) and the one going to the lungs (pulmonary artery). The condition is congenital.

aortorenal bypass A shunt between the aorta and the distal renal artery to circumvent an obstruction of the renal artery.

aortosubclavian Relating to or joining the aorta and the subclavian arteries.

APA American Psychiatric Association.

APACHE Acute Physiology And Chronic Health Evaluation System.

APB Atrial premature beat.

APC Ambulatory Payment Class.

Apert's syndrome Acrocephalo-syndactyly, type I.

apex The tip or end of the root of the tooth.

APG Ambulatory Payment Group.

Apgar score Numerical score evaluating the condition of an infant at birth.

aphakia The absence of the lens of the eye, due to surgical removal, a perforating wound or ulcer, or congenital anomaly.

aphasia An acquired language disorder in which there is an impairment of any language modality. This may include difficulty in producing or comprehending spoken or written language.

apheresis A procedure where whole blood is removed from the body and desired component(s), such as plasma or platelets is retained and the remainder of the blood is returned to the donor.

aphonia Loss of voice; the inability to speak.

apical at the top, tip or end of a structure, terminal.

apical vertebra The most rotated vertebra in a curve; the most deviated vertebra from the patient's vertical axis.

apicoectomy Excision of the apical portion of a tooth through an opening made in the overlying labial, buccal, or palatal alveolar bone.

aplastic anemia An anemia caused by deficient red blood cell production by the bone marrow.

apnea Temporary absence or cessation of breathing.

apo- Separated from, derived from.

aponeurosis A sheet like fibrous membrane, resembling a flattened tendon, that serves as a fascia to bind muscles together or as a means of connecting muscle to bone.

appeal A process whereby the provider and/or beneficiary (or representative) exercises the right to request a review of a contractor determination to deny Medicare coverage or payment for a service in full or in part.

appeals review committee The MCO committee that reviews member appeals related to medical management or coverage determinations.

appendectomy Surgical removal of the appendix.

appendiceal of or referring to the appendix.

appendicitis Inflammation of the vermiform appendix (small tube that extends from the first part of the large intestine). Symptoms may include right lower abdominal pain, nausea, vomiting, constipation or diarrhea, and fever.

appendicular skeleton is composed of 126 bones in the human body. The word appendicular is the adjective of the noun appendage which itself means a part that is joined to something larger. Functionally it is involved in locomotion (Lower limbs) of the axial skeleton and manipulation of objects in the environment (Upper limbs).

appendix A small, fingerlike tube located where the large and small intestines join which has no known function.

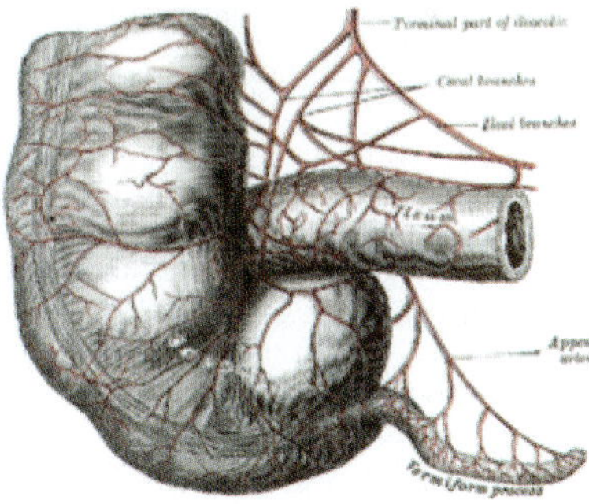

appendix

appropriate care A diagnostic or treatment measure whose expected health benefits exceed its expected health risks by a wide enough margin to justify the measure.

appropriateness review An analysis of health care services with the goal of reviewing the extent to which necessary care was provided and unnecessary care was avoided.

approved amount The fee Medicare sets as reasonable for a covered medical service. This is the amount a physician or supplier is paid by you and Medicare for a service or supply. It may be less than the actual amount charged by a physician or supplier. The approved amount is sometimes called the Approved Charge. (*See* Actual Charge; Assignment.).

approved charge The maximum fee Medicare will pay in a given area for a covered service.

approved health care facility or program Facility or Program that is licensed, certified or otherwise authorized pursuant to the laws of the state to provide health care and which is approved by a health plan to provide the care described in a contract.

appy appendectomy.

APTA American Physical Therapy Association.

aptitude tests Tests designed to determine ability to undertake study or training in a particular field.

aqueous A solution in which the solvent is water.

aqueous humor Clear watery fluid that flows between and nourishes the lens and the cornea. It is secreted by the ciliary processes.

aqueous shunt Devices, usually incorporating unidirectional valves, which are surgically inserted in the sclera to maintain normal intraocular pressure.

arachnoidal Pertaining to the arachnoid membrane.

arachnoiditis Inflammation of the arachnoid membrane, a thin, delicate membrane enclosing the brain and spinal cord.

Aran-Duchenne disease Spinal muscular atrophy.

arbitration A process in which the parties to a dispute submit their dispute to an impartial third party for a final, binding decision.

arborization A collection of branches, as the branching terminus of a nerve-cell process.

ARC AIDS Related Complex.

arch Describes the alignment of the upper or lower teeth.

ARDS Acute Respiratory Distress Syndrome.

area agency on aging State and local programs that help older people plan and care for their lifelong needs. These needs include adult day care, skilled nursing care or therapy, transportation, personal care, respite care, and meals.

areola Any circular area such as the colored skin surrounding the nipple.

arginosuccinic aciduria Presence of arginosuccinic acid in the urine.

This is an inborn error of metabolism and causes mental retardation.

Argyll Robertson pupil Miotic pupil which reacts to accommodation but does not react to light.

Arithmetic Mean Length of Stay (AMLOS) The average number of days patients are assigned to a specific DRG stay in the hospital.

ARI Acute Respiratory Infection.

Arnold ganglion Otic ganglion, situated below the foramen ovale, medial to the mandibular nerve.

Arnold Pick disease A rare and permanent form of dementia that is similar to Alzheimer's disease, except that it tends to affect only certain areas of the brain. People with Pick's disease have abnormal substances (called Pick bodies and Pick cells) inside nerve cells in the damaged areas of the brain. *Synonym:* semantic dementia, frontotemporal dementia.

Arnold-Chiari deformity Congenital anomaly of the cerebellum and medulla oblongata.

arrhythmias Occasional or constant abnormalities in the rhythm of the heartbeat.

arrhythmogenic Producing or promoting arrhythmia.

arteri(o)- of or pertaining to an artery.

arterial of or referring to the arteries.

arterial blood gas A technique used primarily to measure the oxygen level of the blood with precision.

arterial-occlusive disease Total or partial blockage of any large artery.

arteries blood vessels that carry blood away from the heart.

arteriography X-ray examination of arteries.

arteriole A small diameter blood vessel that extends and branches out from an artery and leads to capillaries.

arteriosclerosis Common disorder of the arteries characterized by thickening, loss of elasticity and calcification of artery walls. Results in decreased blood supply to the brain and lower extremities. Condition often develops with aging or with nephrosclerosis, scleroderma, diabetes and hyperlipidemia. *See* Diabetes; nephrosclerosis; scleroderma.

arteriotomy Opening or cut of an artery wall. *Synonym:* arterotomy.

arteriovenous fistula An abnormal connection or passageway between an artery and a vein. It may be congenital, surgically created for hemodialysis treatments, or acquired due to pathologic process, such as trauma or erosion of an arterial aneurysm.

arteriovenous malformation An abnormal connection between veins and arteries, usually congenital.

arteriovenous malfunction Problem at the junction of an artery and vein at the capillary level.

arteriovenous shunt Surgical shunt allowing direct passage of blood from an artery to a vein.

arteritis Inflammation of an artery.

artery Any of the blood vessels that carry blood away from the heart and to the various parts of the body.

arthr(o)- of or pertaining to the joints, limbs.

arthrectomy Surgical removal of a joint.

arthritis Inflammatory condition of the joints, characterized by pain and swelling.

arthrocentesis The clinical procedure of using a syringe to collect synovial fluid from a joint capsule. It is also known as joint aspiration. Used in the diagnosis of gout, arthritis, and synovial infections. *Synonym:* joint aspiration.

arthrodesis Artificial induction of joint ossification between two bones via surgery. This is done to relieve intractable pain in a joint which cannot be managed by pain medication, splints, or other normally-indicated treatments. *Synonym:* artificial ankylosis, syndesis.

arthrography A series of images, often X-rays, of a joint after injection of a contrast medium. The injection is normally done under a local anesthetic.

arthropathy Any disease or abnormal condition affecting a joint.

arthroplasty An operative procedure of orthopedic surgery performed, in which the arthritic or dysfunctional joint surface is replaced with something better or by remodeling or realigning the joint by osteotomy or some other procedure.

arthropod-borne viral diseases, Other viral diseases caused by insects.

arthropods Organisms with jointed appendages and exoskeletons, including insects, spiders, and crustaceans.

arthroscopic Refers to arthroscopy.

arthroscopy A minimally invasive surgical procedure in which an examination and sometimes treatment of damage of the interior of a joint is performed using an arthroscope, a type of endoscope that is inserted into the joint through a small incision.

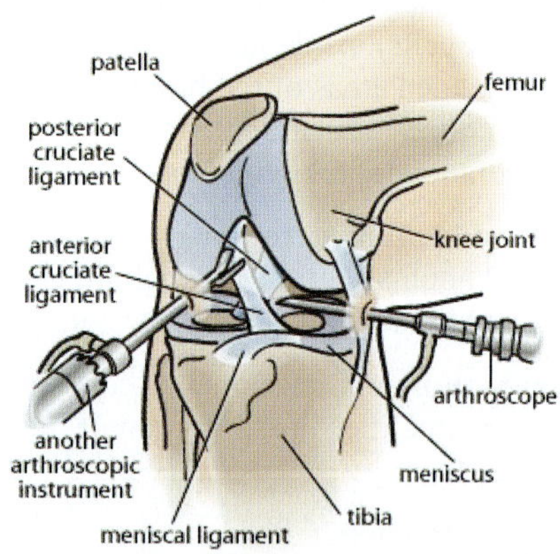

arthroscopy

arthrotomy Incision into a joint. *Synonym:* synosteotomy.

articul(o)- Joint.

articular Relating to or affecting the joints of the body.

artificial insemination The process by which sperm is placed into the reproductive tract of a female for the purpose of impregnating the female by using means other than sexual intercourse.

ARV AIDS-related virus.

-ary Pertaining to.

arytenoidectomy The surgical treatment of bilateral vocal cord paralysis.

arytenoidopexy Surgical fixation of arytenoid cartilage or muscle.

ASA American Society of Anesthesiologists.

ASAP as soon as possible.

asbestosis A condition featuring scarring of the lungs caused by inhaled asbestos fibers.

ASC Ambulatory Surgical or Surgery Center.

a-scan Routine type of diagnostic test used in ophthalmology. The a-scan provides data on the length of the eye, which is a major determinant in common sight disorders.

ascariasis Infestation of the human intestine with Ascaris roundworms.

ascending aortic aneurysm The first portion of the aorta as it exits from the heart is the ascending aorta. Occasionally the aorta will enlarge or dilate. Such areas of dilatation are called aneurysms.

Aschheim-Zondek test Pregnancy test performed by injecting the woman's urine into immature female mice.

Aschoff bodies (nodules) Granuloma specific for rheumatic fever.

ascites Accumulation of serous fluid in the abdominal cavity. It contains large amounts of protcin and electrolytes. May be a complication of cirrhosis, congestive heart failure, nephrosis, cancer, peritonitis or various fungal and parasitic diseases. *See* Cirrhosis; congestive heart failure; nephrosis; cancer; peritonitis.

ascorbic acid deficiency, A deficiency of ascorbic acid (vitamin c). Ascorbic acid is found in citrus fruits, tomatoes, potatoes, and leafy green vegetables and used to prevent scurvy.

ASCVD Arteriosclerotic Cardiovascular Disease.

asd Atrial septal defect.

-ase Enzyme.

aseptic Free or freed from contaminating organism(s).

ASHD Arteriosclerotic Heart Disease.

Ashman phenomenon Aberrant arrhythmia of atrial fibrillation.

ASMI Anteroseptal Myocardial Infarction.

ASOT Antistreptolysin O Titer.

Asperger's syndrome Idiot savant.

aspergillosis An opportunistic infection by a fungus of the genus Aspergillus; characterized by inflammation and lesions of the ear and other organs.

asphyxia Loss of consciousness due to too little oxygen and too much carbon dioxide in the blood. If not corrected, it results in death.

aspiration 1) The act of removing a fluid, as pus or serum, from a cavity of the body, by a hollow needle or trocar connected with a suction syringe. 2) The act of inhaling fluid or a foreign body into the bronchi and lungs, often after vomiting.

ASPVD Arteriosclerotic Peripheral Vascular Disease.

assault to attack someone physically or emotionally.

assay A quantitative or qualitative test of a substance (especially an ore or a drug) to determine its components; frequently used to test for the presence or concentration of infectious agents or antibodies etc.

asset Medicaid term referring to resources such as savings, stocks, bonds, and certain possessions that are considered in determining financial eligibility.

assigned claim A claim submitted for a service or supply by a provider who accepts Medicare assignment.

assignment An arrangement whereby a provider of service or supplier agrees to accept the Medicare approved amount as full payment for services and supplies covered under Medicare Part B. Medicare usually pays 80% of the approved amount directly to the provider of service or supplier after the beneficiary meets the annual Part B deductible.The beneficiary pays the other 20%.

assignment of benefits A procedure whereby the subscriber authorizes the carrier to make payment of allowable benefits directly to the provider.

assistant surgeon A physician who actively assists the operating surgeon in the performance of a surgical procedure. Reported by adding CPT modifier -80 to the main procedure code. *Synonym:* assistant-at-surgery.

assisted circulation Pumping that aids the natural activity of the heart.

assisted living A type of living arrangement in which personal care services such as meals, housekeeping, transportation, and assistance with activities of daily living are available as needed to people who still live on their own in a residential facility. In most cases, the assisted living residents pay a regular monthly rent. Then, they typically pay additional fees for the services they get.

assisted living facility An out-of-home care option for elderly persons who continue to lead relatively active, healthy, and independent lives. Most alfs feature apartment-style living and many services for the elderly.

assistive devices (technology) Any tools that are designed, fabricated, and/or adapted to assist a person in performing a particular task, e.g., cane, walker, shower chair, computer speech recognition, communication device.

association test One based on associative reaction, usually by mentioning words to a patient and noting what other words the patient will think of and give in reply.

AST (SGOT) Aspartate aminotransferase.

-asthenia weakness.

asthma A condition often of allergic origin that is marked by labored breathing accompanied by wheezing and a sense of constriction in the chest, and often by attacks of coughing or gasping.

astigmatic keratotomy A surgical procedure in which microscopic incisions are placed in the peripheral cornea to create a more spherical shape. Similar to Radial Keratotomy.

astigmatism Visual impairment caused by abnormal eye shape.

astragalectomy A surgical operation for removal of the talus bone (astragalus) for stabilization of the ankle.

astragalus The bone in the ankle that articulates with the leg bones to form the ankle joint.

astringents Agents, usually topical, that cause the contraction of tissues for the control of bleeding or secretions.

astrocytomas Brain tumor composed of neuroglial cells (one of the two main kinds of cells that make up the nervous system). Usually grows slowly, but often a highly malignant tumor, called a glioblastoma, develops inside the astrocytoma. Complete surgical removal of an astrocytoma may be possible early in the development of the tumor, but not after it has invaded surrounding tissue.

ASVD Arteriosclerotic Vascular Disease.

ataxia-telangiectasia Severe, hereditary, progressive disease beginning in early childhood. It results in lesion of a blood vessel formed by dilation of a group of small blood vessels (telangiectsias) of the eyes and skin, failure of muscles to coordinate (ataxia), including abnormal eye movements and immunodeficiency. This probably accounts for increased susceptibility to infections. Usually results in shortened life span.

atelectasis The collapse of a part of or the whole lung.

atherectomy A procedure that mechanically removes plaque and other debris that can block arteries throughout the body.

atheroembolism Obstruction of a blood vessel by an atherosclerotic embolism originating from an atheroma in a major artery.

atherosclerosis A condition in which an artery wall thickens as the result of a build up of fatty materials such as cholesterol. It a syndrome affecting arterial blood vessels.

atherosclerotic Pertaining to atherosclerosis.

-ation Process.

atomic absorption spectroscopy a technique for determining the concentration of a particular metal element in a sample.

atonic Without normal muscle tone or strength. An atonic seizure is one in which the person suddenly loses muscle tone and strength and cannot sit or stand upright and, unless supported, falls down.

atony Lack of normal muscular tension or tonus.

atopic dermatitis Chronic inflammatory disease of the skin; often associated with other allergic disorders that affect the respiratory system, such as asthma or hay fever. Symptoms include itchy rash in skin creases, dry, thickened skin in affected areas, uncontrolled scratching and fatigue from loss of sleep due to intense itching.

ATP Adenosine Triphosphate.

ATR Achilles Tendon Reflex.

atraumatic Not causing trauma or damage.

atresia Absence of a normal opening or failure of a structure to be tubular.

atria the two smaller chambers of the heart. The right atrium receives deoxy-genated blood from the body through the vena cava and pumps it into the right ventricle which then sends it to the lungs. The left atrium receives oxygen-ted blood back from the lungs and pumps it down into the left ventricle for relatively high-pressure delivery to the body.

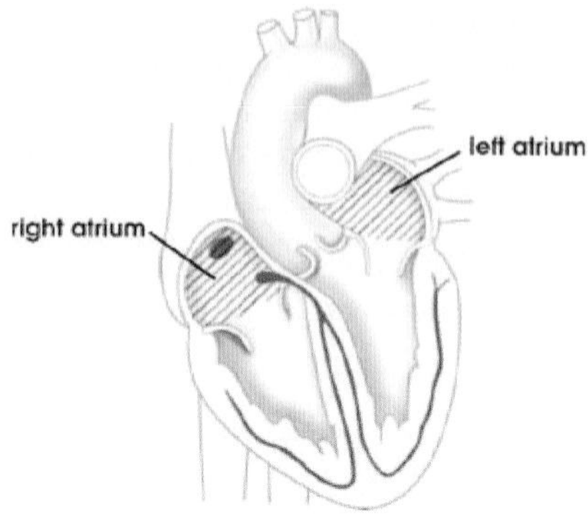

atria

atrial of or pertaining to an atrium, especially the atrium of the heart.

atrial contraction Atrial contraction refers to the part of the heart cycle when the atrium (or upper, low-pressure chamber) squeezes or contracts forcing blood into the ventricle (the main pumping chamber).

atrial fibrillation An abnormal rhythm or heartbeat pattern involving the atria or upper chambers of the heart. It can interrupt the normal flow of blood through the heart, allowing clots to form. These clots can potentially travel through the arteries, lodge in the brain and cause strokes.

atrial flutter An abnormal heart rhythm that occurs in the atria of the heart.

atrial septal defect An opening between the septum (wall) between the right and left atrium, allowing blood to flow in both directions.

atrioseptopexy Surgical correction of a defect in the interatrial septum.

atrioventricular node A part of electrical control system of the heart that co-ordinates heart rate. It electrically connects atrial and ventricular chambers. *Synonym:* av node.

atrioventricular valve Either of two heart valves through which blood flows from the atria to the ventricles; prevents return of blood to the atrium.

atrium see atria.

atrophy Wasting away; diminishing in size such as a cell, tissue, organ or part. May result from disease, lack of use, aging or other influences.

attachment(s) Information, hard copy or electronic, related to a particular claim. Attachments may be structured (such as Certificates of Medical Necessity) or non-structured (such as an Operative Report). Though attachments may be submitted separately, it is common to say the attachment was submitted with the claim.

attending physician The licensed physician who would normally be expected to certify and recertify the medical necessity of the number of services rendered and/or who has primary responsibility for the patient's medical care and treatment.

Attention-Deficit Disorder (ADD) A behavior disorder, usually first diagnosed in childhood, that is characterized by inattention, impulsivity and, in some cases, hyperactivity.

attenuation The property of somehing that has been weakened or reduced in thickness or density.

atticotomy Incision into the tympanic attic.

attrition Loss of tooth structure due to natural wear.

attrition rate Disenrollment or fall-out rate expressed as a percentage of total membership. Off-open enrollment terminations are generally due to subscriber's employment or relocation outside of the MCO's service area, and cannot be controlled. Open enrollment terminations are sometimes due to subscriber dissatisfaction and thus may be controllable.

atypical Not representative of a group, class, or type.

AUD Auditory.

audiometry The testing of hearing ability.

audit controls The mechanisms employed to record and examine system activity.

audiologist Performs duties directly related to problems and disorders of human communication in the process of speech and hearing.

audit of provider treatment Review of the patient's medical record and charges and claims for services to assure that the services provided were consistent with the patient's diagnosis(es) and that documentation in the medical record supports the submitted charges.

auditory of or relating to the process of hearing.

auditory canal A tube running from the outer ear to the middle ear.

auditory reflex Momentary closure of both eyes upon a sudden sound.

auditory system The sensory system for the sense of hearing.

auer bodies Faulty granule formations in myeloblastic and monoblastic leukemia.

Auerbach's plexus Esophageal autonomic nerve plexus.

aur(i)- of or pertaining to the ear.

aura The perceptual disturbance experienced by some migraine sufferers before a migraine headache.

auricle An ear-shaped appendage of the left or right atrium of the heart.

auricular of or pertaining to the outer ear.

auricular prosthesis A removable superficial prosthesis, which restores all or part of the ear.

aut(o)- Self, same.

authoritative approval Method or type of approval that requires a determination that the service is likely to have a diagnostic or therapeutic benefit for the patient for whom it is intended.

authorization As it applies to managed care, authorization is the approval of care, such as hospitalization. Pre-authorization may be required before a patient is admitted or care is given by (or reimbursed to) non-HMO providers.

authorization control The mechanism for obtaining consent for the use and disclosure of health information.

autistic disorder A neurological and developmental disorder that usually appears during the first three years of life. *Synonym:* autism.

auto-assignment A term used with Medicaid mandatory managed care enrollment plans. Medicaid recipients who do not specify their choice for a contracted plan within a specified time frame are assigned to a plan by the state. Can also refer to assignment to primary care physicians.

autogenous Self-generated or self-generating.

autograft Tissue transplanted from one part of the body to another in the same individual. *Synonym:* autotransplant.

autoimmune disease Disease in which the immune system produces antibodies that attack the body's own tissues.

autologous blood Autologous blood (donation) is blood drawn from one individual to be given back to that individual, or a close very blood match designee, as the need for transfusion arises. Exclusive or supplemental use of autologous blood can eliminate or reduce adverse effects of transfusion. Patients who receive their own blood receive the safest possible blood transfusions. Reactions due to components of blood such as white blood cells, platelets and serum protein are eliminated with autologous blood.

automated claim review Claim review and determination made using system logic (edits). Automated claim reviews never require the intervention of a human to make a claim determination.

automated reagin test A modification of the rapid plasma reagin (RPR) test for use with automated analyzers used in clinical chemistry.

autonomic The part of the nervous system responsible for the control of automatic bodily functions.

autonomic agents Agents affecting the function of, or mimicking the actions of, the autonomic nervous system and thereby having an effect on such processes as respiration, circulation, digestion, body temperature regulation, certain endocrine gland secretions, etc.

autonomic nervous system The part of the peripheral nervous system that acts as a control system functioning largely below the level of consciousness, and controls visceral functions. The autonomic nervous system affects heart rate, digestion, respiration rate, salivation, perspiration, diameter of the pupils, micturition (urination), and sexual arousal.

autopagnosia tests The patient is asked to hold up, point to and identify body parts such as fingers, arms, etc. Lesions of the parietal lobe causing autopagnosia, may prompt the patient to fail in the identification of his body parts or even identify the examiners hand as his own.

autopsy A medical procedure that consists of a thorough examination of a corpse to determine the cause and manner of death and to evaluate any disease or injury that may be present. *Synonym:* post-mortem examination.

autosomal anomalies A disorder caused by a non-sex (gender) chromosome.

autotransplant Tissue transplanted from one part of the body to another in the same individual. *Synonym:* autograft.

autotransplantation The transplantation of tissue from one part of the body to another in the same individual.

AV aortic valve • arteriovenous • atrioventricular.

AVA Arteriovenous anastomosis.

availability The property of being accessible and usable upon demand by an authorized entity.

Average Adjusted Per Capita Cost (AAPCC) Payment rates used by the CMS to reimburse managed care organizations for care delivered to Medicare enrollees.

average cost (or average benefit) The average cost (or benefit) for a unit of output (e.g., one day in a hospital for one patient) is the total cost (or benefit) of the total units of output delivered by the total units of output.

Average Length of Stay (ALOS) A standard hospital statistic used to determine the average amount of time between admission and discharge for patients in a diagnosis related group (DRG), an age group, a specific hospital or other factors.

AVH Acute Viral Hepatitis.

AVL Augmented voltage unipolar left arm lead (ECG).

AVM Arteriovenous malformation.

AVR Aortic Valve Replacement

AVS Arteriovenous Shunt • Aortic Valve Stenosis.

AVT Allen Vision Test.

avulsion A forcible tearing or surgical separation of one body part from another.

AW anterior wall.

AWI anterior wall infarction.

axial of or pertaining to an axis; of the nature of, or resembling, an axis; around an axis; Belonging to the axis of the body; as, the axial skeleton.

axial skeleton Consists of the 80 bones in the head and trunk of the human body. It is composed of five parts; the human skull, the ossicles of the inner ear, the hyoid bone of the throat, the rib cage, and the vertebral column.

axill- of or pertaining to the armpit [uncommon as a prefix].

axilla The armpit, or the cavity beneath the junction of the arm and shoulder.

axillary Pertaining to the cavity beneath the junction of the arm and the body.

axis 1) a straight line through a body 2) the 2nd cervical vertebra; serves as a pivot for turning the head.

Ayerza's disease (syndrome) A condition characterised by dyspnea, slowly developing asthma, bronchitis, and chronic cyanosis in association with polycythemia.

B

B scan Ultrasonic procedure used to check for abnormalities or locate foreign bodies within the eye.

BADS Syndrome Oculocutaneous albinism.

Baastrup disease False joint of the lumbar spine. *Synonym:* kissing spine.

Babcock's operation A technique for eradication of varicose veins by extirpation of the saphenous vein.

Babès-Ernst granules Metachromatic granules present in bacterial (bodies) cells, yeasts, fungi and protozoa.

Babington disease Hereditary multiple telangiectasia.

Babinski reflex (sign) Dorsiflexion of the great toe upon plantar stimulation, considered indicative of pyramidal tract disturbance.

bacillary dysentery A food borne illness caused by infection by bacteria of the genus shigella. *Synonym:* shigellosis.

backbench The standard preparation or reconstruction of cadaver or living donor organ allograft prior to transplantation.

bacteremia Bacterial infection of the blood. It is the principal means by which local infections spread to distant organs. Often results from simple cuts or scratches, and elicits a vigorous immune response to keep bacteria from spreading.

bacteria Microscopic unicellular organisms, typically spherical, rod-like, or spiral and threadlike in shape, often clumped into colonies.

bacterial Relating to or caused by bacteria; bacterial infection.

bacterial culture A method of multiplying microbial organisms by letting them reproduce in predetermined culture media under controlled laboratory conditions. Microbial cultures are used to determine the type of organism, its abundance in the sample being tested, or both. It is one of the primary diagnostic methods of microbiology and used as a tool to determine the cause of infectious disease by letting the agent multiply in a predetermined media.

bacterial endocarditis Noncontagious infection of the valves or lining of the heart.

bacterial myocarditis Infection of the heart muscle caused by bacterial germs.

bacterial sepsis *See* Sepsis.

bacterial vaginosis An infection of the female genital tract by bacteria of the Gardnerella vaginalis strain, often in combination with various anaerobic bacteria. *Synonym:* gardnerella vaginalis.

bacteriological of or relating to bacteriology.

BAEP Brain-stem auditory evoked potential.

BAER Brain-stem auditory evoked response.

Baghdad boil Lesion occurring in the cutaneous leishmaniasis.

Baker's cyst Benign tumor on the back of the knee joint. Tumor consists of accumulated fluid that protrudes between two groups of muscles behind the knee.

balance bill or extra bill Physician's charges exceeding the Medicare allowed charge.

Balance Billing A provider's billing of a covered person directly for charges above the amount reimbursed by the health plan (i.e., difference between billed charges and the amount paid). This may or may not be allowed, depending upon the contractual arrangements between the parties.

Balanced Budget Act of 1997 (BBA) This law made sweeping changes in the Medicare and Medicaid programs. Several of the significant provisions of the BBA were payment reductions to health care providers, new prospective payment systems for health care providers, and reduction of coverage of health care services by the Medicare and Medicaid programs.

balance sheet The financial statement that shows an MCO's financial status on a specified date.

balanitis Inflammation of the head of the penis.

balanoplasty Surgical repair of the glans penis.

balanoposthitis Inflammation of both the head of the penis and the foreskin.

balantidiasis A protozoan infection caused by infection with Balantidium coli. Symptoms can be local due to involvement of the intestinal mucosa, or systemic in nature and include either diarrhea or constipation.

Baldy-Webster operation An operation for retroversion of the uterus by shortening the round ligaments.

balloon angioplasty the technique of mechanically widening a narrowed or obstructed blood vessel; typically as a result of atherosclerosis. Tightly folded balloons are passed into the narrowed locations and then inflated to a fixed size using water pressures.

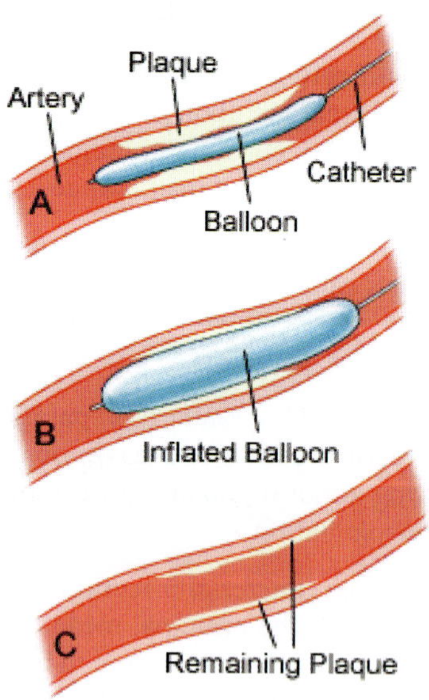

balloon angioplasty

Balser fatty necrosis Gangrenous pancreatitis with omental bursitis and disseminated patches of necrosis of the fatty tissues.

Bamberger-Marie disease Hypertrophic pulmonary osteoarthropathy.

Bankart procedure A surgical technique for the repair of recurrent shoulder joint dislocations. In the procedure, the torn ligaments are re-attached to the proper place in the shoulder joint, with the goal of restoring normal function.

Banks-Dervin rod Multiple level rod that is fixed with the oblique spinous process to contralateral lamina screws.

Banti disease (syndrome) Portal hypertension with congestive splenomegaly.

baresthesia tests In testing for parietal lobe lesions, the patient holds, with eyes closed, two weights that are unequal by one to two grams. Normals can generally discriminate between the weights. Sensation of weight may be lost in the contralateral limb.

bariatric surgery Surgery to reduce the volume of the stomach.

barium enema An X-ray examination of the large intestine.

Barlow disease Infantile scurvy.

Barlow syndrome Mitral valve prolapse syndrome.

Barr body The condensed, inactive X-chromosome found in the nuclei of somatic cells of most female mammals. *Synonym:* sex chromatin.

Barrett's esophagus Chronic peptic ulcer of the lower esophagus.

Bartholin cyst Retention cyst of the major vestibular or Bartholin gland.

Bartholin's gland Either of the two posterior vestibular glands that secrete a lubricating mucus.

Barton fracture Fracture of the distal radius into the wrist joint.

bartonella A genus of Gram-negative bacteria transmitted by insect vectors such as ticks, fleas, sand flies and mosquitoes.

bartonellosis An infectious disease produced by bacteria of the genus Bartonella. Bartonella species cause diseases such as Carrion's disease, trench fever, and cat scratch disease, and other recognized diseases, such as bacillary angiomatosis, peliosis hepatis, chronic bacteremia, endocarditis, chronic lymph-adenopathy, and neurological disorders.

Bartter's syndrome Inherited disease characterized by short stature, mental retardation, hyperaldosteronism and decreased potassium in the blood.

basal metabolism The amount of energy needed to maintain essential physiologic functions when a person is at complete rest, both physically and mentally.

base A set dollar amount to cover the cost of health care per covered person excluding mental health or substance abuse services, pharmacy and administrative charges.

base (dental) Cement placed under a dental restoration to insulate the pulp (nerve chamber).

base capitation A stipulated dollar amount to cover the health care per covered person less mental health or substance abuse services, pharmacy and administrative charges.

base estimate The updated estimate of the most recent historical year.

Base Rate A payment rate per inpatient discharge will be calculated for and assigned to each hospital by the Department of Health and Family Services for the rate year.

Basedow's disease Graves's disease; a form of hyperthyroidism characterized by thyrotoxicosis with diffuse hyperplasia, exophthalmos of pretibial myxedema.

basement membrane A membrane of tissue beneath the epithelium that helps adhere the epithelium to the Bowman's layer or stromal tissue.

basic benefits Basic Benefits includes both Medicare-covered benefits (except hospice services) and additional benefits.

basic benefits (medigap policy) Benefits provided in Medigap Plan A. They are also included in all other standardized Medigap policies. *See* Medigap Policy.

Basic life support (BLS) A level of medical care which is used for patients with life-threatening illness or injury until the patient can be given full medical care. It can be provided by trained medical personnel, including emergency medical technicians, and by laypersons who have received BLS training. BLS is generally used in the pre-hospital setting, and can be provided without medical equipment.

basic metabolic panel A panel of laboratory tests to determine the status of kidneys, blood sugar, and electrolyte and acid or base balance.

basilar artery An unpaired artery; supplies the pons and cerebellum and the back part of the cerebrum and the inner ear.

basophil A type of white blood cell that contains (and which can release) histamine and serotonin during the immune response; elevated in allergic reactions and malignancies.

basophil (absolute count) Represents the total number of basophils in blood based on the percentage of basophils present in the differential and the total white blood cell count.

basophil degranulation test An in vitro test used in the diagnosis of allergies including drug hypersensitivity. The allergen is added to the patient's white blood cells and the subsequent histamine release is measured.

Bassen-Kornzweig syndrome A rare, inherited disease in which a person is unable to fully absorb dietary fats through the intestines.

Bassini operation An operation for the radical correction of inguinal hernia.

Battle sign Discoloration near the tip of the mastoid process which is seen in basilar skull fractures.

BBBB Bilateral bundle branch block.

BC or BS Blue cross or Blue Shield.

BCE Basal-cell epithelioma.

BCG Bacillus Calmette-Guerin.

BCG vaccine Bacillus Calmette-Guérin, a vaccine for tuberculosis.

BDE Bile duct exploration.

BEAM Brain electrical activity mapping.

Bearn-Kunkel syndrome Lupoid hepatitis.

beating heart surgery A way to perform surgery without stopping the heart. Surgeons use a special device to stabilize the part of the heart on which they are operating. The heart continues to beat and circulate blood to heart muscle during the operation. Surgery on a beating-heart helps reduce the risk for complications associated with temporarily stopping the heart during surgery.

Beau Lines Transverse grooves on fingernails after serious illness or trauma.

bed reservations The department in the hospital responsible for bed availability and assignment.

bed reservation benefit In some long-term care policies, a benefit paid to maintain the enrollee's space in a nursing home facility when the enrollee must be hospitalized temporarily.

bed rest Confinement of an individual to bed for therapeutic or experimental reasons.

Beer's Operation A flap method for cataract.

Beevor's sign (see also the Hoover Test and Thigh Adduction Test). In functional paralysis, inability to inhibit the antagonist muscles.

behavior control Manipulation of the behavior of persons or animals by biomedical, physical, psychological, or social means, including for nontherapeutic reasons.

behavioral health care The provision of mental health and substance abuse services.

behavioral therapy A form of psychotherapy that focuses on modifying observable problematic behaviors by manipulating the individual's environment.

Behcet's syndrome Chronic inflammatory disorder involving ulcerations of mucous membranes in the mouth, genitals and eyes, and frequently arthritis.

Békésy audiometry That in which the patient, by pressing a signal button, traces monaural thresholds for pure tones the intensity of the tone decreases as long as the button is depressed and increases when it is released; both continuous and interrupted tones are used.

Bell's palsy Paralysis of the facial nerve.

Belsey Mark IV procedure An operation for gastroesophageal reflux performed through a thoracic incision; the fundus is wrapped 270 degrees around the circumference of the esophagus, leaving its posterior wall free.

Bence Jones protein Abnormal protein found in the urine of patients with multiple myeloma.

Bender visual-motor gestalt A psychological assessment used to evaluate visual-motor functioning, visual-perceptual skills, neurological impairment, and emotional disturbances in children and adults ages three and older.

Benedict's test A qualitative or quantitative test for the determ-ination of glucose content of urine.

beneficiary A person eligible to receive benefits under a health care plan. Under Part B of Medicare, Americans over 65, many disabled individuals, and certain individuals with end-stage renal disease can become beneficiaries by paying a monthly premium.

benefit Amount payable by the insurance company to a claimant, assignee, or beneficiary when the insured suffers a loss.

benefit cap Total dollar amount that a payer will reimburse for covered health care services during a specified period, such as one year.

benefit design The process an MCO uses to determine which benefits or the level of benefits that will be offered to its members, the degree to which members will be expected to share the costs of such benefits, and how a member can access medical care through the health care system.

benefit package Services covered by a health insurance plan and the financial terms of such coverage, including cost sharing and limitations on amounts of services.

benefit payments The amounts disbursed for covered services to beneficiaries after the deductible and coinsurance amounts have been deducted.

Benefit Payment Schedule List of the amounts an insurance plan will pay for covered health care services.

benefit period A benefit period is a way of measuring a beneficiary's use of hospital and skilled nursing facility services covered by Medi-care. A benefit period begins the day the beneficiary is hospital-ized. It ends after the beneficiary has been out of the hospital or other facility that primarily provides skilled nursing or rehab-ilitation services for 60 days in a row. If the beneficiary is hospital-ized after 60 days, a new benefit period begins, most Part A benefits are renewed, and the beneficiary must pay a new inpatient hospital deductible. Benefit periods are unlimited.

benign A mild and nonprogressive illness. The term is most familiar as a description of a non-cancerous (non-malignant) neoplasm, but may also refer to other mild health conditions.

benign neoplasm A localized tumor that has a fibrous capsule, limited potential for growth, a regular shape, and cells that are well differentiated. A benign neoplasm does not invade surrounding tissue or metastasize to distant sites. Some kinds of benign neoplasms are adenoma, fibroma, hemangioma, and lipoma.

Bennett fracture A fracture of the base of the first metacarpal bone which extends into the carpometacarpal joint. It is caused by compression along the metacarpal bone and is often sustained when punching.

benzoyl peroxide An antibacterial medication used to combat the bacteria that aggravate acne.

Berger's disease A kidney disease the affects the part of the kidney that filters blood to make urine (the glomerulus). It may lead to serious kidney damage and kidney failure requiring dialysis and/or kidney transplant. At this time, Berger's is considered to be "idiopathic" meaning that its exact cause is unknown. *Synonym:* immunoglobulin A nephropathy,.

Bernard-Soulier syndrome Hereditary coagulation disorder marked by a mild decrease in the number of platelets circulating in the blood and abnormally shaped platelets. Following trauma and surgery, blood loss may be greater than normal; transfusion may be needed. The use of aspirin may provoke hemorrhage in people with this condition.

Bernheim syndrome Right ventricular failure with left ventricular hypertrophy.

Bernstein test A method to reproduce symptoms of heartburn. It is usually done with other tests to measure esophageal function. *Synonym:* acid perfusion test.

beta hydroxy acid An oil-soluble exfoliant that is commonly found in skin-care products. Beta hydroxy acid (salicylic acid) is used to treat wrinkles, blackheads and photoaging.

beta-blockers Medications that reduce heart or blood vessel overactivity to improve blood circulation. Also used to prevent migraine headaches, hypertension and angina. *See* Hypertension; angina.

BETOS Berenson Eggers Type of Service.

Bezold's abscess Abscess in the neck following a bout of mastoiditis.

bi- Twice, double.

biased selection The phenomena whereby individuals or groups with atypical health risks disproportionately enroll in a specific health plan or type of health plan. Favorable selection occurs when a plan's enrollment predominantly consists of above-average health risks, while plans that disproportionately enroll individuals (and groups) of below-average health risks are said to experience adverse selection. Biased selection may be influenced by individual decisions in response to benefit design and plan characteristics as well as by insurer marketing and rating practices.

biceps A muscle located on the upper arm. The biceps has several functions, the most important being to rotate the forearm (supination) and to flex the elbow.

biceps reflex The tendon of the biceps is tapped. Normally there is a contraction of the bicep muscles accompanied by a jerk of the forearm. In corticospinal tract lesions, the reflex is excessive. In lesions of the peripheral reflex arc or damage to the C5-C6 segments of the cord on the side being tested, there is a depressed or absent response.

bicondylar joint A joint in which two rounded surfaces of one bone articulate with shallow depressions on another bone.

bicuspid Having two flaps or cusps.

bicuspid aortic valve A defect of the aortic valve that results in the formation of two leaflets or cusps instead of the normal three.

bid Twice daily (bis in die).

bifocals Corrective lenses that have two powers of correction. Bifocals and trifocals are normally prescribed for individuals with presbyopia.

bifurcated The splitting of a main body into two parts.

bilateral Affecting both right and left sides of the body or the right and left portions of an organ. The CPT modifier -50 is used to report bilateral procedures performed during the same operative session.

bilateral procedure A procedure performed on both sides of the body during the same operative session.

bile duct A tube that carries bile from the liver to the gallbladder and then to the small intestine.

bile sand Thickened, gritty bile excreted by the liver into the gallbladder and bile ducts. Bile sand usually indicates the presence of infection of the gallbladder.

biliary obstruction Blockage of the common or cystic bile duct, usually by one or more gallstones. Prevents normal bile flow into the small intestine.

biliary tract The system of organs and ducts through which bile is made and transported from the liver. Bile is a liquid produced in the liver whose function is to remove waste from the liver and break down fats as food is digested.

biliopancreatic diversion A surgical procedure which diverts pancreatobiliary secretions via the duodenum and the jejunum into the colon, the remaining small intestine being anastomosed to the stomach after antrectomy.

bilirubin Yellowish red blood cell waste product in bile the blood carries to the liver. It contributes to the yellow color of urine. Can cause jaundice if it builds up in the blood. Formed mainly by the breakdown of hemoglobin in red blood cells after the end of their normal life span.

bilirubin, total Bilirubin is a bile pigment normally found in the blood in trace amounts. Increased levels are seen in liver disease and liver cell injury. Bilirubin is also measured in its direct or conjugated form (linked to protein) and in its indirect form.

bilirubin, unconjugated Bilirubin that is insoluble in water. Bilirubin normally travels in the bloodstream to the liver, where it is converted to a water soluble (conjugated) form and excreted in the bile. Abnormally high levels of unconjugated bilirubin may be caused by liver damage, severe hemolytic anemia or Gilbert's disease. Very high levels in a newborn require treatment with phototherapy or an exchange transfusion to prevent brain damage. Usually someone with a high unconjugated-bilirubin level appears jaundiced. *See* Jaundice.

billed amount The amount charged for each service performed by the provider.

billed claims The fees or costs for health care services provided to a covered person submitted by a health care provider.

Billroth's operation Partial resection of the stomach with anastomosis to the duodenum (Billroth I) or to the jejunum (Billroth II).

bilobectomy Surgical excision of two lobes of the right lung, either right upper and middle or right lower and middle.

bimalleolar Refers to a fracture on both sides of the ankle.

binaural Relating to or having or hearing with two ears.

Binet's test A method of ascertaining a child's or youth's mental age by asking a series of questions adapted to, and standardized on, the capacity of normal children at various ages.

Binet-Simon test Intelligence test used particularly on children aged 3 to 15 years.

Bing test A vibrating tuning fork is held to the mastoid process and the auditory meatus is alternately occluded and left open; an increase and decrease in loudness is perceived by the normal ear and in sensorineural hearing loss, whereas the hearing of no difference occurs in conductive hearing loss.

binocular Both eyes.

binocular microscopy Refers to light microscopes using two eye tubes and eyepieces.

binocular vision The blending of the separate images seen by each of two eyes into a single image. Normal binocular vision yields a stereoscopic image and parallax-induced depth perception.

bio- Life.

biofeedback The process of detecting information about a patient's biological functions, eg. heart rate, breathing rate, skin temperature, and amount of muscle tension, picked up by surface electrodes (sensors) and electronically amplified to provide feedback.

bioimpedance A non-invasive method of determining the composition of body tissues to evaluate the presence of body fluids such as lymph. *Synonym:* bioelectrical impedance analysis.

biological assay A method of measuring the effects of a biologically active substance using an intermediate in vivo or in vitro tissue or cell model under controlled conditions. It includes virulence studies in animal fetuses in utero, mouse convulsion bioassay of insulin.

biological specimen banks Facilities that collect, store, and distribute tissues, e.g., cell lines, microorganisms, blood, sperm, milk, breast tissue, for use by others. Other uses may include transplantation and comparison of diseased tissues in the identification of cancer.

biological therapy Treatment of disease by the administration of substances which produce a biological reaction in the organism. It includes the use of sera, antitoxins, vaccines, cells, tissues, and organs.

biological valves Artificial valves made from humans or animals, rather than from metal. Examples of biological valves are porcine xenografts, human homografts or allografts, and pulmonary autografts.

biologicals Usually a drug or vaccine made from a live product and used medically to diagnose, prevent, or treat a medical condition. For example, a flu or pneumonia shot.

biomedical enhancement The use of technology-based interventions to improve functional capacities rather than to treat disease.

biometric identifier An identifier based on some physical characteristic, such as a fingerprint.

biometry The development and application of statistical methods to biological problems.

biopsy Removal and pathologic examination of specimens in the form of small pieces of tissue from the living body.

bioreactors Tools or devices for generating products using the synthetic or chemical conversion capacity of a biological system. They can be classical fermentors, cell culture perfusion systems, or enzyme bioreactors.

bipolar of or relating to manic depressive illness.

bipolar disorder A mood disorder (formerly called manic-depressive disorder) that is characterized by episodes of major depression and mania.

birthing centers Free-standing facilities that provide prenatal, childbirth, and postnatal care and usually incorporate family-centered maternity care concepts and practices.

bite Relationship of the upper and lower teeth on closure (occlusion).

bite wings Caries (decay) detection devices used during X-rays.

bitemporal hemianopsia Defective vision in which blindness occurs in the outer half of the visual field in each eye.

biventricular Pertaining to or affecting both ventricles of the heart.

BKA Below-knee amputation.

Blackfan-Diamond anemia Congenital hypoplastic anemia.

bladder A hollow, distensible organ with muscular walls that stores urine and expels it through the urethra.

bladder neck The junction between the bladder and the prostate.

Blalock-Taussig operation Surgery to repair the congenital cardiac defect known as the tetralogy of Fallot.

blast(o)- Germ or bud.

blastic phase Immature stage of cell development.

blastogenesis Asexual reproduction by budding.

blastomyces Genus of pathogenic yeast like fungi.

blastomycosis Infectious fungal disease that starts in the lungs. Occasionally it spreads through the bloodstream to other body parts, especially the skin. It is not contagious. Symptoms may include cough, chest pain, shortness of breath, chills, fever and drenching sweats. Usually occurs in the southeastern states and the Mississippi River Valley in the U.S. Fungus can cause severe, debilitating illness that may be fatal without treatment. With intensive treatment, it is usually curable in several weeks.

blastomycotic infection A fungal infection caused by the organism blastomyces dermatitidis. Endemic to portions of north america, blastomycosis causes clinical symptoms similar to histoplasmasis. *Synonym:* north american blastomycosis, blastomycetic dermatitis, Gilchrest's disease.

bleaching Chemical or laser treatment of natural teeth for whitening effect.

bleb A large blister filled with serous fluid.

blended rating For groups with limited recorded claim experience, a method of forecasting a group's cost of benefits based partly on an MCO's manual rates and partly on the group's experience.

blephar(o)- of or pertaining to the eyelid.

blepharitis A chronic inflammatory condition of the eyelids, common in children and adults, which causes redness, burning, itching, swollen and crusty lid margins and dry-eye symptoms.

blepharochalasis an inflammation of the eyelid that is characterized by exacerbations and remissions of eyelid edema, which results in a stretching and subsequent atrophy of the eyelid tissue. It typically affects only the upper eyelids, and may be unilateral as well as bilateral. In blepharochalasis the eyelid skin becomes lax and falls in redundant folds over the lid margins.

blepharoconjunctivitis Inflammation of the eyelid and conjunctiva.

blepharophimosis A condition where the patient has bilateral ptosis with reduced lid size, vertically and horizontally.

blepharoplasty A primarily cosmetic surgical procedure that reduces bagginess from lower eyelids and raises drooping upper eyelids. The procedure involves the removal of excess skin, muscle and underlying fatty tissue.

blepharoptosis An abnormally low position (drooping) of the upper eyelid.

blepharospasm Spasm of the eyelid(s).

blepharotomy Cutting of the eyelid.

blindness The inability to see.

blink rate The number of times per minute that the eyelid automatically closes normally 10 to 30 per minute.

blister A small pocket of fluid within the upper layers of the skin.

block injection Anesthesia of a nerve trunk that covers a large area of the jaw; a mandibular block injection produces numbness of the lower jaw, teeth and half of the tongue.

blood bank A blood Bank place where whole blood or plasma is typed, processed, and appropriately stored for future use in blood transfusion.

blood cells The red (erythrocytes) and white (leukocytes) blood cells which comprise the minor portion of whole blood.

blood circulation time Determination of the shortest time interval between the injection of a substance in the vein and its arrival at some distant site in sufficient concentration to produce a recognizable end result.

blood clot Blood that has been converted from a liquid to a solid state. Also called a thrombus.

blood component removal Any procedure in which blood is withdrawn from a donor, a portion is separated and retained and the remainder is returned to the donor.

blood count The complete blood count, or CBC.

blood culture The normally sterile specimen of a patient's blood that is incubated with a nutrient medium; if bacteria are present, the specimen will become cloudy with germs as they multiply rapidly.

blood dyscrasias Condition caused by or relating to disease in which any component of the blood is abnormal or present in abnormal quantity.

blood flow velocity A value equal to the total volume flow divided by the cross-sectional area of the vascular bed.

blood pressure The pressure (force per unit area) exerted by circulating blood on the walls of blood vessels, and constitutes one of the principal vital signs. The pressure of the circulating blood decreases as it moves away from the heart through arteries and capillaries, and toward the heart through veins.

blood smear A laboratory procedure for examination of a small drop of blood spread over a glass slide.

blood transfusion The process of transferring blood or blood-based products from one person into the circulatory system of another. blood transfusions can be life-saving in some situations, such as massive blood loss due to trauma, or can be used to replace blood lost during surgery.

blood type Everyone's blood falls into one of four groups, or types; A, B, AB or O. The type depends on the presence or absence of certain substances on red blood cells. blood types are inherited.

blood typing Test to determine the type of a person's blood.

blood urea nitrogen A measure of the amount of nitrogen in the blood in the form of urea, and a measurement of renal function.

blood vessel An artery, vein, or capillary that carries blood to and from the heart and body tissues.

blood volume determination Method for determining the circulating blood volume by introducing a known quantity of foreign substance into the blood and determining its concentration some minutes later when thorough mixing has occurred.

blood-factor deficiency Deficiency of one of the blood factors. *See* Factor I through Factor XIII.

BLS Basic life support.

Blue Cross Nonprofit, community service organizations, providing in-hospital health care services to their subscribers. Some Blue Cross plans have converted to for-profit status recently.

Blue Cross and Blue Shield Association An organization that offers information, consultation, representation and operational services for the Blue Cross and Blue Shield plan members across the country for purposes of providing insurance benefits.

Blue Shield Nonprofit voluntary organization which provides subscribers with coverage for expenses (other than hospital costs). May also serve as the carrier for programs like Medicare.

BMAD Part B Medicare annual data files.

BMI Body mass index.

BMQA Board of Medical Quality Assurance.

BMR Basal metabolic rate.

board and care home A type of group living arrangement designed to meet the needs of people who cannot live on their own. These homes offer help with some personal care services.

board certified A physician who has passed examinations given by a medical specialty group and who has, as a result, been certified as a specialist in this area of practice.

board eligible A term used to describe a physician who is eligible to take the specialty board examination by virtue of having graduated from an approved medical school, completed a specific type and length of training and practiced for a specified amount of time.

body mass index A measurement of the relative percentages of fat and muscle mass in the human body.

body record The body or data record contains information on a single OASIS-B1 patient assessment.

Bohman fusion Posterior triple spinous process wiring technique in the cervical spine to secure bone graft.

bolus A round mass of something, especially of chewed food in the mouth or alimentary canal; a single, large dose of a drug, especially one in that form.

bonding Chemically etching the tooth's enamel then covering it by painting a layer of plastic on the tooth to correct stained or damaged teeth.

bone cartilage A tough, elastic, fibrous connective tissue found in various parts of the body, such as the joints, outer ear, and larynx.

bone conduction The conduction of sound to the inner ear through the bones of the skull.

bone disorders Any abnormality or disease of the bone or skeletal system.

bone graft A surgical procedure that replaces missing bone with material from the patient's own body, an artificial, synthetic, or natural substitute. Bone grafting is used to repair bone fractures that are extremely complex, pose a significant health risk to the patient, or fail to heal properly.

bone loss The breakdown and loss of the alveolar bone that supports the teeth; usually caused by infection or long-term wear on chewing areas of the teeth.

bone marrow The tissue that produces blood cells and is found within the hollow cavities of many of the bones of the body. Bone marrow contains the stem cells from which all blood cells are derived.

bone plate Usually a relatively thin metal device which is affixed to bone via screws. Bone plates are used to immobilize bones or bone fragments such that healing can occur.

bone resorption Decrease in bone supporting the roots of teeth, which is a common result of periodontal (gum disease).

bone scan An imaging test in which a radionuclear substance is injected into the veins and taken up by the bones in areas of potential meta-static disease.

bone screw A threaded metal device which is inserted into bone. The functions of bone screws are to immobilize bones or bone fragments or to affix other medical devices, such as metal bone plates, to bones.

bonus A payment a physician or entity receives beyond any salary, fee-for-service payments, capitation or returned withhold.

borderline personality disorder A personality disorder marked by a pattern of instability of interpersonal relationships, self-image, and affects, and marked impulsivity beginning by early adulthood and present in a variety of contexts.

bordetella A genus of small Gram-negative coccobacilli of the phylum proteobacteria.

borrelia A genus of bacteria of the spirochete phylum. It causes borreliosis, a zoonotic, vector-borne disease transmitted primarily by ticks.

Bosworth lumbar fusion A fusion using an H-shaped bone graft in spondylolisthesis.

botox A substance derived from botulinum toxin that works by preventing nerve impulses from reaching the muscle, causing the muscle to relax.

botulism Serious form of food poisoning caused by eating contaminated food containing a toxin that severely affects the nervous system.

boutique hospital A limited service hospital designed to provide one medical specialty such as ortho-pudic or cardiac care.

boutique practice A medical practice set up to provide services to a limited number of patients who pay a premium, in exchange for unlimited and unfettered access to the practice's physicians. A boutique practice is usually comprised of two or three physicians who limit the number of patients they each treat to approximately 600-800 patients. By limiting the number of patients under their care the physicians are able to spend more time with their patients, offer same day appoint-mints, and usually increase their net income in the process. From the patient perspective the annual premium is money well spent in exchange for this personalized and prompt care.

Bowman's layer A layer of cells in the cornea. Between the epithelium and stroma. The Bowman's layer appears to be without specific purpose.

BP Blood pressure.

BPD Borderline personality disorder.

BPH Benign prostatic hypertrophy.

braces Devices used by orthodontists to gradually reposition teeth to a more favorable alignment.

brachi(o)- of or relating to the arm.

brachial of or relating to an arm.

brachial blood vessels Blood vessels in the arm.

brachial neuritis An acute syndrome of unknown cause marked by pain in the shoulder girdle, flaccid weakness of the muscles innervated by the brachial plexus, and mild sensory loss in the affected upper extremity. Brachial neuritis is usually of limited duration with spontaneous recovery. *Synonym:* brachial radiculitis, brachial plexus neuropathy, shoulder-girdle syndrome, shoulder-hand syndrome.

brachial plexus A network of nerves formed by cervical and thoracic spinal nerves and supplying the arm and parts of the shoulder.

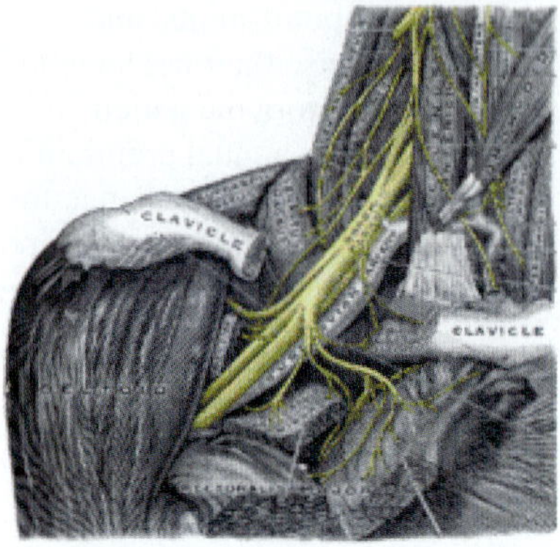

The right brachial plexus with its short branches, viewed from in front.

brachiocephalic artery An artery of the mediastinum that supplies blood to the right arm and the head and neck. It is the first branch of the aortic arch, and soon after it emerges, the brachiocephalic artery divides into the right common carotid artery and the right subclavian artery.

brachioradialis reflex This wrist reflex test is conducted to determine lesions at C5-C6 segments of the cord on the side being tested, there is a depressed or absent response.

brachy- Indicating something as 'short' or less commonly 'little'.

brachycephaly A type of cephalic disorder that occurs when the coronal suture fuses prematurely, causing a shortened front-to-back diameter of the skull. *Synonym:* flat-head syndrome.

brachytherapy A form of radiotherapy where a radioactive source is placed inside or next to the area requiring treatment. Brachytherapy is commonly used to treat localized prostate cancer, cervical cancer and cancers of the head and neck. *Synonym:* sealed source radiotherapy, endocurie-therapy.

Bradford procedure Staged anterior and posterior approach for interbody fusion and correction of deformity.

brady- Indicating something as 'slow'.

bradycardia A slow heart rate, usually defined as less than 60 beats per minute.

brain That part of the central nervous system that is located within the cranium (skull). The brain functions as the primary receiver, organizer and distributor of information for the body. It has two (right and left) halves called hemispheres.

brain infarctions Localized area of brain tissue death resulting from lack of oxygen to that area because of an interruption in blood supply. Severity of symptoms following brain infarction depends on the location of the infarct and the extent of damage. *See* Infarction.

brain stem The part of the central nervous system which houses the nerve centers of the head as well as the centers for respiration and heart control. It extends from the base of the brain to the spinal cord.

branchial of or relating to parts of the body derived from the embryonic branchial arches and clefts.

brand-name drug Prescription drugs marketed with a specific brand name by the company that manufactures it, usually the company which develops and patents it. When patents run out, generic versions of many popular drugs are marketed at lower cost by other companies.

Brattstrom fusion Use of acrylic cement for C-1 to C-2 fusion.

Braxton-Hicks contractions Light, painless uterine contractions during pregnancy.

breast The upper ventral region of the human torso. The breasts of the female contain the mammary glands, which secrete milk used to feed infants.

breast augmentation A surgical procedure done to increase breast size.

breast engorgement Occurs when the breasts fill with milk after delivery and cause breast pain and swelling.

breast implantation Surgical insertion of an inert sac filled with silicone or other material to augment the female form cosmetically.

breast prosthesis Breast forms intended to simulate breasts. There are a number of materials and designs although the most common construction is silicone gel in a plastic skin. Off-the shelf breast prostheses come in a range of shapes and sizes, while customized breast prostheses are molded to fit an individual's chest by taking an impression of both breasts and sculpting a mirror image.

breast reconstruction Surgery that rebuilds the breast contour after mastectomy. A breast implant or the woman's own tissue is used.

breech delivery The position of the baby in the uterus such that it will be delivered buttocks first as opposed to the normal head first position.

breech presentation In the breech presentation the baby enters the birth canal with the buttocks or feet first as opposed to the normal head first presentation.

bridge Stationary dental prosthesis (appliance) fixed to teeth adjacent to a space. A bridge replaces one or more missing teeth, cemented or bonded, to supporting teeth or implants adjacent to the space.

Bright disease A historical classification of kidney diseases that would be described in modern medicine as acute or chronic nephritis. The term is no longer used.

Briquet's syndrome A chronic but fluctuating mental disorder, usually of young women, characterised by frequent complaints of physical illness involving multiple organ systems simultaneously.

Brissaud-Marie syndrome Unilateral spasm of the tongue and lips, of hysterical nature.

broad ligament The broad ligament of the uterus is the wide fold of peritoneum that connects the sides of the uterus to the walls and floor of the pelvis.

Broca's aphasia Patients with Broca's aphasia have difficulty with verbal expression and articulation, but may write or sign well. *Synonym:* ataxic aphasia, expressive aphasia, motor aphasia.

Brock's operation Transventricular valvotomy.

bronch Bronchoscope • bronchoscopy.

bronch(i)- Bronchus.

bronchi Hollow air passageways that branch from the windpipe (trachea) into the lungs. They carry oxygen into the lungs and pass waste gases (mostly carbon dioxide) out of the body.

bronchial Relating to or associated with the bronchi.

bronchial tree The larger air passages of the lungs.

bronchiectasis Lung disease in which bronchial tubes become blocked and accumulate thick secretions. Frequently secondary infections occur. Not contagious unless associated with tuberculosis. *See* Tuberculosis. Symptoms may include cough, shortness of breath, malaise, fatigue and anemia.

bronchioles The smallest branches of the airways in the lungs. They connect to the alveoli (air sacs).

bronchiolitis Inflammation of the bronchioles.

bronchitis Acute or chronic inflammation of the bronchial tubes. Acute bronchitis is usually caused by a virus, although secondary bacterial infection is common. May also be caused from breathing chemical irritants (fumes, smoke, dust). Symptoms include cough, fever, chest discomfort and sometimes wheezing.

bronchoalveolar carcinoma a type of non-small cell lung cancer. The World Health Organization (WHO) classifies it as a subtype of adenocarcinoma. Bronchoalveolar cancer may be spread throughout the lungs more than other types of cancer.

bronchoalveolar lavage Washing out of the lungs with saline or mucolytic agents for diagnostic or therapeutic purposes. It is very useful in the diagnosis of diffuse pulmonary infiltrates in immunosuppressed patients.

bronchodilation A widening of the lumen of the bronchi, allowing increased airflow to and from the lungs.

bronchodilator Any member of a group of drugs that dilates bronchial tubes and makes air passage in and out of the lungs easier.

bronchogenic carcinoma Malignant tissue growth in the lung, which may be caused by cigarette smoking, air pollution, metastasis from another cancer site or an unknown cause. Symptoms may include persistent cough, wheezing, chest pain, blood in the sputum, weakness, fatigue and weight loss.

bronchography The x-ray examination of the tracheo-bronchial tree following the injection of a radiopaque material.

bronchoplasty Surgical repair of a defect in the bronchus.

bronchopneumonia A pneumonia characterized by acute inflammation of the walls of the bronchioles.

bronchopulmonary Pertaining to both the air passages (bronchi) leading to the lungs and the lungs (pulmonary) themselves.

bronchoscope An instrument with a small light and camera which is inserted through the nose or mouth. When a suspicious area is seen, an instrument is channeled through the bronchoscope to take a lung or bronchial biopsy (tissue samples taken to diagnose or rule out a disease.

bronchoscopy A technique of visualizing the inside of the airways for diagnostic and therapeutic purposes. An instrument (bronchoscope) is inserted into the airways, usually through the nose or mouth, or occasionally through a tracheostomy. This allows the practitioner to examine the patient's airways for abnormalities such as foreign bodies, bleeding, tumors, or inflammation.

bronchospasm A spasm of the bronchi that makes exhalation difficult and noisy; associated with asthma and bronchitis.

bronchus A passage of airway in the respiratory tract that conducts air into the lungs.

Brooks and Jenkins fusion Loops of wire around lamina of C-1 and C-2 to hold bone graft between lamina.

brow lift A surgical procedure in which the skin of the forehead and eyebrows is tightened to eliminate sagging eyebrows or correct frown lines in the forehead.

Browne operation A type of urethroplasty for hypospadias repair, in which an intact strip of epithelium is left on the ventral surface of the penis to form the roof of the urethra, and the floor of the urethra is formed by epithelialization from the lateral wound margins.

brucellosis Illness caused by the brucella bacteria, which is transmitted to humans from animals. Characterized by fever, severe sweating, anxiety, generalized aching and abscesses in the bones, spleen, liver, kidney or brain. With treatment, it is rarely fatal, although complications can cause permanent disability. *Synonym:* undulant fever, Malta fever.

Brudzinski's sign When the neck is flexed, flexion of the knees also occurs (present in meningeal irritation).

Brunner glands Duodenal glands.

Brunschwig operation Pancreatoduodenectomy performed in two stages.

bruxism Tooth grinding, often caused by stress; most often done unconsciously at night.

bruxomania Persistent nervous grinding of the teeth while the patient is awake.

BSA Body surface area.

BSO Bilateral salpingo-oophorectomy.

BSR Blood sedimentation rate.

b-thalassemia Hemolytic anemia caused by decreased production of beta chains of hemoglobin in red blood cells. *See* Anemia, hemolytic; thalassemia.

bucc(o)- of or pertaining to the cheek.

buccal Toward the inside of the cheek.

Budd Chiari syndrome Thrombosis of the (hepatic) veins coming from the liver, usually presenting with abdominal pain, enlargement of the liver and fluid in the abdomen.

budget neutrality For the Medicare program, adjustment of payment rates when policies change so that total spending under the new rules is expected to be the same as it would have been under the previous payment rules.

buffy coat A thin grayish white layer of white blood cells (leuko-cytes) and platelets covering the top of the packed red blood cells of a hematocrit.

bulbocavernosus transplant Surgical transplant of the bulbocarvernosus muscle for the purpose of creating a blood supply to a vaginal fistula site.

bulbourethral gland One of two small exocrine glands present in the reproductive system of human males. They are homologous to bartholin's glands in females. *Synonym:* cowper's gland.

bulbus cord Anomalies of cardiac septal closure, bulbus corda transitory dilation in the embryonic heart where the arterial trunk joins the ventral roots of the aortic arches.

bulimia Episodic binge eating. The episodes may be associated with the fear of not being able to stop eating, depressed mood, or self-deprecating thoughts (binge-eating disorder) and may frequently be terminated by self-induced vomiting (bulimia nervosa).

bullous dermatoses A skin disease, especially one that is not accompanied by inflammation.

BUN Blood urea nitrogen.

bun or creatinine ratio Blood urea nitrogen (BUN) and creatinine tests can be used together to find the BUN-to-creatinine ratio (BUN creatinine). A BUN-to-creatinine ratio can help your doctor check for problems, such as dehydration, that may cause abnormal BUN and creatinine levels.

Bundle Branch Block (BBB) A condition in which the electrical impulses traveling through the heart are slowed or blocked completely from traveling along their normal route through the ventricles. The condition tends to produce no symptoms, although a complete heart block can cause a person to feel either faint (syncope) or as if they are going to faint (presyncope).

bundle of HIS A collection of heart muscle cells specialized for electrical conduction that transmits the electrical impulses from the AV node to the point of the apex of the fascicular branches. *Synonym:* AV bundle, atrioventricular bundle.

bundling payment The use of a single payment for a group of related services. *Synonym:* bundled payment.

bundled rate Payments that represent an amalgamation of services.

bundled services A single comprehensive group of related services. Payments for bundled services have become the norm in recent years and unbundled services are investigated closely by CMS and other payers for evidence of fraud.

bundling The use of a single payment for a group of related procedures or services.

buphthalmos A congenital open-angle glaucoma of the eye.

Burkitt's lymphoma Malignant lymphoma usually found in Africa, but also seen elsewhere including the United States, that may involve the facial bones, ovaries, or abdominal lymph nodes.

burr hole A small opening in the skull made with a surgical drill.

burs(o)- Bursa.

bursa Any of the many small fluid-filled sacs located at the point where a muscle or tendon slides across bone. These sacs serve to reduce friction between the two moving surfaces.

bursectomy Surgical removal of a bursa.

bursitis The inflammation of one or more bursae (small sacs) of synovial fluid in the body.

bursocentesis Drainage of bursa by aspiration.

business associate Under HIPAA, a person or organization that performs a function or activity on behalf of a covered entity, but is not part of the covered entity's workforce. A business associate can also be a covered entity in its own right.

buttock The rump or fleshy masses on the posterior aspect of the lower trunk, formed primarily by the gluteal muscles.

bx Biopsy.

BX/BS Blue Cross/Blue Shield.

bypass graft A medical procedure in which a vein graft from another part of the body or a graft made from artificial material is used to create a detour around a blocked artery.

C

CA Cancer.

CAAT Computer assisted axial tomography.

CABG Coronary artery bypass graft.

cabulance A taxi cab that also functions as an ambulance.

cachexia General poor health and malnutrition, including weakness and muscle wasting. Usually associated with serious disease.

CAD Coronary artery disease.

cadaveric transplant A transplant from a deceased and usually unrelated donor.

cafeteria plan Flexible benefit plan under which the employer provides a range of taxable and nontaxable benefits options from which each eligible employee can make a limited number of selections. Options that may be available to employees through these plans include life insurance, health programs, retirement plans, vacation time, and stock options. Nontaxable benefits can include group term life insurance up to a specified amount of coverage, disability benefits, accident and health benefits, and group legal services to the extent that such benefits are excludable from gross income. A cafeteria plan that includes taxable and nontaxable benefits must meet certain requirements under the Internal Revenue Code. The term "Cafeteria Plan" may also describe a health benefit program that allows employees to select among various cost, coverage, or provider options.

CAH Critical access hospital.

calcaneal Relating to the heel bone or heel.

calcaneal spur A bony spur projecting from the back or underside of the heel bone that often makes walking painful. A calcaneal spur is also called a heel spur. *Synonym:* heel spur.

calcaneus A large bone that forms the foundation of the rear part of the foot. The calcaneus connects with the talus and cuboid bones. The connection between the talus and calcaneus forms the subtalar joint. This joint is important for normal foot function. *Synonym:* heel bone.

calcerous degeneration Degeneration of tissue with deposit of calcareous material.

calcification Process by which calcium from the blood is deposited abnormally into tissues from injury, infection or aging. Often it is part of healing and not a sign of active disease.

calcium Component of blood that helps regulate the heartbeat, transmit nerve impulses, contract muscles and form bone and teeth.

calcium channel blockers A class of drugs that act by selective inhibition of calcium influx through cell membranes or on the release and binding of calcium in intracellular pools.

calcium disorders Imbalance in the amount of calcium in the blood. Too much or too little can cause serious, sometimes life-threatening, medical problems.

calculi Stones formed of mineral salts. Usually found within hollow organs or ducts. They can cause obstruction and inflammation. Kinds of calculi include gallstones and kidney stones.

Caldwell-Luc procedure A surgical procedure where the maxillary sinus is entered by making an opening under the upper lip above the teeth.

calf A pair of muscles--the gastrocnemius and soleus--at the back of the lower human leg.

calibration Determination, by measurement or comparison with a standard, of the correct value of each scale reading on a meter or other measuring instrument.

Callahan fusion Individual wire fixation of a strut bone graft to involved facets.

Calmette Guerin bacillus vaccine A vaccine against tuberculosis that is prepared from a strain of the attenuated (weakened) live bovine tuberculosis bacillus, Mycobacterium bovis, that has lost its virulence in humans by being specially cultured in an artificial medium for years.

caloric test Irrigation of the normal ear with warm water produces a rotatory nystagmus toward that side; irrigation with cold water produces a rotatory nystagmus away from that side.

caloric vestibular test A test of the vestibulo-ocular reflex that involves irrigating cold or warm water or air into the external auditory canal. *Synonym:* caloric reflex test.

calorimetry The measurement of the quantity of heat involved in various processes, such as chemical reactions, changes of state, and formations of solutions, or in the determination of the heat capacities of substances.

calycoplasty Plastic repair of a calix, usually designed to increase its lumen at the infundibulum.

canaliculitis A relatively rare disorder that predominantly affects individuals over the age of 50. Complaints center on a chronic, recalcitrant unilateral red eye, and often epiphora. The discharge may range from a simple watery consistency to full-blown mucopurulence.

canaliculus A small canal or duct in the body.

canaloplasty A procedure intended to restore the natural drainage of fluid from the eye, thus reducing intraocular pressure in persons with glaucoma.

canalplasty A procedure used to repair defects of the external auditory canal by removing abnormal bone growth, e.g., anterior overhang or exostosis, removal and replacement of intract-ably infected mucocutaneous tissue in the canal and enlargement or straightening of a stenotic or tortuous external auditory canal.

cancer a class of diseases in which a group of cells display uncontrolled growth (division beyond the normal limits), invasion (intrusion on and destruction of adjacent tissues), and sometimes metastasis (spread to other locations in the body via lymph or blood). *Synonym:* malignant neoplasm.

candidiasis Infection caused by a species of the yeast candida, usually candida albicans. Candidiasis is a common cause of vaginal infections in women. *Synonym:* moniliasis.

canine tooth The second tooth from the large front tooth, commonly called the eye tooth or cuspid.

canker sore Mouth sore appearing whitish, often with a red halo, of ten to fourteen day duration.

cannula Tube for insertion into a vessel or body cavity.

cannulation Insertion of a cannula into a bodily cavity, duct, or vessel, for the drainage of fluid or the administration of medication.

canthopexy Surgery to tighten the lower eyelids and raise the external corners of the eyes.

canthoplasty A surgical procedure that involves tightening the muscles or ligaments that provide support to the outer corner of a patient's eyelid.

canthorrhaphy The surgical shortening of the palpebral fissure of the eyelids by suturing the either corner of the eye where the upper and lower eyelids meet (canthus).

canthotomy An incision of either corner of the eye where the upper and lower eyelids meet (canthus).

canthus Demarcation between the sclera and nasal corner of the eye.

CAO Chronic airway obstruction.

cap Another term for crown; usually referring to a crown for a front tooth.

CAPD Continuous ambulatory peritoneal dialysis.

capill- of or pertaining to hair.

capillary Any of the minute blood vessels connecting arterioles into the veins. Capillaries distribute oxygenated blood from arteries to the tissues of the body and feed deoxygenated blood from the tissues back into the veins.

capillary precipitation Settling of solid substances formerly in solution in the bloodstream.

capit- Pertaining to the head (as a whole).

capitation A set dollar payment per patient per unit of time (usually per month) that is paid to cover a specified set of services and administrative costs without regard to the actual number of services provided. The services covered may include a physician's own services, referral services or all medical services. The set dollar payment may be a percent of the premium that the managed care organization collects for a beneficiary; the capitation received from CMS would be considered a premium for this purpose.

Capner procedure Draining of thoracic spinal abscess through an anterolateral approach.

capped rental item Durable medical equipment (like nebulizers or manual wheelchairs) that costs more than $150, and the supplier rents it to people with Medicare more than 25 percent of the time.

capsulectomy Excision of a capsule (as of a joint, kidney, or lens).

capsulitis Inflammation of a ligament. Capsulitis can occur at any joint in the human body and may occur in a number of places on the foot.

capsulodesis Tightening the tissue around a joint to make it more stable.

capsulorrhaphy Suture of a tear in a capsule, especially of a joint capsule to prevent recurring dislocation.

capsulorrhexis A technique used to remove the lens capsule during cataract surgery. It generally refers to removal of a part of the anterior lens capsule, but in situations like a developmental cataract a part of the posterior capsule is also removed by a similar technique.

capsulotomy Incision into a capsule, especially that of the crystalline lens of the eye, as to remove cataracts by surgery.

carbohydrates and hypoglycemic agents A collective term for carbohydrates and agents used to lower the level of glucose in the blood.

carbuncle An abscess larger than a boil, usually with one or more openings draining pus onto the skin. It is usually caused by bacterial infection, most commonly staphylococcus aureus.

carcin(o)- Cancer.

carcinoid syndrome A syndrome due to carcinoid tumor which secretes large amounts of the hormone serotonin.

carcinoid tumor A small tumor (benign or malignant) arising from the mucosa of the gastrointestinal tract; usually associated with excessive secretion of serotonin.

carcinoma Malignant tumor that tends to invade surrounding tissue; it may travel to distant regions of the body. *See* Cancer.

carcinoma in situ A cluster of malignant cells that has not yet invaded the deeper epithelial tissue or spread to other parts of the body.

cardi(o)- of or pertaining to the heart.

cardiac of or relating to the heart.

cardiac arrhythmia A term for any of a large and heterogeneous group of conditions in which there is abnormal electrical activity in the heart.

cardiac catheterization A procedure to examine blood flow to the heart and test how well the heart is pumping. A catheter is inserted into an artery or vein in the arm or leg. From there it can be advanced into the chambers of the heart or into the coronary arteries.

cardiac distress Any condition causing difficulty in heart's normal functioning.

cardiac dysrhythmias A term for any of a large and heterogeneous group of conditions in which there is abnormal electrical activity in the heart. The heart beat may be too fast or too slow, and may be regular or irregular.

cardiac glycosides Family of drugs used to treat heart disease. Digitalis is the outstanding cardiac glycoside.

cardiac pacing, artificial Regulation of the rate of contraction of the heart muscles by an artificial pacemaker.

cardiac surgery Surgery on the heart and/or great vessels performed by a cardiac surgeon. Frequently, it is done to treat complications of ischemic heart disease (for example, coronary artery bypass grafting), correct congenital heart disease, or treat valvular heart disease created by various causes including endocarditis. It also includes heart transplantation.

cardiac tamponade Compression of the heart due to collection of blood in the sac enclosing the heart (pericardium). Usually caused by a ruptured blood vessel in the heart muscle or by a penetrating wound. *Synonym:* pericardial tamponade.

cardiectomy Excision of the cardiac portion of the stomach.

cardiogenic shock Shock that results from low cardiac output in heart disease.

cardiomegaly An abnormal enlargement of the heart.

cardiomyopathy A weakening of the heart muscle or a change in heart muscle structure. It is often associated with inadequate heart pumping or other heart function problems.

cardiomyoplasty An operation that uses stimulated latissimus dorsi muscle (skeletal muscle ventricle) to assist cardiac function. The latissimus dorsi muscle is mobilized from the chest wall and moved into the thorax through the bed of the resected 2nd or 3rd rib. The mu.

cardiomyotomy Surgical splitting of the muscular ring at the junction of the stomach and esophagus to relieve achalasia.

cardioplasty A surgical procedure to correct a defect in the cardiac sphincter of the esophagus.

cardioplegic solutions Solutions which, upon administration, will temporarily arrest cardiac activity. They are used in the performance of heart surgery.

cardiopulmonary of or relating to the heart and lungs.

cardiopulmonary bypass Diversion of the flow of blood from the entrance of the right atrium directly to the aorta (or femoral artery) via an oxygenator thus bypassing both the heart and lungs. *Synonym:* heart-lung machine.

cardiorespiratory disease Any disease affecting the heart and lungs.

cardiospasm A spasm of the cardiac sphincter (between the esophagus and the stomach); if the cardiac sphincter does not relax during swallowing the passage of food into the stomach is obstructed. *Synonym:* achalasia.

cardiothoracic surgery The specialty of treating heart, lung and other problems in the chest with surgery.

cardiotomy Surgical incision of the heart.

cardiotonic agents Agents that have a strengthening effect on the heart or that can increase cardiac output. They may be cardiac glycosides, sympathomimetics, or other drugs. They are used after myocardial infarct, cardiac surgical procedures, in shock, or in congestive heart failure.

cardiovascular agents Agents that affect the rate or intensity of cardiac contraction, blood vessel diameter, or blood volume.

cardiovascular disease General term for any disease of the cardiovascular (heart and blood vessels) system.

cardiovascular monitoring services Diagnostic medical procedures using face-to-face and remote monitoring technology to record cardiovascular data and assess the effectiveness of treatment.

cardiovascular services Refers to the study and treatment of diseases of the heart and vascular (arteries and veins) system.

cardiovascular syphilis The involvement of the cardiovascular system in late syphilis usually resulting in aortitis aneurysm formation, and aortic valvular insufficiency.

cardiovascular system The group of organs responsible for moving blood and nutrients throughout the body. The organs in the system include the heart, veins, arteries, capillaries, and the plasma and cells that make up the blood.

cardioversion Restoration of normal rhythm of the heart by electrical shock.

carditis Inflammation of the heart.

care coordination benefit A benefit in newer long-term care policies that pays consultation fees for a professional, such as a registered nurse or a medical social worker, to periodically assess and make recommendations about the enrollee's care program. The purpose is to adjust services when and if the individual's care needs change. *Synonym:* personal care advisor benefit, personal care advocate benefit.

care plan A written plan for a patient's health care. It describes what services the patient will receive in order to maintain their best physical, mental, and social well being.

care plan oversight services Care plans prepared and/or reviewed by a physician.

caregiver Someone who provides assistance, generally in the home environment, to an aging parent, spouse, other relative, or unrelated person, or to an ill or disabled person of any age. A caregiver can be a family member, friend, volunteer, or paid professional.

caries Cavities or tooth decay.

carotid artery An artery that supplies the head and neck with oxygenated blood; it divides in the neck to form the external and internal carotid arteries.

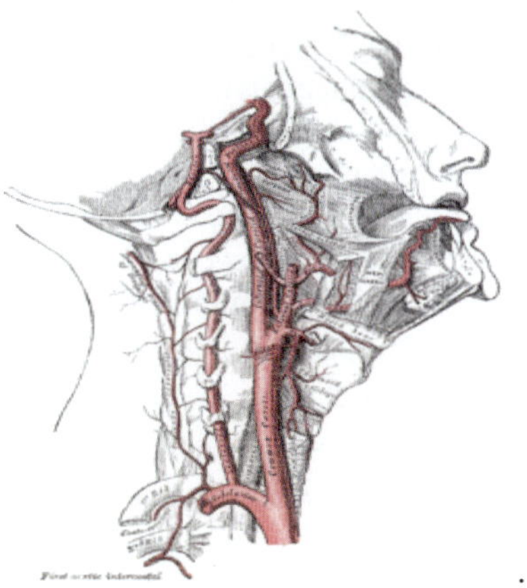

carotid artery

carotid body A small neurovascular structure lying in the bifurcation of the right and left carotid arteries, containing chemoreceptors that monitor oxygen content in blood and help to regulate respiration.

carotid sinus syndrome A localized dilation of the internal carotid artery at its origin, the common carotid artery bifurcation.

carp(o)- of or pertaining to the wrist.

carpal bone One of the wrist bones. There are eight carpal bones that are arranged in two rows.

carpal joint Any of the joints between the carpal bones. *Synonym:* intercarpal joint.

carpal tunnel syndrome A painful progressive condition caused by compression of a key nerve in the wrist.

carpectomy Surgical excision of a carpal bone.

carpometacarpal joint A joint in the wrist that connects the carpal bones and the metacarpals.

carrier The health insurance company which writes and administers the health insurance policy.

carrier (Medicare) A private contractor who administers claims for Part B Medicare services.

carryover That provision in medical plans that allows individuals who have not satisfied their deductible in a given calendar year to apply expenses incurred in the last quarter of that calendar year to the next year's deductible.

carry-over lines Are always indented more than two spaces from the level of the preceding line.

cartilage A type of dense connective tissue existing within many joints. It is composed of specialized cells called chondrocytes. Cartilage is found in many areas in the body, including the articular surface of the bones, the rib cage, the ear, the nose, the bronchial tubes and the intervertebral discs.

caruncle A small fleshy eminence, often abnormal.

carve-out Specialty health service that an MCO obtains for members by contracting with a company that specializes in that service.

carve-out companies Organizations that have specialized provider networks and are paid on a capitation or other basis for a specific service, such as mental health, chiropractic, and dental. *See* also carve-out.

case management Monitoring and coordinating the delivery of health services for individual patients to enhance care and manage costs. Often used for patients with specific diagnoses or who require high-cost or extensive health care services.

case manager An experienced health professional that works with patients, providers and insurers to coordinate all services deemed necessary to provide the patient with a plan of medically necessary and appropriate health care. Often used for patients with specific diagnoses or who require high-cost or extensive health care services.

case mix The distribution of patients into categories reflecting differences in severity of illness or resource consumption.

case mix index The average DRG relative weight for all Medicare admissions.

case mix report (HHA) a graphical or tabular document that provides average values for patient attributes at start of care. Comparative data are provided for either (1) agency case mix for a prior time period, (2) case mix for a reference sample of patients from other agencies, or (3) both of the above. The case mix differences are taken into consideration in producing risk-adjusted outcome reports.

case-mix adjustment Risk-adjustment.

case rate Flat fee paid for services based on client characteristics (such as diagnosis). For this fee the provider covers all of the services the client requires for a specific period of time. Also called bundled rate, or flat fee-per-case. Very often used as an intermediate step prior to capitation.

cash basis The costs of the service when payment was made rather than when the service was performed.

cash indemnity benefits Payments to subscribers for covered services that require submission of an health insurance claim. Subscribers may assign such payments directly to providers.

CASS Coronary artery surgery study.

cast A protective shell which is used to help heal broken bones by holding the limb in place.

cast application The process of applying a cast.

castration Surgical removal or artificial destruction of gonads.

casts Gelled protein particles on the walls of kidney tubules that break off and are washed out by urine. The presence of casts in urine is an abnormal finding caused by kidney disease.

CAT Computerized axial tomography.

cata- Down.

cataplexy A sudden loss of muscle tone and reflexes that leads to muscle weakness, paralysis or postural collapse. Usually caused by an outburst of emotion such as laughter.

cataract Clouding of the eye lens. A common cause of vision loss. Most commonly occurs in people over age 70. Congenital cataracts occur in newborns as genetic defects or from the mother having rubella (German measles) during the first 3 months of pregnancy. Other causes are rare. Usually curable with surgical removal of the lens. Special eyeglasses or contact lenses are needed after surgery.

cataract extraction Surgical removal of a cataractous lens.

catastrophic case A catastrophic case is any medical condition where total cost of treatment (regardless of payment source) is expected to exceed an amount designated by the HMO contract with the medical group.

catastrophic coverage Insurance protection for extremely high health care costs.

catastrophic health insurance Health insurance which provides protection against the high cost of treating severe or lengthy illnesses or disability. Generally such policies cover all, or a specified percentage of, medical expenses above an amount that is the responsibility of another insurance policy up to a maximum limit of liability. It is also used to describe those services covered by reinsurance in a capitated program.

catastrophic illness A very serious and costly health problem that could be life threatening or cause life-long disability. The cost of medical services alone for this type of serious condition could cause financial hardship.

catastrophic limit The highest amount of money you have to pay out of your pocket during a certain period of time for certain covered charges. Setting a maximum amount you will have to pay protects you.

catatonic disorder A group of symptoms characterized by disturbances in motor (muscular movement) behavior that may have either a psychological or a physiological basis. The best-known of these symptoms is immobility, which is a rigid positioning of the body held for a considerable length of time.

catchment area Geographical region where the majority of health care providers customers are located. Also see market area.

categorically needy Persons who are aged, blind, or disabled (as defined under the Supplemental Security Income program - SSI) or a member of a family with dependent children where one parent is absent, incapacitated or unemployed (as defined under the Aid to Families with Dependent Children program - AFDC).

category In the ICD-9-CM refers to diagnoses codes listed within a specific three-digit category, for example category 250, Diabetes Mellitus.

Category II, performance measurement CPT codes CPT codes designed to facilitate outcomes research.

Category III emerging technology codes Temporary CPT codes for emerging technology, services and procedures. These codes are designed to permit data collection and assessment of new technologies.

cath catheterization.

catheter Hollow tube used to introduce fluids into the body or to drain fluids from the body.

catheterization Insertion of a tubular device into a duct, blood vessel, hollow organ, or body cavity for injecting or withdrawing fluids for diagnostic or therapeutic purposes.

cauda equina A structure within the lower end of the spinal column of most vertebrates, that consists of nerve roots and rootlets from above. The cauda equina is the part of the spinal cord where a lumbar puncture is performed in order to obtain a sample of cerebrospinal fluid (csf) for diagnostic purposes.

cauda equina syndrome A serious neurologic condition in which there is acute loss of function of the neurologic elements (nerve roots) of the spinal canal below the termination (conus) of the spinal cord.

cause That which brings about any condition or produces any effect.

cauterization The burning of part of a body to remove or close off a part of it in a process called cautery, which destroys some tissue, in an attempt to mitigate damage, remove an undesired growth, or minimize other potential medical harmful possibilities such as infections, when antibiotics are not available.

cautery The application of a caustic substance, a hot instrument, an electric current, or other agent to destroy tissue.

CAVB Complete atrioventricular block.

cavernosography Radiographic visualization of the corpus cavernosum of the penis.

cavernosometry Measurement of the vascular pressure in the corpus cavernosum.

CAVH Continuous arteriovenous hemodialysis.

Cavitron Dental tool that uses high frequency ultrasonic waves to clean teeth.

CBBB Complete bundle branch block.

CBC Complete blood count.

CBS Chronic brain syndrome, current beneficiary survey.

CBSAs Core Based Statistical Areas.

CBV Circulating blood volume.

CC Complication or comorbidity.

CCI Correct coding initiative.

CCPD Continuous cycling peritoneal dialysis.

CCU Cardiac care unit, coronary care unit, critical care unit.

CDC The Centers for Disease Control and Prevention is a government health care agency, located in Atlanta, GA, whose mission is the prevention and treatment of disease.

CDT Current dental terminology.

CEA Carcinoembryonic antigen.

cecostomy Surgical formation of a permanent artificial opening into the cecum.

-cele Pouching, hernia.

celiac artery Also known as the celiac trunk, is the first major branch of the abdominal aorta. The celiac artery supplies oxygenated blood to the liver, stomach, abdominal esophagus, spleen and the superior half of both the duodenum and the pancreas. *Synonym:* celiac trunk.

celiac disease Congenital disorder caused by an intolerance for gluten, a protein present in most grains. Gluten triggers an allergic reaction in the small intestine, which prevents the intestine from absorbing nutrients. Symptoms include poor appetite, abdominal bloating, fatigue and pale, bad-smelling stool that floats on water. Treatment includes a high protein, high calorie, gluten-free diet and vitamin-mineral supplements. Recovery is usually complete with treatment. *Synonym:* non-tropical sprue.

celioscopy Examination of the abdominal cavity by surgical insertion of an endoscope through the abdominal wall.

celiotomy Incision of the abdomen. *Synonym:* abdominal section, laparotomy, ventrotomy.

cellulitis Infection of the finger or toe, usually caused by normal skin bacteria that get under the top layer of skin. Signs of infection include red, warm, tender skin, swelling, fever, and/or chills.

celotomy The surgical correction of a hernia by cutting through a band of tissue that constricts it. *Synonym:* herniotomy.

cement A special type of glue used to hold a crown in place. It also acts as an insulator to protect the tooth's nerve.

cementation The joining of objects by means of a cement (e.g., in fracture fixation, such as in hip arthroplasty for joining of the acetabular component to the femoral component).

cementum The very thin, bonelike structure that covers the root of the tooth.

Center for Medicare and Medicaid Services (CMS) Formerly known as HCFA (Health Care Financing Administration), this branch of the Department of Health and Human Services oversees the Medicare and Medicaid programs.

Centers for Disease Control and Prevention An organization that maintains several code sets included in the HIPAA standards, including the ICD-9-CM codes.

-centesis Surgical puncture for aspiration.

central nervous system the portion of the vertebrate nervous system consisting of the brain and spinal cord.

central nervous system agents A class of drugs producing both physiological and psychological effects through a variety of mech-anisms. They can be divided into specific agents, e.g., affecting an identifiable molecular mechanism unique to target cells bearing receptors for that agent.

central nervous system assessments Services provided during testing of the cognitive function of the central nervous system.

central nervous system depressants A very loosely defined group of drugs that tend to reduce the activity of the central nervous system. The major groups included here are ethyl alcohol, anesthetics, hypnotics and sedatives, narcotics, and tranquilizing agents.

central nervous system stimulants A loosely defined group of drugs that tend to increase behavioral alertness, agitation, or excitation. They work by a variety of mechanisms, but usually not by direct excitation of neurons.

central retinal artery The blood vessel that carries blood into eye; supplies nutrition to the retina.

central retinal vein The blood vessel that carries blood from the retina.

central vision Clearness of vision. The ability to distinguish details and shapes of objects. *Synonym:* visual acuity.

centrifugation Process of using a rotating machine to generate centrifugal force to separate substances of different densities, remove moisture, or simulate gravitational effects.

centrum The body of a vertebra.

cephal(o)- of or pertaining to the head (as a whole).

cephalic of or relating to the head.

cephalocele The protrusion of a part of the brain through an opening in the skull. The opening may be congenital or may result from an injury.

cephalogram An x-ray image of the structures of the head; cephalometric radiograph.

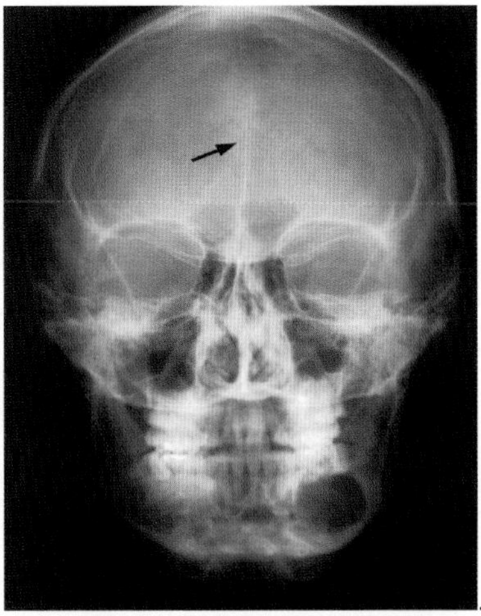

cephalogram

cephalopelvic disproportion Obstetric condition in which an infant's head is too large or the birth canal is too small to permit normal labor and delivery. A Cesarean operation is necessary to deliver the infant, unless the CPD is mild, then vaginal delivery may be possible.

cerat(o)- of or pertaining to the cornu; a horn.

cerclage The surgical closure of the incompetent cervix uteri with suture material.

cerebell(o)- of or pertaining to the cerebellum.

cerebellum A region of the brain that plays an important role in the integration of sensory perception, coordination and motor control.

cerebr(o)- of or pertaining to the brain.

cerebral of or relating to the brain or cerebrum.

cerebral aneurysm A cerebrovascular disorder in which weakness in the wall of a cerebral artery or vein causes a localized dilation or ballooning of the blood vessel.

cerebral artery Any of the arteries supplying blood to the cerebral cortex.

cerebral cortex A thin mantle of gray matter about the size of a formal dinner napkin covering the surface of each cerebral hemisphere. The cerebral cortex is crumpled and folded, forming numerous convolutions (gyri) and crevices (sulci). It is made up of six layers.

cerebral decortication Partial or total removal, ablation, or destruction of the cerebral cortex; may be chemical. It is not used with animals that do not possess a cortex, i.e., it is used only with mammals.

cerebral embolism A brain attack that occurs when a wandering clot (embolus) or some other particle forms in a blood vessel away from the brain usually in the heart.

cerebral infarction The blockage of the flow of blood to the cerebrum, causing or resulting in brain tissue death.

cerebral laceration A type of traumatic brain injury that occurs when the tissue of the brain is mechanically cut or torn.

cerebral revascularization Microsurgical revascularization to improve intracranial circulation. It usually involves joining the extracranial circulation to the intracranial circulation but may include extracranial revasc-ularization.

cerebrospinal fluid A clear bodily fluid that occupies the subarachnoid space and the ventricular system around and inside the brain.

cerebrospinal fluid shunt A tubes inserted to create communication between a cerebral ventricle and the internal jugular vein. The shunt permits draining of cerebrospinal fluid for relief of hydrocephalus or other condition leading to fluid accumulation in the ventricles.

cerebrovascular disease A disease of the blood vessels, especially, the arteries that supply the brain. Cerebrovascular disease is usually caused by atherosclerosis and can lead to a stroke.

cerebrovascular system Refers to the blood vessels of the cerebrum or brain.

certificate of authority A certificate issued by a state government licensing the operation of an HMO.

certificate of coverage A document given to an insured that describes the benefits, limitations and exclusions of coverage provided by an insurance company.

certificate of **insurance** The printed description of the benefits and coverage provisions forming the contract between the carrier and the customer. Discloses what it covered, what is not, and dollar limits.

certificate of medical necessity A form required by Medicare that allows the use of certain durable medical equipment prescribed by the physician or one of the physician's office staff.

certified registered nurse anesthetist A nurse who is trained and licensed to give anesthesia.

cerumen A soft yellow wax secreted by glands in the ear canal. *Synonym:* earwax.

cervic- of or pertaining to the neck, the cervix.

cervical spondylosis Degenerative changes of bones in the neck that place pressure on nerves and muscles to the arms, legs and bladder. May be caused by arthritis, injury or outgrowths of bone that may occur with aging. Symptoms include pain in neck and shoulders, numbness and tingling in arms, hands and fingers, muscle weakness, dizziness, headache and double vision. Loss of bladder control and leg weakness may occur with advanced disease. Treatment usually relieves symptoms; rarely, surgery is required.

cervicalgia Discomfort or more intense forms of pain that are localized to the cervical region. This term generally refers to pain in the posterior or lateral regions of the neck. *Synonym:* neck pain.

cervicectomy Surgical removal of the cervix, the lower portion of the uterus that protrudes into the vagina. Cervicectomy is also called trachelectomy. *Synonym:* trachelectomy.

cervicitis Inflammation of the uterine cervix.

cervicography A technique, equivalent to colposcopy , for photographing part or all of the uterine cervix.

cervicoplasty Reconstructive surgical procedures in the neck region to restore or improve form and function.

cervix The lower, narrow portion of the uterus where it joins with the top end of the vagina. *Synonym:* neck of the uterus.

cesarean delivery A surgical procedure in which incisions are made through a the abdomen uterus to deliver one or more babies. *Synonym:* c-section.

cestode infection Infestation by any of various parasitic flatworms of the class cestoda, including the tapeworms.

CF Conversion Factor •cystic fibrosis.

CG Centigram.

CGH Chorionic gonadotropic hormone.

Chadwick sign Blue discoloration of vaginal mucosa that indicates pregnancy.

chain of trust A term used in the HIPAA Security NPRM for a pattern of agreements that extend protection of health care data by requiring that each covered entity that shares health care data with another entity require that that entity provide protections comparable to those provided by the covered entity, and that that entity, in turn, require that any other entities with which it shares the data satisfy the same requirements.

chain of trust partner agreement Contract entered into by two business partners in which it is agreed to exchange data and that the first party will transmit information to the second party, where the data transmitted is agreed to be protected between the partners.

chalazion A cyst in the eyelid that is caused by inflammation of a blocked meibomian gland, usually on the upper eyelid.

CHAMPUS Civilian Health and Medical Program of the Uniformed Services (see Tricare).

CHAMPVA Civilian Health and Medical Program of the Veterans Administration.

chancroid Infectious venereal ulcer.

CHAP Child Health Assessment Program.

Charcot's syndrome Amyotrophic lateral sclerosis.

Charcot-Marie-Tooth disease Peroneal muscular atrophy.

Charcot's disease Chronic, progressive degeneration of a joint, which is the result of an underlying neurological disorder. Characterized by swelling, heat, bleeding into the joint and instability of the joint. Early treatment may prevent further damage to the joint. Extensive disease may require amputation. *Synonym:* Neuropathic joint disease.

charge reduction (Medicare) The percentage difference between a provider's billed charge and the Medicare allowed charge.

CHB Complete heart block.

CHC Community health center.

CHD Congenital heart disease, coronary heart disease.

cheilectomy 1) Excision of a portion of the lip. 2) The chiseling away of bony irregularities on the lips of a joint cavity that interfere with movements of the joint.

cheiloplasty The technical term for surgery of the lip. It includes lip reduction, the process of surgically reducing the size of the lip or lips in order to reduce the appearance of abnormally large or protruding lips and the process of forming an artificial tip or part of the lips by using a piece of healthy tissue from some neighboring part.

chem(o)- Chemistry, drug.

chemexfoliation A process in which a chemical solution is applied to the skin to remove dead skin cells and stimulate the production of new skin cells. *Synonym:* chemical peel.

chemical inhibition Process of retarding, arresting or restraining a chemical reaction.

chemical profile (smac) A profile of tests is performed on an electronic machine and includes from 12 to 36 blood-chemistry determinations, including those listed in other profiles.

chemocauterization The corroding or burning of living tissue by a caustic chemical substance, such as potassium hydroxide. *Synonym:* chemocautery.

chemodenervation Refers to the use of chemical agents to produce neuromuscular blockade for the purpose of selective weakening of specific muscles, or muscle groups.

chemonucleolysis A non-surgical treatment for a bulging disc that involves the injection of an enzyme into the vertebral disc with the goal of dissolving the inner part of the disc, the nucleus pulposus.

chemoprevention Use of chemotherapeutic agents as the means of preventing the development of a specific disease.

chemosurgery Selective destruction of tissue by use of chemicals, as for removing malignant skin lesions. *Synonym:* Mohs surgery.

chemotherapy Treatment of cancer with medication that kills cancer cells without harming healthy tissue. Used to treat cancers that cannot be completely cured or treated with surgery or radiation.

cherry picking The practice of seeking only healthy customers.

chest The region of the body between the neck and the abdomen, along with its internal organs and other contents. It is mostly protected and supported by the ribcage, spine, and shoulder girdle.

chest cavity The cavity in the vertebrate body enclosed by the ribs between the diaphragm and the neck and containing the lungs and heart.

chest wall The bony and muscular structures that form the outer framework of the thorax and move during breathing.

chevron procedure Surgical procedure used to treat a large bunion deformity in which there minimal angulation of the great toe.

chewing reflex When a tongue depressor is placed in the mouth, the patient chews or clenches his teeth on the depressor. Reflex chewing is seen in diffuse bilateral lesions of the frontotemporal cortex and is frequently seen in cases of dementia, incomplete paralysis (generalized paresis) and brain injury related to a lack of oxygen.

Cheyne-Stokes respiration Recurrent episodes of rapid breathing alternating with apnea, often seen in coma resulting from affection of the nervous centers.

CHF Congestive heart failure.

chickenpox Acute contagious disease caused by herpes varicella zoster virus; causes a rash of vesicles on the face and body.

chicf complaint Λ concise statement describing the symptoms, problems, conditions, diagnoses or other factors that is the reason for the encounter, usually stated in the patient's words.

Children's Health Insurance Program A program, established by the Balanced Budget Act, designed to provide health assistance to uninsured, low-income children either through separate programs or through expanded eligibility under state Medicaid programs.

CHIP Children's health insurance program, comprehensive health insurance plan.

chir(o)-, cheir(o)- of or pertaining to the hand.

chiropractic A health care discipline and profession that emphasizes diagnosis, treatment and prevention of mechanical disorders of the musculoskeletal system, especially the spine, under the hypothesis that these disorders affect general health via the nervous system.

Chiropractic Manipulation Treatment (CMT) A form of manual treatment applied by a chiropractic physician to eliminate or alleviate somatic dysfunction and related disorders.

chlamydia A type of bacteria one species of which causes an infection very similar to gonorrhea in the way that it is spread, the symptoms it produces, and the long-term consequences.

chlamydia trachomatis An organism that lives in the conjunctivae of the eye and the epithelium of the urethra and cervix and is responsible for conjunctivitis, lymphogranuloma venereum, and trachoma.

chlor(o)- Denoting a green color.

chloride, serum Chloride is another electrolyte and is involved in maintaining the normal amount of water and the acid-base balance in body fluids. In general, the serum level of chloride is closely associated with the level of sodium. Abnormal levels may be associated with diseases of the gastrointestinal tract, kidney and adrenal gland.

chol(e)- of or pertaining to bile.

cholangiopancreatography Radiographic examination of the bile ducts and pancreas following administration of a radiopaque contrast medium.

cholangiotomy Incision into a bile duct.

cholangitis Infection or inflammation of the bile ducts (biliary tract) that drain bile from the gallbladder to the small intestine. Usually caused by gallstone formation and bile duct blockage. Symptoms include fever, belching, nausea, vomiting and pain in the upper right abdomen.

cholecyst(o)- of or pertaining to the gallbladder.

cholecystectomy The surgical removal of the gallbladder.

cholecystitis Gallbladder inflammation usually caused by a gallstone that cannot pass through the cystic duct. *See* Gallstones.

cholecystoenterostomy Surgical anastomosis of the gallbladder and intestinal tract, usually indicated if the common bile duct has been disrupted by injury or neoplasia.

cholecystography X-ray of the gallbladder following injection or ingestion of a radiopaque substance excreted.

cholecystostomy Establishment of an opening into the gallbladder either for drainage or surgical communication with another part of the digestive tract, usually the duodenum or jejunum.

choledochoenterostomy The surgical formation of a communication between the common bile duct and any part of the intestine.

choledocholithiasis Stone formed in the biliary tract. May lead to cholangitis if stone cannot pass spontaneously into small intestine. *See* Cholangitis. *Synonym:* biliary calculus, biliary stone.

choledochoplasty Plastic repair of the common bile duct.

choledochoscopy Surgical inspection of the common bile duct.

choledochostomy Surgical formation of an opening (stoma) into the common bile duct for drainage or for direct communication with a site in the small intestine, primarily the duodenum or jejunum.

choledochotomy Incision into the common bile duct.

choledochus The ductus choledochus, or bile duct.

cholelithiasis Stones in the gallbladder that may or may not cause symptoms. If symptoms occur, surgery to remove the gallbladder is recommended to prevent complications of cholecystitis or cholangitis. Symptoms may include colicky pain in upper right abdomen or between shoulder blades, nausea, vomiting, belching or bloating, intolerance for fatty foods and jaundice. *Synonym:* gallstones.

choleperitonitis Inflammation of the peritoneum which is caused by the escape of bile into the peritoneal cavity.

cholera Infectious gastroenteritis caused by enterotoxin-producing strains of the bacterium vibrio cholerae. *Synonym:* asiatic cholera, epidemic cholera.

cholestasis intrahepatic Interruption in the flow of bile to the biliary tract. May be caused by hepatitis, drug and alcohol use, pregnancy and metastatic liver cancer.

cholesteatoma A destructive and expanding keratinizing squamous epithelium in the middle ear and/or mastoid process.

cholesterol A blood fat related in part to eating animal fats such as eggs, cheese, cream, liver, pork, beef, etc. Increased values may indicate a tendency to have hardening of the arteries. Values of 180 or less are associated with least risk of heart disease.

cholesterol, total Cholesterol is a lipid compound produced in the liver that's normally found in the blood. Increased cholesterol levels are seen in familial lipid disorders and hypothyroidism and are considered a risk factor for heart disease.

chondr(i)o- Cartilage, gristle, granule, granular.

chondritis Any inflammatory condition affecting the cartilage.

chondrocalcinosis A rheumatologic disorder with varied clinical manifestations due to precipitation of calcium pyrophosphate dihydrate crystals in the connective tissues.

chondrodystrophy A group of disorders in which there is abnormal conversion of cartilage to bone, particularly in the epiphyses of the long bones.

chondromalacia Abnormal softening of cartilage.

chondromalacia patellae Occurs after knee injury. Characterized by swelling, pain and degenerative changes in the kneecap that are revealed by an X-ray examination.

chondroplasty Surgical repair of cartilage.

chondrosteoma A cartilage capped by knobby projection of the sternal surface of endochondral bone.

Chopart's amputation Transtarsal amputation of the forefoot.

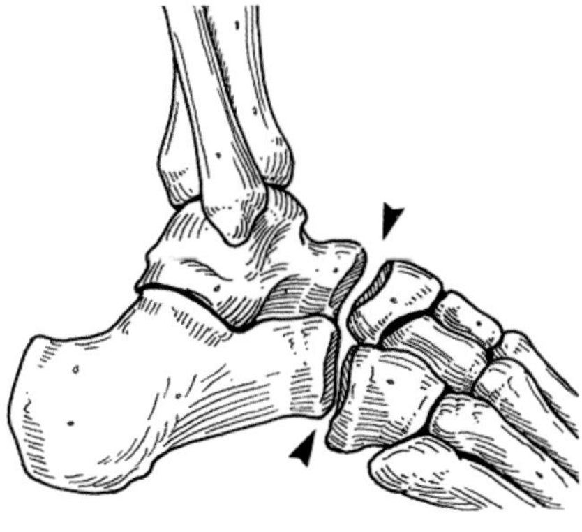

Chopart's amputation

chordae tendineae Thread-like bands of fibrous tissue which attach on one end to the edges of the tricuspid and mitral valves of the heart and on the other end to the papillary muscles, small muscles within the heart that serve to anchor the valves.

chordee A condition in which the head of the penis curves downward (that is, in a ventral direction) or upward, at the junction of the head and shaft of the penis.

chordotomy Surgical division of a spinal nerve tract to relieve severe intractable pain.

chorea An abnormal involuntary movement disorder, one of a group of neurological disorders called dyskinesias.

chorioamnionitis An inflammation of the fetal membranes (amnion and chorion) due to a bacterial infection.

chorioangioma A benign vascular tumor of the placenta.

choriocarcinoma Malignancy arising in the uterus associated with pregnancy, abortion or hydatidiform mole.

Chorionic Villus Sampling (CVS) A form of prenatal diagnosis to determine chromosomal or genetic disorders in the fetus.

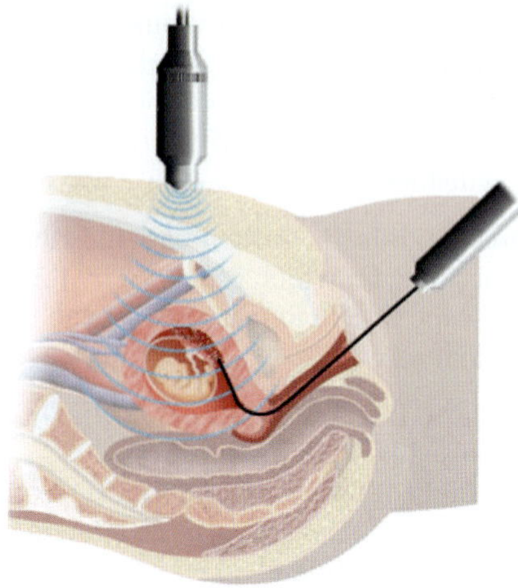

Chorionic Villus Sampling

chorioretinal inflammations Scars and other disorders of choroid inflammation affecting the choroid and the retina of the eye.

chorioretinitis An inflammation of the choroid and retina of the eye. *Synonym:* choroid retinitis.

choroid The vascular layer containing connective tissue, of the eye lying between the retina and the sclera. *Synonym:* choroidea, choroid coat.

choroideremia A rare inherited disorder that causes progressive loss of vision due to degeneration of the choroid and retina. It occurs almost exclusively in males.

choroiditis An inflammation of the layer of the eye behind the retina, either in its entirely (multifocal choroiditis) or in patches (focal choroiditis). Usually the only symptom is blurred vision.

CHP Comprehensive health plan.

Christmas disease Hemophilia B; caused by hereditary deficiency of Factor IX. *Synonym:* Factor IX deficiency.

chrom(ato)- Color.

chromatin mass Portion of the cell nucleus that carries the genes of inheritance.

chromatin test Determination of genetic sex of an individual by examination of somatic cells for the presence of sex chromatin.

chromatography Laboratory techniques for the separation of mixtures.

chromoblastomycosis A chronic fungal infection of the skin and the subcutaneous tissue caused by traumatic inoculation of a specific group of dematiacious fungi.

chromophobe adenoma Tumor of the anterior portion of the pituitary gland; cells do not stain with acid or basic dyes. These tumors are usually not malignant and are associated with decreased function of the pituitary gland.

chromosomal anomalies Refer to changes in the normal structure or number of chromosomes; often resulting in physical or mental abnormalities.

chromosome Structures inside the nucleus of living cells that contain hereditary information. Defects in chromosomes cause many birth defects and inherited diseases.

chromosome analysis A procedure in which cells of fetal origin are obtained, either by chorionic villus biopsy, or amniocentesis, and grown in a tissue culture, to detect major chromosome defects.

chromatin test Determination of genetic sex of an individual by examination of somatic cells for the presence of sex chromatin.

chromotubation The injection of fluid containing a colored dye at the time of laparoscopy to determine if there is any blockage of the fallopian tubes.

chronic Long-term; continuing. Chronic illnesses are usually not curable, but they can often be prevented from worsening. Symptoms usually can be controlled.

chronic airway obstruction A pulmonary disorder, such as emphysema or chronic bronchitis, in which the upper or lower airway is chronically obstructed.

chronic bronchitis Inflammation caused by repeated irritation or infection of the bronchial tubes. Causes them to thicken, narrow and lose elasticity. Symptoms include frequent cough, shortness of breath and sputum that is thick and difficult to cough up. Treatment includes stopping cigarette smoking and avoiding air pollution and other irritants, taking expectorants, bronchial drainage and deep breathing exercises.

chronic care Care and treatment rendered to individuals whose health problems are of a long-term and continuing nature. Rehabilitation facilities, nursing homes, and mental hospitals may be considered chronic care facilities.

chronic case A patient with one or more medical conditions that persist for long periods of time or for the patient's lifetime.

chronic disease A disease which has one or more of the following characteristics (1) is permanent, leaves residual disability; (2) is caused by nonreversible pathological alternation; (3) requires special training of the patient for rehabilitation, or may be expected to require a long period of supervision, observation, or care.

chronic kidney disease A progressive loss of renal function over a period of months or years. *Synonym:* chronic renal disease.

chronic maintenance dialysis Dialysis that is regularly furnished to an ESRD patient in a hospital based independent (non-hospital based), or home setting.

chronic rheumatic pericarditis Inflammation of the pericardium resulting from rheumatic heart disease.

chronic thromboembolic pulmonary hypertension High blood pressure in the lungs that occurs in a small percentage of those who have had pulmonary embolism. The problem usually progresses but may be cured with surgery.

chronotherapy The adaptation of the administration of drugs to circadian rhythms. The concept is based on the response of biological functions to time-related events, such as the low point in epinephrine levels between 10 p.m. and 4 a.m.

Chvostek's sign Spasm of the facial muscles caused by tapping the facial nerve near the parotid gland.

chyle Lymph and droplets of triglyceride fat in a stable emulsion. Lymph forms a milky fluid taken up by special structures in the intestinal tract during digestion of food.

CIBD Chronic inflammatory bowel disease.

CICU Cardiac (coronary) intensive care unit.

-cidal, -cide Killing, destroying.

cili- of or pertaining to the cilia, the eyelashes; eyelids.

ciliary body The circumferential tissue inside the eye composed of the ciliary muscle and ciliary processes.

ciliary muscles The muscles that relax the zonules to enable the crystalline lens to change shape for focusing.

ciliary processes The extensions or projections of the ciliary body that secrete aqueous humor.

cineplasty Cineplasty is the surgical isolation of a loop of muscle of chest or arm, covering it with skin, and attaching to it a prosthetic device to be operated by contraction of the muscle in the loop.

cineradiography A diagnostic technique in which a movie camera is used to film the images, as of internal body structures, produced through radiography or fluoroscopy.

cingulotomy A form of psychosurgery, first introduced in 1952 as an alternative to lobotomy. Currently it is mainly used as a last resort for the treatment of obsessive-compulsive disorder and chronic pain.

circle of **Willis** Network of blood vessels at the base of the brain, formed by the interconnection of several arteries that supply blood to the brain.

circum- Denoting something as 'around' another.

circumcision The removal of some or all of the foreskin (prepuce) from the penis.

cirrhosis Chronic scarring of the liver, leading to loss of normal liver function.

cis- On this side.

cisternography X-ray of the basal cistern of the brain after subarachnoid injection of a contrast medium.

cis-trans test A test in microbial genetics to determine whether two mutations that have the phenotypic effect, in a haploid cell or a cell with single phage infection, are located in the same gene or in different genes; the test depends on the independent behavior of two alleles of a gene in a diploid cell or in a cell infected with two phages carrying different alleles.

citrullinuria Presence of large amounts of citrulline in the urine, plasma and cerebrospinal fluid. Citrulline is involved in producing urea.

CKD Chronic kidney disease.

Clagett procedure A two-stage surgical procedure for expediting treatment of chronic empyema.

claim An itemized statement of health care services and their costs provided by a hospital, physician's office, or other provider facility. Claims are submitted to the insurer or managed care plan by either the plan member or the provider for payment of the costs incurred.

claim adjustment reason codes A national administrative code set that identifies the reasons for any differences, or adjustments, between the original provider charge for a claim or service and the payer's payment for it.

claim attachment Any of a variety of hardcopy forms or electronic records needed to process a claim in addition to the claim itself.

claim form A form used to present claim information in an organized manner to the carrier. *See* CMS1500.

claim status category codes A national administrative code set that indicates the general category of the status of health care claims. This code set is used in the X12 277 Claim Status Notification transaction, and is maintained by the Health Care Code Maintenance Committee.

claims administration The process of receiving, reviewing, adjudicating, and processing claims.

claims analysts Claims examiners.

claims audit Review of health care claims for the purpose of determining the liability of the payer, eligibility of the beneficiary and provider, and the accuracy of the amounts involved.

claims examiners The carrier's employee who is responsible for handling claims as they are received from patients and medical offices. *Synonym:* claims analysts.

claims investigation The process of obtaining all the information necessary to determine the appropriate amount to pay on a given claim.

claims review The method by which an enrollee's health care service claims are reviewed before reimbursement is made. The purpose of this monitoring is to validate the medical appropriate-ness of the provided service and to be sure the cost of the service is not excessive.

classification Protection of data from unauthorized access by the designation of multiple levels of access authorization clearances to be required for access, dependent upon the sensitivity of the information.

clast Break.

clavicle A bone that links the scapula (shoulder blade) and sternum (breastbone). The clavicle is located just above the first rib on either side of the neck, and has the form of a narrow elongated S. *Synonym:* collarbone.

clavicular of or relating to the clavicle.

claviculectomy Surgical removal of all or part of a clavicle.

CLBBB Complete left bundle branch block.

cleaning Removal of plaque and calculus (tartar) from teeth, generally above the gum line.

clearing house A public or private entity that processes or facilitates the processing of nonstandard data elements of health information into standard data elements.

cleft lip The presence of one or two vertical fissures (clefts) in the upper lip. Cleft lip is one of the most common physical birth defects. *Synonym:* cheiloschisis.

cleft palate A congenital fissure in the roof of the mouth, resulting from incomplete fusion of the palate during embryonic development. Cleft lip a congenital deformity characterized by a vertical cleft or pair of clefts in the upper lip, with or without involvement of the palate. *Synonym:* palatoschisis.

clenching The forceful holding together of the upper and lower teeth, which places stress on the ligaments that hold the teeth to the jawbone and the lower jaw to the skull.

CLIA Clinical Laboratory Improvement Act.

clinical chemistry tests Laboratory tests demonstrating the presence of physiologically significant substances in the blood, urine, tissue, and body fluids with application to the diagnosis or therapy of disease.

clinical integration A type of operational integration that enables patients to receive a variety of health care services from the same organization or entity, which streamlines administrative processes and increases the potential for the delivery of high-quality health-care.

Clinical Laboratory Improvement Act (CLIA) A Federal law designed to set national quality standards for laboratory testing. The law covers all laboratories that engage in testing for assessment, diagnosis, prevention or treatment purposes.

clinical laboratory techniques Techniques used to carry out clinical investigative procedures in the diagnosis and therapy of disease.

clinical pathology Clinical pathology focuses on microbiology (including bacteriology, mycology, parasitology, and virology), immunopathology, blood banking or transfusion medicine, chemical pathology, cytogenetics, hematology, coagulation, toxicology, and medical microscopy.

clinical performance measure This is a method or instrument to estimate or monitor the extent to which the actions of a health care practitioner or provider conform to practice guidelines, medical review criteria, or standards of quality.

clinical practice guideline A utilization and quality management mechanism designed to aid providers in making decisions about the most appropriate course of treatment for a specific clinical case.

clinical protocols Precise and detailed plans for the study of a medical or biomedical problem and/or plans for a regimen of therapy.

clinical status A type of outcomes measure that relates to biological health outcomes.

clinic-without-walls A practice setting designed to preserve physician autonomy or independence while taking advantage of the benefits inherent in a large group practice. Results when several independent practices combine into one corporate entity.

clitoroplasty Plastic repair of the clitoris.

clomiphene citrate challenge test Measurement of fertility potential in a woman by examination of the response of follicle-stimulating hormone level to administration of clomiphene citrate early in the menstrual cycle.

clonic seizure A seizure in which there are generalized clonic contractions with the entire body jerking, but without a preceding tonic phase.

closed access A provision which specifies that plan members must obtain medical services only from network providers through a primary care physician to receive benefits.

closed dislocation A dislocation not complicated by an external wound.

closed formulary The provision that only those drugs on a preferred list will be covered by a PBM or MCO.

closed fracture A broken bone when the skin over the fracture site is in tact.

closed panel Medical services delivered in the Health Insuring Corporation owned health center or satellite clinic by physicians who belong to a specially formed, but legally separate, medical group that only serves the HIC.

closed PHO A type of physician-hospital organization that typically limits the number of participating specialists by type of specialty.

closed plans According to the NAIC's Quality Assessment and Improvement Model Act, managed care plans that require covered persons to use participating providers.

closed treatment Refers to the treatment of fractures in which the skin is intact, i.e. not surgically open. A closed reduction re-aligns a bone by manipulation without surgery.

closed-panel HMO An HMO whose physicians are either employees or belong to a group of physicians that contract with the HMO.

closure The closing of a surgical opening by the use of sutures, staples, tape or other means.

clotting disorders A term used to describe a group of conditions in which there is an increased tendency, often repeated and over an extended period of time, for excessive clotting.

clotting factor Substances in the blood that act in sequence to stop bleeding by forming a clot.

clysis Hypodermoclysis.

cm Cubic centimeter.

CMG Cystometrogram.

CMIT Current Medical Information and Terminology.

CMS Center for Medicare and Medicaid Services.

CMS agent Any individual or organization, public or private, with whom CMS has a contractual arrangement to contribute to or participate in the Medicare survey and certification process.

CMS directed improvement process Any project where CMS specifies the subject, size, pace, data source, analytic techniques, educational intervention techniques, or impact measurement model. These projects may be developed by CMS in consultation with.

CMS1450 The uniform institutional claim form.

CMS1500 A universal health insurance claim form that is mandated for Medicare billing and generally accepted by all health insurance carriers. Formerly referred to as the HCFA1500.

CMP Competitive Medical Plan.

CMT Chiropractic manipulative treatment.

CMV Cytomegalovirus.

coagulation The process of blood clotting.

coagulation defects Disruption of blood clotting mechanisms, resulting in hemorrhaging or internal bleeding. Complication of an underlying disorder. *Synonym:* coagulopathy, clotting disorder, bleeding disorder.

coagulation factors Chemical compounds necessary for blood to clot. *See* Factor I through Factor VIII.

coagulation time The time required for blood clotting to begin in a capillary tube, normally 2 to 8 minutes. A coagulation time three times normal is a definite danger sign.

coagulometer A device used to measure the INR for warfarin monitoring.

coagulopathy A disorder in which blood is either too slow or too quick to coagulate (clot).

coal workers' pneumoconiosis A diseases characterized by fibrosis and scarring of the lungs caused by repeated inhalation of occupationally associated dust, such as silica, asbestos, and coal dust.

coarctation A congenital condition whereby the aorta narrows in the area where the ductus arteriosus (ligamentum arteriosum after regression) inserts.

COB Coordination of benefits.

COBRA Consolidated omnibus budget reconciliation act (1985).

COC Certificate of coverage.

coccidioidin test An intracutaneous test for determining the presence of infection with the fungus Coccidioides immitis; a reaction of delayed hypersensitivity indicates a positive test and is interpreted as meaning past or present infection with the fungus.

coccidioidomycosis Infection caused by breathing spores of a fungus found in soil. It is not contagious. The disease is most common in desert areas of California, Arizona and Texas. Symptoms often resemble a common cold or influenza. Spontaneous recovery usually occurs in 3 to 6 weeks. Rarely, the infection can spread throughout the body and brain causing a life-threatening illness. *Synonym:* Valley fever.

coccygeal of or relating to or near the coccyx.

coccygectomy Surgery to remove the coccyx for patients with coccyx pain (tailbone pain).

coccyx A series of small bones below the sacrum. *Synonym:* tailbone.

cochlea The snail-shaped tube (in the inner ear coiled around the modiolus) where sound vibrations are converted into nerve impulses by the organ of Corti.

cochlear of or relating to the cochlea.

cochlear device A surgically implanted electronic device that provides a sense of sound to a person who is profoundly deaf or severely hard of hearing. *Synonym:* bionic ear.

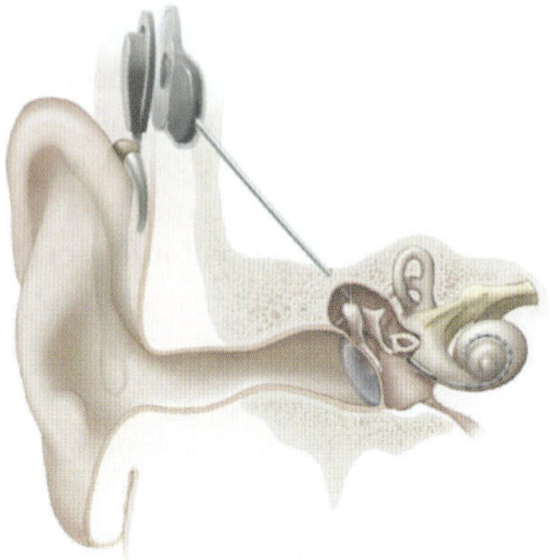

cochlear device

Code of Federal Regulations The official compilation of federal rules and requirements.

code set Under HIPAA, this is any set of codes used to encode data elements, such as tables of terms, medical concepts, medical diagnostic codes, or medical procedure codes. This includes both the codes and their descriptions.

code set maintaining organization Under HIPAA, this organization that creates and maintains the code sets adopted by the Secretary for use in the transactions for which standards are adopted.

coding A mechanism for identifying and defining physicians' and hospitals' services. Coding provides universal definition and recognition of diagnoses, procedures and level of care. Coders usually work in medical records departments and coding is a function of billing. Medicare fraud investigators look closely at the medical record documentation which supports codes and looks for consistency. Lack of consistency of documentation can earmark a record as "upcoded" which is considered fraud.

coding errors Documentation errors in which a treatment is miscoded or the codes used to describe procedures do not match those used to identify the diagnosis.

codominance The situation in which two different alleles for a trait are expressed unblended in the phenotype of heterozygous individuals. Neither allele is dominant or recessive, so that both influence the phenotype. Type AB blood is an example. Such traits are said to be codominant.

cognitive disorders The class of disorders consisting of significant impairment of cognition or memory that represents a marked deterioration from a previous level of functioning.

cognitive impairment A loss of mental capacity demonstrated by a person's inability to think, perceive, reason or remember. Such impairment results in a person's inability to care for him or herself without ongoing supervision from another person and is due to a mental or nervous condition with an organic cause.

cognitive impairment reinstatement provision A provision in some long-term care policies that allows a policy that has lapsed because the enrollee did not pay the premium to be reinstated for full benefits, if the premiums are paid within six months after the lapse. Typically, the enrollee's physician must certify that the enrollee suffered a cognitive impairment that presumably caused the individual to fail to pay the premium on time.

cognitive therapy A method of treating psychiatric disorders that focuses on revising a person's thinking, perceptions, attitudes and beliefs.

cognitive-behavioral therapy A method of treating psychiatric disorders based on the idea that the way we think about the world and ourselves (our cognitions) affects our emotions and behavior.

cohort A population group that shares a common property, characteristic, or event, such as a year of birth or year of marriage. The most common one is the birth cohort, a group of individuals born within a defined time period, usually a calendar year or a five-year interval.

coinsurance A cost-sharing requirement under a health insurance policy that provides that the insured will assume a portion or percentage of the costs of covered services. After the deductible is paid, this provision obligates the subscriber to pay a certain percentage of any remaining medical bills, usually 20 percent.

col-, colo-, colono- Colon.

cold agglutinins Antibodies that cause red blood cells to clump together at low temperatures. Mycoplasma pneumonia and infectious mononucleosis are two of several illnesses that cause a high number of cold agglutinins in the blood.

colectomy Excision of a portion of the colon or of the whole colon.

colitis Inflammatory condition of the large intestine. It can occur in episodes, such as irritable bowel syndrome, or it can be one of the more serious, chronic, progressive, inflammatory bowel diseases, such as ulcerative colitis. Irritable bowel syndrome is characterized by bouts of colicky abdominal pain, bloating, diarrhea or constipation, and fatigue, often due to emotional stress. Treatment includes stress reduction, diet changes and sometimes medication.

collagen A fibrous protein which is a major constituent of connective tissue, such as skin, tendons, ligaments, cartilage, and bones.

collagen injection Injection of collagen into a part of the face or body to make it larger, most often performed on the lips. The effects are long lasting but not permanent. Collagen injections are normally done by a plastic surgeon.

collagen-vascular disease *See* Connective tissue disease.

collar bone *See* clavicle.

collarette Color ring around the pupil.

Colles' fracture Fractured distal radius with posterior displacement.

colloids Two-phase systems in which one is uniformly dispersed in another as particles small enough so they cannot be filtered or will not settle out. The dispersing or continuous phase or medium envelops the particles of the discontinuous phase.

colon The part of the large intestine between the cecum and the rectum.

colon & rectal surgery The specialty of treating problems of the small and large intestine, the rectum and anus with surgery.

colonography CT colonography is a procedure used for the screening of colorectal cancer. The test involves an examination of your colon and rectum using pictures obtained using a CT (cat) scanner.

colonoscopy The endoscopic examination of the large colon and the distal part of the small bowel with a CCD camera or a fiber optic camera on a flexible tube passed through the anus.

coloproctostomy The surgical formation of a communication between the rectum and a discontinuous segment of the colon.

color vision The ability to perceive differences in color, including hue, saturation and brightness.

colorectal Relating to or affecting the colon and the rectum.

colorrhaphy Suture of the colon.

colostomy A surgical procedure that involves connecting a part of the colon onto the anterior abdominal wall, leaving the patient with an opening on the abdomen called a stoma.

colotomy A surgical incision into the colon, usually performed through the abdominal wall.

colp(o)- of or pertaining to the vagina.

colpocentesis Surgical puncture of the vagina.

colpocleisis Surgical obliteration of the lumen of the vagina.

colpohysterectomy Removal of the uterus through the vagina.

colpoperineorrhaphy Suture of the ruptured vagina and perineum.

colpopexy Fixation of the vagina by suturing it to the adjacent abdominal wall.

colporrhaphy A surgical procedure which repairs a defect in the wall of the vagina. It is the surgical intervention for both cystocele (protrusion of bladder into the vagina) and rectocele (protrusion of rectum into the vagina).

colposcopy A diagnostic procedure to examine an illuminated, magnified view of the cervix and the tissues of the vagina and vulva.

colpotomy An incision in the vagina. *Synonym:* culdocentesis.

colpo-urethrocystopexy Surgical procedure for treatment of genuine primary stress incontinence, frequently done with hysterectomy.

com- With, together.

coma Profound state of unconsciousness. A comatose person cannot be awakened, fails to respond normally to pain or light, does not have sleep-wake cycles, and does not take voluntary actions.

combination code An ICD-9-CM code that combines a diagnosis with an associated secondary process or combination.

combined modality therapy The treatment of a disease or condition by several different means simultaneously or sequentially. Chemoimmunotherapy, radio-immunotherapy, chemoradio-therapy, cryochemotherapy, and salvage therapy are seen most frequently.

commercial MCO A health maintenance organization, an eligible organization with a contract under 11876 or a Medicare-Choice organization; a provider sponsored organization.

comminuted fracture A fracture in which a bone is broken into more than two pieces. Often internal or external fixation devices are used to maintain proper alignment of the fragments.

Commission on Accreditation of Rehabilitation Facilities (CARF) Nationally recognized independent review organization that accredits disability service organizations.

Commission on Health Care Quality (CHCQ) National Commission charged with improving health care quality.

commissure A site of union of corresponding parts, as the angle of the lips or eyelids; used also with specific reference to the sites of junction between adjacent cusps of the heart valves.

commissurotomy A surgical incision of a commissure in the body, as one made in the heart to relieve constriction of the mitral valve or one made in the brain to treat certain psychiatric disorders.

common working file A CMS data reporting system which combines Part A and Part B claims in a common file.

community based care The blend of health and social services provided to an individual or family in their place of residence (or nearby) for the purpose of promot-ing, maintaining, or restoring health or minimizing the effects of illness and disability.

community care networks Systems of health care providers organized to provide access to a compre-hensive range of personal health services to members of a geo-graphic area. The "network" may act as a health insurance plan offering its services for a specified premium. In this setting, primary care physicians and mid-level professionals are usually used as the entry and referral point for services and a range of services tailored to the needs of the specific community.

Community Health Center (CHC) An ambulatory health care program usually serving a geographic area which has scarce or nonexistent health services or a population with special health needs (sometimes known as the neighborhood health center). Community Health Centers attempt to coordinate Federal, state, and local resources into a single organization capable of delivering both health and related social services to a defined population. While such a center may not directly provide all types of health care, it usually takes responsibility to arrange all medical services needed by its patient population.

Community Health Information Network (CHIN) An information network for providers and insurers to record, access and share health information.

Community Health Purchasing Alliance (CHPA) Established by the Health Care and Insurance Reform Act of 1993. CHPAs are responsible for assisting their members and particularly small employers to be prudent purchasers of health care by analyzing and disseminating data on prices, quality and patient satisfaction. CHPAs annually solicit bids for a variety of state mandated insurance products.

community health services Diagnostic, therapeutic and preventive health services provided for individuals in the community.

community mental health center A facility that provides the following services; Outpatient services, including specialized outpatient services for children, the elderly, individuals who are chronically ill, and residents of the CMHC's mental health services area who have been discharged from inpatient treatment at a mental health facility.

community rating method of establishing health insurance premiums on a communitywide rather than group-specific basis. The premium is based on a blend of the average cost of actual and anticipated health services use by all enrollees in a geographic area or industry and does not consider variables such as claims experience, age, sex, or health status of the covered population. Community rating spreads the cost of illness more evenly over the whole community. Federally qualified HMOs must community rate.

community rating area Under community rating, a defined geographic area for which each insurer must establish a single set of health insurance premiums.

community rating by class Modifies community rating principles to establish different premiums based upon the age, sex, marital status, or industry of the individual group. The 1981 amendments to the Federal HMO Act allowed Federally qualified HMOs to community rate by class. Defined under the Tax Equity and Fiscal Responsibility Act of 1982 (TEFRA), a competitive medical plan (CMP) resembles a health maintenance organization but is not qualified under the Federal HMO Act; it must be state-licensed; to be eligible to participate in Medicare, the CMP must be Federally approved.

comorbidity Presence of a second disease or condition influencing the care or treatment of a patient, and in the hospital setting is expected to increase the length of stay by at least one day for most patients.

comparability Requirement that the state must ensure that the same Medicaid benefits are available to all people who are eligible. Exceptions include benefits approved under Medicaid waiver programs for special sub populations of Medicaid eligibles.

compensatory curve A curve, which can be structural, above or below a major curve that tends to maintain normal body alignment.

Competitive Medical Plan (CMP) A mechanism created in TEFRA to enable organized provider groups, in addition to Federally qualified HMOs, to participate in Medicare; these may be hospitals, medical group practices, PPOs, non-Federally qualified HMOs or other entities that meet certain financial solvency requirements. The CMP must be Federally approved to participate in Medicare.

complaint (of fraud or abuse) A statement, oral or written, alleging that a provider or beneficiary received a Medicare benefit of monetary value, directly or indirectly, overtly or covertly, in cash or in kind, to which he or she is not entitled under current Medicare law, regulations, or policy. Included are allegations of misrepresentation and violations of Medicare requirements applicable to persons or entities that bill for covered items and services.

complement Series of enzymes in normal blood that interacts with antigens and antibodies.

complication A medical condition that arises during treatment and in the hospital setting that is expected to increase the length of stay by at least one day for most patients.

component blood is made up of different parts or components; red blood cells, plasma, platelets and several types of white blood cells. Donated blood is often separated into components so that patients can be transfused only with the part of blood needed.

composite A tooth-colored filling made of plastic resin.

composite resin Material composed of plastic with small glass or ceramic particles that is usually cured with filtered light or chemical catalyst.

comprehensive inpatient rehabilitation facility A facility that provides comprehensive rehabilitation services under the supervision of a physician to inpatients with physical disabilities. Services include physical therapy, occupational therapy, speech pathology, social or psychological services, and orthotics and prosthetics services.

comprehensive major medical coverage A health insurance plan that combines basic health benefits with higher benefit maximums to help cover the costs of major claims. The maximum benefit may range up to $500,000 or have no limit. This coverage usually includes a deductible and coinsurance.

comprehensive MCO A MCO is a health maintenance organization, an eligible organization with a contract under 1876 or a Medicare-Choice organization. These MCOs provides comprehensive services to both commercial and/or Medicare, as well as Medicaid enrollees.

comprehensive medical insurance A policy designed to give the protection offered by both a basic and a major medical health insurance policy.

comprehensive medical review A thorough analysis of a sample of processed claims and all pertinent data (such as medical records, beneficiary payment history, etc.), for selected providers, for a specified time period.

comprehensive metabolic panel The Comprehensive Metabolic Panel (CMP) is a group of 13 specific tests. The CMP is a frequently ordered panel that gives your doctor important information about the current status of your kidneys, liver, and electrolyte and acid or base balance as well as of your blood sugar and blood proteins.

comprehensive outpatient rehabilitation facility A facility that provides comprehensive rehabilitation services under the supervision of a physician to outpatients with physical disabilities. Services include physical therapy, occupational therapy, and speech pathology services.

compression fracture A collapse of a vertebra. It may be due to trauma or due to a weakened vertebra in a patient with osteoporosis or osteogenesis imperfecta.

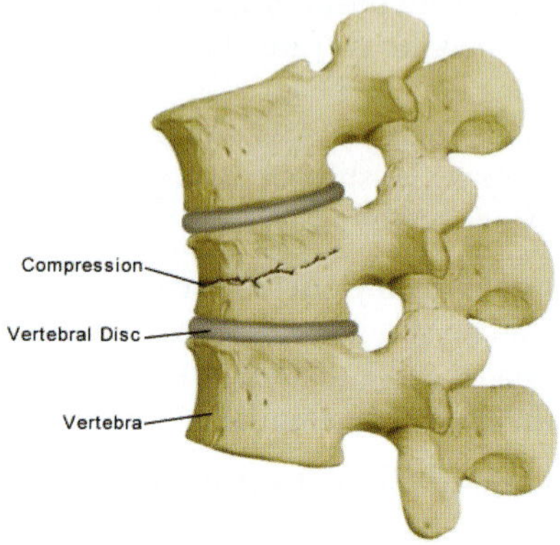

compression fracture

compulsive personality disorder A personality disorder characterized by an emotionally constricted manner that is unduly conventional, serious, formal, and stingy, by preoccupation with trivial details, rules, order, organization, schedules, and lists, by stubborn insistence on having t.

computed tomography An x-ray procedure that uses the help of a computer to produce a detailed picture of a cross section of the body. *Synonym:* CT scan, CAT scan.

computer-assisted diagnosis Application of computer programs designed to assist the physician in solving a diagnostic problem.

computer-based patient record Electronic medical record.

concomitant An event or situation that happens at the same time as or in connection with another.

concurrent When a patient is being treated by more than one provider for different care conditions at the same time.

concurrent authorization Authorization to deliver health care service that is generated at the time the service is rendered.

concurrent review Assessment of a patient's need for inpatient hospital services at admission and at specified intervals throughout the inpatient stay, using objective criteria to determine the medical necessity of acute inpatient care. Includes admission review, continued stay review, and utilization review.

concussion A trauma-induced change in mental status, with confusion and amnesia, and with or without a brief loss of consciousness.

conditional payment A payment made by Medicare for services for which another payer is responsible.

conduction disorder Interference with the normal electrical conduction in the heart.

conductive hearing loss Occurs when there is a problem conducting sound waves through the outer ear, tympanic membrane (eardrum) or middle ear (ossicles).

conductive keratoplasty A refractive surgery procedure for hyperopia and astigmatism that uses a probe to apply high frequency radio waves into the corneal tissue, causing shrinkage. This controlled shrinkage will reshape the cornea to accommodate refractive error.

condylar of or relating to or resembling a condyle.

condylar process The articular process of the ramus of the mandible.

condyle A round bump on a bone where it forms a joint with another bone.

condylectomy Surgical removal of a rounded prominence at the end of a bone (condyle).

condyloma Wart-like growth on the mucous membrane or skin of the external genitals or around the anus.

cone cells One type of specialized light sensitive cells (photoreceptors) in the retina that provides sharp central vision and color vision.

confidence interval (Home Health) an agency's rate is calculated from a sample of patients at one point in time. If we were to repeatedly pick a different sample of patients, or repeatedly collect the data at different points in time, we would likely get different rates-some higher and some lower. The confidence interval takes into account this error in measurement. It is a range of scores that has a certain probability of containing the true score.

confidentiality The property that information is not made available or disclosed to unauthorized individuals, entities or processes.

congenital Present at, and existing from, the time of birth.

congenital anomalies Abnormality of the body present at birth; a birth defect. May be inherited or caused by conditions occurring while the fetus grows in the uterus.

congenital hypothyroidism Deficiency or lack of thyroid hormone secretion during fetal development. In infants it is characterized by breathing difficulties, jaundice and hoarse crying. Infants diagnosed and treated before age 3 months usually grow and develop normally. If left untreated, child will suffer irreversible mental retardation, stunted growth and bone and muscle dystrophy. *Synonym:* cretinism.

congestive heart failure (CHF) Compli-cation of many serious diseases in which the heart loses its full pumping capacity. blood backs up into other organs, especially the lungs and liver.

conization Surgery to remove a cone-shaped piece of tissue from the cervix and cervical canal. Conization may be used to diagnose or treat a cervical condition. *Synonym:* cone biopsy.

conjunctiva The thin transparent mucous membrane that lines the inner surface of the eyelid and covers the white surface of the eye.

conjunctival Refers to the conjunctiva.

conjunctivitis Inflammation of the lining of the eyelids and the covering of the white part of the eye. Caused by infection, allergy or chemical irritation. Usually lasts 2 to 3 weeks but can become a chronic condition.

conjunctivochalasis Condition in which redundant bulbar conjunctiva billows over the eyelid margin or covers the lower punctum.

conjunctivocystorhinostomy Surgical creation of a tunnel between the conjunctival sac and the nasal cavity where the drainage of tears is possible through a hollow tube made from allogenic material implanted into the tunnel.

conjunctivodacryocystostomy Surgical creation of a conduit through the conjunctiva into the lacrimal sac to restore drainage.

conjunctivoplasty Plastic repair of the conjunctiva.

conjunctivorhinostomy A surgical procedure to construct a passageway through the conjunctiva into the nasal cavity.

connective tissue A type of tissue made up of fibers forming a framework and support structure for body tissues and organs.

connective-tissue disease Any one of many abnormal conditions characterized by diffuse immunologic and inflammatory changes in small blood vessels and connective tissue. Some collagen diseases include systemic lupus erythematosus, scleroderma, polymyositis and rheumatic fever. *Synonym:* collagen disease.

Conn's syndrome Disorder of the adrenal cortex. Usually a non-cancerous tumor that causes primary aldosteronism.

conscious sedation An alternative to general anesthesia in patients for whom general anesthesia is refused or considered inadvisable. It involves the administering of an antianxiety drug (minor tranquilizer) and an analgesic or local anesthetic.

consent and authorization A covered entity may use or disclose PHI only With the consent of the individual for treatment, payment, or health care operations; With the authorization of the individual for all other uses or disclosures; As permitted under this rule for certain public policy purposes.

consolidated medical group A large single medical practice that operates in one or a few facilities rather than in many independent offices. The single-specialty or multi-specialty practice group may be formed from previously independent practices and is often owned by a parent company or a hospital. *Synonym:* medical group practice, clinic model.

Consolidated Omnibus Budget Reconciliation Act A federal act which requires each group health plan to allow employees and certain dependents to continue their group coverage for a stated period of time following a qualifying event that causes the loss of group health coverage. Qualifying events include reduced work hours, death or divorce of a covered employee, and termination of employment.

constriction A narrowing that reduces the flow through a channel.

consultation A consultation is the process of taking a history, performing a physical examination, and ordering and interpreting appropriate diagnostic tests, for the purpose of rendering an expert opinion about a patient's illness and/or injury.

consumer self-report data Data collected through survey or focus group. Surveys may include Medicaid beneficiaries currently or previously enrolled in a MCO or PHP. The survey may be conducted by the state or a contractor to the state.

consumer survey data Data collected through a survey of those Medicaid beneficiaries who are enrolled in the program and have used the services. The survey may be conducted by the state or by the managed care entity (if the managed care entity reports the results to the state).

contact dermatitis A skin reaction resulting from exposure to allergens (allergic contact dermatitis) or irritants (irritant contact dermatitis). Phototoxic dermatitis occurs when the allergen or irritant is activated by sunlight.

contact lens Lens made of glass or plastic designed to maintain contact on the surface of the cornea. Usually used to correct refractive error.

contingency plan A plan for responding to a system emergency. The plan includes performing backups, preparing critical facilities that can be used to facilitate continuity of operations in the event of an emergency, and recovering from a disaster.

continuation of enrollment Allows MCOs to offer enrollees the option of continued enrollment in the M + C plan when enrollees leave the plan's service area to reside elsewhere. CMS has interpreted this to be on a permanent basis. M + C Organizations that choose the continuation of enrollment option must explain it in marketing materials and make it available to all enrollees in the service area. Enrollees may choose to exercise this option when they move or they may choose to disenroll.

continuing care retirement community A housing community that provides different levels of care based on what each resident needs over time. This is sometimes called life care and can range from independent living in an apartment to assisted living to full-time care in a nursing home.

Continuing Medical Education (CME) The continuing education of practicing physicians through refresher courses, medical journals and texts, educational programs and self-study courses. In some states CME is required for continued licensure.

continuous ambulatory peritoneal dialysis A type of dialysis where the patient's peritoneal membrane is used as the dialyzer. The patient dialyzes at home, using special supplies, but without the need for a machine. *See* peritoneal dialysis.

continuous cycling peritoneal dialysis A type of dialysis where the patient generally dialyzes at home and utilizes an automated peritoneal cycler for delivering dialysis exchanges.

continuous quality improvement A process, which continually monitors program performance. When a quality problem is identified, CQI develops a revised approach to that problem and monitors implementation and success of the revised approach. The process includes involvement at all stages by all organizations, which are affected by the problem and/or involved in implementing the revised approach.

continuum of care A range of clinical services provided to a patient that may reflect the treatment rendered during a single hospitalization or may include care for multiple conditions spanning the patient's lifetime.

contra Against.

contraception Intentional prevention of conception or impregnation through the use of various devices, agents, drugs, sexual practices, or surgical procedures.

contraceptive of or referring to contraception.

contraceptive agents Chemical substances that prevent or reduce the probability of conception.

contraceptive devices Devices that diminish the likelihood of or prevent conception.

contract management system An in- formation system that incorporates membership data and reimbursement arrangements, and analyzes transactions according to contract rules.

contraction The tightening and shortening of a muscle.

contraction stress test The monitoring of the response of the fetal heart rate to spontaneous or induced uterine contractions by cardiotocography, with deceleration indicating possible fetal hypoxia.

contractor policy Policy developed by CMS contractors (PSC, AC, FI, or carrier) and used to make coverage and coding determinations. It is developed when there is an absence of national coverage policy for a service or all of the uses of a service, there is a need to interpret national coverage policy, or local coding rules are needed.

contracture scar A type of scar in which a permanent tightening of skin occurs, often in response to a burn. This type of scar may affect the underlying muscles and tendons, limiting mobility and possibly damaging the nerves.

contraindication A condition which makes a particular treatment or procedure inadvisable. A contraindication may be absolute or relative.

contrast Short for contrast media. Contrast media are X-ray dyes used to provide contrast, for example, between blood vessels and other tissue.

contrast sensitivity The ability to perceive differences between an object and its background.

contributory program A method of payment for group coverage in which part of the premium is paid by the employee and part is paid by the employer or union.

contusion An injury caused by a blow to the muscle, tendon or ligament; occurs when blood pools around the injury and discolors the skin. *Synonym:* bruise.

convalescence Gradual return to health and strength after illness.

convalescent care Term often used for short-term custodial care and refers to a "recovery" period after an illness or injury when some assistance may be needed that does not require skilled care.

conventional bypass surgery Surgery performed on a stopped or arrested heart through a 10-12 incision down the middle of the chest. Patients are placed on cardiopulmonary bypass, which functions as the patient's heart and lungs during the operation.

conventions Refers to the use of certain abbreviations, punctuation, symbols, type faces, and other instructions that must be clearly understood in order to use ICD-9-CM.

convergence or divergence The turning of the eyes inward or outward so that they are both aimed toward the object being viewed.

conversion In group health insurance, the opportunity given the insured and any covered dependents to change his or her group insurance to some form of individual insurance, without medical evaluation upon termination of his or her group insurance.

conversion disorder A disorder whose predominant feature is a loss or alteration in physical functioning that suggests a physical disorder but that is actually a direct expression of a psychological conflict or need.

conversion factors The dollar amount that, when multiplied by Relative Value Scale (RVS) unit values, estimate the average cost per service. The unit values vary by medical procedure according to the relative complexity or cognitive value of the different procedures. Conversion factors can be used to measure physician fee levels and they may be by area and the period being used for experience. The term also is used for any factor which is multiplied by a standard value to adjust payments. Also see relative value scales.

conversion factor update Annual percentage change in each Medicare Fee Schedule conversion factor, established by the Congress or the default formula under Volume Performance Standards.

conversion privilege The right of an individual insured under a group plan to convert to an individual plan if the individual leaves the group.

convulsion An intense, paroxysmal, involuntary muscular contraction.

Coombs' test A test for the detection of red cell antibodies.

coordinated care Links the treatmints or services necessary to obtain an optimum level of medical care required by a patient and provided by appropriate providers. It is also another term for managed care used by federal government officials.

coordinated care plan A plan that includes a CMS-approved network of providers that are under contract or arrangement with the M + C organization to deliver the benefit package approved by CMS. Coordinated care plans include plans offered by health maintenance organizations (HMOs), provider-sponsored organizations (psos), preferred provider organizations (ppos), as well as other types of network plans.

coordination of benefits An insurance provision whereby responsibility for primary payment for medical services is allocated among carriers when a person is covered by more than one employer-sponsored health benefit program. This prevents beneficiaries from being reimbursed for more than 100% of allowable charges.

coordination of coverage *See* coordination of benefits..

coordination period A period of time when the employer group health plan pays first and Medicare pays second. If the employer group health plan doesn't pay 100% of health care bills during the coordination period, Medicare may pay the remaining costs.

copayment A type of cost-sharing which requires the insured or subscriber to pay a specified flat dollar amount, usually on a per-unit-of-service basis, with the third-party payer reimbursing some portion of the remaining charges.

COPD Chronic Obstructive Pulmonary Disease.

coproporphyria *See* porphyria.

cor- With, together.

cor pulmonale An alteration in the structure and function of the right ventricle caused by a primary disorder of the respiratory system.

cor triatriatum A congenital heart defect where the left atrium or right atrium is subdivided by a thin membrane, resulting in three atrial chambers.

cor-, core-, coro- of or pertaining to eye's pupil.

coracoacromial of or relating to the coracoid and the acromial processes.

coracoclavicular ligament A band joining the coracoid process of the scapula and the acromial extremity of the clavicle, consisting of two ligaments, the conoid and trapezoid.

coracohumeral ligament A broad ligament which strengthens the upper part of the capsule of the shoulder joint.

coracoid process A curved process arising from the upper neck of the scapula and overhanging the shoulder joint.

cordectomy 1) Surgical removal of a vocal cord. 2) Surgical removal of part of the spinal cord.

cordi- of or pertaining to the heart [uncommon as a prefix].

cordocentesis A diagnostic test that examines blood from the fetus to detect fetal abnormalities. *Synonym:* percutaneous umbilical cord blood sampling.

cordotomy A surgical procedure that disables selected pain-conducting tracts in the spinal cord, in order to achieve loss of pain and temperature perception. This procedure is commonly performed on patients experiencing severe pain due to cancer or other diseases for which there are currently no cure.

corectomy The surgical removal of part of the iris of the eye. *Synonym:* iridectomy.

coronal Refers to a section that divides the body into anterior and posterior portions.

CORF Comprehensive outpatient rehabilitation facilities.

cornea The transparent front part of the eye that covers the iris, pupil, and anterior chamber.

corneal Refers to the cornea.

corneal abrasion A scratch or similar trauma to the outer surface of the cornea.

corneal opacity A cloudy spot in the cornea, which is normally transparent. Causes include corneal scar tissue and infection.

corneal refractive therapy A temporary non-surgical process of wearing rigid gas permeable contact lenses in an attempt to reshape the cornea and reduce the need for corrective lenses. Essentially orthokeratology.

corneal topography Measurement of the anterior surface of the cornea, its curvature and shape. It is used often to diagnose keratoconus and other corneal diseases, and corneal changes after keratotomy and keratoplasty.

corneal transplant A surgical procedure in which part or all of a damaged or diseased cornea is replaced by healthy corneal tissue from a donor. *Synonym:* keratoplasty.

corneoscleral flaccidity Abnormal softness of the cornea and sclera of the eye.

corneoscleral junction The point at which the sclera's opaque, wavy fibers join the more neatly arranged and transparent corneal fibers. Called also limbus.

corneoscleral rigidity Abnormal inflexibility of the cornea and sclera of the eye.

corns and callosities Especially toughened area of skin which has become relatively thick and hard in response to repeated friction, pressure or other irritation.

cornu- Applied to processes and parts of the body describing them likened or similar to horns.

coronal plane divides the body into front and rear sections. Synonym: frontal plane.

coronary Surrounding like a crown, especially of the blood vessels surrounding the heart.

coronary artery Either of two arteries that originate in the aorta and supply blood to the muscular tissue of the heart.

coronary artery bypass graft (CABG) A surgical procedure performed to relieve angina and reduce the risk of death from coronary artery disease. Arteries or veins from elsewhere in the patient's body are grafted to the coronary arteries to bypass atherosclerotic narrowing and improve the blood supply to the coronary circulation supplying the myocardium (heart muscle).

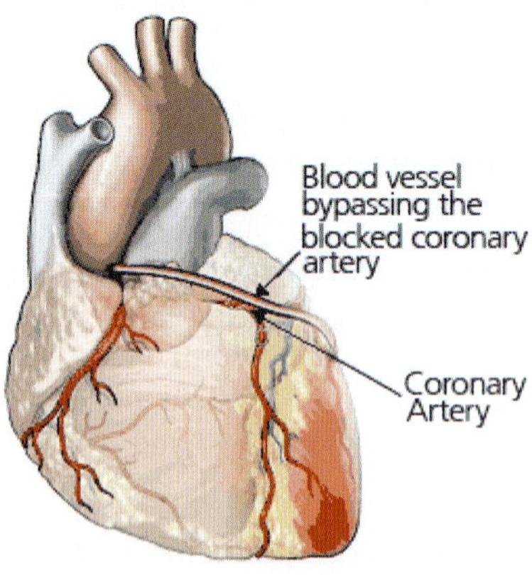

coronary artery bypass graft.

coronary artery disease (CAD) Hardening and narrowing of the coronary arteries that provide blood to the heart muscle. The blood supply is decreased due to narrowing of the arteries; heart cells do not receive adequate oxygen. This disease often results in angina pectoris or myocardial infarction. Treatment can prolong life and improve its quality. Treatment may include medication, diet change, an exercise program and sometimes surgery.

coronary artery vessels A network of vessels that deliver blood, which carries oxygen and nutrients to the heart tissue.

coronary atherosclerosis An inflammatory disease characterized by the accumulation of white blood cells, cell debris, fatty substances (cholesterol and fatty acids), calcium, and fibrous tissue (plaque or atheromas) on the walls of the coronary arteries that supply the heart muscle.

coronary endarterectomy A surgical procedure to remove the atheromatous plaque material, or blockage, in the lining of an artery constricted by the buildup of soft or hardening movements deposits. It is carried out by separating the plaque from the arterial wall.

coronary insufficiency Condition of the main arteries in the heart in which they supply an insufficient amount of oxygen to the cells of the heart. This is a serious increase in symptoms that, without intervention, may lead to myo-cardial infarction. Acute coronary insufficiency is also called unstable angina, preinfarction angina or intermediate syndrome. *See* Myocardial infarction.

coronary occlusion Hardening and narrowing of one or more of the coronary arteries that provide blood supply to the heart. Narrowing is usually caused by atherosclerosis and sometimes spasms of the artery. When this occurs, adequate oxygen can no longer be provided to the heart muscle cells.

coronary-risk profile Blood tests performed to determine coronary risk. The tests include Total Cholesterol and Triglycerides.

coronoidectomy The surgical removal of the coronoid process of the mandible.

corpectomy A surgical procedure that involves removing part of the vertebral body, usually as a way to decompress the spinal cord and nerves.

corporation A type of organizational structure that is an artificial entity, invisible, intangible, and existing only in contemplation of the law.

corpus The body of the uterus (womb).

corpus callosotomy A surgical procedure that disconnects the cerebral hemispheres, resulting in a condition called split-brain.

corpus cavernosa One of two chambers in the penis which run the length of the organ and are filled with spongy tissue. blood flows in and fills the open spaces in the spongy tissue to create an erection.

corpus uteri That part of the uterus above the isthmus and below the orifices of the uterine tubes.

Correct Coding Initiative (CCI) The national rebundling initiative that ensures comprehensive and component, and mutually exclusive procedures are not separately paid.

cortex The outer portion of an organ.

cortical of or relating to a cortex.

cortical audiometry An objective method of determining auditory acuity by recording and averaging electric potentials evoked from the cortex of the brain in response to stimulation by pure tones.

cortical bone Bone tissue which has been depleted of its minerals; e.g. calcium and phosphorous.

cortisol The body's natural stress-fighting and anti-inflammatory hormone.

cosmetic techniques Procedures for the improvement or enhancement of the appearance of the visible parts of the body.

cost-based reimbursement A method of paying hospitals for actual costs incurred by patients. Those costs must conform to explicit principles defined by third-party payers.

cost-benefit analysis A comparison of the cost of an action and the economic benefits it produces through elimination of other direct and indirect costs.

cost containment Efforts by purchasers and by providers to control health care costs through mechanisms such as benefit design, pre-admission certification, pre-admission testing, and concurrent review programs; second opinion programs; discharge planning; claims audits, case management, and employee education.

cost effectiveness Usually considered as a ratio, the cost effectiveness of a drug or proce-dure, for example, relates the cost of that drug or procedure to the health benefits resulting from it. In health terms, it is often expressed as the cost per year per life saved or as the cost per quality-adjusted life-year saved.

cost of practice index (Medicare) A measurement of the differences across geographic areas of the cost of operating a medical practice.

cost outlier An individual whose service costs are significantly higher than the average. In Medicare, it refers to a patient who is more costly to treat compared with other patients in a particular diagnosis related group. Also see day outlier.

cost reimbursement Method of provider reimbursement based on actual costs incurred.

cost report The report required from providers on an annual basis in order to make a proper determination of amounts payable under the Medicare program.

cost sharing The portion of payment for health expenses that the beneficiary must pay, including the deductibles, copayments, coinsurance, and extra bill.

cost shifting When rates are set higher than actual costs to recover unreimbursed costs from government, uninsured, underinsured and other payers.

cost shifting, employer Initiating or increasing employee financial participation in the health benefit cost through premium sharing, co-payments, co-insurance, or deductibles.

cost shifting, Medicare A provision of COBRA, shifting primary coverage for eligible claims from Medicare to employer health plans for employees and their spouses.

cost shifting, provider Charging some patients, or classes of patients, more than others for the same services in order to recover unreimbursed costs from government and other payers.

cost(o)- of or pertaining to the ribs.

cost-based health maintenance organization A type of managed care organization that will pay for all of the enrollees or members' medical care costs in return for a monthly premium, plus any applicable deductible or co-payment.

Costen's syndrome A complex of symptoms that includes loss of hearing, tinnitus, dizziness, headache, and a burning sensation of the throat, tongue, and side of the nose; its anatomical and physiological causes are uncertain but was originally believed to be the result of temporomandibular joint syndrome.

costochondral Pertaining to a rib and its cartilage.

costotransversectomy Excision of a part of a rib along with the transverse process of a vertebra.

costovertebral of or relating to the ribs and the thoracic vertebrae with which they articulate; vertebrocostal.

Cotrell-Dobousset instrumentation Posterior fixation device for spinal deformity, fracture, tumor, and degenerative conditions.

Cotte's Operation Removal of the presacral nerve.

counseling A discussion with a patient and/or family concerning one or more of the following areas diagnostic results, impressions, and/or recommended diagnostic studies; prognosis; risks and benefits of management (treatment) options; and/or instructions.

counterpulsation A technique for assisting the circulation by decreasing the afterload of the left ventricle and augmenting the diastolic pressure.

Coverage Promise by a third party to pay for all or a portion of expenses incurred for specified health care services.

coverage basis The M + C Plan charge schedule used to base the maximum dollar coverage or coinsurance level for a service category (e.g., a $500 annual coverage limit for a prescription drug benefit may be based on a

Published Retailed Price schedule, or 20% coinsurance for DME benefit may be based on a Medicare FFS fee schedule).

coverage decision A decision by a health plan or insurer whether to pay for or provide a medical service or technology for particular clinical indications.

covered benefit A health service or item that is included in a health plan, and that is partially or fully paid by the health plan.

covered charges Services or benefits for which a health plan makes either partial or full payment.

covered employee An individual who is (or was) provided coverage under a group health plan. *See* also Group Health Plan, Retiree.

covered employment All employment and self-employment creditable for Social Security purposes. Almost every kind of employment and self-employment is covered under the program.

covered entity Under HIPAA, this is a health plan, a health care clearinghouse, or a health care provider who transmits any health information in electronic form in connection with a HIPAA transaction.

covered person An individual who meets eligibility requirements and for whom premium payments are paid for specified benefits of the contractual agreement.

covered services Services for which SMI pays, as defined and limited by statute. Covered services include most physician services, care in outpatient departments of hospitals, diagnostic tests, DME, ambulance services, and other health services.

covered worker A person who has earnings creditable for Social Security purposes on the basis of services for wages in covered employment and/or on the basis of income from covered self-employment..

Cowper cyst Retention cyst of the bulbourethral glands.

cowpox and paravaccinia A mild contagious skin disease of cattle, usually affecting the udder that is caused by a virus and characterized by the eruption of a pustular rash. When the virus is transmitted to humans, as by vaccination, it can confer immunity to smallpox.

cox- of or relating to the hip, haunch, or hip-joint.

coxsackie virus Any of various Enteroviruses that are associated with a variety of illnesses including herpangina, epidemic pleurodynia, and a disease resembling poliomyelitis but without paralysis.

CPAP Continuous (constant) Positive Airway Pressure.

CPID Chronic Pelvic Inflammatory Disease.

CPK The CPK isoenzymes test measures the different forms of creatine phosphokinase (CPK) in the blood. CPK is an enzyme found mainly in the heart, brain, and skeletal muscle.

CPM Clinical performance measure.

CPPB Continuous (constant) positive-pressure breathing.

CPR 1) cardiopulmonary resuscitation 2) customary, prevailing and reasonable (charge).

CPT A system of procedure codes and descriptions published annually by the American Medical Association. This procedure coding system is accepted by virtually all commercial health insurance carriers and is required by Medicare and Medicaid.

CQI Continuous Quality Improvement.

CRA Community Rating Area.

crani(o)- Belonging or relating to the cranium.

cranial of or referring to the cranium.

cranial nerve Nerves arising from the base of the brain or the brainstem that provide sensory and motor function to the eyes, nose, ears, tongue, and face.

craniectomy Surgical removal of a portion of the cranium.

craniocervical Junction of the cranium and the cervical spine.

craniofacial Pertaining to the head (skull) and face.

craniopharyngeal Relating to the cranium and the pharynx.

craniopharyngiomas Congenital pituitary tumor appearing most often in children and adolescents. Characterized by increased pressure on the brain, vomiting, severe headaches, stunted growth, defective vision, change in behavior and infant-like genitals (in children). Development of the tumor after puberty results in cessation of menstruation in women and impotence and loss of sex drive in men.

cranioplasty Surgical repair of a defect or deformity of a skull.

craniorachischisis Congenital fissure of the skull and vertebral column.

craniosynostosis A condition in which some or all of the sutures in the skull of an infant or child close too early, causing problems with normal brain and skull growth.

craniotomy Any operation on the cranium or incision into the cranium.

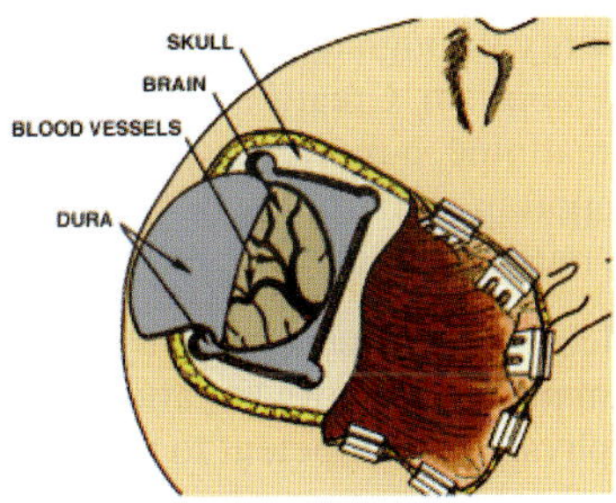

craniotomy.

cranium The upper portion of the skull, which protects the brain. The bones of the cranium include the frontal, parietal, occipital, temporal, sphenoid, ethmoid, lacrimal, and nasal bones; the concha nasalis; and the vomer.

craterization Surgical excision of part of a bone so that a crater remains.

CRBBB Complete Right Bundle Branch Block.

C-reactive protein The CRP test measures inflammation in the body. As an inflammatory marker, the CRP level is elevated in connective tissue diseases, infection, heart disease, and other inflammatory conditions.

creatine An amino acid that does not occur in proteins but is found in the muscle tissue of vertebrates both in the free form and as phosphocreatine; supplies energy for muscle contraction.

creatinine, serum Creatinine and creatinine tests measure the level of the waste product creatinine in your blood and urine. These tests tell how well your kidneys are working. The substance creatine is formed when food is changed into energy through a process called metabolism. Creatine produces Creatinine, a molecule of major importance for energy production in muscles.

credentialing The process by which a managed care organization deems a physician competent to provide medical services to plan members.

credibility A measure of the statistical predictability of a group's experience.

credible coverage Previous health coverage, such as group health plan (including COBRA continuation coverage), an HMO, an individual health insurance policy, Medicare or Medicaid, where the prior coverage was not interrupted by a significant break in coverage. The time period of this prior coverage must be applied toward any pre-existing condition exclusion imposed by a new health plan.

creditable coverage Any previous health insurance coverage that can be used to shorten the pre-existing condition waiting period. *See* HIPPA.

cremasteric reflex (males) A pin is used to stroke the inside of the thighs. In normal individuals, the testis will rise on the same side. The reflex is lost with males with damage to the corticospinal tract at or above L1-L2.

crenation A process by which red blood cells shrink or shrivel, giving a notched appearance to the cells' profiles.

crepitus Crunching sound similar to the sound made when tissue paper is crushed.

crest a narrow prominent ridge.

cretinism Deficiency of thyroid hormone secretion during fetal development or early infancy. In children over age 2, it results from chronic autoimmune thyroiditis. Characterized by breathing difficulties, jaundice and hoarse crying in infants and stunted growth and mental deficiency in children. Without treatment, irreversible mental retardation occurs.

Creutzfeldt-Jakob disease A disease (also known as Classic CJD) that creates a protein plaque on the brain and eventually leads to a rapid death. It usually occurs in patients over the age of 60.

CRF Chronic renal failure.

-crine To secrete.

crisis intervention refers to the methods used to offer immediate, short-term help to individuals who experience an event that produces emotional, mental, physical, and behavioral distress or problems. A crisis can refer to any situation in which the individual perceives a sudden loss of his or her ability to use effective problem-solving and coping skills. A number of events or circumstances can be considered a crisis life-threatening situations, such as natural disasters (such as an earthquake or tornado), sexual assault or other criminal victimization; medical illness; mental illness; thoughts of suicide or homicide; and loss or drastic changes in relationships (death of a loved one or divorce, for example).

criteria The expected levels of achievement or specifications against which performance can be assessed.

critical access hospital A small facility that gives limited outpatient and inpatient hospital services to people in rural areas.

critical care The provision of life support or organ support systems in patients who are critically ill and who usually require intensive monitoring.

critical care services Includes the care of critically ill patients in a variety of medical emergencies that requires the constant attention of the physician.

CRNA Certified Registered Nurse Anesthetist.

Crohn's disease An inflammatory disease of the intestines that may affect any part of the gastro-intestinal tract from anus to mouth, causing a wide variety of sympt-oms. Crohn's disease is an autoimmune disease, in which the body's immune system attacks the gastrointestinal tract, causing inflammation. *Synonym:* granu-lomatous colitis, regional enteritis.

Cronkite-Canada syndrome Juvenile polyposis and ectodermal lesions.

crossbite Reverse biting relationship of upper and lower teeth also known as underbite, as in Class III malocclusion (prognathic jaw).

crossmatch Refers to the testing that is performed to determine the compatibility of a donated unit of blood with its intended recipient.

cross-over patient A patient who has both Medicare and Medicaid coverage.

croup Any obstructive condition of the larynx or trachea, characterised by a hoarse, barking cough and difficult breathing. It occurs chiefly in infants and children.

crown The portion of a tooth that is covered by enamel; also coverage for a decayed or damaged tooth made of porcelain and/or metal.

crown lengthening A surgical procedure exposing more of the tooth for restorative purposes.

crows feet The fine lines found around the eyes. They are often caused by sun exposure. However, smoking also contributes to their formation.

cry(o)- Cold.

cryoablation A procedure in which tissue is frozen to destroy abnormal cells.

cryocautery Application of a substance that destroys tissue by freezing it.

cryoglobulins Abnormal blood proteins that separate from blood at low laboratory temperatures and redissolve when warmed. Cryoglobulins in blood are usually associated with immunologic disease.

cryosurgery The use of freezing as a special surgical technique to destroy or excise tissue.

cryotherapy The local or general use of low temperatures in medical therapy or the removal of heat from a body part. Its goal is to decrease cellular metabolism, increase cellular survival, decrease inflammation, decrease pain and spasm, promote vasoconstriction, and when using extreme temperatures, to destroy cells by crystallizing the cytosol.

cryptectomy Excision or obliteration of an anatomical pit or depression or a simple tubular gland crypt, especially a tonsillar crypt.

cryptococcosis A fungal infection characterized by nodular lesions, first in the lungs and spreading to the nervous system.

cryptosporidiosis A protozoa infection usually affecting the gastrointestinal tract caused by Cryptosporidium. The most common symptom is diarrhea along with cramping abdominal pain, especially in the right side. *Synonym:* crypto.

crystal arthropathies A type of arthropathy characterized by accumulation of crystals in joints.

crystal-induced arthritis Inflammation of a joint charact-erized by crystallization of fluids in a joint space.

crystalline lens The natural lens of the eye, located behind the iris, which helps bring rays of light to focus on the retina. The original state of the lens is transparent, but the lens becomes cloudy with age (cataract).

CSBO Complete small bowel obstruction.

C-section Cesarean section.

CSF Cerebrospinal fluid.

CT scan Images of structures within the body created by a computer that takes the data from multiple X-ray images and turns them into images on a screen. CT stands for computerized tomography.

CUG Cystourethrogram.

culdocentesis Refers to the extraction of fluid from the rectouterine pouch posterior to the vagina through a needle.

culdoscopy Endoscopic examination of a woman's pelvic organs by the insertion of a culdoscope through the vagina.

cure provision A provider contract clause which specifies a time period (usually 60--90 days) for a party that breaches the contract to remedy the problem and avoid termination of the contract.

curettage A scraping, usually of the interior of a cavity or tract, for removal of new growth or other abnormal tissue, or to obtain material for tissue diagnosis. It is performed with a curet (curette), a spoon-shaped instrument designed for that purpose.

Current Dental Terminology (CDT) A medical code set of dental procedures, maintained and copyrighted by the American Dental Association (ADA), and adopted by the Secretary of HHS as the standard for reporting dental services on standard transactions.

Current Procedural Terminology (CPT) A medical code set describing procedures, services and supplies published by the American Medical Association. Used to bill insurance carriers.

curvature of **spine** Abnormal curving of the spine, especially in a lateral direction. *Synonym:* scoliosis.

Cushing's syndrome Condition due to tumors of the adrenal cortex or the anterior lobe of the pituitary gland. More common in women. Symptoms include fatness of the face, neck and trunk, softening of the spine, absence of menstruation, dusky complexion with purple markings, hypertension, muscular weakness and other serious symptoms. *Synonym:* hyperadrenocorticism, hypercorticism.

cusp The protruding portion of a tooth's chewing surface.

custodial care Nonskilled, personal care, such as help with activities of daily living like bathing, dressing, eating, getting in or out of a bed or chair, moving round, and using the bathroom. It may also include care that most people do themselves, like using eye drops. In most cases, Medicare doesn't pay for custodial care.

custodial care facility A facility, which provides room, board, and other personal assistance services, generally on a long-term basis and which does not include a medical component.

customary charge The provider's standard charge for a given service. Typically calculated by health insurance carriers as the provider's median charge for the service over a prior 12 month period.

customary, prevailing and reasonable (Medicare) Current method of payment for physician services by Medicare. Payment for service is limited to the lowest of 1) the billed charge, 2) the customary charge, or 3) the prevailing charge in the community.

cutane- Skin.

cutaneous of or relating to the skin.

CV Cardiovascular.

CVA Cerebrovascular Accident.

CVP Central Venous Pressure.

CVS Chorionic Villi Sampling.

CWF Common Working File.

CXR Chest x-ray.

CY Calendar year.

cyan(o)- Denotes a blue color.

cyanosis Bluish discoloration of skin, lips and nails. Caused by lack of oxygen.

cycl- Circle, cycle.

cyclectomy Excision of a piece of the ciliary body or a portion of the ciliary border of the eyelid.

cyclodialysis Surgical opening of a passage between the anterior chamber and the suprachoroidal space in order to reduce pressure within the eye in glaucoma.

cyclophoria A strabismus in which the eye or eyes rotate inward or outward.

cyclosporiasis Cyclosporiasis is an illness caused by an infection with a microscopic one-celled parasite named Cyclospora cayetanensis.

cyclosporine An immuno-suppressant drug widely used in postallogeneic organ transplant to reduce the activity of the patient's immune system.

cyclothymia A mood disorder of at least two years' duration viewed as a mild variant of bipolar disorder. Cyclothymia is characterized by numerous periods of mild depressive symptoms not sufficient in duration or severity to meet the criteria for major depression interspersed with periods of hypomania.

cyclothymic disorder A chronic bipolar disorder consisting of short periods of mild depression and short periods of hypomania.

cyph(o)- Denotes something as bent [uncommon as a prefix].

cyst Sac or cavity filled with fluid or disease matter.

cyst(o)-, cyst(i)- of or pertaining to the urinary bladder.

cystectomy Surgical removal of a cyst.

cystic fibrosis Inherited disease in which mucus-producing glands throughout the body, especially in the pancreas and lung, fail to produce normal enzymes and mucus.

cystic tumors Tumors with cavities or sacs containing a semisolid or liquid material.

cystinuria Abnormal presence of cystine (an amino acid) in the urine. Also inherited defect in the kidney, characterized by excessive excretion of cystine and other amino acids in the urine. Can result in kidney or bladder stones.

cystitis Inflammation of the urinary bladder and ureters.

cystocele A hernia in which the urinary bladder protrudes through the wall of the vagina; sometimes occurs after childbirth.

cystogram An x-ray examination of the urinary bladder.

cystography A detailed study of the bladder, which uses a dye and X-rays.

cystolithotomy Surgical removal of a urinary calculus from the bladder through an incision in its wall.

cystometrogram A graphic recording of a cystometric measurement.

cystoplasty Surgical repair of a defect in the urinary bladder.

cystorrhaphy Suturing of a wound or defect in the urinary bladder.

cystoscopy Examination of the urinary bladder through the urethra.

cystostomy Surgical creation of an opening (stoma) for drainage of the urinary bladder. *Synonym:* vesicostomy.

cystotomy Surgical removal a calculus from the urinary bladder.

cystourethrocele Bulging of the bladder neck into the vagina.

cystourethroplasty Surgical revision of the urinary bladder and urethra, usually applied to creation of a urethral sling in the treatment of urinary.

cystourethroscope An instrument for examining the posterior urethra and bladder.

cystourethroscopy Examination with a narrow, flexible tube-like instrument passed through the urethra to examine the bladder and urinary tract for structural abnormalities or obstructions, such as tumors or stones.

cyt(o)- Cell.

-cyte Cell.

cytodiagnosis Diagnosis of the type and, when feasible, the cause of a pathologic process by means of microscopic study of cells in an exudate or other form of body fluid.

cytogenetic study A laboratory evaluation of the chromosomes of cells from the blood, bone marrow, or lymph nodes.

cytology The branch of biology that studies the structure and function of cells.

cytomegalovirus (CMV) A virus that resides in leukocytes. In certain patient populations, CMV infection can cause fever, hepatitis, pneumonia, and severe brain damage and can ultimately lead to death. In North America, 50% or more of the adult population has been exposed to the virus, making transfusion-transmitted CMV a high risk.

cytopathology The study of changes at the cellular level caused by disease.

cytoscopy Endoscopy of the urinary bladder via the urethra.

cytotoxic Having a negative effect upon cells.

cytotoxic agents Medications used to destroy cancerous cells with minimal harm to healthy cells.

cytotoxicity tests, immunologic The demonstration of the cytotoxic effect on a target cell of a lymphocyte, a mediator released by a sensitized lymphocyte, an antibody, or complement.

D

D & C Dilation and curettage.

D or W Dextrose in water.

D5W 5% dextrose in water.

Da Vinci® surgery Minimally invasive surgery using a state-of-the-art robotic platform, enabling surgeons to perform highly complex and delicate procedures through extremely small incisions and with a very high level of precision.

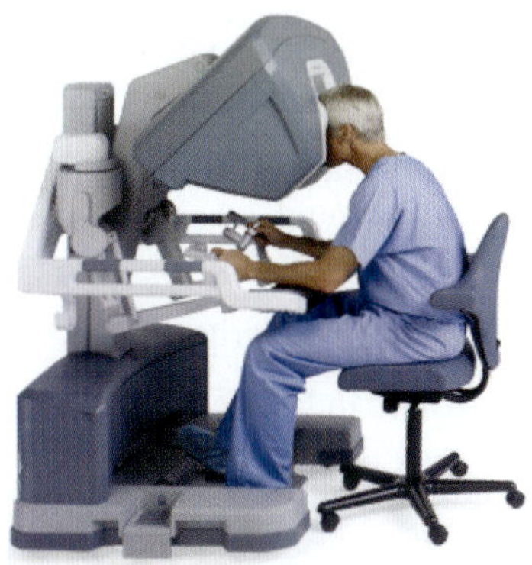

Da Vinci surgery apparatus

dacryo- Tear.

dacryoadenectomy Excision of a lacrimal gland.

dacryoadenitis A viral or bacterial infection and inflammation of the lacrimal gland.

dacryocystectomy Excision of the wall of the lacrimal sac.

dacryocystitis Inflammation of the lacrimal sac causing obstruction of the tube draining tears into the nose.

dacryocystogram A radiograph of the lacrimal apparatus obtained after injection of contrast material for the purpose of determining the presence of and localizing a site of obstruction; this procedure has been largely replaced by the CT and MRI.

dacryocystography An x ray of the tear duct after injection of a dye that is used to help locate a blockage in the duct.

dacryocystorhinostomy Surgical fistulization of the lacrimal sac for external drainage of an obstructed nasolacrimal duct.

dacryocystostomy An operation on a lacrimal sac to form a new opening.

dacryocystotomy Incision of the lacrimal sac.

dacryolith A concretion in a lacrimal sac or duct.

dactyl(o)- of or pertaining to a finger, toe.

daily benefit amount In a long-term care policy the specific amount of insurance the policy pays for each covered day of long term care as defined in the policy. The enrollee may choose from a wide range of daily benefit amounts and, under some policies, different amounts for different types of care, such as a higher daily benefit for nursing home care and a somewhat lower benefit for home care.

Dakin solution (fluid) Antiseptic of diluted sodium hypochlorite used to irrigate wounds.

dark adaptation The adjustment of the eye occurring under reduced illumination in which the sensitivity to light is greatly increased or the light threshold is greatly reduced.

dark field examination A microscopy method for diagnosing syphilis that creates a dark field around a specimen.

data [HIPAA] A sequence of symbols to which meaning may be assigned.

data authentication [HIPAA] The corroboration that data has not been altered or destroyed in an unauthorized manner. Examples of how data corroboration may be assured include the use of a check sum, double keying, a message authentication code, or digital signature.

data backup [HIPAA] A retrievable, exact copy of information.

data backup plan [HIPAA] A documented and routinely updated plan to create and maintain, for a specific period of time, retrievable exact copies of information.

data content [HIPAA] All the data elements and code sets inherent to a transaction, and not related to the format of the transaction.

data dictionary [HIPAA] A document or system that characterizes the data content of a system.

data element [HIPAA] The smallest named unit of information in a transaction.

data integrity [HIPAA] The property that data has not been altered or destroyed in an unauthorized manner.

data storage [HIPAA] The retention of health care information pertaining to an individual in an electronic format.

date of filing and date of submission The day of the mailing (as evidenced by the postmark) or hand-delivery of materials, unless otherwise defined.

date of receipt The date on the return receipt of return receipt requested mail, unless otherwise defined.

date of service The date services were actually performed.

Daviel's operation Extraction of a cataract through a corneal incision without cutting the iris.

daw Dispense as written.

day outlier In Medicare, this refers to a patient with an atypically long length of stay compared with other patients in a particular diagnosis related group. Also see cost outlier..

dc Discharge.

D-codes A subset of the HCPCS Level II medical code set with a high-order value of D that has been used to identify certain dental procedures..

DDD Degenerative Disc Disease.

DDS Doctor of Dental Surgery.

D-dimers A breakdown product of fibrin, a substance present in a blood clot. D-dimers are not generally present in the blood unless a clot has begun to form. However, the presence of D-Dimers does not guarantee that a clot is present. If D-dimers are absent, it is very unlikely that a clot has begun to form.

de- Away from, cessation.

de Andrade and Mcnab fusion Anterior approach for cervical occipital fusion.

de Quervain's syndrome An inflammation or a tendinosis of the sheath or tunnel that surrounds two tendons that control movement of the thumb.

deafness The inability to hear.

death benefit In some long-term care policies, a benefit payable to the enrollee's survivors or estate if the enrollee dies before a specified age, often 65 or 70. The benefit amount is a refund of premiums the enrollee paid minus the amount of any benefits the enrollee received while living.

debridement The removal of foreign material and devitalized or contaminated tissue from or adjacent to a traumatic or infected lesion until surrounding healthy tissue is exposed.

debulking procedure The surgical removal of part of a malignant tumor which cannot be completely excised, so as to enhance the effectiveness of radiation or chemotherapy. It is used only in specific malignancies, as generally partial removal of a tumor is not considered a worthwhile intervention.

decay Destruction of tooth structure caused by toxins produced by bacteria.

deciduous teeth Commonly called "baby teeth," the first set of permanent teeth.

decision for surgery refers to E/M services resulting in a decision to perform surgery. Reported by adding CPT modifier -57 to the main procedure code.

decision making capacity and incapacity Decision making capacity is typically defined under state law as the ability of a patient to understand and appreciate the nature and consequences of health care decisions and to make an informed choice. If a person loses this ability, he or she is said to be incapacitated; and if a court determines that a person has become incapacitated, he/she is referred to as being legally incompetent.

decompression A surgical operation for the relief of pressure in a body compartment or on a body part.

decortication Removal of part or all of the outer surface of an organ such as the lung, kidney, or brain.

decretion Termination of membership in a Medicare HMO; always the last day of the month.

decubitus ulcer A skin ulcer that comes from lying in one position too long so that the circulation in the skin is compromised by the pressure, particularly over a bony prominence such as the sacrum (sacral decubitus).

deductible Required out-of-pocket expenditure by the covered individual before the insurer pays towards the allowable charges for a covered service. Deductibles may be specified in dollar amounts or units of service.

deductible carryover A feature whereby covered charges in the last three months of the year may be carried over to be counted toward the next year's deductible.

deemed status Designation that an M + C organization has been reviewed and determined fully accredited by a CMS-approved accrediting organization for those standards within the deeming categories that the accrediting organization has the authority to deem.

deeming authority The authority granted by CMS to accrediting organizations to determine, on CMS's behalf, whether a M + C organization evaluated by the accrediting organization is in compliance with corresponding Medicare regulations.

deep reflex A sharp tap on a tendon or muscle produces a brief stretch of the muscle.

deep vein thrombosis A blood clot anywhere in the deep veins of the legs, pelvis or arms. A DVT occurs most often in the legs, and may break off and travel to other parts of the body, most commonly the lungs.

defensive medicine Use of unnecessary treatments, procedures or other medical services by doctors to minimize the threat of a malpractice lawsuit.

defibrillation A process in which an electronic device gives an electric shock to the heart.

defibrillator A device used to correct a dangerously abnormal heart rhythm, usually ventricular fibrillation, or to restart the heart by depolarizing its electrical conduction system and delivering brief measured electrical shocks to the chest wall or the heart muscle itself.

defibrination Removal of fibrin from the blood, usually by means of constant agitation while the blood is collected in a container with glass beads or chips.

Deficit Reduction Act of 1984 (DefRA) Federal law with a number of implications, including the provision that requires companies to give employee spouses over 65 the opportunity to enroll under employer group health plans.

defined contribution coverage A funding mechanism for health benefits whereby employers make a specific dollar contribution toward the cost of insurance coverage for employees, but make no promises about specific benefits to be covered.

DefRA Deficit Reduction Act.

dehiscence Release of material by splitting open of an organ or tissue.

dehydration A serious condition where your body's loss of fluid is more than your body's intake of fluid.

dehydroepiandrosterone sulfate (DHEA) DHEA is made in the human body and secreted by the adrenal gland. DHEA serves as precursor to male and female sex hormones. DHEA levels in the body begin to decrease after age 30, and are reported to be low in some people with anorexia, end-stage kidney disease, type 2 diabetes (non-insulin dependent diabetes), AIDS, adrenal insufficiency, and in the critically ill. DHEA levels may also be depleted by a number of drugs, including insulin, corticosteroids, opiates, and danazol.

delayed-action preparations Dosage forms of a drug that act over a period of time by controlled-release processes or technology.

delirium tremens Acute, sometimes fatal, psychotic reaction caused by excessive intake of alcoholic beverages over a long period of time. Usually seen after withdrawal from heavy alcohol intake. Symptoms include mental confusion, excitement, hallucinations, anxiety, tremors of the tongue and extremities, fever, sweating and stomach and chest pain. An episode of DTs is considered a medical emergency.

delirium, dementia, amnestic, cognitive disorders Cognitive disorders including delirium, dementia, and other cognitive disorders. These may be the result of substance use, trauma, or other causes.

delivery, obstetric Delivery of the fetus and placenta under the care of an obstetrician or a health worker. Obstetric deliveries may involve physical, psychological, medical, or surgical interventions.

Delmege's sign Flattening of the deltoid muscles seen as an early sign of tuberculosis.

delusional disorders Any mental disorder in which delusions play a significant role.

demand management The use of strategies designed to reduce the overall demand for and use of health care services, including any benefit offered by a plan that encourages preventive care, wellness, member self-care, and appropriate utilization of health services.

dementia A group of mental disorders involving a general loss of intellectual abilities, including memory, judgment and abstract thinking. Dementias may be associated with poor impulse control and personality changes.

demographic data Data that describe the characteristics of enrollee populations within a managed care entity. Demographic data include but are not limited to age, sex, race or ethnicity, and primary language.

demonstrations Projects and contracts that CMS has signed with various health care organizations. These contracts allow CMS to test various or specific attributes such as payment methodologies, preventive care, social care, etc., and to determine if such projects or pilot.

demyelinating disease Outer wrapping (myelin sheath) of the nerves or nerve fibers is destroyed. One example is multiple sclerosis.

denervation The resection or removal of the nerve to an organ or part. *Synonym:* sympathectomy.

dengue fever Acute febrile and sometimes hemorrhagic disease endemic to the tropics, caused by any of four species of the virus genus flavivirus, and primarily transmitted to humans from mosquitoes, though human-to-human transmission is also well documented.

denial of claim Refusal by a health insurance company to honor a request by an individual (or his or her provider) to pay for health care services obtained from a health care professional.

Denis-Browne splint A rigid or flexible appliance for fixation of displaced or movable parts.

dent- of or pertaining to teeth.

dental care The total of dental diagnostic, preventive, and restorative services provided to meet the needs of a patient.

dental debonding Techniques used for removal of bonded orthodontic appliances, restorations, or fixed dentures from teeth.

Dental Health Maintenance Organization (DHMO) An organization that provides dental services through a network of providers to its members in exchange for some form of prepayment.

dental health services Services designed to promote, maintain, or restore dental health.

dental hygienist A dental profess-ional specializing in cleaning the teeth by removing plaque, calculus and diseased gum tissue. The hygienist acts as the patients guide in establishing a proper oral hygiene program.

dental implant An artificial tooth root replacement used in prosthetic dentistry to support restorations that resemble a tooth or group of teeth.

dental occlusion The relationship between the maxillary (upper) and mandibular (lower) teeth when they approach each other, as occurs during chewing or at rest.

dental pins Small cylindrical pieces of metal used to enhance retention.

dental point of service A dental service plan that allows a member to use either a DHMO network dentist or to seek care from a dentist not in the HMO network.

dental point of service option A dental service plan that allows a member to use either a DHMO network dentist or to seek care from a dentist not in the HMO network.

dental polishing Creation of a smooth and glossy surface finish on a denture or amalgam.

dental PPO Dental preferred provider organization.

dental preferred provider organization An organization that provides dental care to its members through a network of dentists who offer discounted fees to the plan members.

dental stress analysis The description and measurement of the various factors that produce physical stress upon dental restorations, prostheses, or appliances, materials associated with them, or the natural oral structures.

dentin The part of the tooth that is under the enamel that covers the crown and the cementum which covers the root.

dentition The arrangement of natural or artificial teeth in the mouth.

dentoalveolar structures Relating to the teeth and/or any part of the surrounding alveolar bone.

dentofacial of or pertaining to the teeth and alveolar process and the face.

dentofacial anomalies A misalignment of teeth and/or incorrect relation between the teeth of the two dental arches.

denture A dental appliance that artificially replaces missing teeth.

Department of Health and Human Services (DHHS) The Federal department which regulates and administers health and human service programs in the United States. It was created in 1953 and was known as the Department of Health, Education, and Welfare until 1980 when the U.S. Department of Education was created as a separate department. The Secretary of HHS advises the President on the health, welfare, and income security plans, policies, and programs of the Federal government.

denture A removable appliance used to replace teeth. A complete denture replaces all of the upper and/or teeth.

denturism The production of dentures dispensed directly by laboratory technicians.

dependent personality disorder A personality disorder characterized by a pervasive and excessive need to be taken care of that leads to submissive and clinging behavior and fears of separation, beginning by early adulthood and present in a variety of contexts.

dependents The spouse and children of the insured as defined in the health insurance contract.

depilation The act of removing hair from the body.

depression 1) Movement in an inferior direction, the opposite of elevation. 2) a mental state characterized by a pessimistic sense of inadequacy and a despondent lack of activity.

depressive disorder An affective disorder manifested by either a dysphoric mood or loss of interest or pleasure in usual activities. The mood disturbance is prominent and relatively persistent.

dermabrasion Planing of the skin by mechanical means, as by fine sandpaper, wire brushes, or other abrasive materials. It is used to remove acne scars and dermal nevi.

dermal of or referring to the skin.

dermalogen A product derived from human donor tissue that is used in lip augmentation to produce a look of fuller lips.

dermat(o)-, derm(o)- of or pertaining to the skin.

dermatitis Inflammatory condition of the skin, characterized by redness and pain or itching. The type of skin rash or lesions that occur may suggest a particular allergy, disease or infection. The condition may be chronic or acute; treatment is specific to the cause.

dermatofibromas Fibrous, tumor like nodule of the skin most commonly found on the arms or legs. Requires no treatment. It is sometimes associated with systemic lupus erythematosus. *See* Lupus erythematosus, systemic.

dermatoglyphics The study of the patterns of ridges of the skin of the fingers, palms, toes, and soles.

dermatologic agents Drugs used to treat or prevent skin disorders or for the routine care of skin.

dermatologist A physician who specializes in the treatment and diagnosis of skin and skin-related problems.

dermatology The branch of medicine dealing with the skin and its diseases.

dermatomycosis A superficial fungal infection of the skin or its appendages.

dermatomyositis Inflammation of connective tissue, with degenerative changes in muscles and skin. This causes weakness and muscle wasting, especially in the arms and legs. Cause is unknown.

dermatophytosis A disease that can affect the scalp (tinea capitis), body (tinea corporis), nails (tinea unguium), feet (tinea pedis), groin (tinea cruris), and bearded skin (tinea harbae). *Synonym:* tinea, ringworm.

dermatoplasty The use of skin grafts in plastic repair to correct defects or replace skin destroyed by injury or disease.

dermatoses Other skin diseases, especially those not accompanied by inflammation.

dermis The deep vascular inner layer of the skin.

dermoid cyst A cystic tumor (usually benign) with a wall lined with epithelium and a cavity containing other material.

DES Diethylstilbestrol.

Descemet's layer Layer of cells in the cornea above the corneal endothelium.

descriptor The text defining a code in a code set.

desensitization The reduction of sensitivity to a drug by administering a small amount and gradually increasing the dose.

designated code set A medical code set or an administrative code set that is required to be used by the adopted implementation specification for a standard transaction.

designated facility A facility which has an agreement with a health insurance plan to render approved services (Organ transplants are the most common example.). The facility may be outside a covered person's geographic area.

-desis Binding.

destruction 1) the removal of lesions by laser surgery, electro-surgery, cryosurgery, chemo-surgery, or surgical curettement. 2) To destroy all or part of an organ.

detached retina Separation or tear of the light-sensitive tissue at the back of the eye (retina) from the eye. Symptoms include light flashes or floating spots in the field of vision, blurred vision, partial loss of vision or gradual vision loss. Often curable with prompt surgical treatment.

determination A decision made to either pay in full, pay in part, or deny a claim.

DEU Disability Evaluation Unit.

Developmental Disability (DD) A severe, chronic disability which is attributable to a mental or physical impairment or combination of mental and physical impairments; is manifested before the person attains age 22; is likely to continue indefinitely; results in substantial functional limitations in three or more of the following areas of major life activity self-care, receptive and expressive language, learning, mobility, self-direction, capacity of independent living, economic self-sufficiency; and reflects the person's needs for a combination and sequence of special, interdisciplinary, or generic care treatments of services which are lifelong or extended duration and are individually planned and coordinated.

deviated nasal septum Abnormal shift in location of the nasal septum; a common condition causing obstruction of the nasal passages and difficulty in breathing and recurrent nosebleeds.

device removal Removal of an implanted therapeutic or prosthetic device.

DEXA Dual energy X-ray absorptiometry.

dextr(o)- Right, on the right side.

DHEA Dehydroepiandrosterone sulfate.

DHEW Department of Health, Education and Welfare.

DHHS Department of Health and Human Services.

DHMO Dental health maintenance organization.

di- Apart, separation.

dia- Through, throughout, completely.

diabetes Any of various diseases characterized by an excessive discharge of urine.

diabetes insipidus Disorder of the hormone system caused by a deficiency of antidiuretic hormone (ADH) normally secreted by the pituitary gland. Usually a temporary condition. Characterized by passage of large amounts of diluted, colorless urine (up to 15 quarts a day), unquenchable thirst, dry skin and constipation.

diabetes mellitus A condition in which the pancreas no longer produces enough insulin or cells stop responding to the insulin that is produced, so that glucose in the blood cannot be absorbed into the cells of the body. Symptoms include frequent urination, lethargy, excessive thirst, and hunger.

diabetic ketoacidosis Serious complication of diabetes mellitus in which the body produces acids that cause fluid and electrolyte disorders, dehydration and sometimes coma.

diabetic retinopathy A complication of diabetes that results from damage to the blood vessels of the light-sensitive tissue at the back of the eye (retina). At first, diabetic retinopathy may cause no symptoms or only mild vision problems. Eventually, however, diabetic retinopathy can result in blindness. In the United States, diabetic retinopathy is a leading cause of blindness in adults.

diagnosis A written description of the reason(s) for the procedure, service, supply or encounter.

diagnosis code Refers to the ICD-9-CM code that describes the reason(s) for the encounter, procedure, service or diagnostic test. There are diagnoses codes for accidents, injuries, illnesses, signs, symptoms, and ill-defined conditions. There may be more than one diagnosis code per encounter.

Diagnosis-Related Group (DRG) A classification system that groups patients according to diagnosis, type of treatment, age, and other relevant criteria. Under the prospective payment system, hospitals are paid a set fee for treating patients in a single DRG category, regardless of the actual cost of care for the individual.

diagnostic equipment Refers to non-expendable items used in examination.

diagnostic errors Incorrect diagnoses after clinical exami-nation or technical diagnostic procedures.

diagnostic guidelines A practice guideline targeted at evaluating patients with particular symptoms for the presence of diseases that would benefit from intervention. They are also used to guide the screening of asymptomatic patient populations for early stages of disease.

diagnostic radiology The branch of medicine that deals with the use of radioactive substances in diagnosis and treatment of disease.

Diagnostic Related Group (DRG) A Medicare-developed health care cost schedule in which medical service providers are assigned a uniform payment for specific services.

Diagnostic Related Group (DRG) creep The illegal practice of manipulating and relabeling case mix into a higher reimbursement group.

diagnostic techniques and procedures Methods, procedures, and tests performed to diagnose disease, disordered function, or disability.

diagnostic tests blood testing utilized when a specific disease is suspected, to verify the presence and severity of that disease.

diagnostic ultrasound Use of ultrasound to obtain images for medical diagnostic purposes.

dialysate Dialysate or the dialysate fluid is the solution used in dialysis to remove excess fluids and waste products from the blood.

dialysis A process by which dissolved substances are removed from a patient's body by diffusion from one fluid compartment to another across a semi-permeable membrane. The two types of dialysis that are currently commonly in use are hemodialysis and peritoneal dialysis.

dialysis center A hospital unit that is approved to furnish the full spectrum of diagnostic, therapeutic, and rehabilitative services required for the care of the ESRD dialysis patients (including inpatient dialysis) furnished directly or under arrangement.

dialysis station A portion of the dialysis patient treatment area, which accommodates the equipment necessary to provide a hemodialysis or peritoneal dialysis treatment.

diaphoresis Profuse perspiration.

diaphragm Large, thin muscle that separates the chest cavity from the abdominal cavity.

diaphragmatic of or referring to the diaphragm.

diaphragmatic paralysis Complete loss of function of the diaphragm.

diaphysectomy The partial or complete removal of the shaft of a long bone.

diastema Space between teeth.

diastole Diastole is the portion of the heart's pumping cycle during which the muscle relaxes to let the heart fill. The portion of the cycle when the heart empties is called systole.

diastolic The period of time when the heart fills with blood after contraction.

diathermy The therapeutic generation of local heat in body tissues by high-frequency electromagnetic currents.

Dick test An intracutaneous test for determination of susceptibility to scarlet fever.

dietary services Services provided by dietitians or nutritionists to meet the nutritional needs of individuals, including consultation with other professional personnel.

dif- Apart, separation.

differential The out-of-pocket (or payroll deduction) difference that an eligible individual may be required to pay.

differential count Part of a complete blood count (CBC) the differential or diff count measures the percent of each white blood cell subtype within 100 cells.

differential diagnosis Determination of which one of two or more diseases or conditions a patient is suffering from by systematically comparing and contrasting results of diagnostic measures.

Digeorge's syndrome Congenital disorder characterized by severe immunodeficiency, birth defects and absence of the thymus and parathyroid glands. Death usually occurs by age 2, often caused by infection.

digestive system The organs that are responsible for getting food into and out of the body and for making use of it. These organs include the salivary glands, the mouth, esophagus, stomach, small intestine, liver, gallbladder, pancreas, colon, rectum, and anus.

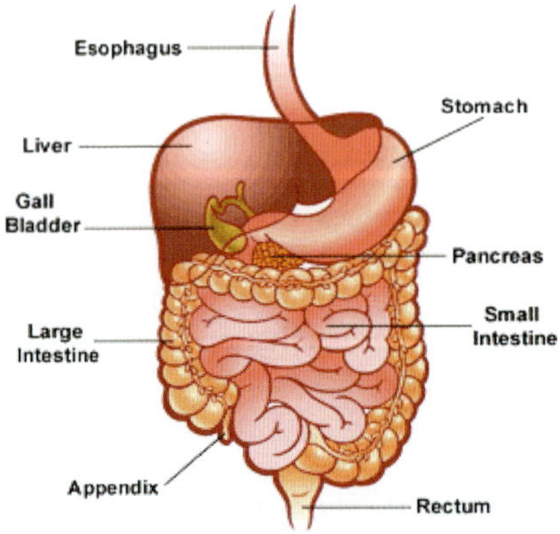

Organs of the digestive system.

digit- of or pertaining to the finger [rare as a root].

digital signature An electronic signature based upon cryptographic methods of originator authentication, computed by using a set of rules and a set of parameters such that the identity of the signer and the integrity of the data can be verified.

dilatation The process of enlargement or expansion.

dilation The act of expanding an aperture or opening.

Dilation and Curettage (D & C) A procedure used to diagnose or treat many conditions that cause abnormal bleeding from the uterus. The cervix is dilated and the contents of the uterus removed.

dilutional coagulopathy Usually seen in patients with trauma after receiving multiple red blood transfusions. The transfusions dilute the body's own platelets and coagulation factors, which may predispose to bleeding. These individuals may require platelet and plasma transfusions.

diphtheria Highly contagious infection, primarily affecting the mucous membranes of the nose, throat and larynx. May lead to difficulty breathing, airway obstruction and shock. The bacteria that causes diphtheria produces poisons that spread to the heart and central nervous system. Usually curable with prompt treatment. Delayed treatment may result in death or long-term heart disease.

diplegia Paralysis of corresponding parts on both sides of the body.

diploidy Having two full sets of chromosomes.

diplopia A condition in which a single object is perceived as two. Usually with both eyes open as in binocular diplopia, but can be with only one eye as in monocular diplopia. *Synonym:* double vision.

direct contracting Providing health services to members of a health plan by a group of providers contracting directly with an employer, thereby cutting out the middleman or third party insurance carrier. The provider is usually at full risk in this situation.

direct contract HMO An HMO that contracts with each participating physician directly.

direct cost Costs that are wholly attributable to the service in question, for example, the services of professional and paraprofess-ional personnel, equipment, and materials.

direct data entry Under HIPAA, this is the direct entry of data that is immediately transmitted into a health plan's computer.

direct fluorescent antibody Serologic test for syphilis using direct immunofluorescence.

direct pulp cap The procedure in which the exposed pulp is covered with a dressing or cement that protects the pulp and promotes healing and repair.

direct spending on health The amount directly paid for health insurance premiums by a household, as well as other out-of-pocket expenses for health care services.

directed donation Blood donated by a friend or family member for use by a designated patient.

directly observed therapy A treatment method in which patients are under direct observation when they take their medication or receive their treatment. This method is designed to reduce the risk of treatment interruption and to ensure patient compliance.

dis- Separation, taking apart.

disability For Social Security purposes, the inability to engage in substantial gainful activity by reason of any medically determinable physical or mental impairment that can be expected to result in death or to last for a continuous period of not less than 12 months. Special rules apply for workers aged 55 or older whose disability is based on blindness. The law generally requires that a person be disabled continuously for 5 months before he or she can qualify for a disabled worker cash benefit. An additional 24 months is necessary to qualify under Medicare.

disability income insurance A form of health insurance that provides periodic payments to replace income when the insured is unable to work as a result of illness, injury or disease.

disabled enrollee An individual under age 65 who has been entitled to disability benefits under Title II of the Social Security Act or the Railroad Retirement system for at least 2 years and who is enrolled in the SMI program.

disarticulation The amputation of a limb through a joint, without the cutting of bone.

disaster recovery plan Part of an overall contingency plan. The plan for a process whereby an enterprise would restore any loss of data in the event of fire, vandalism, natural disaster, or system failure.

disc (intervertebral) The tough, elastic structure that is between the bodies of spinal vertebrae. The disc consists of an outer annulus fibrosus enclosing an inner nucleus pulposus.

disc degeneration The loss of the structural and functional integrity of the disc.

discectomy The surgical removal of herniated disc material that presses on a nerve root or the spinal cord.

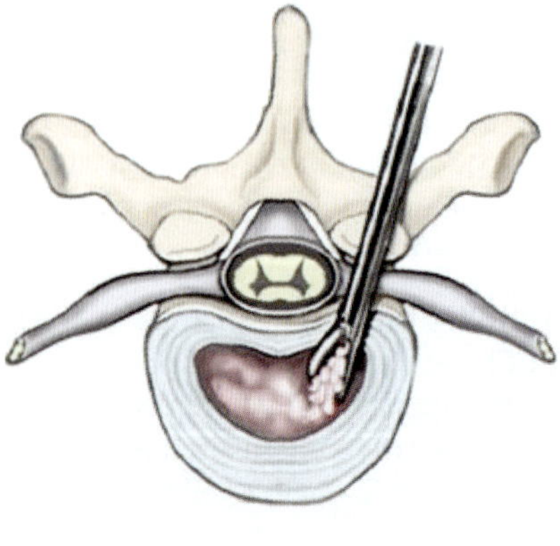

Discectomy.

discharge planning A process used to decide what a patient needs for a smooth move from one level of care to another. This is done by a social worker or other health care professional. It includes moves from a hospital to a nursing home or to home care. Discharge planning may also include the services of home health agencies to help with the patient's home care.

discharge status Refers to how the patient left the acute care facility; for example, discharge to home, transferred to a skilled nursing facility, left the hospital against medical advice, or expired.

discission An incision of the capsule of the lens of the eye.

disclosure Release or divulgence of information by an entity to persons or organizations outside of that entity.

disclosure history Under HIPAA this is a list of any entities that have received personally identifiable health care information for uses unrelated to treatment and payment.

discography A diagnostic tool for the evaluation of spinal radicular or referral pain by injection of a contrast agent into the nucleus of the disc.

discolysis The dissolving of the nucleus pulposus of a displaced intervertebral disk, usually by the direct injection of a proteolytic enzyme, especially chymopapain, into the diseased disk.

discontinued procedure Under certain circumstances, a surgical or diagnostic procedure may be terminated without completion. This is reported by adding modifier -53 to the procedure code.

discount drug list A list of certain drugs and their proper dosages. The discount drug list includes the drugs the company will discount.

discounted fee-for-service An agreed upon rate for service that is usually less than the provider's full fee. This may be a fixed amount per service, or a percentage discount. Providers generally accept such contracts because they represent a means to increase their volume or reduce their chances of losing volume. Also see preferred provider organization or exclusive provider organization.

disease Process representing a departure from normal health.

disease management A coordinated system of preventive, diagnostic, and therapeutic measures intended to provide cost-effective, quality health care for a patient population who have or are at risk for a specific chronic illness or medical condition. *Synonym:* disease state management.

Disenrollment Terminating coverage with a health plan or insurance.

disk diffusion test A test for antibiotic sensitivity in bacteria; agar plates are inoculated with a standardized suspension of a microorganism. Antibiotic-containing disks are applied to the agar surface. Following overnight incubation, the diameters of the zones of inhibition are interpreted as sensitive (susceptible), indeterminate (intermediate), or resistant.

diskography The radiographic examination of individual intervertebral disks after introduction of a radiopaque contrast medium into the center of the disk.

dislocation The displacement of bones that form a joint, often resulting from trauma.

disposal The final disposition of electronic data, and/or the hardware on which electronic data is stored.

disproportionate share Refers to providers who serve a disproportionately high percentage of low-income, uninsured, or otherwise underserved patients.

Disproportionate Share Hospital (DSH) A hospital that provides care to a high number of patients who cannot afford to pay and/or do not have insurance.

disseminated intravascular coagulation Serious disruption of blood clotting mechanisms, resulting in hemorrhaging or internal bleeding. Condition is a complication of an underlying disorder.

dissociative disorders Sudden temporary alterations in the normally integrative functions of consciousness.

distal Situated away from the center of the body.

distribution The activities and systems designed to make products or services available so that consumers can buy them.

diverticula Small, pouch-like projections in the wall of the colon. *Synonym:* diverticulum.

diverticulectomy Surgery to remove an abnormal pouch.

diverticulitis Inflammation of diverticula. During periods of inflammation, person experiences crampy pain and fever. White blood cells increase to fight off infection.

division To separate into parts.

DKA Diabetic ketoacidosis.

DLE Disseminated lupus erythematosus.

DM Diabetes Mellitus.

DMD Doctor of Dental Medicine.

DME Durable Medical Equipment.

DMEPOS Durable Medical Equipment, Prosthetics, Orthotics, and Supplies.

DMERC Durable medical equipment regional carriers. Four contracted regional carriers, which process Medicare claims for DME, orthotics, prosthetics and supplies. Providers are required to obtain supplier numbers and disclose ownership prior to submitting claims.

DMSO Dimethyl sulfoxide.

DNR Do Not Resuscitate.

Do Not Resuscitate (DNR) An advance directive that patients may make to forego cardiopulmonary resuscitation or other resuscitative efforts (see advance directive).

DO Doctor of Osteopathy.

DOB Date of Birth.

documentation 1) refers to entries in the patient's medical record that explain medical services and procedures provided and the reasons that the services were necessary. 2) written security plans, rules, procedures, and instructions concerning all components of an entity's security. (HIPAA).

DOI Date of Injury.

domiciliary, rest home or custodial care services Services provided to a new or established patient in domiciliary, rest home or custodial care facility.

Donohue's syndrome A rare genetic disorder characterized by mental and physical retardation, emaciation, endocrine disorders, hirsutism, and facial features dominated by large wide-set eyes and large low-set ears. *Synonym:* Leprechaunism.

Doppler Scan A special ultrasound test that gives information about blood flow.

dors(o)-, dors(i)- of or pertaining to the back.

dorsal Relating to the back or posterior of a structure. *Synonym:* posterior.

dorsiflexion Flexion of the entire foot superiorly, as if taking one's foot off an automobile pedal.

dosimeter A measuring instrument for measuring doses of ionizing radiation (X-rays or radioactivity).

Douglas' Abscess Abscess in the rectouterine pouch.

down coding A process used by health insurance carriers to reduce the value of billed procedures by changing the codes submitted to ones of lower value. Procedure code and procedure description mismatch, and diagnosis code not supporting the level of care are the two most common opportunities for health insurance carrier down-coding.

Down's syndrome Condition associated with a chromosome abnormality, usually trisomy of chromosome 21. *See* Trisomy. Symptoms and findings include a small, flattened skull, short, flat-bridged nose, an abnormal fold at the inner edge of the eyes, short fingers and toes, and moderate to severe mental retardation. *Synonym:* trisomy 21, (formerly) mongoloidism.

DPH Department of Public Health.

DPM Doctor of Podiatric Medicine.

DPT Diphtheria, pertussis and tetanus toxoid.

drainage The systematic withdrawal of fluids and discharges from a wound, sore, or cavity.

drawer tests Tests for the integrity of the cruciate ligaments of the knee; with the knee flexed 90 degrees, if the tibia can be drawn too far forward there is rupture of the anterior ligaments (anterior drawer t.), if too far back then the rupture is of the posterior ligaments (posterior drawer t.).

DRG Diagnosis Related Group.

DRG Coding The DRG categories used by hospitals on discharge billing.

drug administration routes The various ways of administering a drug or other chemical to a site in a patient or animal from where the chemical is absorbed into the blood and delivered to the target tissue.

drug administration schedule Time schedule for administration of a drug in order to achieve optimum effectiveness and convenience.

drug formulary A listing of prescribed drugs covered by an insurance plan or used within a hospital. A positive formulary lists eligible products while a negative one lists exclusions. Some insurers will not reimburse for prescribed drugs not listed on the formulary; others may have limited reimbursement for non-formulary drugs.

drug list A list of drugs covered by a health insurance plan. *Synonym:* formulary.

drug maintenance list A catalog of a limited number of prescription medications, as designated by a managed health care organization, commonly prescribed by health care providers for their long-term patient use. This list is usually modified on a regular basis. Also referred to as an additional drug benefit list.

drug therapy electric counter-shock An electric shock applied to the heart to terminate a disturbance of its rhythm.

drug use evaluation (DUE) An evaluation of prescribing patterns of physicians to specifically determine the appropriateness of drug therapy. There are three forms of DUE Prospective (before or at the time of prescription dispensing), concurrent (during the course of drug therapy), and retrospective (after the therapy has been completed).

drug utilization review An evaluation of prescribing patterns or targeted drug use to specifically determine the appropriateness of drug therapy.

drug-induced mental disorders A drug-induced psychological or behavioral pattern that occurs in an individual and is thought to cause distress or disability that is not expected as part of normal develoment or culture.

drusen Tiny yellow or white deposits in the retina or optic nerve head.

dry socket A localized inflammation of the tooth socket following an extraction due to infection or loss of a blood clot.

DSH Disproportionate Share Hospital.

DSM Diagnostic and Statistical Manual of Mental Disorders.

DSM-IV Diagnostic & Statistical Manual of Mental Disorders, 4th Edition.

DTAP Diphtheria and tetanus toxoid and acellular pertussis vaccine.

DTP Diphtheria toxoid-tetanus toxoid-pertussis vaccine.

dual choice A health benefit offered by an employer which permits eligible employees a choice of health plans.

dual choice provisions Provisions in the HMO Act of 1973 that required employers that offered health care coverage to more than 25 employees to offer a choice of traditional indemnity coverage or managed health care coverage under either a closed-panel HMO or an open-panel HMO.

dual diagnosis (psychiatry) The coexistence of a substance abuse disorder with a psychiatric disorder. The diagnostic principle is based on the fact that it has been found often that chemically dependent patients also have psychiatric problems of various degrees of severity.

dual eligibles Medicare beneficiaries who also receive the full range of Medicaid benefits offered in their state.

Dubois' abscess Abscess of the thymus in congenital syphilis.

Duchenne muscular dystrophy Abnormal congenital condition characterized by progressive weakness and wasting of the leg and pelvic muscles. Often involves the heart muscle. Affects only male children. Symptoms usually begin between the ages of 3 and 5.

Duchenne paralysis 1) Progressive bulbar paralysis; 2) pseudohypertrophic muscular dystrophy.

duct A bodily passage or tube lined with epithelial cells and conveying a secretion or other substance.

ductogram A special type of mammogram used for imaging the breast ducts. It can aid in diagnosing the cause of abnormal nipple discharges. *Synonym:* galactogram.

ductus arteriosus A shunt connecting the pulmonary artery to the aortic arch. It allows most of the blood from the right ventricle to bypass the fetus' fluid-filled lungs, protecting the lungs from being overworked and allowing the left ventricle to strengthen.

ductus deferens The excretory duct of the testis which joins the excretory duct of the seminal vesicle to form the ejaculatory duct.

due process clause A provider contract provision which gives providers that are terminated with cause the right to appeal the termination.

Duhamel procedure An operation used in the treatment of Hirschsprung's disease in which normally ganglionated bowel is anastomosed to the aganglionic segment by a side to side anastomosis.

Dührssen's operation Vaginal fixation of the uterus.

dumping syndrome Group of symptoms that is a complication of surgical removal of all or part of the stomach. Often experienced 1 to 6 months after surgery. It becomes a serious problem in 1 to 2% of all patients. Symptoms include weakness, faintness, decreased blood pressure, abdominal cramping, diarrhea, sweating and anxiety.

Dunn procedure Use of a contouring L-rod for posterior stabilization with myelomeningocele spinal deformity.

duodenal In or relating to the duodenum.

duodenal lesions Abnormalities in the duodenum, such as ulcers, tumors or inflammatory reactions.

duodenal ulcer Peptic ulcer located in the duodenum, which is the first segment (about 10-inches long) of the small intestine that leads from the stomach.

duodenectomy Surgical removal of the duodenum.

duodenitis Inflammation of mucous membrane lining of the duodenum.

duodeno- Duodenum - upper part of the small intestine, connects to the stomach.

duodenography X-ray examination of the duodenum and pancreas.

duodenoileostomy Anastomosis of the duodenum to the ileum.

duodenojejunostomy The surgical formation of a passage between the duodenum and the jejunum.

duodenostomy The surgical establishment of an opening into the duodenum.

duodenotomy Incision of the duodenum.

duodenum First portion of the small intestine.

duplex scan A type of vascular ultrasound study done to assess the blood flow of the arteries that supply blood from the heart through the neck to the brain.

duplex ultrasound This method combines two kinds of ultrasound. The conventional ultrasound shows the structure of blood vessels and the Doppler ultrasound shows the movement of red blood cells through the vessels. It produces images that can be color coded to show physicians where blood flow is severely blocked as well as the speed and direction of blood flow.

duplicate coverage inquiry A request to an insurance company or group plan by another insurance company or plan to determine whether other coverage exists for purposes of coordination of benefits.

duplication of benefits Overlapping or identical coverage of an insured person under two or more health plans, usually the result of contracts with different insurers.

Dupuy-Dutemps operation Blepharoplasty of the lower lid with tissue from the upper lid.

Dupuytren's contracture Flexure of the 4th and 5th fingers due to contracture of palmar fascia.

dura matter The tough fibrous membrane covering the brain and the spinal cord and lining the inner surface of the skull. It is the outermost of the three meninges that surround the brain and spinal cord.

Durable Medical Equipment (DME) Purchased or rented items such as hospital beds, iron lungs, oxygen equipment, seat lift equipment, wheelchairs, and other medically necessary equipment prescribed by a health care provider to be used in a patient's home which are covered by Medicare.

durable medical equipment regional carrier A private company that contracts with Medicare to pay bills for durable medical equipment.

durable power of **attorney** A legal document that enables you to designate another person, called the attorney-in-fact, to act on your behalf, in the event you become disabled or incapacitated.

dural of or relating to the dura mater.

duraplasty A reconstructive operation on the open dura mater that involves a primary closure or secondary closure with another soft tissue material (muscle, fascia, allograft dura).

DUS Doppler ultrasound stethoscope.

Duvries operation A surgical procedure for the correction of hallux valgus.

DVT Deep vein thrombosis.

dwarfism Underdevelopment of the body.

Dwyer instrumentation Anteriorly placed screws and band device for correction of spinal deformities.

Dwyer procedure A surgical procedure performed to change the position of the heel.

Dwyer-Hartsill procedure Pedicle screws wired to a rectangular frame along with posterolateral fusion.

dx Diagnosis.

dynam(o)- Force, energy, power.

dynamometry A test for motor impairment.

-dynia Pain.

dys- Bad, difficult.

dyschromia Any disorder of pigmentation of skin or hair.

dysentery Inflammation of the intestine, especially the colon; may be caused by chemical irritants, bacteria, viruses, parasites or protozoa. Characterized by frequent, bloody stools, abdominal pain and ineffective, painful straining to have a bowel movement (tenesmus).

dysfibrinogenemia Congenital disorder in which fibrinogen is present in the blood, but does not function normally. *See* Fibrinogen.

dysfunction Impaired or abnormal functioning.

dyshidrosis A skin condition that is characterized by small blisters on the hands or feet. It is an acute, chronic, or recurrent dermatosis of the fingers, palms, and soles, characterized by a sudden onset of many deep-seated pruritic, clear vesicles; later, scaling, fissures and lichenification occur. *Synonym:* dyshidrotic eczema.

dyslexia A learning disorder that manifests itself primarily as a difficulty with reading and spelling.

dyspepsia Symptoms of poor digeston including heartburn, nausea, bloating and gas.

dysphagia Medical terms for the symptom of difficulty in swallowing.

dysphasia A partial or complete impairment of the ability to communicate resulting from brain injury.

dysphonia Speech disorder attributable to a disorder of phonation.

dyspnea Shortness of breath. It is a common symptom of numerous medical disorders, particularly those involving the cardiovascular and respiratory systems.

dysproteinemia Derangement of the protein content of the blood.

dysthymia A mood disorder characterized by chronic mildly depressed or irritable mood often accompanied by a loss of interest or pleasure in normal activities that is present most of the time for at least two years. Many people with dysthymia experience major depressive episodes at times. *Synonym:* dysthymic disorder.

dystocia Pathologic or difficult labor, which may be caused by an obstruction or constriction of the birth passage or abnormal shape, size, position, or condition of fetus.

dystonia A neurological movement disorder in which sustained muscle contractions cause twisting and repetitive movements or abnormal postures. The disorder may be inherited or caused by other factors such as birth-related or other physical trauma, infection, poisoning or reaction to drugs, particularly neuroleptics.

dystrophy Any condition of abnormal development, often denoting the degeneration of muscles.

E

E codes Specific ICD-9-CM codes used to identify the cause of injury, poisoning and other adverse effects.

E coli Escherichia coli.

-eal Pertaining to.

Early and Periodic Screening, Diagnosis, and Treatment (EPSDT) A program which covers screening and diagnostic services to determine physical or mental defects in recipients under age 21, as well as health care and other measures to correct or ameliorate any defects and chronic conditions discovered.

early diagnosis Methods to determine in patients the nature of a disease or disorder at its early stage of progression. Generally, early diagnosis improves prognosis and treatment outcome.

early pregnancy test A do-it-yourself immunological test for pregnancy, performed as early as one day after menstruation was expected (missed period); a variety of tests exist, all based on an increase in urinary levels of human chorionic gonadotropin after fertilization.

EBS Electric Brain Stimulator.

ec- Out, away.

ECCE Extracapsular cataract extraction.

ECF Extended Care Facility.

ECG Electrocardiogram, electrocardiography.

echinococcosis A potentially fatal parasitic disease resulting from infection by tapeworm larvae of the genus echinococcus. *Synonym:* hydatid disease, hydatid cyst, unilocular hydatid disease, cystic echinococcosis.

ECHO Echoencephalogram, echoencephalography.

echocardiogram An ultrasound of the heart. Using standard ultrasound techniques, two-dimensional slices of the heart can be imaged.

echoencephalogram A diagnostic procedure which uses ultrasound to test for abnormalities in the eye. The ultrasound helps evaluate the farthest part of the eyeball when there are cataracts. The test may help diagnose retinal detachment or other disorders and evaluate orbital lesions and intraocular lesions.

echography Refers to ultrasonography; the use of ultrasound as a diagnostic aid.

echotomography Visualization of deep structures of the body by recording the reflections of echoes of pulses of ultrasonic waves directed into the tissues.

eclampsia Extremely serious disturbance in blood pressure, kidney function and the central nervous system, including seizure and coma. May occur from the 20th week of pregnancy until 7 days after delivery. Cause is unknown. *Synonym:* toxemia of pregnancy.

ECMO Extracorporeal membrane oxygenation.

economic credentialing Hospital practice of determining whether to front physicians admitting privileges based on their ability to generate revenues and/or their cost-effectiveness.

economy class syndrome The occurrence of deep vein thrombosis (DVT) in airline travelers due to cramped conditions compounded by inactivity, especially on long haul flights. The term was first coined in the late 1980's when it was observed that people who had traveled long distances by plane were at an increased risk for blood clots, especially DVT, resulting often in a pulmonary embolism.

ECP External counter-pulsation.

ECT Electroconvulsive Therapy.

ect(o)- Outer, outside.

ectasia Dilation or distention of a tubular structure.

-ectasis Expansion, dilation.

ectodermal of or referring to the outer germ layer that develops into skin and nervous tissue.

-ectomy Denotes a surgical operation or removal of a body part.

ectopic ACTH production Adrenocorticotropic hormone production (ACTH) at some site other than the pituitary gland.

ectopic pregnancy Pregnancy that develops outside the uterus. The most common site is one of the narrow tubes that connect each ovary to the uterus (Fallopian tube). Other sides include the ovary or abdominal cavity.

ectropion An outward turning or sagging of the eyelid.

eczema A skin condition characterized by itchy, irritated, inflamed skin. Eczema comes in many forms and can be triggered by a variety of factors, including allergies, environmental factors or family history.

Eddowes disease Osteogenesis imperfecta. (syndrome).

edema Accumulation of fluid under the skin (swelling), in the lungs or elsewhere.

edentulism The absence or complete loss of all natural dentition (teeth).

EDI Electronic data interchange.

EDI enrollment form A CMS agreement stating that the supplier is responsible for the Medicare claims sent by itself, its employees, or its agents. Each provider of health care services, physician, or supplier that intends to submit electronic media claims (EMC) must execute this agreement.

edit Logic within the Standard Claims Processing System (or PSC Supplemental Edit Software) that selects certain claims, evaluates or compares information on the selected claims or other accessible source, and depending on the evaluation, takes action on the claims, such as pay in full, pay in part, or suspend for manual review.

Edwards instrumentation Posterior rod and sleeve device used in destabilization of traumatic spinal conditions.

EEG Electroencephalogram, electroencephalography.

EEG brain mapping A term commonly used for several quantitative (computerized) EEG techniques. These include (a) EEG frequency analysis, (b) topographic display, (c) statistical comparisons to a normative database and (d) other similar computer-based calculations based on EEG or evoked potentials.

EENT Eye, Ear, Nose and Throat..

EERP Extended endocardial resection procedure.

effective date The date health insurance coverage begins.

effectiveness The net health benefits provided by a medical service or technology for typical patients in community practice settings.

efficacy The net health benefits provided by a medical service or technology under ideal conditions, usually in controlled, expert settings with carefully selected patients.

effusion The escape of fluid from the blood vessels or lymphatics into the tissues or a cavity.

EFM Electronic fetal monitoring.

EFT Electronic funds transfer.

eg For example.

EGD Esophagogastroduodenoscopy.

EGG Electrogastrogram.

EGHP Employer Group Health Plan.

EHIP Employee health insurance plan.

Ehlers-Danlos syndrome A group of inherited connective tissue disorders producing over elasticity and friability of the skin, excessive extensibility of the joints, and fragility of the cutaneous blood vessels, due to deficient quality or quantity of collage. *Synonym:* cutis hyperelastica.

ehrlichiosis A bacterial illness transmitted by ticks. Ehrlichiosis causes flu-like symptoms.

ejaculatory duct A canal in the male formed by union of the vas deferens and the duct from the seminal vesicle. The ejaculatory duct passes through the prostate. Semen passes through them at the time of ejaculation.

EKG Electrocardiogram.

EKY Electrokymogram.

eldercare A relatively new and growing area of health care concerned with providing medical and other services for the rapidly growing, aging population (most often persons 65 and older).

election periods Time when an eligible person may choose to join or leave the Original Medicare Plan or a Medicare + Choice plan.

elective surgery Surgery that is subject to choice (election). The choice may be made by the patient or doctor.

electric stimulation Emergency and, if delayed, would not result in death or permanent impairment of health.

electroanalgesia The reduction of pain by electrical stimulation of a peripheral nerve or the dorsal column of the spinal cord.

electrocardiogram A test used for diagnosing heart conditions by recording the small electric waves generated during heart activity.

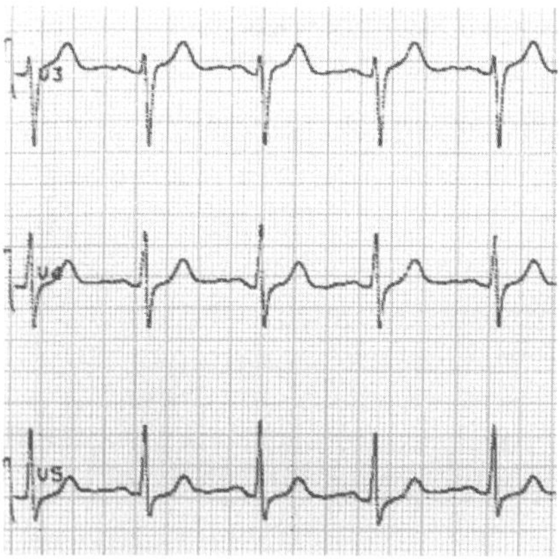

Electrocardiogram tracing.

electrocardiography Diagnostic procedure consisting of recording the activity of the heart electronically with a cardiograph (and producing a cardiogram).

electrocautery Application of a needle heated by an electric current to destroy tissue (as to remove warts).

electrocoagulation A procedure that uses an electrical current to stop bleeding.

electrocochelographic audiometry Measurement of electrical potentials from the middle ear or external auditory canal (cochlear microphonics and eighth nerve action potentials) in response to acoustic stimuli.

electrocochleography A test that measures the electrical potentials generated in the inner ear in response to stimulation by sound. Electrocochleography may be ordered to confirm the diagnosis of Meniere disease.

electroconversion The process of restoring sinus rhythm by application of electric current.

electroconvulsive therapy A treatment method usually reserved for very severe or psychotic depressions or manic states that often are not responsive to medication treatment. A low-voltage alternating electric current is sent to the brain on an anesthetized patient to induce a convulsion or seizure, which has a therapeutic effect.

electrocorticogram A record of the electrical activity of the cerebral cortex.

electrocortiogram An electroencephalogram made with the electrodes in direct contact with the brain.

electrodermal audiometry Audiometry in which the subject is conditioned by harmless electric shock to pure tones, thereafter anticipating a shock when hearing a pure tone; the anticipation results in a brief electrodermal response, which is recorded; the lowest intensity at which the response is elicited is taken to be the hearing threshold.

electrodes Mediums used between an electric conductor and the object to which the current is to be applied. In electrotherapy, electrodes are instruments with a point or surface from which to transmit electric current to the body of a patient or to another instrument.

electrodesiccation Use of an electric current to destroy cancerous tissue and control bleeding.

electroejaculation Induction of ejaculation by application of a gradually increasing electrical current delivered through a probe inserted into the rectum.

electroencephalogram (EEG) A graphical record of electrical activity of the brain; produced by an electro-encephalograph.

electroencephalography Recording of electric currents developed in the brain by means of electrodes applied to the scalp, to the surface of the brain, or placed within the substance of the brain.

electrofulguration A procedure to destroy tissue (such as a tumor) using an electric current. *Synonym:* fulguration.

electrogastrography (EGG) A noninvasive method for the measurement of gastric myoelectrical activity using abdominal surface electrodes.

clcctrogram Any rccord produced by changes in electric potential.

electrolysis A hair removal procedure in which chemicals or heat is used to destroy the hair follicle.

electrolyte panel A laboratory test frequently ordered as part of a routine physical, either by itself or as components of a basic metabolic panel or comprehensive metabolic panel. It is used to screen for an electrolyte or acid-base imbalance and to monitor the effect of treatment on a known imbalance that is affecting bodily organ function.

electrolytes Electrolytes are a large category of substances dissolved in plasma. The balance of water and salt is critical to good health. Electrolyte testing reveals important indicators of the amount of water and salt in your body, including; sodium, potassium, calcium, chloride, bicarbonate (carbon dioxide) and magnesium. These chemicals are essential in many bodily functions including fluid balance, nerve conduction, muscle contraction (including the heart), blood clotting and ph balance.

electromyogram (EMG) A graphical record of electric currents associated with muscle contractions.

electromyography A technique for evaluating and recording the activation signal of muscles. EMG is performed using an instrument called an electromyograph, to produce a record called an electromyogram. An electro-myograph dctccts thc clcctrical potential generated by muscle cells when these cells are both mechanically active and at rest.

electronarcosis Profound stupor produced by passing an electric current through the brain.

electroneuronography (ENG) A test of facial nerve integrity and function in which the compound muscle action potential resulting from transdermal supramaximal electrical stimulation of the facial nerve near the stylomastoid foramen is recorded from surface electrodes over the perioral muscles.

electronic claim A claim form which is processed and delivered from one computer to another via some form of magnetic media (magnetic tape, diskette) or via telecommunications (telephone link).

Electronic Data Interchange (EDI) The automated exchange of data and documents in a standardized format. In health care, some common uses of this technology include claims submission and payment, eligibility, and referral authorization.

Electronic Funds Transfer (EFT) Movement of funds from one bank account to another using communications networks to activate banking transactions.

electronic health care network accreditation commission An organization that tests transactions for consistency with the HIPAA requirements, and that accredits health care clearinghouses.

electronic media claims (EMC) Transmitting claims by computer rather than submitting them on paper.

electronic media questionnaire A process that large employers can use to complete their requirements for supplying IRS or SSA or CMS data match information electronically.

electronic medical record (EMR) Computerized system providing real-time data access and evaluation in medical care. Together with clinical workstations and clinical data repository technologies, the EMR provides the mechanism for longitudinal data storage and access. A motivation for health care providers to implement this technology derives from the need for medical outcome studies, more efficient care, speedier communication among providers and management of health plans. *Synonym:* computerized patient record, computerized medical record.

electronic remittance advice A provider who submits claims electronically can choose to receive their Medicare Remittances electronically. ERA allows providers to systemically maintain accounts receivable when used with appropriate accounting software.

electronic signature The attribute that is affixed to an electronic document to bind it to a particular entity. An electronic signature process secures the user authentication (proof of claimed identity, such as by biometrics – fingerprints, retinal scans, hand written signature verification—tokens or passwords) at the time the signature is generated; creates the logical manifestation of signature (including the possibility for multiple parties to sign a document and have the order of application recognized and proven) and supplies additional information such as time stamp and signature purpose specific to that user; and ensures the integrity of the signed document to enable transportability, interoperability, independent verifiability, and continuity of signature capability. Verifying a signature on a document verifies the integrity of the document and associated attributes and verifies the identity of the signer. There are several technologies available for user authentication, including passwords, cryptography, and biometrics.

electrooculography (EOG) A technique for measuring the resting potential of the retina.

electroretinography (ERG) A test that measures the electrical responses of various cell types in the retina, including the photoreceptors (rods and cones), inner retinal cells (bipolar and amacrine cells), and the ganglion cells.

electroshock The administration of a strong electric current that passes through the brain to induce convulsions and coma.

electrostimulation Refers to electrical shocks administered in nonconvulsive doses.

electrosurgery Division of tissues by a high-frequency current applied locally with a metal instrument or needle.

electrothermal of or pertaining to the production of heat by electricity.

electrothrombosis The formation of intravascular thrombosis by application of direct current to intravascularly placed electrodes.

electroversion The act of electrically terminating a cardiac dysrhythmia.

elephantiasis A disease that is characterized by the thickening of the skin and underlying tissues, especially in the legs, male genitals and female breasts.

elevation Movement in a superior direction.

eligibility Refers to the process whereby an individual is determined to be eligible for health care coverage through the Medicaid program. Eligibility is determined by the state. Eligibility data are collected and managed by the state or by its Fiscal Agent.

eligibility date The defined date a covered person becomes eligible for benefits under an existing contract.

eligibility guarantee An assurance of reimbursement to the health care provider for services/goods provided to a member who subsequently is found to be ineligible for benefits. *Synonym:* presumptive eligibility.

eligibility period Time following the eligibility date (usually 31 days) during which a member of an insured group may apply for insurance without evidence of insurability. Also, in insurance policies, a period after the onset of an illness or injury during which no benefits are paid, effectively providing for a deductible. Common in long-term care policies, although some insurers offer policies with no elimination period. Sometimes incorrectly called a waiting period.

eligible One who is qualified to receive benefits.

eligible cases (HHA) episodes of care in which the patient had the potential to improve for a specific quality measurement. Eligible cases for the improvement outcomes are those patients whose status at SOC or ROC is not optimal. Cases eligible for stabilization outcomes are those whose status at the SOC or ROC are not at the most severely impaired level for the outcome under consideration.

eligible dependent A dependent of a covered person (spouse, child, or other dependent) who meets all requirements specified in the contract to qualify for coverage and for who premium payment is made.

eligible expenses The lower of the reasonable and customary charges or the agreed upon health services fee for health services and supplies covered under a health plan.

ELISA Enzyme-Linked Immuno-Sorbent Assay.

Elliot's operation A surgical procedure in which the eyeball is trephined at the corneoscleral margin to relieve tension in glaucoma.

elliptocytosis Hereditary disorder in which red blood cells (erythrocytes) are oval in shape, instead of round, and have pale centers. Disorder may occur in a variety of anemias.

Eloesser procedure Transposition of a pedicled skin flap from the chest wall into the depths of an incision that communicates with an empyema or peripheral lung abscess. Used to prevent scar closure of the tract to insure long-term mandatory dependent drainage.

EM Evaluation and management services.

embolectomy Surgical removal of an obstructing clot or foreign material which has been transported from a distant vessel by the bloodstream. Removal of a clot at its original site is called thrombectomy.

embolism A sudden interruption in arterial blood flow to an organ or body extremity. The blockage is caused by a blood clot or foreign object. A thrombosis is the formation or presence of a thrombus (a clot of coagulated blood) in a blood vessel.

embolization A non-surgical, minimally-invasive procedure performed by an interventional radiologist and interventional neuroradiologist. It involves the selective occlusion of blood vessels by purposely introducing emboli.

embolus A blood clot that moves through the bloodstream until it lodges in a narrowed vessel and blocks circulation.

EMC Electronic Media Claim.

EMD Electromagnetic dissociation.

emergency department A hospital or primary care department that provides initial treatment to patients with a broad spectrum of illnesses and injuries, some of which may be life-threatening and requiring immediate attention.

emergency department services Services provided to new or established patients in the emergency department. The emergency department is defined as a facility for the treatment of patients with emergent conditions.

emergency medical services (EMS) Services specifically designed, staffed, and equipped for the emergency care of patients.

emergency medical technician (EMT) A person certified to provide on-site or in-transit emergency medical treatment.

emergency mode operation Access controls in place that enable an enterprise to continue to operate in the event of fire, vandalism, natural disaster, or system failure.

emergency mode operation plan Part of an overall contingency plan. The plan for a process whereby an enterprise would be able to continue to operate in the event of fire, vandalism, natural disaster, or system failure.

emergency room A portion of a hospital where emergency diagnosis and treatment of illness or injury is provided.

emergency treatment First aid or other immediate intervention for accidents or medical conditions requiring immediate care and treatment before definitive medical and surgical management can be procured.

emergi-center A health care facility whose primary purpose is the provision of immediate, short-term medical care for minor but urgent medical conditions.

emesis The reflex act of ejecting the contents of the stomach through the mouth.

-emesis Vomiting condition.

emetics Agents that cause vomiting. They may act directly on the gastrointestinal tract, bringing about emesis through local irritant effects, or indirectly, through their effects on the chemoreceptor trigger zone in the postremal area near the medulla.

EMG Electromyogram, electromyography.

EMGN Extra-membranous glomerulonephritis.

EMI Electromagnetic interference.

-emia blood condition.

Emmet's operation A surgical procedure for repair of a lacerated perineum or ruptured uterine cervix.

emollients Oleaginous substances used topically to soothe, soften or protect skin or mucous membranes. They are used also as vehicles for other dermatologic agents.

emphysema A chronic respiratory disease where there is over-inflation of the air sacs (alveoli) in the lungs, causing a decrease in lung function, and often, breathlessness.

emphysematous A pathological condition of the lungs marked by an abnormal increase in the size of the air spaces, resulting in labored breathing and an increased susceptibility to infection. It can be caused by irreversible expansion of the alveoli or by the destruction of alveolar walls.

employee For purposes of the Medicare Secondary Payer (MSP) provisions, an employee individual who works for an employer, whether on a full- or part-time basis, and receives payment for his or her work.

employee assistance programs Workplace programs designed to help identify, educate, rehabilitate, and return the physically or emotionally impaired individual to the job. These programs may include helping employees gain access to health, legal and social services and to control specific conditions (e.g., chemical dependency, gambling, hypertension, stress, etc.).

employee benefits consultant A specialist in employee benefits and insurance who is hired by a group buyer to provide advice on a health plan purchase.

Employee Retirement Income Security Act (ERISA) A Federal law that exempts self-insured health plans from state laws governing health insurance, including contribution to risk pools, prohibitions against disease discrimination, and other state health reforms.

employer contribution The amount an employer contributes toward the premium costs of the contract. Employer contributions can be based on dollar amounts, percentages, employment status, length of service, single or family status, or other variables or combinations of the above.

employer group health plan Group health plan provided by a single employer of 20 or more employees or provided by an employee organization associated with that employer.

employer mandate The requirement that all employers above a minimum size provide a standard level of health insurance benefits to their employees.

employment-based health insurance plan A group health plan that is sponsored by an employer for its employees and their dependents.

employment-model IDS An IDS that generally owns or is affiliated with a hospital and establishes or purchases physician practices and retains the physicians as employees.

empyema A collection of pus within a naturally existing anatomical cavity.

empyemectomy Extrapleural enucleation of empyema.

EMR Electronic Medical Record.

EMS Emergency Medical Services.

EMT Emergency Medical Technician.

enamel Hard tissue covering the portion of tooth above the gum line.

encephal(o)- of or pertaining to the brain.

encephalitis Acute inflammation of the brain, usually caused by a contagious viral infection. May also be caused by lead poisoning, leukemia or as a vaccine reaction. Symptoms in severe cases may include impairment of vision, speech and hearing, vomiting, headache, personality changes, seizures and coma.

encephalocele A rare type of neural tube birth that affects the brain. Encephalocele happens when the neural tube does not close completely during pregnancy. The result is an opening in the midline of the upper part of the skull, the area between the forehead and nose, or the back of the skull.

encephalography X-ray of the brain after spinal fluid has been replaced by a gas (usually oxygen); produces an encephalogram.

encephalomyelitis Inflammation of the brain and spinal cord.

encephalopathy Any diffuse disease of the brain that alters brain function or structure. Depending on the type and severity of encephalopathy, common neurological symptoms are progressive loss of memory and cognitive ability, subtle personality changes, inability to concentrate, lethargy, and progressive loss of consciousness.

encounter A face-to-face meeting between a covered person and a health care provider where services are provided or rendered.

encounter data Detailed data about individual services provided by a capitated managed care entity. The level of detail about each service reported is similar to that of a standard claim form.

encryption Transforming confidential plain text into cipher text to protect it. Also called encipherment. An encryption algorithm combines plain text with other values called keys, or ciphers, so the data becomes unintelligible. Once encrypted, data can be stored or transmitted over unsecured lines. Decrypting data reverses the encryption algorithm process and makes the plain text available for further processing.

endarterectomy A surgical procedure to remove the plaque material, or blockage, in the lining of an artery constricted by the buildup of soft or hardening movements deposits. It is carried out by separating the plaque from the arterial wall.

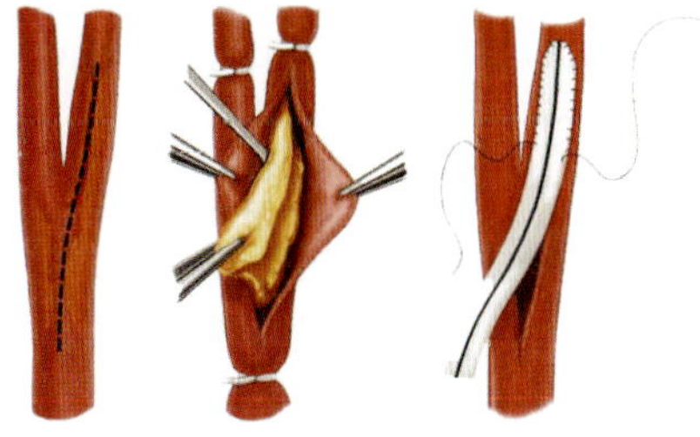

Endarterectomy.

endo- Denotes something as 'inside' or 'within'.

endobronchial Within the bronchial tubes.

endocardial of or referring to the endocardium.

endocarditis Infection of the lining of the heart chambers and heart valves that is caused by bacteria, fungi, or other infectious substances.

endocardium The membrane that lines the cavities of the heart and forms part of the heart valves.

endocervicitis Inflammation of the mucous lining of the uterine cervix.

endocervix The mucous membrane of the uterine cervical canal.

endocrine disorders Any disorder involving the endocrine system. The endocrine system is made up of organs that secrete hormones into the blood to regulate basic functions of cells and tissues. Endocrine organs are pituitary, thyroid, parathyroid, adrenal glands, pancreas, ovaries (in women) and testicles (in men).

endocrine glands Glands of the endocrine system that secrete their products, hormones, directly into the blood rather than through a duct. The main endocrine glands include the pituitary gland, pancreas, ovaries, testes, thyroid gland, and adrenal glands.

endocrine surgical procedures Surgery performed on any endocrine gland.

endocrine system A system of glands that release hormones. The endocrine system is instrumental in regulating metabolism, growth, development and puberty, and tissue function and also plays a part in determining mood.

endocrinology A branch of medicine dealing with disorder of the endocrine system and its specific secretions called hormones.

endodontics Refers to a dental specialty that deals with the tooth pulp and the tissues surrounding the root of a tooth.

endogenous Arising within or derived from the body.

endolymphatic shunt Surgical fistulization of the membranous labyrinth of the inner ear with mastoid, subarachnoid or cochlear shunt. This procedure is used in the treatment of Ménière's disease.

endometrial of or pertaining to the endometrium.

endometrioma A type of cyst formed when endometrial tissue grows in the ovaries. It affects women during the reproductive years and may cause chronic pelvic pain associated with menstruation.

endometriosis Disorder in women in which tissue resembling inner lining of the uterus (endometrium) is found at unusual locations in the lower abdomen. Tissue may be found on the outside of the ovaries, behind the uterus, low in the pelvic cavity, on the intestinal wall and rarely, at other sites far away.

endometritis Inflammation of the lining of the uterus (of the endometrium).

endometrium The cells that line the uterus. This tissue is shed monthly in response to the hormonal changes of the menstrual period.

endomyocardial Pertaining to the endocardium and the myocardium.

endosseous implant An implant into alveolar bone inserted through the prepared root canal of a tooth in order to increase effective root length.

endophthalmitis An inflammation within the eye. Inflammations may be caused by organisms such as bacteria or may be sterile as in immune disorders. Endophthalmitis usually indicates an infectious disease, but occasionally occurs as a complication of surgery.

endoprosthesis A prosthesis that is used internally.

endopyelotomy An incisional procedure to correct a stenosed ureteropelvic junction using an instrument inserted through an endoscope.

endoscope A medical device for viewing internal portions of the body. It is usually comprised of fiber optic tubes and video display instruments.

endoscopic of or relating to endoscopy.

endoscopy Procedures of applying endoscopes for disease diagnosis and treatment. Endoscopy involves passing an optical instrument along either natural body pathways such as the digestive tract, or through keyhole incisions to examine the interior parts of the body.

endothelium 1) The lining of a blood vessel. 2) The inner layer of cells on the inside surface of the cornea.

end-stage renal disease Permanent kidney failure. That stage of renal impairment that appears irreversible and permanent, and requires a regular course of dialysis or kidney transplantation to maintain life.

end-stage renal disease treatment facility A facility, other than a hospital, which provides dialysis treatment, maintenance, and/or training to patients or caregivers on an ambulatory or home-care basis.

ENG Electronystagmography.

engraftment The process by which transplanted or transfused cells (for example, after a bone marrow transplant) begin to grow and reproduce themselves within the recipient.

enophthalmos Recession of the eyeball within the orbit.

enroll To join a health plan.

enrollee The person who is the primary insured. Under an individual or family policy, this person is the applicant. Under an employer-sponsored group health policy, this person is the employee.

enrollment Purchasing health care coverage from a health plan or insurance. Individuals who purchase coverage are known as enrollees. Also refers to the total number of enrolled covered persons in a health plan. Also see open enrollment, and disenroll-ment..

ENT ear, nose and throat.

entamoeba histolytica An anaerobic parasitic protozoan, part of the genus Entamoeba. Infection can lead to amebic dysentery or amebic liver abscess. Symptoms can include dysentery, bloody diarrhea, weight loss, fatigue, and abdominal pain.

enter(o)- of or pertaining to the intestine.

enterectomy Surgical removal of a segment of the intestine.

enteritis Inflammation of the mucous membrane lining of the small intestine.

enterobiasis Or pinworm infection, is an intestinal infection caused by the parasitic roundworm called Enterobius vermicularis.

enterocele A hernial protrusion through a defect in the rectovaginal or vesicovaginal pouch.

enteroclysis A fluoroscopic X-ray of the small intestine.

enterococcus A genus of lactic acid bacteria of the phylum Firmicutes. Clinical infections caused by Enterococcus include urinary tract infections, bacteremia, bacterial endocarditis, diverticulitis, and meningitis.

enterocolitis Inflammation of the mucous membrane lining of the small and large intestine.

enterocystoplasty The most common type of augmentation cystoplasty, using a portion of intestine for the graft.

enteroenterostomy Surgical anastomosis of two parts of the intestine with creation of an opening between them.

enterolysis The surgical division or removal of intestinal adhesions.

enteropancreatostomy Surgical anastomosis of the pancreatic duct, or the divided end of the transected pancreas, with the jejunum.

enterorrhaphy Surgical suture of the intestine.

enteroscopy The use of a flexible instrument to examine the small intestine.

enterostomy A surgical operation that opens the small intestine and brings it through the abdominal wall to create a new opening (a stoma) to permit intestinal draining.

enterotomy An incision into the intestine.

enterprise liability The assumption of liability by a health care organization for all negligent injuries to patients under its care, thereby relieving individual practitioners of all personal liability for such injuries.

enterprise scheduling system An information system that permits physician groups, hospitals, and other facilities within an enterprise to function as a single organization in arranging access to facilities and resources.

enthesopathy A disease occurring at the site of attachment of muscle tendons and ligaments to bones or joint capsules.

entitlement The first date that a Medicare beneficiary can receive benefits under the Medicare program (the date of entitlement begins at age 65 for most beneficiaries).

entropion A malposition resulting in inversion of the eyelid margin.

enucleation The surgical removal of the eyeball leaving the eye muscles and remaining orbital contents intact.

enuresis Inability to control the flow of urine and involuntary urination.

Environmental Protection Agency (EPA) A Federal and State agency responsible for programs to control air, water and noise pollution, solid waste disposal and other environmental concerns.

EOB Explanation of Benefits.

EOC Episode of Care.

EOG Electro-oculogram, electro-oculography.

EOI Evidence of Insurability.

EOL End-of-life.

EOMB Explanation of Medicare Benefits.

eosinophil A type of white blood cell. Eosinophils often rise above the normal range due to allergic reactions and/or parasitic infections.

eosinophil (absolute count) The absolute eosinophil count is a measure of the total number of eosinophils present in blood based on the differential measurement of eosinophils and the total white blood cell count. The absolute eosinophil count is increased in allergic and hypersensitivity reactions and in parasitic infections.

EP test *See* erythrocyte protoporphyrin test.

EPCG Endoscopic pancreato-cholangiography.

ependymomas Tumor in the brain or spinal cord that is usually benign and slow growing.

epi- A prefix suggesting that the structure lies, grows, or points above or out from the root structure (e.g. epidermis).

epicardial of or pertaining to the epicardium.

epicondylar of or referring to the epicondyle.

epicondyle A projection on a bone above a condyle serving for the attachment of muscles and ligaments.

epicondylitis An inflammation of the inside or outside of the elbow, resulting from tiny tears in the tendons that attach the muscles of the lower arm to the elbow. It is commonly caused by repeated movement requiring a twisting arm motion, such as bowling, pitching a baseball, swinging a racket, or using a hammer. *Synonym:* tennis elbow.

epidermal Pertaining to the epidermis, the outermost layer of the skin.

epididymectomy Surgical removal of the epididymis.

epididymis A structure within the scrotum attached to the backside of the testis. The epididymis is a coiled segment of the spermatic ducts that serves to store, mature and transport spermatozoa between the testis and the vas deferens.

epididymitis Painful inflammation of the epididymis.

epididymogram Radiograph of the epididymis.

epididymoplasty Surgical repair of the epididymis.

epididymovasostomy The surgical severing of the vas deferens with anastomosis to the epididymis.

epidural 1) Regional anesthesia resulting from injection of an anesthetic into the epidural space of the spinal cord; sensation is lost in the abdominal and genital and pelvic areas; used in childbirth and gynecological surgery. 2) Situated outside the thin, tough dural membrane that surrounds the brain and spinal cord.

epidurography Radiographic visualization of the epidural space following the introduction of a radiopaque contrast medium.

epigastric of or relating to the anterior walls of the abdomen.

epiglottidectomy Surgical removal of the epiglottis.

epiglottis A flap of cartilage that covers the windpipe while swallowing.

epiglottitis Inflammation of the epiglottis. Swelling of the epiglottis can interfere with breathing and constitutes a medical emergency. The infection can cause the epiglottis to either obstruct or completely close off the windpipe.

epikeratoplasty A surgical procedure on the cornea aimed at correcting ametropia.

epilation The act of removing hair.

epilepsy Disorder of brain function. There are several forms of epilepsy, each with its own characteristics. Cause is usually unknown (75% of the time) but may be due to brain damage at birth, severe head injury, drug or alcohol abuse, brain infection or brain tumor. It is incurable, except in rare cases where brain tumor or infection is treatable. Anti-seizure drugs can prevent most seizures and allow a nearly normal life.

epilepsy, focal Small part of the body begins twitching uncontrollably. The twitching (seizure) spreads until it may involve the entire body. The person does not lose consciousness.

epilepsy, grand mal Affects all ages. Person loses consciousness, stiffens, then twitches and jerks uncontrollably and may lose bladder control. Seizure may last several minutes and is often followed by a deep sleep or mental confusion.

epilepsy, petit mal Affects children mostly. Child stops activity and stares blankly around for a minute or so and is unaware of what is happening.

epilepsy, temporal lobe Person suddenly behaves out of character or inappropriately, such as becoming suddenly violent or angry, laughing for no reason or making bizarre body movements, including odd chewing movements.

epinephrine A hormone and neurotransmitter that participates in the fight or flight response of the sympathetic nervous system. *Synonym:* adrenaline.

epiphora An overflow of tears, usually caused by insufficient drainage of the tear film from the eye. The most common cause is a blockage of the lacrimal ducts, but the condition may also result from the excessive production of tears. Epiphora is a symptom rather than a disease and may be caused by a variety of conditions.

epiphyseal Pertaining to or resembling the epiphysis.

epiphysiodesis A Pediatric surgical procedure in which the epiphyseal (growth) plate of a bone is removed. The procedure is use to lengthen or shorten abnormally short or long legs and to limit growth of a normal leg to allow a shorter leg time to match in length.

epiphysis The end of a long bone; initially separated from the main bone by a layer of cartilage that eventually ossifies so the parts become fused.

epiploectomy Surgical removal or the excision of the upper part of the omentum.

episcleral Situated on the sclera of the eye.

episcleritis Inflammation of the episclera that occurs without an infection.

episi(o)- of or pertaining to the pubic region, the loins.

episiotomy A surgical incision through the perineum made to enlarge the vagina and assist childbirth.

episode 60-day unit of payment for Home Health PPS.

episode of care The health care services given during a certain period of time, usually during a hospital stay.

episodic mood Disorders are psychological disorders that may include depression, bipolar disorder (manic-depression), major depression, dysthymia, and cyclothymia.

epispadias A congenital abnormality in males in which the urethra is on the upper surface of the penis.

epistaxis Bleeding from the nose.

epithelial of or belonging to the epithelium; epithelial layer.

epitheliopathy Refers to diseases of the epithelium.

epithelium A tissue composed of cells that line the cavities and surfaces of structures throughout the body.

EPO Exclusive Provider Organization.

eponyms Medical procedures or conditions named after a person or a place.

Epstein's anomaly Rare congenital heart defect in which an abnormal tricuspid valve prevents backward blood flow from the right ventricle to the right atrium.

Epstein's syndrome Nephrotic syndrome.

Equal Employment Opportunity Commission (EEOC) The EEOC was created by the Civil Rights Act of 1964. The purpose of the EEOC is to eliminate discrimination on the basis of race, color, religion, sex, national origin, disability or age in hiring, promoting, firing, wages, testing, training, apprenticeship, and all other terms and conditions of employment.

EQRO organization Federal law and regulations require States to use an External Quality Review Organization (EQRO) to review the care provided by capitated managed care entities. Eqros may be Peer Review Organizations (pros), another entity that meets PRO requirements, or a private accreditation body.

equilibrating operation Tenotomy of the direct antagonist of a paralyzed eye muscle.

equivalency review The process CMS employs to compare an accreditation organization's standards, processes and enforcement activities to the comparable CMS requirements, processes and enforcement activities.

ER Emergency room.

Erb-Goldflam disease Myasthenia gravis.

ERCP Endoscopic retrograde cholangiopancreatography.

ERD Evoked response detector.

ERG Electroretinogram, electroretinography.

ergometry Any method of measuring the amount of work done by an organism, usually during exertion. Ergometry also includes measures of power. Some instruments used in these determinations include the hand crank and the bicycle ergometer.

ERIA Electro radioimmunoassay.

ERO External review organization.

ERP Endoscopic retrograde pancreatography.

ERT Estrogen replacement therapy.

eruption The process of teeth protruding through the gums.

ERV Expiratory reserve volume.

erysipelas Acute febrile disease that is associated with intense often vesicular and edematous local inflammation of the skin and subcutaneous tissues and that is caused by a hemolytic streptococcus.

erythema Abnormal redness of the skin resulting from dilation of blood vessels (as in sunburn or inflammation).

erythematosquamous dermatosis A skin disease, especially one that is not accompanied by inflammation.

erythematous conditions Conditions causing diffuse or patchy redness of skin.

erythr(o)- Denotes a red color.

erythremia A chronic form of polycythemia of unknown cause, characterized by an increase in blood volume and red blood cells, bone marrow hyperplasia, redness or cyanosis of the skin, and enlargement of the spleen.

erythroblastosis fetalis Incompatibility between an infant's blood type and that of its mother. Results in destruction of the infant's red blood cells (hemolytic anemia) after birth by antibodies from mother's blood. Treatment includes an exchange transfusion. *Synonym:* Rh-incompatibility.

erythrocytapheresis An apheresis procedure where red blood cells are collected.

erythrocyte A mature blood cell that contains hemoglobin to carry oxygen to the bodily tissues; a biconcave disc that has no nucleus.

erythrocyte protoporphyrin test Determination of erythrocyte protoporphyrin levels as a screening test for lead toxicity; levels are increased in lead poisoning and iron deficiency.

erythrocytes The relatively large red cells in blood that transport oxygen from the lungs to all of the living tissue in the body. Normally, 40% to 45% of human blood volume consists of erythrocytes.

erythroleukemia A form of acute myeloid leukemia (AML) involving the cells that give rise to the erythrocytes (the red blood cells). In this type of leukemia, the body produces large numbers of abnormal, immature red blood cells.

erythromelalgia A rare disorder characterized by burning pain and warmth and redness of the extremities.

erythropoiesis The process by which red blood cells (erythrocytes) are produced.

erythropoietic porphyrias Inherited disorder in which there is an abnormal increase in the production of porphyrins (chemicals in all living things). Erythropoietic porphyria is characterized by production of large quantities of porphyrins in the blood-forming tissue of bone marrow. Symptoms include sensitivity to light, abdominal pain and neuropathy.

erythropoietin A glycoprotein secreted by the kidneys that stimulates the production of red blood cells.

escharotomy A surgical procedure used to treat full thickness (third-degree) circumferential burns. An escharotomy is used primarily to combat compartment syndrome.

escherichia coli A Gram negative bacterium that is commonly found in the lower intestine. Most E. Coli strains are harmless, but some can cause serious food poisoning.

ESG Electrospinogram.

esophageal Refers to the esophagus.

esophageal hemorrhage Bleeding of the esophagus.

esophageal rings Muscular fibers that surround the esophagus.

esophageal varices Extremely dilated sub-mucosal veins in the lower esophagus. They are most often a consequence of portal hypertension, commonly due to cirrhosis; patients with esophageal varices have a strong tendency to develop bleeding.

esophagectomy Excision of part (partial) or all (total) of the esophagus.

esophagitis Inflammation of the mucous-membrane lining of the esophagus. May be caused by infection, irritation, or most commonly, from the backflow of stomach acid.

esophagoenterostomy The surgical formation of a direct communication between the esophagus and intestine.

esophagogastromyotomy *See* esophagomyotomy.

esophagogastrostomy The surgical formation of an artificial communication between the esophagus and the stomach.

esophagojejunostomy The surgical formation of an artificial communication between the esophagus and the jejunum.

esophagomyotomy Treatment of esophageal achalasia by a longitudinal division of the lowest part of the esophageal muscle down to the submucosal layer.

esophagoplasty A plastic operation on the esophagus.

esophagorrhaphy Radiographic visualization of the esophagus using a swallowed radiopaque contrast medium.

esophagoscopy Examination of the interior of the esophagus by means of an esophagoscope.

esophagostomy Surgical formation of an external opening (stoma) into the esophagus.

esophagotomy An incision through the wall of the esophagus.

esophagus The muscular membranous tube for the passage of food from the pharynx to the stomach. *Synonym:* gullet.

esophoria A tendency of the eyes to deviate inward.

esotropia Strabismus in which one or both eyes turn inward toward the nose.

ESR Erythrocyte sedimentation rate.

ESRD End Stage Renal Disease.

ESRD eligibility requirements To qualify for Medicare under the renal provision, a person must have ESRD and either be entitled to a monthly insurance benefit under Title II of the Act (or an annuity under the Railroad Retirement Act), be fully or currently insured under Social Security (railroad work may count), or be the spouse or dependent child of a person who meets at least one of the two last requirements. There is no minimum age for eligibility under the renal disease provision.

ESRD facility A facility, which is approved to furnish at least one specific, ESRD service. These services may be performed in a renal transplantation center, a renal dialysis facility, self-dialysis unit, or special purpose renal dialysis facility.

ESRD network All Medicare approved ESRD facilities in a designated geographic area specified by CMS.

ESRD network organization The administrative governing body of the ESRD Network and liaison to the Federal Government.

ESRD patient A person with irreversible and permanent kidney failure who requires a regular course of dialysis or kidney transplantation to maintain life.

ESRD services The type of care or service furnished to an ESRD patient. Such types of care are transplantation, dialysis, outpatient dialysis, staff assisted dialysis, home dialysis, and self-dialysis and home dialysis training.

Essential Community Providers Those organizations in a community that specialize in serving low income persons or provide unique services that cannot be provided by others. MCOs are sometimes required by public payers to contract with these providers to ensure a comprehensive continuum of care.

essential hypertension Hypertension without known cause.

EST Electroshock therapy.

established patient A patient who has received any professional services from the physician or another physician of the same specialty who belongs to the same group practice within the past three years.

Estes operation Transposition of one ovary to the uterine cavity.

esthesio- Sensation.

Estlander procedure A procedure to transfer a full-thickness flap of the lip from one side of the lip to the same side of the opposite lip.

estradiol (men's panel) Often mislabeled a female hormone, Estradiol is also present in males; it represents the major estrogen in humans. Estradiol has not only a critical impact on reproductive and sexual functioning, but also affects other organs including bone structure.

estradiol (women's panel) Estradiol levels are used to help evaluate ovarian function. Estradiol is also sometimes used to monitor menopausal hormone replacement therapy. Its main use has been in the differential diagnosis of amenorrhea (for example, to determine whether the cause is menopause, pregnancy, or a medical problem).

ESWL Extracorporeal shock wave lithotripsy.

et al And others.

ethics in patient referrals act A federal act and its amendments, commonly called the Stark laws, which prohibit a physician from referring patients to laboratories, radiology services, diagnostic services, physical therapy services, home health services, pharmacies, occupational therapy services, and suppliers of durable medical equipment in which the physician has a financial interest.

ethmoid bone Bone in the skull that separates the nasal cavity from the brain.

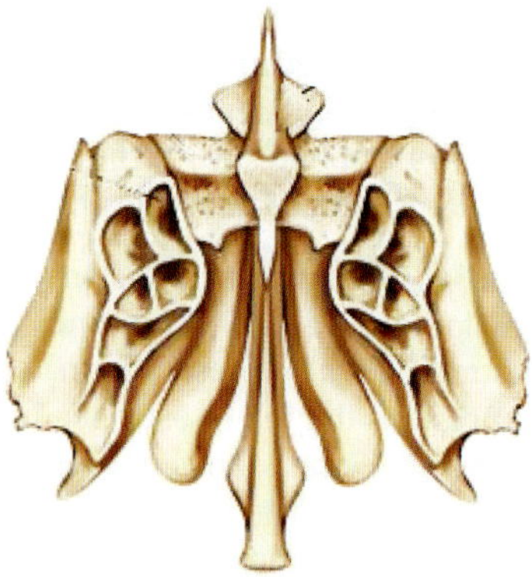

ethmoid bone

ethmoidectomy Surgical removal of the ethmoid bone.

etiology The cause(s) or origin of a disease.

eu- Good, well.

eunuchoidism Deficiency of male hormone, which results in abnormal tallness, small testes and deficient development of secondary sex characteristics, sex drive and potency.

eustachian tube A tube that links the pharynx to the middle ear.

eutelegenesis Artificial insemination by semen from a donor selected because of certain desirable characteristics.

evaluation and management services Nontechnical services provided by most physicians for the purpose of diagnosing and treating diseases and counseling and evaluating patients.

eventration Anatomical or functional deficiency of part of the diaphragm, allowing abdominal contents to herniate into the chest.

Evercare Medicare managed care demonstration for nursing home residents. A geriatric Nurse Practitioner acts as a case manager.

eversion The movement of the sole of the foot away from the median plane.

evidence Signs that something is true or not true. Physicians can use published studies as evidence that a treatment works or does not work.

evidence of **funding** Proof that sufficient funds are available for completion of the project. Usually a copy of the face sheet of the grant, contract, or cooperative agreement is sufficient.

evidence of **insurability** Proof of physical condition. This may be provided through physician records or by the results of an examination.

evisceration The act of removing the bowels or viscera.

evocative or suppression testing Evocative or suppression testing involves administration of agents to determine a patient's response to those agents.

EVR Evoked visual response.

Ewart's procedure Elevation of the larynx between the thumb and forefinger to elicit tracheal tugging.

Ewing sarcoma Malignant bone tumor usually found in children.

ex- Out of, away from.

exacerbation Action that makes a problem or a disease (or its symptoms) worse.

exam Examination, examiner.

examination the process by which a physician investigates the body of a patient for signs of disease. It generally follows the taking of the medical history. Together with the medical history, the physical examination aids in determining the correct diagnosis and devising the treatment plan. This data then becomes part of the medical record.

exanthema Eruption on the skin occurring as a symptom of a disease.

excess charges For patients in the original Medicare Plan, this is the difference between a physician's or other health care provider's actual charge (which may be limited by Medicare or the state) and the Medicare-approved payment amount.

exchange transfusion Introduction of whole blood in exchange for 75 to 85% of an infant's circulating blood. blood is repeatedly with-drawn in small amounts and replaced with equal amounts of donor blood. This procedure is performed in infants to treat erythroblastosis fetalis. *See* Erythroblastosis fetalis.

excision The complete removal of an organ, tissue, or tumor.

exclusion period A period of time when an insurance company can delay coverage of a pre-existing condition. Sometimes this is called a pre-existing condition waiting period.

exclusions Specific services or conditions which the policy will not cover or which are covered at a limited rate.

exclusions (Medicare) Items or services that Medicare does not cover, such as most prescription drugs, long-term care, and custodial care in a nursing or private home.

exclusions and limitations Medical services that are either not covered or limited in benefit by a health insurance policy.

Exclusive Provider Organization (EPO) A provider network similar to a PPO wherein a patient must pay the entire cost of any care obtained outside the EPO network of providers. EPO providers typically are paid for services rendered instead of by capitation.

exclusive remedy doctrine A rule which states that employees who are injured on the job are entitled to workers' compensation benefits, but they cannot sue their employers for additional amounts.

exclusivity clause A part of a contract which prohibits a health care provider from contracting with more than one managed care organization.

exenteration Surgical removal of the organs within a body cavity.

exercise tests Any of various stress tests in which exercise is used in the electrocardiographic assessment of cardiovascular health and function, particularly in the diagnosis of myocardial ischemia. The most widely used forms are the treadmill and bicycle ergometer exercise tests; they are usually graded, consisting of a series of incrementally increasing workloads sustained for defined intervals.

exfoliation To remove the top layer of skin. Chemical peels and dermabrasion are examples of methods in which the skin is exfoliated.

exo- Denotes something as 'outside' another.

exogenous Originating outside of the body.

exophoria The position of the eyes in an over diverged position compensated by the external eye muscles so that the eyes do not appear turned outward.

exophthalmos Protrusion of the eyeball from the socket.

exostectomy Removal of the medial prominence, a lateral release and sometimes other soft tissue releases and medial capsular reinforcements are done.

exostosis The formation of new bone on the surface of a bone. Exostosis can cause chronic pain ranging from mild to debilitating, depending on where they are located and what shape they are.

exotropia A condition in which only one eye fixes on an object while the other turns outward.

expenditure In the context of health care, monies spent on the acquisition of health care coverage and/or services.

expenditure limits Includes various mechanisms which limit the amounts that may be spent to acquire health care coverage and services (e.g., negotiated fee schedules, hospital global operating budgets).

expenditure targets Voluntary or involuntary limits on health care spending. This may refer to spending for specific types of service (e.g., physician care), multiple types of service (e.g., hospital, physician, drugs), or all health care services.

experience rating A system used by insurers to set premium levels based on the insured's past loss history. For example, rating may be based on service utilization for health insurance or on liability experience for professional liability insurance.

explanation of benefits (EOB) Statement sent by health plans to persons who have experienced a claim under the health plan. The explanation of benefits (EOB) details the charges for the services received, the amount the health insurance company will pay for those services, and the amount the insured person will be responsible for paying.

exploration An active examination, usually involving endoscopy or a surgical procedure, to determine conditions present as an aid in diagnosis.

exploratory laparotomy A method of abdominal exploration via a large incision made into the abdomen.

exploratory operation Incision into a body area to determine the cause of unexplained symptoms.

exstrophy Congenital condition in which part of an internal organ is present outside the body (eg bladder, intestine).

Extended Care Facility (ECF) A nursing home-type setting that offers skilled, intermediate, or custodial care.

extended care services Refers to skilled nursing facility services.

extension The opposite of flexion; a straightening movement that increases the angle between body parts. In a conventional handshake, the fingers are fully extended. When standing up, the knees are extended. Extension of the hip or shoulder moves the limb backward (towards the posterior side of the body).

extension of benefits A provision of many policies which allows medical coverage to be continued past the termination date of the policy for employees not actively at work and for dependents hospitalized on that date. Such extended coverage usually applies only to the specific medical condition that has caused the disability and continues only until the employee returns to work or the dependent leave the hospital.

external ocular muscles The six muscles that turn the eyes to position them for viewing.

External Quality Review Organization (EQRO) The organization with which the state contracts to evaluate the care provided to Medicaid managed eligibles. Typically the EQRO is a peer review organization. It may conduct focused medical record reviews (for example, reviews targeted at a particular clinical condition) or broader analyses on quality. While most EQRO contractors rely on medical records as the primary source of information, they may also use eligibility data and claims or encounter data to conduct specific analyses.

external rotation A motion of the shoulder or hip that points the toes or the flexed forearm outwards (away from the midline). *Synonym:* lateral rotation.

extirpation To destroy or remove completely.

extra- Outside.

extracapsular Situated outside of a capsule, esp. Outside the capsular ligament of a joint.

extracapsular cataract extraction A surgical procedure that removes the cataractous lens of the eye but leaves the posterior lens capsule intact.

extracavitary Outside of a cavity.

extracoronal The outside of the crown of the tooth.

extracorporeal blood circulation occurring outside of the body, for example, in an apheresis machine during donation.

extracorporeal membrane oxygenation An extracorporeal technique of providing both cardiac and respiratory support oxygen to patients whose heart and lungs are so severely diseased or damaged that they can no longer serve their function.

extracranial Outside the cranium.

extraction The removal of a tooth from the mouth. Extractions are performed for a wide variety of reasons, including tooth decay that has destroyed enough tooth structure to prevent restoration.

extradural On or outside the dura mater.

extranasal On or outside the nose.

extranet A private computer network that incorporates Web-based technologies and links selected resources of an MCO to external entities or individuals.

extranodal Refers to an area or organ outside of the lymph nodes.

extraocular Situated outside the eye.

extraoral Pertaining to the outside of the mouth.

extrapelvic On or outside the pelvis.

extraperitoneal Located or taking place outside the peritoneal cavity.

extrapleural Situated or occurring outside the pleural cavity.

extrapulmonary Outside of or unrelated to the lungs.

extrapyramidal disease A general term for a number of disorders caused by abnormalities of the basal ganglia or certain brain stem or thalamic nuclei; characterised by motor deficits, loss of postural reflexes, bradykinesia, tremor, rigidity, and various involuntary movements.

extrascleral Situated or occurring outside the sclera of the orbit.

extraspinal Outside or not part of the spine or spinal cord.

extratemporal Outside or not part of the temporal lobe.

extrauterine pregnancy A pregnancy that is not in the usual place and is located outside the inner lining of the uterus. A fertilized egg settles and grows in any location other than the inner lining of the uterus.

extravaginal Located outside the vagina.

extravasation Refers to the leakage of a fluid out of its container. In the case of inflammation, it refers to the movement of white blood cells from the capillaries to the tissues surrounding them. In the case of malignant cancer metastasis it refers to cancer cells exiting the capillaries and entering organs.

extremity Refers to the arms or legs.

extrinsic allergic alveolitis Inflammation of the alveoli in the lungs caused by inhaling dust.

exudate Matter that penetrates through vessel walls into adjoining tissue. Production of pus or serum. Accumulation of fluid in a cavity.

eye movements Voluntary or reflex-controlled movements of the eye.

eyeteeth The four upper and lower canine (cuspid) teeth.

F

Faber's syndrome Hypochromic anemia.

Fabere's sign The hip is rotated internally and externally then placed in an external position with the foot resting on the opposite knee. Pain denotes hip disease rather than lumbar disc pathology.

face lift A surgical procedure to improve visible signs of aging in the face and neck.

facing Tooth colored overlay on the visible portion of a crown that is made of acrylic, composite or porcelain.

facet A posterior structure of a vertebra which articulates with a facet of an adjacent vertebra to form a facet joint that allows motion in the spinal column. Each vertebra has two superior and two inferior facets.

facetectomy Excision of a facet, a surgical procedure which involves decompression of a spinal nerve root.

face-to-face time Refers to time that a physician spends face-to-face with the patient and/or family. This includes time involved in history taking, examination and counseling.

faci(o)- of or pertaining to the face.

facial nerve disorders A disorder resulting from a weakness of the facial nerve. Bell's palsy example of a facial nerve disorder.

facility charge Some plans may vary cost shares for services based on place of treatment; in effect, charging a cost for the facility in which the service is received.

facility security plan A plan to safeguard the premises and building(s) (exterior and interior) from unauthorized physical access, and to safeguard the equipment therein from unauthorized physical access, tampering, and theft.

factitious disorders Disorders characterized by physical or psychological symptoms that are not real, genuine, or natural.

Factor I Fibrinogen needed for blood to clot.

Factor II Prothrombin needed for blood to clot.

Factor III Tissue thromboplastin needed for blood to clot.

Factor IV Calcium needed for blood to clot.

Factor IX Plasma thromboplastin component needed for blood to clot.

Factor V Proaccelerin needed for blood to clot.

Factor V deficiency An inherited bleeding disorder in which the clotting factor V (five) is low. The disorder is very rare, occurring in only 1 in 1,000,000 people.

Factor V Leiden An inherited blood clotting disorder that is found in 5% of Caucasian Americans and 1.2% of African-Americans. One can be heterozygous (have one abnormal gene), homozygous (have two abnormal genes) or normal (not have any abnormal genes).

Factor VI Accelerin needed for blood to clot.

Factor VII Proconvertin needed for blood to clot.

Factor VII deficiency Deficiency of normal clotting factor. Can be inherited or acquired. This deficiency commonly causes nosebleeds, easy bruising and bleeding gums.

Factor VIII Anti-hemophilic factor needed for blood to clot.

Factor VIII rich cryoprecipitate Contains extra clotting factor used to control bleeding in hemophiliacs.

Factor X Stuart factor (auto-prothrombin C) needed for blood to clot.

Factor XI Plasma thromboplastin antecedent needed for blood to clot.

Factor XII Hageman factor needed for blood to clot.

Factor XIII A clotting factor that stabilizes blood clots.

fallopian tube Tubes that transport the egg from the ovary to the uterus.

false negative (blood test) A blood test result that is incorrectly normal in a person who has the suspected disease.

false negatives Occur when the medical record contains evidence of a service that does not exist in the encounter data. This is the most common problem in partially or fully capitated plans because the provider does not need to submit an encounter in order to receive payment for the service, and therefore may have a weaker incentive to conform to data collection standards.

false positive (blood test) A blood test result that is incorrectly abnormal in a person who does not have the suspected disease.

false positives Occurs when the encounter data contain evidence of a service that is not documented in the patient's medical record. If we assume that the medical record contains complete information on the patients medical history, a false positive may be considered a fraudulent service. In a fully capitated environment, however, the provider would receive no additional reimbursement for the submission of a false positive encounter.

familial hypoproteinemia Inherited abnormal decrease in the amount of protein in the blood.

familial myoglobinuria Inherited condition in which myoglobin appears in urine. Causes include vigorous, prolonged exercise and severe injuries, such as a broken bone. *See* myoglobin.

familial xanthurenic aciduria Inherited deficiency disorder of xanthine oxidase that causes physical and mental retardation.

family of codes Refers to CPT codes followed by one or more indented CPT codes. The first CPT code descriptor includes a semi-colon. The portion of the descriptor of the first code in the family preceding the semicolon is a common part of the descriptor for each subsequent code of the family.

Family Medical Leave Act (FMLA) 1993 Federal law requiring that employers of 50 or more (and public employers of any size) allow employees to take leave to care for ill family members and to return to substantially similar employment conditions following the leave.

Fanconi's syndrome Rare, usually congenital disorder characterized by aplastic anemia, bone abnormalities, olive-brown skin pigmentation, abnormally small head, small gonads and kidney-function abnormalities. Adults can get a form of the syndrome as a result of heavy-metal poisoning. It also may occur after a kidney transplant.

faq Frequently asked question.

Farr test A radioimmunoassay for DNA antibodies in the context of autoimmune disease.

Fasanella-Servat procedure A surgical procedure used for the repair of mild to moderate ptosis.

fascia Strong connective tissue which performs a number of functions, including enveloping and isolating the muscles of the body, providing structural support and protection.

fascial of or referring to fascia.

fasciectomy Surgical excision of strips of fascia.

fasciitis An inflammation of the fascia.

fascioliasis An infection caused by flukes of the class Trematoda, most often characterized by fever, eosinophilia, and abdominal pain.

fasciolopsiasis Infestation with the large intestinal fluke Fasciolopsis buski; common in eastern Asia.

fasciotomy A surgical procedure where the fascia is cut to relieve tension or pressure, and treat the resulting loss of circulation to an area of tissue or muscle.

FAT Fluorescent Antibody Test.

fatigue fracture A fracture that occurs in bone or in other materials, including metal, as a result of repeated stress as opposed to a single injury.

Favorable Selection Strategy that encourages the enrollment of the healthier persons while discouraging the enrollment of sicker persons. Also see cherry picking, adverse selection, and risk selection.

FB Foreign body.

FBG Fasting blood glucose.

FBS Fasting blood sugar.

FCE Functional capacity evaluation.

FDA Food and Drug Administration.

febrile non-hemolytic transfusion reaction A transfusion complication defined as a rise in temperature by one degree Celsius or more during or within 24 hours of the completion of a blood transfusion.

fecal of or relating to feces.

fecal impaction A large mass of dry, hard stool that can develop in the rectum due to chronic constipation.

Federal Employee Health Benefits Program (FEHBP) A voluntary health insurance program administered by the Office of Personnel Management (OPM) for federal employees, retirees, and their dependents and survivors.

Federal HMO Act Federal law regulating HMOs. Under the Federal HMO act, an entity must have three characteristics to call itself an HMO (1) an organized system for providing health care or otherwise assuring health care delivery in a geographic area, (2) an agreed upon set of basic and supplemental health maintenance and treatment services, and (3) a voluntarily enrolled group of people.

Federal Qualified Health Center (FQHC) A Federal payment option that enables qualified providers in medically underserved areas to receive cost-based Medicare and Medicaid reimbursement and allows for the direct reimbursement of nurse practitioners, physician assistants and certified nurse midwives. Many outpatient clinics and specialty outreach services are qualified under this provision.

Federal Register An official publication of the Federal government that provides final and proposed regulations of Federal legislation.

federally qualified HMO An HMO that has satisfied certain federal qualifications pertaining to organizational structure, provider contracts, health service delivery information, utilization review or quality assurance, grievance procedures, financial status, and marketing information.

Federation of American Health Systems (FAHS) A trade association comprised of proprietary or investor-owned hospitals.

fee disclosure Physicians and caregivers discussing their charges with patients prior to treatment.

fee for service Refers to paying medical providers for individual services rendered. UCR, CPR and Fee Schedules are examples of fee for service systems.

fee hr service equivalency Quantitative measures of the difference between the amount a provider receives from an altern-ative reimbursement system (e.g., capitation) compared to fee-for-service reimbursement.

fee schedule 1). A list of certain services and payable amounts indicating the maximum Medicare payment for the service. Method of payment is calculated by the Resource Base Relative Value Unit Scale by which Medicare reimburses physician and non-physician services. 2) A complete listing of fees used by health plans to pay physicians or other providers.

fee schedule payment areas Geographic areas within which payment under the fee schedule will be equal. Analogous to localities under current payment policies. *See* Geographic Adjustment Factor.

fee-for-service A payment system for health care where the provider is paid for each service rendered rather than a pre-negotiated amount for each patient.

fee-screen year A specified period of time in which SMI-recognized fees pertain. The fee-screen year period has changed over the history of the program.

FEF Forced Expiratory Flow.

FEHBP Federal Employees Health Benefits Program.

female genital system Consists of internal and external genital organs involved in sexual reproduction. The internal genital organs include the ovaries, uterine tubes, uterus and vagina.

female infertility The biological inability of the female to contribute to conception.

femoral of or relating to or near the femur or thigh.

femoral artery A large artery that starts in the lower abdomen and goes down into the thigh The femoral artery starts as a continuation of the external iliac artery which comes from the abdominal aorta.

femoral vein A vein which returns blood in the leg to the heart via the iliac veins.

femur The longest and thickest bone of the human skeleton; extends from the pelvis to the knee.

fenestration The surgical creation of an artificial opening in the bony part of the inner ear so as to improve or restore hearing.

FEP Free erythrocyte protoporphyrin.

ferritin An iron-carrying protein which is a more accurate monitor of long term body iron status than the blood iron level, which varies with diet.

fertility agents Drugs used to increase fertility or to treat infertility.

fertilization The union of a human egg and sperm, usually occurring in the ampulla of the fallopian tube. It is also the initiation of prenatal development.

FES Functional electrical stimulation.

fetal hypoxia Absence of sufficient oxygen to sustain life in a fetus.

fetal monitoring Physiologic or biochemical monitoring of the fetus. It is usually done during labor, obstetric and may be performed in conjunction with the monitoring of uterine activity. It may also be performed prenatally as when the mother is undergoing surgery.

fetus A developing human from two months after conception to birth.

FEV Forced expiratory volume.

fever Common term for an increase in internal body temperature to levels above normal. *Synonym:* pyrexia.

FFS Fee-for-Service.

FI Fiscal Iintermediary.

FIA Fluorescence immunoassay.

FIB Fibrillation.

fiberscope A flexible fiber optic bundle with an eyepiece at one end, and a lens at the other.

fibr(o) Fiber.

fibrillation Commonly refers to the rapid, irregular, and unsynchronized contraction of the muscle fibers of the heart.

fibrin Protein formed from fibrinogen by the action of blood clotting.

fibrin split products *See* FSP.

fibrinogen A protein involved in coagulation. Fibrinogen reacts with other molecules to produce blood clots.

fibrinolysis Breakdown of fibrin by enzyme action.

fibrinolysis, secondary Process by which connective tissue is dissolved by the action of enzymes as a result of some disease process.

fibrinolytic agents Fibrinolysin or agents that convert plasminogen to fibrinolysin (PLASMIN).

fibrinolytic disorders Disease process characterized by dissolution of connective tissue by the action of enzymes.

fibroadenoma A benign growth in the breast that is solid, firm, smooth and usually painless or only slightly tender.

fibroadenosis A benign neoplasm composed of glandular and fibrous tissues, with a relatively large proportion of glands.

fibroblastoma A tumor derived from a fibroblast, now differentiated as a fibroma or a fibrosarcoma.

fibrocystic disease Disorder of the female breast characterized by nonmalignant lumps. Cause is unknown. Lumps may be accompanied by generalized breast pain, especially before menstrual periods. Lumps often enlarge before menstrual periods, then shrink afterward. *Synonym:* breast lumps.

fibroids Abnormal growth of cells in the muscular wall of the uterus (myometrium). Uterine fibroids are composed of abnormal muscle cells and are almost always benign. Cause is unknown. Usually decreases in size without treatment after menopause.

fibromas Benign neoplasm of fibrous or fully developed connective tissue.

fibromatosis Refers to a group of benign soft tissue tumors (fibromas) which have certain characteristics in common.

fibromyalgia Defined as muscle and connective tissue pain, is an unexplained syndrome characterized by chronic widespread pain and a painful response to pressure.

fibromyoma A benign tumor that contains a large amount of fibrous tissue. *Synonym:* uterine fibroid, uterine leiomyoma.

fibrosis The formation of scar tissue due to injury or long-term inflammation.

fibrositis Inflammation of white fibrous tissues (especially muscle sheaths).

fibrous ankylosis Immobility and consolidation of a joint from disease caused by fibrous tissue.

fibrous tissue Tissue that is made up of fibers.

fibula The outer and thinner of the two bones of the human leg between the knee and ankle.

FICA Federal insurance contribution act.

fifth-digit subclassifications Refers to the highest specificity of diagnosis coding in which five-digit code numbers are reported if available.

filariasis Disease caused by the presence of parasitic worms or larvae in body tissue. Worms are round, long and threadlike. They are common in tropical and subtropical regions. They enter the body as microscopic larvae through the bite of a mosquito or other insect then infest the lymph glands and channels. Treatment is not very effective. After many years, this disease usually results in elephantiasis, characterized by tremendous swelling of the external genitals and legs.

filli- Fine, hair like.

filling Restoration of lost tooth structure with metal, porcelain or resin materials.

filtering surgery A surgical procedure used in treatment of glaucoma in which an opening is created through which aqueous fluid may pass from the anterior chamber into a sac created beneath the conjunctiva, thus lowering the pressure within the eye.

fimbria A fringe of tissue around the ostium of the Fallopian tube, in the direction of the ovary.

fimbrioplasty Reconstructive or corrective surgery on the fimbria of a damaged or blocked fallopian tube.

finger-nose test A test for coordinated limb movements; with upper limb extended to one side the patient is asked to try to touch the end of the nose with the tip of the index finger.

Finn chamber test A type of patch test in which the materials being tested are held in shallow aluminum cups (Finn chambers) that are taped against the skin, usually for a few days.

Finney operation Gastroduodenostomy that creates, by the technique of closure, a large opening to ensure free emptying from the stomach.

first degree burn A burn usually limited to redness, a white plaque and minor pain at the site of injury. These burns involve only the epidermis.

first dollar coverage Refers to not having to meet a calendar year deductible prior to receiving reimbursement or payment for a medical service.

first responder The first responder uses a limited amount of equipment to perform initial assessment and intervention and is trained to assist other Emergency Medical Services (EMS) providers. Example At the scene of a cardiac arrest, the First Responder would be expected to notify EMS (if not already notified) and initiate CPR with an oral airway and a barrier device.

Fiscal Intermediary (FI) A regional administrator of payment or reimbursement for government programs.

fiscal year The accounting year of the U.S. Government. Since 1976, each fiscal year has begun October 1 of the prior calendar year and ended the following September 30th. For example, fiscal year 2008 began October 1, 2008 and ended September 30, 2009.

Fishberg concentration test Determination of the ability of the kidneys to maintain excretion of solids under conditions of reduced water intake and a high protein diet, in which urine samples are collected and tested for specific gravity.

fissure A long narrow slit or groove that divides an organ into lobes.

fissurectomy Surgical removal of a fissure.

fissures 1) Cleft or groove on the surface of an organ, often marking division of the organ into parts, as the fissures of the brain. 2) Crack-like lesion of skin.

fistula An abnormal connection or passageway between two epithelium-lined organs or vessels that normally do not connect. It is generally a disease condition, but a fistula may be surgically created for therapeutic reasons.

fistulectomy Surgical removal of a fistula.

fistulization Surgical production of an artificial channel Fixation The act or operation of holding, suturing or fastening in a fixed position.

fistulotomy The surgical opening or removal of a fistulous tract performed by excision of the tract and surrounding tissue, simple division of the tract, or gradual division and assisted drainage of the tract by means of a seton.

fitted elastic compression stockings Elastic stockings that provide counter-pressure to veins and help return fluid that has leaked out back into circulation. Ideally, they exert a pressure of at least 30 to 40 mm Hg at the ankle with less pressure at the knee.

fixation A chemical process by which biological tissues are preserved from decay.

flap A movable piece of tissue partly connected to the body.

flap operation 1. Any operation involving the raising of a flap of tissue. 2. In periodontics, an operation to secure greater access to granulation tissue and osseous defects, consisting of detachment of the gingivae, the alveolar mucosa, and/or a portion of the alveola.

flat foot A common term for a medical condition in which the arch of the foot collapses. *Synonym:* pes planus, fallen arches.

Fletcher factor deficiency A rare blood coagulation abnormality which does not cause bleeding problems and is usually an incidental finding.

flexible benefit plan A benefits package allowing an employee to choose from a range of benefit choices.

flexion Bending movement that decreases the angle between two parts. Bending the elbow, or clenching a hand into a fist, are examples of flexion. When sitting down, the knees are flexed. Flexion of the hip or shoulder moves the limb forward (towards the anterior side of the body).

flexorplasty A surgical procedure to restore elbow flexion.

flicker fusion threshold The point or frequency at which all flicker of an intermittent light stimulus disappears.

flocculation test Any serologic test in which a flocculent agglomerate is formed; usually applied to a variant form of the precipitin reaction.

flow cytometry A test that can be used to measure the amount of DNA in cells.

fluorescein angiography A test to examine blood vessels in the retina, choroid, and iris. A special dye is injected into a vein in the arm and pictures are taken as the dye passes through blood vessels in the eye.

fluorescein staining A tiny amount of a fluorescein dye is placed in the tear film. The color will make microscopic dots appear where the eye has become dry. Excessive staining is an indication of dry eye.

fluorescent antibody test A test for the distribution of cells expressing a specific protein by binding antibody specific for the protein and detecting complexes by fluorescent labeling of the antibody.

fluorescent treponemal antibody absorption test The standard treponemal antigen serologic test for syphilis, using fluorescein-labeled antihuman globulin to demonstrate specific treponemal antibodies in patient serum.

fluoride A chemical compound used to prevent dental decay, utilized in fluoridated water systems and/or applied directly to the teeth.

fluorophotometry Measurement of light given off by fluorescein in order to assess the integrity of various ocular barriers. The method is used to investigate the blood-aqueous barrier, blood-retinal barrier, aqueous flow measure-mints, corneal endothelial permeability, and.

fluoroscopy An imaging technique used to obtain real-time moving images of the internal structures through the use of a fluoroscope.

FLAP (Federal Medical Assistance Percentage) The portion of the Medicaid program which is paid by the Federal government.

FMLA Family and Medical Leave Act.

FOB Fecal Occult Blood test.

FOC Functional Ovarian Cyst.

focal epilepsy *See* Epilepsy, focal.

focal seizures Convulsions brought about by a disease process or injury to an identifiable part of the brain. Such seizures usually affect only one side or a specific area of the body as opposed to a generalized seizure, which is likely to involve all muscle groups in the body.

focused studies State required studies that examine a specific aspect of health care (such as prenatal care) for a defined point in time. These projects are usually based on information extracted from medical records or MCO or PHP administrative data such as enrollment files and encounter or claims data.

folate A B-vitamin.

fontanelle Any membranous gap between the bones of the cranium in an infant or fetus.

Food and Drug Administration (FDA) An agency within the Federal government that is responsible for regulations pertaining to food and drugs sold in the United States.

food poisoning Any illness resulting from the consumption of contaminated food.

foramen A natural opening or perforation through a bone or a membranous structure.

foraminotomy A surgical procedure used to relieve pressure on nerves that are being compressed by the intervertebral foramina.

forensic dentistry The practice of gathering legal evidence for body identification or judicial issues.

Forestier disease Ankylosing spinal hyperostosis.

-form, -iform Used to form adjectives indicating 'having the form of'.

formal mechanism for processing records Documented policies and procedures for the routine, and non-routine, receipt, manipulation, storage, dissemination, transmission, and/or disposal of health information.

format Under HIPAA, this is those data elements that provide or control the enveloping or hierarchical structure, or assist in identifying data content of, a transaction.

formed elements The red and white blood cells and platelets found in whole blood.

formulary The panel of drugs chosen by a hospital or managed care organization that is used to treat patients. Drugs outside of the formulary are not used, unless in rare, specific circumstances.

fossa The valley found on the surface of posterior teeth.

Fothergill operation An operation for uterine prolapse by fixation of the cardinal ligaments.

fovea A part of the eye, located in the center of the macula region of the retina. The fovea is responsible for sharp central vision.

Fowler-Stephens orchiopexy A special technique for surgical correction of an undescended testicle inside the scrotum.

FP Family Practice.

FPG Fasting Plasma Glucose.

FPMP Federal Preventive Medicine Program.

FPP Faculty Practice Plan.

FQHC Federally Qualified Health Centers.

fractionation The process by which blood plasma is separated into some of its different component parts.

fracture A complete or incomplete break in a bone resulting from the application of excessive force.

Franco's operation Suprapubic cystotomy.

fraud The intentional deception or misrepresentation that an individual knows, or should know, to be false, or does not believe to be true, and makes, knowing the deception could result in some unauthorized benefit to himself or some other person(s).

fraud and abuse Fraud To purposely bill for services that were never given or to bill for a service that has a higher reimbursement than the service produced. Abuse Payment for items or services that are billed by mistake by providers, but should not be paid for by Medicare. This is not the same as fraud.

Frazier-Spiller operation Trigeminal rhizotomy using an approach through the middle cranial fossa.

FRC Functional residual capacity.

Fredet-Ramstedt operation *See* pyloromyotomy.

free look provision An insurance policy provision required by most states, allowing the policy owner to inspect the policy for a specified period of time. If desired the owner may return the policy to the insurer for a refund of the entire premium.

free standing emergency medical service center A health care facility that is physically separate from a hospital and whose primary purpose is the provision of immediate, short-term medical care for minor but urgent medical conditions. Also called urgent care center.

free standing facility Usually a specialty facility that is not part of a comprehensive care system. For example, a free-standing surgery facility or a free-standing assisted living facility.

free standing outpatient surgical center A health care facility that is physically separate from a hospital, that provides pre-scheduled, outpatient surgical services. Also called surgicenter or ambulatory surgical facility..

free testosterone (direct) Free testosterone is the testosterone that is not bound to proteins in the body and is bioavailable or circulating free in the blood.

Freedom of Choice (FOC) In general, laws that permit enrollees to choose any provider and receive substantial reimbursement from their health plan. Also refers to a Federal Medicaid rule requiring states to ensure that Medicaid beneficiaries are free to obtain services from any qualified provider. Exceptions are possible through waivers of Medicaid and special contract options. Also see any willing provider and point of service.

frenectomy The removal or reshaping of thin muscle tissue that attaches the upper or lower lips to the gum, or the tongue to the floor of the mouth.

frenoplasty The surgical alteration of a frenulum when its presence restricts range of motion between interconnected tissues. Two of the most common sites for a frenulo-plasty are the penis and the tongue.

frenotomy Incision of a frenum, especially of the frenulum of the tongue.

frenulectomy The surgical removal of a frenulum.

frenuloplasty The surgical alteration of a frenulum when its presence restricts range of motion between interconnected tissues.

frenulotomy Excision of a frenum.

frenum A fold of tissue or muscle connecting the lips cheek or tongue to the jawbone.

frenumectomy *See* frenectomy.

frequency The number of times a service was provided.

fresh frozen plasma This is used to reverse warfarin by replacing clotting factors.

Frickman operation Abdominal proctopexy.

Friedländer bacillus The bacteria that causes pneumonia. *Synonym:* klebsiella pneumoniae.

Friedreich ataxia An autosomal recessive disease usually beginning in childhood with sclerosis of the posterior and lateral columns of the spinal cord and ataxia of the lower extremities, followed by paralysis and contractures. *Synonym:* hereditary spinal ataxia.

front- of or pertaining to the forehead.

frontal bone forms the forehead, the roofs of the orbits, and most of the anterior part of the cranial floor.

frontal plane Divides the body into dorsal and ventral (back and front, or posterior and anterior) portions. *Synonym:* coronal plane.

Frost-Lang operation Insertion of a gold ball in place of an enucleated eyeball.

FRV Functional Residual Volume.

FSB Fetal Scalp Blood.

FSH Follicle-Stimulating Hormone.

FSP Results from the breakdown of fibrinogen by plasmin (an enzyme). *See* Fibrin.

FT Full-term.

FU Followup.

fulguration A procedure to destroy tissue (such as a tumor) using an electric current. *Synonym:* electro-fulguration.

full capitation The plan or Primary Care Case Manager is paid for providing services to enrollees through a combination of capitation and fee-for-service reimbursements.

full denture A removable dental prosthesis (appliance) that replaces all upper or lower teeth.

full mouth reconstruction Extensive restorations of natural teeth with crowns and/or fixed bridges to manage bite problems.

Fuller's operation Perineal incision and drainage of the seminal vesicles.

full-time student Under a health plan, an eligible dependant child student (typically age 19 or older) who meets the health plan's criteria of full-time. Such criteria normally typically includes minimum credit hour requirements (such as 12 credit hours in a semester).

fully accredited Designation that all the elements within all the accreditation standards for which the accreditation organization has been approved by CMS have been surveyed and fully met or have otherwise been determined to be acceptable.

fully capitated A stipulated dollar amount established to cover the cost of all health care services delivered for a person.

fully funded plan A health plan under which an insurer or MCO bears the financial responsibility of guaranteeing claim payments and paying for all incurred covered benefits and administration costs.

fulminating infection Infection that occurs suddenly, with great intensity.

functional digestive disorders Are a group of disorders, which include irritable bowel syndrome or ibs, dyspepsia, gerd, and chronic constipation or diarrhea.

functional status A patient's ability to perform the activities of daily living.

functionally disabled An inability to live independently or to perform ADLs or IADLs independently.

funding level The amount of revenue required to finance a medical care program. Under an insured program, this is usually premium rate. Under a self-funded program, this amount is usually assessed per expected claim cost, plus stop-loss premium, plus all related fees.

funding method The means by which an employer pays for the employee health benefit plan. The most common methods are 1) prospective and/or retrospective, 2) refunding products, 3) self-funding, and 4) shared risk management.

funding vehicle In a self-funded plan, the account into which the money that an employer and employees would have paid in premiums to an insurer or MCO is deposited until the money is paid out.

fundoplasty A procedure performed to reinforce the cardiac sphincter of the distal esophagus for treatment of reflux disease.

fundoplication Mobilization of the lower end of the esophagus and plication of the fundus of the stomach around it (fundic wrapping) in the treatment of gastroesophageal reflux that may be associated with various disorders, such as hiatal hernia.

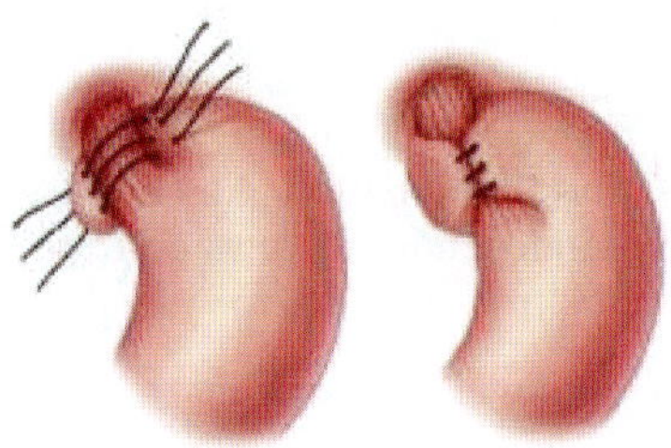

Fundoplication.

fundus The bottom or base of anything; the bottom or base of an organ, or the part of a hollow organ farthest from its mouth.

fungus A type of organism that includes molds, mildews, yeasts, and mushrooms.

fuo Fever of undetermined origin • Fever of unknown origin.

furuncle A skin disease caused by the infection of hair follicles, resulting in the localized accumulation of pus and dead tissue. Individual boils can cluster together and form an interconnected network of boils called carbuncles.

fusion 1) A procedure to join bones together permanently so there is no longer movement between them. 2) Union or healing of bone.

FX Fracture.

FY Fiscal year.

G

g-6-pd (glucose-6-phosphate dehydrogenase) Enzyme normally found in most body cells. Deficiency is inherited and makes red blood more prone to destruction.

GAF Geographic Adjustment Factor.

gag rule laws Special laws that make sure that health plans let doctors tell their patients complete health care information. This includes information about treatments not covered by the health plan.

gait A person's manner of walking.

gait training Refers to helping a patient relearn to walk safely and efficiently. Gait training is usually done by rehabilitation specialists and often incorporates the use of such assistive devices as parallel bars, walkers or canes to promote safe and proficient ambulation.

galact(o)- Milk.

galactocele A cystic tumor containing milk or a milky substance that is usually located in the mammary.

galactogram A special type of mammogram used for imaging the breast ducts. It can aid in diagnosing the cause of abnormal nipple discharges. *Synonym:* ductogram.

galactorrhea Breast milk flow not associated with childbirth or breast feeding. It may be a symptom of a pituitary gland tumor.

galactosemia Inherited disease of infants in which milk cannot be digested. Milk should be eliminated from the infant's diet to prevent malnutrition, liver disease, kidney disease and mental retardation.

gallbladder A small, pear-shaped muscular sac, located under the right lobe of the liver, in which bile secreted by the liver is stored until needed by the body for digestion.

gallbladder disease Any disease involving the gallbladder or biliary tract. The gallbladder is a reservoir for bile; the biliary tract is the passageway that transports bile to the small intestine. Gallbladder disease is a common, often painful condition requiring surgery. It is commonly associated with gallstones and inflammation.

Gallie fusion Wire around lamina of C-1 and C-2.

gallstones Calculus or stone formed in the gallbladder. *Synonym:* cholelithiasis.

gaming Gaining advantage by using improper means to evade the letter or intent of a rule or system.

gamma globulin 1) A protein fraction of blood serum containing many antibodies that protect against bacterial and viral infectious diseases. 2) A solution of gamma globulin prepared from human blood and administered for passive immunization against measles, German measles, hepatitis A, poliomyelitis, and other infections.

ganglia An encapsulated neural structure consisting of a collection of cell bodies or neurons.

ganglion A swelling that often appears on or around joints and tendons in the hand or foot. The size of the cyst can vary over time. It is most frequently located around the wrist and on the fingers.

ganglioneuroblastoma Tumor of nerve cells.

ganglioneuroma Benign tumor composed of nerve fibers.

gangrene The decay or death of an organ or tissue caused by a lack of blood supply. It a complication resulting from infectious or inflammatory processes, injury, or degenerative changes associated with chronic diseases, such as diabetes mellitus.

gardnerella vaginalis An infection of the female genital tract by bacteria of the Gardnerella vaginalis strain, often in combination with various anaerobic bacteria. *Synonym:* bacterial vaginosis.

Gasserian ganglion A sensory ganglion of the trigeminal nerve. *Synonym:* trigeminal ganglion.

gastr(o)- of or pertaining to the stomach.

gastrectomy Excision of the whole (total gastrectomy) or part (subtotal gastrectomy, partial gastrectomy, gastric resection) of the stomach.

gastric Refers to the stomach.

gastric balloon An inflatable device implanted in the stomach as an adjunct to therapy of morbid obesity.

gastric ulcer A hole in the lining of the stomach corroded by the acidic digestive juices which are secreted by the stomach cells.

gastrin Hormone that stimulates the production of gastric acid or stomach acid.

gastrinoma Benign or malignant gastrin-secreting islet-cell tumor of the pancreas. There is an overproduction of gastric acid often resulting in an ulcer.

gastritis Irritation, inflammation or infection of the stomach lining. Cause is sometimes unknown but may be due to excess stomach acid, food allergy, viral infection or adverse reaction to alcohol, caffeine or some drug. Symptoms may include nausea, diarrhea, abdominal pain, cramps, fever, weakness, belching, bloating and loss of appetite.

gastrocnemius muscle The muscle in the back part of the leg that forms the greater part of the calf; responsible for the plantar flexion of the foot.

gastroduodenitis Inflammation of the stomach and duodenum. It is one of the most frequent causes of jaundice.

gastroduodenostomy The surgical formation of a communication between the stomach and the duodenum.

gastroenteritis Inflammation of the stomach and intestines accompanying many digestive-tract disorders.

Causes may include bacterial, viral or parasitic infections, food poisoning, food allergy, excess alcohol consumption or emotional upset. Symptoms are the same as gastritis.

gastroenterology The study and treatment of diseases of the stomach and digestive system.

gastroenterostomy A variety of surgical reconstructive procedures devised to restore gastrointestinal continuity, The two major classes of reconstruction are the Billroth I (gastroduodenostomy) and Billroth II (gastrojejunostomy) procedures.

gastroesophageal reflux disease A condition in which food or liquid travels backwards from the stomach to the esophagus. This can irritate the esophagus, causing heartburn and other symptoms.

gastrointestinal of or referring collectively to the stomach and small and large intestines.

gastrointestinal agents Drugs used for their effects on the gastro-intestinal system, as to control gastric acidity, regulate gastro-intestinal motility and water flow, and improve digestion.

gastrointestinal disease Any disorder of the gastrointestinal tract, which includes the mouth, esophagus, stomach, duodenum, small intestine, cecum, appendix, the ascending colon, transverse colon, descending colon, sigmoid colon, rectum and anus.

gastrointestinal disorders Any condition or disease relating to any part of the digestive system, including the mouth, esophagus, stomach, small intestine, large intestine and rectum. May also include some conditions relating to the liver, gallbladder and pancreas.

gastrointestinal hemorrhage Bleeding in any segment of the gastrointestinal tract from esophagus to rectum.

gastrointestinal mucositis The inflammation of a mucous membrane of the gastrointestinal system.

gastrointestinal symptoms Any symptoms relating to the stomach or intestine. Some common GI symptoms include vomiting, diarrhea, constipation, bloating and heartburn.

gastrojejunal of or relating to the stomach and jejunum.

gastrojejunostomy Surgical establishment of an anastomosis between the jejunum and the anterior or posterior wall of the stomach.

gastroplasty Surgical treatment of the stomach or lower esophagus used to decrease the size of the stomach. The procedure is used mainly in the treatment of morbid obesity and to correct defects in the lower esophagus or the stomach.

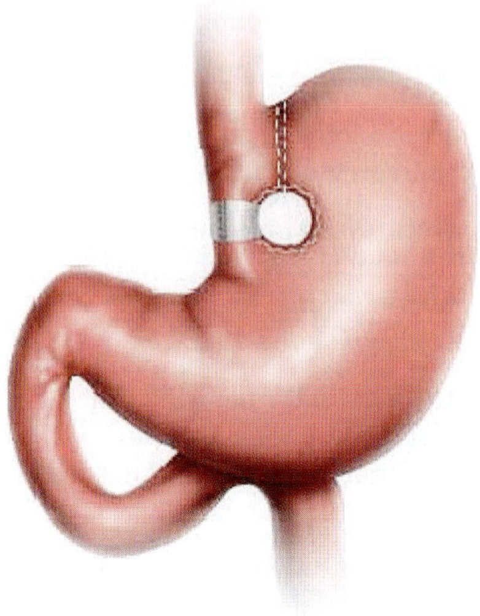

Gastroplasty

gastroptosis The abnormal downward displacement of the stomach. The condition frequently causes digestive symptoms and constipation, and is much more prominent in women than men.

gastrorrhaphy Suture of a perforation of the stomach.

gastroschisis A type of inherited congenital abdominal wall defect in which the intestines and sometimes other organs develop outside the fetal abdomen through an opening in the abdominal wall.

gastrostomy Creation of an artificial external opening into the stomach for nutritional support or gastrointestinal compression.

gastrotomy Surgical incision into the stomach.

gatekeeper A primary care physician in an HMO who reviews and evaluates patients for referral to specialists. The gatekeeper's mission is to reduce unnecessary services and costs.

Gaucher's disease Rare familial disorder of fat metabolism characterized by an enlarged spleen, enlarged liver and abnormal bone growth in early childhood.

GC Gonococcus, gonococcal.

-gen (1) denotes the sense 'born in, from' (2) denotes the sense 'of a certain kind'.

general agent This typically refers to a middle man agent who facilitates business between retail agents and the insurance company.

general anesthesia A state of total unconsciousness resulting from general anesthetic drugs. A variety of drugs are given to the patient that have different effects with the goal of ensuring unconsciousness, amnesia and analgesia.

General Practitioner (GP) A physician whose practice is based on a broad understanding of all illnesses and who does not restrict his/her practice to any particular field of medicine.

general surgery The specialty of treating common abdominal problems such as hernias and appendicitis with surgery.

generic drug In cases in which the patent on a specific pharmaceutical product expires and drug manufacturers produce generic versions of the original branded product, the generic version of the drug (which is theorized to be exactly the same product manufactured by a different firm) is dispensed even though the original product is prescribed. Some managed care organizations and Medicaid programs mandate generic substitution because of the generally lower cost of generic products.

generic substitution The dispensing of a drug that is the generic equivalent of a drug listed on a pharmacy benefit management plan's formulary. In most cases, generic substitution can be performed without physician approval.

genetic counseling Genetic counseling is the process of helping people understand and adapt to the medical, psychological and familial implications of genetic contributions to disease. It includes interpreting family and medical histories to assess the chance of disease occurring or recurring; educating about inherited risk, testing, management, prevention, resources and research; and counseling to promote informed choices and adaptation to the risk or condition.

genetic testing Tests on blood and other tissue to find genetic disorders. Genetic testing is performed to confirm genetic diseases before birth, determine if people carry a gene for a genetic disorder, screen embryos for disease, and to confirm a diagnosis in a person with disease symptoms.

-genic Formation.

genioplasty Commonly known as chin repositioning, a surgical procedure to correct receding chins, chin misalignment or chin excess.

genital herpes Viral infection of the genitals transmitted by intercourse or oral sex. Genital herpes may increase the risk of cervical cancer. Symptoms include painful blisters on the genitals that can cause painful urination, fever, malaise and enlarged lymph glands. Currently incurable, but treatment can relieve symptoms.

genital prolapse A condition in which the vaginal wall or uterus descend below their normal positions; part of the bladder or rectum may protrude from the vagina.

genitalia The external organs of the reproductive system.

genitourinary of or related to the genital and urinary organs or their functions.

genitourinary system of or related to the genital and urinary organs or their functions.

genu- of or pertaining to the knee.

geographic accessibility Health plan accessibility, generally determined by drive time or number of primary care providers in a service area.

geographic adjustment factor The adjustment made to a service's fee in the Medicare Fee Schedule to determine the correct payment in each fee schedule payment area. The GAF is composed of three components; work, cost of practice and malpractice cost.

geographic availability The number of primary care providers within a given radius of a particular target.

Geographic Cost of Practice Index (GCPI) An index summarizing the prices of inputs to physician services in an area relative to national average prices. The GCPI is based on three components reflecting the opport-unity cost of physician work, the costs of goods and services that comprise practice expenses, and malpractice expenses.

geographic multiplier A factor used to make geographic adjustments to the Medicare Fee Schedule or any other fee schedule.

Geometric Mean Length of Stay (GMLOS) A statistically adjusted value for all cases for a specific DRG which adjusts for outliers, transfer cases and negative outlier cases. The GMLOS is used to determine payment for transfer cases.

GERD Gastroesophageal reflux disease.

geriatrics Medical field specializing in care for the elderly.

geriatrician A physician who specializes in the diagnosis and treatment of diseases of older persons.

gerontology Social Science field studying the biological, psychological and social aspects of aging.

germ cell tumors One of three types of cancer of the ovary. Arises in the ovum (egg). Prognosis is often poor because tumors tend to progress rapidly. Advances in chemotherapy may improve outcome. Rarely may occur in children.

Gestalt therapy A form of psychotherapy with emphasis on the interplay of organism and environment. Basic to this therapy is the development of awareness and maturity, as well as self-confidence.

Getty procedure Excision of lamina and a portion of the facet for decompression of lumbar spinal stenosis.

GG Gamma globulin.

GI Gastrointestinal.

giardia A parasite that is the common cause of giardiasis.

giardiasis Infection of the intestines with protozoa found in contaminated food and water; characterized by diarrhea and nausea and flatulence and abdominal discomfort.

Gifford sign Inability to evert the upper eyelid in Graves' disease.

gigantism Condition in which the body or a body part grows excessively, sometimes due to an overactive pituitary gland.

Gilbert's disease (syndrome) Benign hereditary condition characterized by jaundice and high bilirubin levels in the blood. *See* Jaundice. No treatment is required.

Gill lumbar fusion Removal of the posterior spinal arch in spondylolisthesis.

gingiv- of or pertaining to the gums.

gingiva The tissue (covered by mucous membrane) of the jaws that surrounds the bases of the teeth.

gingival of or relating to the gingiva (gums).

gingivectomy Surgical excision of the gingiva at the level of its attachment, thus creating new marginal gingiva. This procedure is used to eliminate gingival or periodontal pockets or to provide an approach for extensive surgical interventions.

gingivitis An inflammation of infection of the gingiva (gum tissue) caused by plaque and or tartar build-up. Precursor to periodontitis if not treated.

gingivoplasty Surgical reshaping of the gingivae and papillae for correction of deformities (particularly enlargements) and to provide the gingivae with a normal and functional form, the incision creating an external bevel.

gingivostomatitis A viral or bacterial infection of the mouth and gums that leads to swelling and sores.

Girdlestone procedure Complete resection or excision of the head and neck of the femur.

Glabella reflex The forehead is tapped lightly between the eyes. If the patient responds with persistent spasm of the eye muscles and closing of the eyes, the Glabella is positive. This may indicate damage to the connections between the frontal cortex and the facial nerve complex in the pons. The reflex is seen in Parkinson's disease, frontal lobe tumors and frequently appears with dementia.

gland An organ that synthesizes a substance for release such as hormoncs or breast milk, into the bloodstream or into cavities inside the body or its outer surface.

glanders An infectious disease that occurs primarily in horses, mules, and donkeys that can be transmitted to humans. Glanders is endemic in Africa, Asia, the middle east, central and South America.

glandular of or referring to gland(s).

Glanzmann's thromboasthenia Rare, inherited hemorrhagic disease. *See* Hemorrhagic disease. Platelet cells cannot cluster normally; clots do not form and hemorrhage occurs. Transfusion with platelets is usually effective in stopping any bleeding.

glauc(o)- Denoting a grey, bluish-grey color.

glaucoma Abnormally increased pressure within the eyeball that may produce severe, permanent vision defects. It is the most preventable cause of blindness. If diagnosed and treated early, it rarely results in permanent loss of vision.

Glenn procedure A palliative (temporary) treatment used to improve the flow of blood to the lungs in complex conditions where only one ventricle is working properly and not enough blood is getting to the lungs.

global service A group of clinically related services that are treated as a single unit for the purpose of coding, billing and payment.

global surgery policy The payment policy in the Medicare Fee Schedule that specifies the surgical procedure and the related services and visits that are included in a global surgical fee.

globulin Globulin helps to combat infection on a normal level. It is the total protein value minus albumin value.

globulin, total Globulin is a type of protein used for the production of antibodies. Proteins are made from amino acids and are important parts of all cells and tissues. There are many different kinds of proteins in the body with many different functions. Examples of proteins are enzymes, some hormones, hemoglobin (oxygen transport), LDL (cholesterol transport), fibrinogen (blood clotting), collagen (structure of bone and cartilage), and immunoglobulins (antibodies).

globulins Class of proteins that are insoluble in water but soluble in saline solutions.

glomerular of or pertaining to a glomerulus.

glomerulonephritis A form of nephritis with inflammation of the capillary loops in the renal glomeruli. The acute form is characterized by proteinuria, edema, hematuria, renal failure, and hypertension, sometimes preceded by tonsillitis or febrile pharyngitis.

glomerulus Tiny structure composed of blood vessels. One of several structures that make up a nephron in the kidney.

gloss(o)-, glott(o)- of or pertaining to the tongue.

glossectomy Partial or total surgical excision of the tongue.

glossitis Inflammation of the tongue.

glossodynia Pain in the tongue.

glossopexy An adhesion of the tongue to the lip.

glossopharyngeal neuralgia Irritation of the glossopharyngeal nerve, a cranial nerve that provides feeling to the tongue and throat.

glossorrhaphy Suture of a wound of the tongue.

glottis The middle part of the larynx.

glucagonoma Glucagon-secreting tumor of the islet cells of the pancreas. Glucagon increases blood sugar.

gluco- Glucose.

glucocorticoid deficiency Decreased amount of hormone from the adrenal gland that increases production of glycogen.

glucose Glucose is the primary blood sugar test and indicates blood sugar level at the time blood was drawn. High values are seen in diabetics. In addition to pancreatic functions, glucose may be altered by diet and medication.

glucose tolerance test A test of the body's ability to utilize carbohydrates by measuring the plasma glucose level at stated intervals after ingestion or intravenous injection of a large quantity of glucose.

glucose, serum Glucose is the primary energy source for the body. This test measures the sugar level in your blood. High values are associated most often with diabetes mellitus and sometimes with other metabolic diseases.

glyco- Sugar.

glycogen Substance formed from glucose, stored chiefly in the liver. When the blood-sugar level is too low, glycogen is converted back to glucose for the body to use as energy.

glycogen-storage disease Any of a group of inherited disorders of glycogen metabolism. An enzyme deficiency causes glycogen to accumulate in abnormally large amounts in the body. *Synonym:* glycogenosis.

glycosuria The presence of abnormally high levels of sugar in the urine.

glycosylated hemoglobin test Measurement of the percentage of hemoglobin A molecules that have formed a stable keto–amine linkage between their terminal amino acid position of the β-chains and a glucose group; in normal persons this is about 7 per cent of the total, in diabetics about 14.5 per cent.

gm Gram.

gnath(o)- of or pertaining to the jaw.

GNB Gram negative bacillus.

goiter Enlargement of the thyroid gland, which causes a swelling in the front part of the neck.

gon(o)- *See*d, semen; also, reproductive.

gonadal Pertaining to gonads.

gonadal impairment Decreased function of the gonads.

gonadectomy Surgical removal of an ovary or testis.

gonadotropin Hormone secreted by the anterior pituitary gland and placenta; stimulates the gonads and controls reproductive activity.

gonads Parts of the reproductive system that produce and release eggs (ovaries in the female) or sperm (testes in the male).

Gonin's operation Thermocautery of the fissure in the retina, performed through an opening in the sclera, for retinal detachment.

goniophotography Ocular photography for medical evaluation and documentation.

gonioscopy A diagnostic procedure using a mirror or lens device placed directly upon the cornea that is used to view the drainage area through which aqueous fluid exits the eyeball.

goniosynechiae Focal iris synechiae to the spur or posterior meshwork.

goniotomy Surgical opening of Schlemm's canal by way of the angle of the anterior chamber of the eye to treat congenital glaucoma.

gonococcal infection A sexually transmitted disease caused by gonococcal bacteria that affects the mucous membrane chiefly of the genital and urinary tracts and is characterized by an acute purulent discharge and painful or difficult urination, though women often have no symptoms.

gonorrhea Infectious disease of the reproductive organs and other body structures that is sexually transmitted (venereal disease). The most prominent symptom is a thick, green-yellow discharge from the penis or vagina. Antibiotics usually effect a cure.

Goodpasture syndrome Acute glomerulonephritis with intra-pulmonary hemorrhage, hemo-ptysis and anemia, usually progressing to renal failure.

gout A painful inflammation of the big toe and foot caused by defects in uric acid metabolism resulting in deposits of the acid and its salts in the blood and joints.

GP General practice.

GPCI Geographic Practice Cost Index.

GPWW Group Practice Without Walls.

Grace Period A set number of days past the due date of a premium payment during which medical coverage may not be canceled and through which the premium payment may be made.

Graduate Medical Education (GME) Medical education as an intern, resident or fellow after graduating from a medical school.

graft Created by using portions of another artery or vein from the patient's body to reroute blood around a blockage.

grafting A procedure in which healthy skin and/or muscle is moved from one area of the body to another area damaged by disease or injury.

Graft-Versus-Host Disease (GVHD) A disease caused by the infusion or transplantation of immune cells from one individual into another.

-gram Record or picture.

grand mal epilepsy A form of epilepsy characterized by tonic-clonic seizures. Involving two phases -- the tonic phase in which the body becomes rigid, and clonic phase in which there is uncontrol-led jerking.

granulocytes A type of white blood cell that attacks and destroys foreign substances. These are leukocytes which have specific granules. The three different types of granulocytes have different types of specific granules. Granulocytes are spherical in shape, contain nuclei and include neutrophils, eosinophils, and basophils. These cells are part of the formed elements of whole blood.

granulomas Nodule of firm tissue formed as a reaction to chronic inflammation, such as from foreign bodies or bacteria.

granulomatosis Formation of multiple granulomas. Each has nodules of granulated tissue forming a tumor like mass.

-graph Record or picture.

graphism tests Two point discrimination and numbers written on the skin assist in the detection of parietal brain lesions.

-graphy Process of recording.

grasp reflex The palm is stroked. If the patient grasps the examiner's finger and frequently is unable to release the examiner's finger, the test is termed positive. This reflex disappears in the infant by the age of nine months, but is seen in the adult with frontal lobe injury, anoxic and severe toxic states. *Synonym:* Palmer reflex.

Graves' disease Disorder of the thyroid gland occurring most often in women. Characterized by bulging eyes, rapid pulse rate, profuse sweating, restlessness, irritability and weight loss.

gravid In an advanced stage of pregnancy.

greater saphenous veins Veins in the leg often used as a source for a bypass graft to be placed during open heart surgery.

GRH Growth hormone-releasing hormone.

grievance Request made to a health plan to reconsider coverage of a health care service that the health plan has not interpreted to be a covered benefit.

group contract A contract between an HMO and a subscribing group of beneficiaries which specifies rates, performance, relationships, schedule of benefits, and other conditions, usually for a 12 month period.

group health insurance Health insurance purchased through a group that exists for some purpose other than buying insurance, such as a workplace, labor union, or professional association.

group health plan A health plan that provides health coverage to employees, former employees, and their families, and is supported by an employer or employee organization.

group home A residence, with shared living areas, where clients receive supervision and other services such as social and/or behavioral services, custodial service, and minimal services (e.g., medication administration).

group insurance Any insurance policy or health services contract by which groups of employees (and often their dependents) are covered under a single policy or contract, issued by their employer or other group entity.

group model HMO An HMO that contracts with a multi-specialty medical group to provide care for HMO members; members are required to receive medical care from a physician within the group unless a referral is made outside the network.

group practice association A formal arrangement of three or more physicians or other health professionals providing health services. Income is pooled and redistributed to the members of the group according to a prearranged plan.

group practice HMO model An HMO model in which the HMO contracts with one or more medical group(s) on a capitation basis for the provision of services. The physicians practice in a common facility and use common staff. Income is pooled and distributed according to an agreed-upon plan.

group practice without walls A legal entity that combines multiple independent physician practices under one umbrella organization and performs certain business operations for the member practices or arranges for these operations to be performed.

group provider identification number A provider identification number assigned to an entity where more than one practitioner is rendering services. This number allows payment to be made under one name and one tax identification number.

Group Purchasing Organization (GPO) An organization that pools purchasers working together to provide larger potential purchases and therefore lower costs.

GROUPER A software program used to group medical records for acute hospital stays into Diagnostic Related Groups (DRGs) and Major Diagnostic Categories (MDCs) for case mix purposes. The grouping is based on both clinical information (diagnoses and procedures) and demographic information such as age and sex. The clinical information is coded using ICD-9-CM.

growth hormone deficiency Deficiency of hormone that results in dwarfism.

GSW Gunshot wound.

GT Gait training.

GTT Glucose Tolerance Test.

GU Genitourinary.

guaiac test One for occult blood; glacial acetic acid and a solution of gum guaiac are mixed with the specimen; on addition of hydrogen peroxide, the presence of blood is indicated by a blue tint.

guaranteed issue The requirement that an insurer or health plan accept everyone, regardless of health, income or age, that applies for coverage and guarantees the renewal of that coverage as long as the premium is paid.

guaranteed renewability The requirement that each insurer and health plan continue to renew health policies purchased by individuals as long as the person continues to pay the premium for the policy.

guidelines Guidelines are systematically developed by appropriate groups to assist practitioners and patient decisions about appropriate health care for specific clinical circumstances.

Guillain-Barré syndrome Acute idiopathic polyneuritis; rapidly progressing ascending motor neuron paralysis usually beginning with the feet and spreading to the legs, arms, trunk and face.

gull disease Atrophy of the thyroid with myxedema (hypothyroidism).

gum recession The exposure of dental roots due to shrinkage of the gums as a result of abrasion, periodontal disease or surgery.

gyn Gynecologic, gynecology, gynecologist.

gyn(ec)o- Woman.

gynecologic surgery The specialty of treating problems with the female reproductive system with surgery.

gynecomastia Excessive development of the breasts in males; usually the result of hormonal imbalance or treatment with certain drugs (including some antihypertensives).

H

H & P History and physical.

H reflex A monosynaptic reflex elicited by stimulating a nerve, particularly the tibial nerve, with an electric shock.

Hageman factor Deficiency of this factor results in prolonged bleeding. *Synonym:* Factor XII.

hai Hemagglutination inhibition.

hair follicle Part of the skin that grows hair by packing old cells together.

Halifax fusion Clamp across lamina of C-1 and C-2.

hallux valgus Lateral displacement of the great toe, producing deformity of the first metatarso-phalangeal joint with callous, bursa, or bunion formation over the bony prominence.

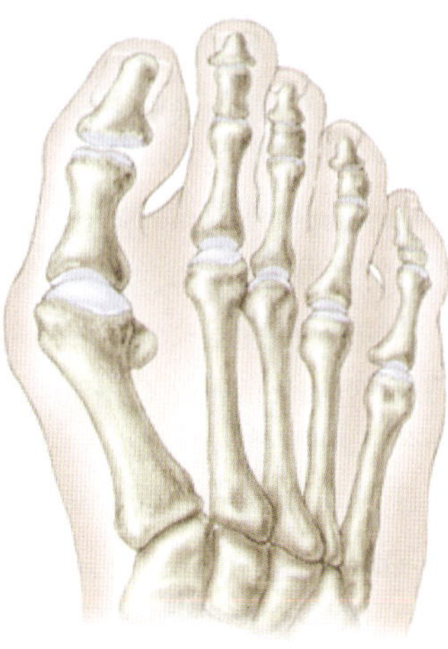

Hallux valgus

Halsted mastectomy Removal of the breast, pectoral muscles, axillary lymph nodes, and associated skin and subcutaneous tissue.

hamartoses A benign focal malformation resembling a neoplasm, composed of an overgrowth of mature cells and tissues that normally occur in the affected area.

Hand-Schueller-Christian disease Group of three symptoms that may occur in any of several disorders. Symptoms include marked protrusion of eyeballs (exophthalmos), diabetes insipidus and bone destruction.

Hansen's disease Leprosy.

hantavirus A virus transmitted to humans from the dried droppings, urine, or saliva of mice and rats. The disease begins as a flu-like illness characterized by fever, chills, and muscle aches, but can rapidly progress to a life-threatening condition marked by respiratory failure as the lungs fill with fluid.

haplotypes The genetic constitution of individuals with respect to one member of a pair of genes; sets of single alleles or closely linked genes that tend to be inherited together, such as those of the major histocompatibility complex; portions of phenotypes determined by genes located on one of a pair of chromosomes.

haptoglobin test A test for the evaluation of hemolytic anemia.

harelip *See* cleft palate.

Harii procedure A procedure for insertion of a vascular pedicle into a carpal bone.

Harrington rod Instrumentation and fusion using a straight, stiff rod for distraction or compression; associated with a posterior spinal fusion in the thoracic or thoraco-lumbar spine for scoliosis or trauma.

Hartmann pouch Abnormal pouch formed at the neck of the gallbladder.

Hartmann solution Intravenous lactated Ringer's solution.

Hartmann's operation Resection of a diseased portion of the colon, with the proximal end of the colon brought out as a colostomy and the distal stump or rectum being closed by suture.

Hartnup disease Hereditary disease that causes skin rash, unsteady gait and excess amino acids in the urine.

Harvard Relative Value Study A study completed at Harvard University to develop a resource-based relative value scale.

HASHD Hypertensive Arteriosclerotic Heart Disease.

Hashimoto's thyroiditis One of several kinds of thyroid gland inflammation.

HASP Hospital Admission and Surveillance Program.

Hauser procedure A surgical procedure for recurrent dislocation of the patella.

HAV Hepatitis A Virus.

HCEC Hospital Care Evaluation Committee.

HCFA Health Care Financing Administration, former name of the Center for Medicare & Medicaid.

HCFA1450 HCFA's name for the institutional uniform claim form, or UB-92.

HCFA1500 Uniform health insurance claim form used for billing services to Medicare and other insurance carriers.

HCG Human Chorionic Gonadotropin.

HCM Hypertrophic cardiomyopathy.

HCPCS Health care Common Procedure Coding System. A two-level coding system, consisting of CPT, and National or Level II codes used to report and bill services provided to Medicare patients.

HCQIA Health Care Quality Improvement Act.

HCQIP Health Care Quality Improvement Program.

HCS Human Chorionic Somatomammotropin.

HCT Hematocrit.

HCVD Hypersensitive Cardiovascular Disease.

HDL High Density Lipoprotein.

health alliances Nonprofit agencies that act as the health insurance purchasing agent for consumers under a system of managed competition, organized at either the state or regional level, or by employer groups. These alliances negotiated with provider networks to get the best plan at the lowest cost and would serve defined regions or classes of customers.

Health and Human Services (HHS) The federal government department that has overall responsibility for implementing HIPAA.

Health and Welfare Fund Health care benefit funds established under provisions of the Taft-Hartley Act, financed through employer and employee contributions, and administered by a board composed equally of representatives from labor and management.

health benefits manager Independent organization that provides functions to assist enrollees. This may include information, acting as an enrollment broker, handling complaints and grievances etc.

health care clearinghouse Under HIPAA, this is an entity that processes or facilitates the processing of information received from another entity in a nonstandard format or containing nonstandard data content into standard data elements or a standard transaction, or that receives a standard transaction from another entity and processes or facilitates the processing of that information into nonstandard format or nonstandard data content for a receiving entity.

health care coalition Voluntary alliance of discrete interests sharing the principal objective of improving access to high quality health care services provided in a cost effective manner.

health care data base Collection of information on health care episodes, such as utilization, costs, or charges.

health care decision counseling Services, sometimes provided by insurance companies or employers, that help individuals weigh the benefits, risks and costs of medical tests and treatments. Unlike case management, health care decision counseling is non-judgmental. The goal of health care decision counseling is to help individuals make more informed choices about their health and medical care needs, and to help them make decisions that are right for the individual's unique set of circumstances.

health care delivery system That combination of insurance companies, employer groups, providers of care and government agencies that work together to provide health care to a population.

Health Care Financing Administration (HCFA) Former name of the agency within the U.S. Department of Health and Human Services that is responsible for the administration of the Medicare and Medicaid programs. Now known as the Center for Medicare and Medicaid Services (CMS).

health care prepayment A health plan with a Medicare cost contract to provide only Medicare Part B premiums. Some administrative requirements for these plans are less stringent than those of risk contracts or other cost contracts.

Health Care Prepayment System (HCPP) A cost contract with HCFA that prepays a health plan a flat amount per month to provide Medicare-eligible Part B medical services to enrolled members. Members pay premiums to cover the Medicare coinsurance, deductibles and co-payments, plus any additional non-Medicare covered services that the plan provides. The HCPP does not arrange for Part A services.

health care provider An individual or institution that provides medical services.

health care provider taxonomy committee An organization administered by the NUCC that is responsible for maintaining the Provider Taxonomy coding scheme used in the X12 transactions.

health care proxy A health care proxy is recognized in some states as an alternate method for naming a person to act on one's behalf in health care decision making. In a few states, a health care proxy may be included as part of a living will.

Health Care Quality Improvement Act (HCQIA) A federal act which exempts hospitals, group practices, and HMOs from certain antitrust provisions as they apply to credentialing and peer review so long as these entities adhere to due process standards that are outlined in the Act.

health care quality improvement program A program which supports the mission of CMS to assure health care security for beneficiaries. The mission of HCQIP is to promote the quality, effectiveness, and efficiency of services to Medicare beneficiaries by strengthening the community of those committed to improving quality, by monitoring and improving quality of care; by communicating with beneficiaries and health care providers, practitioners; and by plans to promote informed health choices, to protect beneficiaries from poor care, and to strengthen the infrastructure.

health care reform Changes in the organization, delivery and financing of health care to improve access, quality and to reduce the cost of care.

Health Employer Data and Information Set (HEDIS) A set of standard performance measures that provides information about the quality of a health plan. These measures are used to compare managed care plans.

health information Health information, under HIPAA, means any information, whether oral or recorded in any form or medium, that is created or received by a health care provider, health plan, public health authority, employer, life insurer, etc.

health information network An electronic system that uses telecommunications devices to link various health care entities within a geographic region in order to exchange patient, clinical, and financial information in an effort to reduce costs and practice better medicine.

health insurance A mechanism to spread the risk of unforeseen expenditures across a broad base to protect the individual from personal expenditures for health care services. Health insurance may be purchased individually or on a group basis. It may be custom designed to cover specific services and procedures and include requirements to control the level of use and payment for these services. An employee health insurance benefit is a nontaxable form of compensation to the employee in lieu of taxable salary or wages, provided through employment.

Various types of insurance, such as accident, disability income, medical expense, dental, vision, hearing, and accidental death and dismemberment may be made available through employment. Benefits may be available to dependents of active employees, retirees, spouses, survivors, and dependents through employment. Benefits for classes of active and retired employees and their dependents need not be uniform. The employer may purchase benefits or the costs may be shared between the employer and employee.

Health Insurance Association of **American (HIAA)** A corporate member trade association of health and accident insurance companies; based in Washington, D.C.

Health Insurance Claim Number (HICN) The number listed on the beneficiary's Medicare card consisting of nine digits followed by one or more letters. The nine digits represent the Social Security number of either the beneficiary or their spouse depending upon whose income it is based upon.

Health Insurance Portability and Accountability Act (HIPAA) The 1996 Federal legislation that makes long-term care insurance premiums tax deductible if non-reimbursable medical expenses, including part or all of long-term care premiums, exceed 7.5% of an individual's gross income. HIPPA also excludes long-term care insurance benefits from taxable income. Not all long-term care insurance coverage qualifies for this benefit.

health insurance trust fund The Federal hospital insurance trust fund is a fund of the Treasury of the United States in which the monies collected from taxes on the annual earnings of employees, employers, and self-employed people covered by Social Security are deposited. Disbursements from the fund are made to help pay for benefit payments and administrative expenses incurred by the hospital insurance program (Medicare Part A).

health insuring organization A hybrid of a state-funded health plan and a health maintenance organization. It is usually a public corporation that pays for medical services provided to recipients in exchange for payment of a premium or subscription charges paid for by the corporation that assumes the underwriting risk.

health maintenance organization A public or private organization providing, either directly or through arrangements with others, a comprehensive range of health services to enrolled members who live within a specified service area. Payment is based on a predetermined periodic rate, or periodic per capita rate, without regard to the frequency or extent of covered services furnished to any particular member. The HMO must also meet statutory requirements.

health maintenance organization or federally qualified A public or private organization that contracts on a prepaid capitated risk basis to provide a comprehensive set of services and is federally qualified.

health maintenance organization or state plan defined A public or private organization that contracts on a prepaid capitated risk basis to provide a comprehensive set of services and is state plan defined.

Health Manpower Shortage Area (HMSA) An area or group which the U.S. Department of Health and Human Services designates as having an inadequate supply of health care providers. HMSAs can include (1) an urban or rural geographic area, (2) a population group for which access barriers can be demonstrated that prevent members of the group from using local providers, or (3) public or non-profit private residential facilities. Also see health professional shortage area.

health plan An organization that acts as an insurer for an enrolled population. May be structured as a fee-for-service or managed care plan.

Health Plan Employer Data and Information Sets (HEDIS) A set of performance measures designed to standardize the way health plans report data to employers. HEDIS measures five major areas of health plan performance quality, access and patient satisfaction, membership and utilization, finance, and descriptive information on health plan management.

health plan purchasing cooperative A health insurance purchasing entity advanced by some health system reform proposals to enroll individuals, collect premiums, purchase enrollee's health insurance from participating health plans, and enforce the rules that manage health plan competition.

Health Professional Shortage Area (HPSA) A geographic area, population group, or medical facility that DHHS determines to be served by too few health professionals of particular specialties. Physicians who provide services in HPSAs qualify for the Medicare bonus payments, repayment of medical school loans or other incentives. Also see health manpower shortage area.

health promotion programs Preventive care programs designed to educate and motivate members to prevent illness and injury and to promote good health through lifestyle choices, such as smoking cessation and dietary changes. *Synonym:* wellness programs.

health risk appraisal Health risk assessment.

health risk assessment A process by which an MCO uses inform-ation about a plan member's health status, personal and family health history, and health-related behaviors to predict the member's likelihood of experiencing specific illnesses or injuries. *Synonym:* health risk appraisal.

Health Savings Account (HSA) Operating similarly to iras, hsas are tax-advantaged savings accounts for health care services. A person must enroll in a qualified High-Deductible Health Plan (HDHP) before they can establish an HSA.

health services The health care services or supplies covered under the plan contract.

Health Services Corporation (HSC) General term to refer to a provider of an array of health services. Sometimes used in the insurance field to designate organizations that are required to meet special licensure require-ments.

health services for the aged Services for the diagnosis and treatment of diseases in the aged and the maintenance of health in the elderly.

health services misuse Excessive or unnecessary utilization of health services by patients or physicians.

Health care Common Procedural Coding System (HCPCS) Federal coding system for medical procedures. HCPCS includes CPT (Current Procedural Terminology) codes and national alpha-numeric codes. The national codes are developed by HCFA to supplement CPT codes. They include physical services not included in CPT as well as non-physician services such as ambulance, physical therapy and durable medical equipment. HCPCS codes are 5-digit codes, the first digit a letter followed by four numbers.

Health care Financial Management Association (HFMA) The nation's leading personal member-ship organization for more than 35,000 financial management professionals employed by hospitals, integrated delivery systems, long-term and ambulatory care facilities, managed care organizations, medical group practices, public accounting and consulting firms, insurance companies, government agencies, and other health care organizations.

Health Care Information Management Systems Society A professional organization for health care information and management systems professionals.

health care provider taxonomy codes An administrative code set that classifies health care providers by type and area of specialization. The code set will be used in certain adopted transactions.

health care quality The degree to which health services for individuals and populations increase the likelihood of desired health outcomes and are consistent with current professional knowledge.

Healthy Start A Medicaid program that provides health care for pregnant women and children who are at or below a specified level of income and age.

hearing A procedure that gives a dissatisfied claimant an opportunity to present reasons for the dissatisfaction and to receive a new determination based on the record developed at the hearing.

hearing loss The partial or complete loss of hearing.

heart The muscle that pumps blood received from veins into arteries throughout the body. It is positioned in the chest behind the sternum and above the diaphragm muscle.

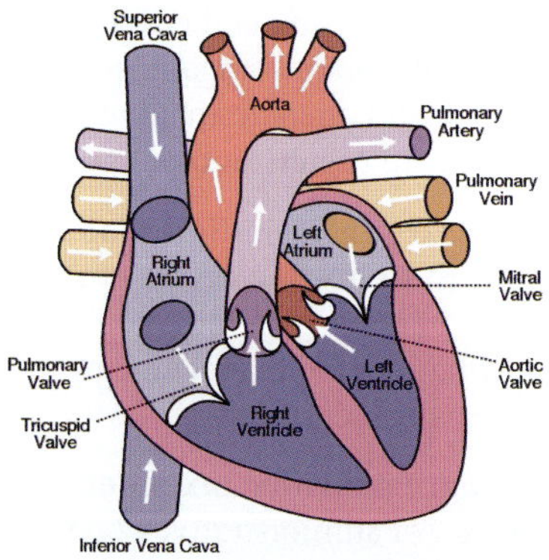

heart attack A heart attack occurs when the heart does not get enough blood flow leading to the death of the heart muscle. *Synonym:* myocardial infarction.

heart failure Heart failure is a degenerative condition that occurs when the heart muscle weakens and the ventricle no longer contracts normally. The heart can then no longer pump enough blood to the body. This may limit exercise tolerance, or may cause fluid retention.

heart rate The number of heart beats per unit time, usually per minute. The heart rate is based on the number of contractions of the ventricles (the lower chambers of the heart). The heart rate may be too fast (tachycardia) or too slow (bradycardia).

heart valve prosthesis implantation Surgical insertion of synthetic material to repair injured or diseased heart valves.

heart-assist devices Small pumps, often implantable, designed for temporarily assisting the heart, usually the left ventricle, to pump blood; they consist of a pumping chamber and a power source, which may be partially or totally external to the body.

heart-lung machine Functions as the patient's heart and lungs during the conventional bypass surgery. *Synonym:* cardiopulmonary bypass.

Heberden nodes Bony prominence and flexion deformities of the finger joints associated with osteoarthritis.

HEDIS Health plan Employer Data and Information Set.

HEENT Head, Eyes, Ears, Nose and Throat.

Heimlich maneuver Method of dislodging a foreign body from the airway by applying quick thrust pressure to the subdiaphragmatic area.

Heine operation Surgical opening of a passage between the anterior chamber and the suprachoroidal space in order to reduce pressure within the eye in glaucoma.

Heinz bodies Granular deposits in red blood cells from precipitation of proteins. They are present in certain hemolytic anemias. *See* Anemia, hemolytic.

helicobacter pylori A Gram-negative, microaerophilic bact-erium that can inhabit various areas of the stomach and duo-denum. It causes a chronic low-level inflam-mation of the stomach lining and is strongly linked to the development of duodenal and gastric ulcers and stomach cancer.

helminthiasis A disease in which a part of the body is infested with worms such as pinworm, round-worm or tapeworm. Typically, the worms reside in the gastrointestinal tract but may also burrow into the liver and other organs.

hema or hemo- blood.

hemagglutination The agglutination of red blood cells caused by an antibody either for red blood cell antigens or for antigens that coat red blood cells or by the presence of viruses or other microbes.

hemangioma Benign tumor made up of a mass of blood vessels.

hemapheresis *See* apheresis.

hemarthrosis A bleeding into joint spaces.

hemat-, hem- of or pertaining to blood.

hematemesis The vomiting of blood.

hematocele Swelling caused by blood collecting in a body cavity (especially a swelling of the membrane covering the testis).

hematochezia The passage of maroon colored stool.

hematocrit The measure of packed red blood cells to plasma in the blood reported as a percentage. Low levels (<30%) are seen in anemia and blood loss. A high hematocrit (e.g., 70%) produces problems as well, but is uncommon.

hematologic of the blood.

hematologic agents Drugs that act on blood and blood-forming organs and those that affect the hemostatic system.

hematologic tests Tests used in the analysis of the hemic system.

hematologic, gastrointestinal, and renal agents A collective grouping for agents that act on the hematopoietic, gastrointestinal, and renal systems.

hematologist A physician special-izing in the treatment of blood disorders.

hematology The study of blood, the blood-forming organs, and blood diseases. Hematology includes the study of etiology, diagnosis, treatment, prognosis, and prevention of blood diseases.

hematoma Collection of blood that has escaped from a blood vessel and is localized in an organ or tissue.

hematopoiesis The process of formation, development, and differentiation of the formed elements of whole blood. *Synonym:* hemopoiesis.

hematuria Abnormal presence of blood in the urine. May be gross (can actually see the blood) or microscopic (seen only under a microscope). Is usually a sign of kidney disease or urinary tract disorder.

hemeralopia Day blindness. Often caused by clouding or opacity of one or more of the normally clear ocular tissues.

hemi- One-half.

hemiarthroplasty A surgical procedure which replaces one half of the joint with an artificial surface and leaves the other part in its natural. This procedure is most commonly performed on the hip after a hip fracture.

hemic of or relating to the blood.

hemicrania A headache affecting only one side of the head, usually migraine.

hemiepiphyseal arrest A surgical procedure using a screw and plate device to treat knee and ankle deformities in children.

hemiglossectomy The surgical removal of half of the tongue.

hemilaminectomy Removal of a vertebral lamina on one side only.

hemilaryngectomy Excision of one lateral half of the larynx.

hemiparesis Muscle weakness on one side of the body.

hemipelvectomies Amputation of an entire leg together with one lateral half of the pelvis on the same side. *Synonym:* interpelviabdominal amputation.

hemiphalangectomy Excision of part of a digital phalanx.

hemiplegia Paralysis or loss of voluntary motion, on one side of the body; may include head and neck, trunk and/or limbs. Hemiparesis is weakness on one side of the body.

hemiplegic Of, pertaining to, or afflicted with hemiplegia.

hemispherectomy A surgical procedure where one cerebral hemisphere (half of the brain) is removed or disabled. This procedure is used to treat a variety of seizure disorders where the source of the epilepsy is localized to a broad area of a single hemisphere of the brain.

hemochromatosis A hereditary disorder that causes your body tissues to absorb and store too much iron. One cannot catch Hemochromatosis. It is a hereditary condition, primarily. The disease (which is actually many diseases) has also been known to develop as a result of dietary iron intake in sufficient quantity. Its worst effects are preventable, by early diagnosis and treatment, but, if the patient is not found in time, it is crippling and potentially fatal.

hemoconcentration Decrease of the fluid content of the blood, with resulting increase in concentration of blood cells.

hemocytoblast A stem cell derived from the embryonic mesenchyme and considered to be capable of developing into any type of blood cell.

hemodiafiltration Simultaneous hemodialysis and hemofiltration which involves the removal of large volumes of fluid and fluid replacement to maintain hemodynamic stability.

hemodialysis A method of dialysis in which blood from a patient's body is circulated through an external device or machine and then returned to the patient's bloodstream.

hemodilution Increase in fluid content of blood, with resulting decrease in concentration of blood cells.

hemodynamic The study of the forces involved in the circulation of blood.

hemofiltration Fluid removal.

hemoglobin The molecule in the red blood cell that carries oxygen. Hemoglobin combines with oxygen in the lungs and releases it in the tissues. It is what makes blood red.

hemoglobin-c disease Inherited blood disorder characterized by a moderate, chronic hemolytic anemia and associated with the presence of hemoglobin C, an abnormal form of the red cell pigment.

hemogram A graphic representation of the differential blood count.

hemolysin Any substance that can cause lysis (destruction) of erythrocytes (red blood cells) and the release of their hemoglobin.

hemolysis Process by which red blood cells breakdown and hemoglobin is released. Occurs normally at the end of the life span of a red blood cell. It may also occur abnormally with certain diseases or conditions such as hemolytic anemia.

hemolytic Condition in which red blood cells break down and release the hemoglobin they contain.

hemolytic disease Disorder characterized by the premature destruction of red blood cells. May or may not result in anemia, depending on the ability of the bone marrow to increase production of red blood cells.

hemolytic episode Separation of hemoglobin from red blood cells.

hemolytic jaundice Jaundice caused by severe hemolytic anemia, which results in high levels of unconjugated bilirubin. Leads to a jaundiced appearance.

hemoperfusion A medical process used to remove toxic substances from a patients blood. The technique involves passing large volumes of blood over an adsorbent substance.

hemopericardium Refers to blood in the pericardial sac of the heart. It is a cause of pericardial effusion, and can also cause cardiac tamponade.

hemoperitoneum The presence of blood in the peritoneal cavity.

hemophilia Inherited deficiency of a blood clotting factor that may result in bleeding episodes. Characterized by bleeding into joints, muscles and skin, excessive bleeding from minor cuts, nosebleeds and blood in urine.

hemophilus influenzae Bacteria that causes numerous diseases in children. Two of these diseases are especially serious. Meningitis (infection of the brain and spinal cord) can cause death or permanent brain damage. Epiglottitis is a condition of the throat in which the child can choke to death.

hemoptysis Coughing up blood from the respiratory tract. blood-streaked sputum can occur with minor upper respiratory tract infections. A greater amount of blood may indicate a serious disease or infection.

hemorrhage Flow of blood from a ruptured blood vessels.

hemorrhagic of or relating to a hemorrhage.

hemorrhagic disease Medical problem accompanied by uncontrolled bleeding.

hemorrhagic fever A group of viral infections characterized by fever, chills, headache, malaise, and respiratory or gastrointestinal symptoms, followed by capillary hemorrhages and, in severe infection, by oliguria, kidney failure, hypotension, and possibly death.

hemorrhagic gastritis Inflammation of stomach accompanied by bleeding from stomach lining.

hemorrhoid A swollen blood vessel in and around the anus that cause itching, pain, and sometimes bleeding.

hemorrhoidectomy Surgical removal of a hemorrhoid.

hemorrhoidopexy A surgical procedure for the treatment of prolapsing hemorrhoids.

hemorrhoids Dilated (varicose) veins of the rectum or anus. Usually caused by straining during bowel movements, although pressure from a rectal tumor or pregnancy may cause them. Symptoms may include rectal bleeding, pain, itching or mucus discharge after bowel movements and a lump that can be felt in the anus.

hemostasis Surgical procedure of stopping the flow of blood.

hemostatic techniques Techniques for controlling bleeding.

hemothorax Accumulation of blood in the pleural cavity (the space between the lungs and the walls of the chest).

Henoch-Schonlein purpura Allergic or anaphylactic purpura (an inflammation of small blood vessels of the skin, joint, gastro-intestinal tract and kidneys).

heparin An anticoagulant medicine (blood thinner) routinely prescribed for the treatment of clotting disorders.

heparin therapy Course of treatment with medication that prolongs blood clotting time. Used to prevent or treat blood clots.

heparinized To render blood nonclottable with heparin. For example, tubes used to collect blood often have heparin in them so blood does not coagulate.

hepat- of or pertaining to the liver.

hepatectomy Excision of all or part of the liver.

hepatic of or relating to the liver.

hepatic coma Stupor or coma caused by waste products in the blood that are toxic to the brain. Normally, waste products are neutralized by the liver, but due to extensive liver damage they continue to circulate in the blood.

hepatic disease Any disease involving the liver, including many types of hepatitis and cirrhosis.

hepatic dysfunction Poor liver function.

hepaticodochotomy Incision into the common bile duct and the hepatic duct.

hepaticoenterostomy The surgical formation of a communication between a hepatic duct and the intestine.

hepaticostomy The surgical formation of an opening into a hepatic duct.

hepaticotomy Incision into a hepatic duct.

hepatitis Inflammatory liver condition characterized by jaundice, enlarged liver, loss of appetite, abdominal discomfort, abnormal liver function, dark urine and clay-colored stool. Can be caused by bacterial or viral infection, parasites, alcohol, drugs or blood transfusions with incompatible blood. Symptoms may be mild, severe or life-threatening.

hepatitis B Form of viral hepatitis caused by the hepatitis-B virus. Characterized by rapid onset of acute signs and symptoms. *See* Hepatitis. Usually enters the body through blood transfusions contaminated with the virus or by the use of contaminated needles or instruments. Infection may be very severe and result in prolonged illness, cirrhosis or death. *See* Cirrhosis.

hepatitis Bsurface antigen An indicator of a probable hepatitis B carrier (serum hepatitis.).

hepatitis C In the United States, the most common blood-borne infection and a major cause of liver damage. HCV is spread primarily through contact with infected blood. It is responsible for 8,000 to 10,000 deaths in the United States annually. Many people have the disease for years before it is detected.

hepatitis panel A blood test used to find markers of hepatitis infection.

hepatobiliary of or relating to the liver plus the gallbladder, bile ducts, or bile.

hepatocellular carcinoma The most common primary malignant tumor of the liver.

hepatocellular injury Injury of liver cells.

hepatomas Malignant tumor that begins in the liver (primary site of cancer), as opposed to liver cancer that has spread from another site. *Synonym:* malignant liver tumor, hepatocellular carcinoma.

hepatomegaly Abnormal enlargement of the liver.

hepatorenal syndrome A life-threatening medical condition that consists of rapid deterioration in kidney function in individuals with cirrhosis or fulminant liver failure.

hepatorrhaphy Suture of a wound of the liver.

hepatotomy Incision into the liver.

hepatotoxicity Tendency of a substance, usually a medication or alcohol, to have a destructive effect on the liver.

hereditary Transmitted genetically from generation to generation.

hereditary anti-edema Inherited condition that prevents accumulation of fluid.

hereditary spherocytosis Inherited disorder characterized by small, spherical red blood cells, leading to anemia because abnormal cells are fragile. *See* Anemia.

hernia Protrusion of an internal organ through a weakness or abnormal opening in the muscle around it. The most common types are inguinal hernia (in groin), femoral hernia (in groin), incisional hernia (at surgery site), umbilical hernia (at navel) and hiatal hernia. Umbilical hernias rarely require surgery. Other hernias are usually curable with surgery.

herniated disc Extrusion of part of the nucleus pulposus material through a defect in the annulus fibrosus.

hernioplasty Surgical correction of a hernia.

herniorrhaphy The surgical repair of a hernia.

herniotomy The surgical correction of a hernia by cutting through a band of tissue that constricts it. *Synonym:* celotomy.

herpes Herpes type-1 causes common cold sores, which appear around the mouth. Herpes type-2 (HSV-2) is a viral infection of the genitals transmitted by sexual intercourse. Type-2 herpes infection can be transmitted to a newborn from an actively infected mother. It can be fatal to the child.

herpes simplex Infection caused by the herpes simplex virus; affects the skin and nervous system; produces small temporary blisters on the skin and mucous membranes.

herpes zoster A viral disease characterized by a painful skin rash with blisters in a limited area on one side of the body, often in a stripe.

heter(o)- Denotes something as 'the other' (of two), as an addition, or different.

heterocyclic compounds Ring compounds having atoms other than carbon in their nuclei.

heterograft A type of tissue graft in which the donor and recipient are of different species.

heterophoria An eye condition where the motion of the eyes are not parallel to each other.

heterotropia *See* strabismus.

heterozygous A genotype consisting of two different alleles of a gene for a particular trait (Aa). Individuals who are heterozygous for a trait are referred to as heterozygotes.

Hey's hernia An encysted hernia.

Heyman capsule A method of treating uterine cancer with intracavitary radium sources.

Heyman procedure A surgical procedure for the treatment of slipped upper femoral epiphysis.

HFMA Health care financial management association.

HGB Hemoglobin.

HHA Home Health Agency.

HHD Hypertensive Heart Disease.

HHQI Home Health Quality Initiative.

HI Health insurance.

hiatal hernia Abnormal weakness or opening in the diaphragm. Allows a portion of the stomach to protrude through the diaphragm. If symptoms occur (often there are none), they usually appear at least 1 hour after eating and may include heartburn, belching and sometimes difficulty swallowing. Treatment usually relieves symptoms. Surgery is rarely required.

HIB Hospital Insurance Benefits.

Hibbs spinal fusion Lumbar spinal fusion that includes fusing the spinous process, lamina, and facet for stabilization.

Hickman catheterization An intravenous catheter most often used for the administration of chemotherapy or other medi-cations, as well as for the with-drawal of blood for analysis.

hidr(o)- Sweat.

hidradenitis A chronic condition characterized by swollen, painful, inflamed lesions in the axillae, groin, and other parts of the body that contain apocrine glands.

hierarchy A system that ranks items one above another.

high risk area A potential flaw in management controls requiring management attention and possible corrective action.

high risk pregnancy One in which some condition puts the mother, the developing fetus, or both at higher-than-normal risk for complications during or after the pregnancy and birth.

high-purine diet Diet of foods that are high in purines, including anchovies and sardines, organ meats, legumes and poultry. *See* Purine. Increased intake of purines may lead to development of uric acid stones (a type of kidney stone). *See* Kidney stones.

Hill-Burton Program Federal program created in 1946 to provide funding for the construction and modernization of health care facilities. Hospitals which receive Hill-Burton funds must provide specific levels of charity care.

Hill procedure A surgical procedure for the treatment of reflux esophagitis.

HIMSS Health Care Information Management Systems Society.

HINN Hospital Issued Notice of Non-Coverage.

HIPP Health Insurance Premium Program.

HIPPA Health Insurance Portability and Accountability Act of 1996. There are two sections to the Act. HIPAA Title I deals with protecting health insurance coverage for people who lose or change jobs. HIPAA Title II includes an administrative simplification section which deals with the standardization of health care-related information systems.

hippocampus An area buried deep in the forebrain that helps regulate emotion and memory. Functionally, the hippocampus is part of the olfactory cortex, that part of the cerebral cortex essential to the sense of smell.

HIPPS Health Insurance Prospective Payment System. Procedural coding used in the HCPCS or Accommodation Rates or HIPPS Rate Codes field on institutional claim formats in association with certain CMS prospective payment systems (skilled nursing facility, home health).

Hirschberg sign Adduction reflex of the foot.

Hirschsprung's disease Congenital megacolon.

HIS Hospital Information Service.

hist(o)-, histio- Tissue.

histamine test 1. Subcutaneous injection of 0.1 per cent solution of histamine to stimulate gastric secretion. 2. After rapid intravenous injection of histamine phosphate, normal persons experience a brief fall in blood pressure, but in those with pheochromocytoma, after the fall, there is a marked rise in blood pressure.

histidinemia Hereditary defect of metabolism marked by excess histidine (an amino acid) in the blood and urine. Many people with this defect show mild mental retardation and improper speech development.

histiocytosis A rare blood disease that is caused by an excess of white blood cells called histiocytes.

histochemistry The study of the chemical components of cells and tissues.

histocompatibility testing Identification of the major histocompatibility antigens of transplant donors and potential recipients, usually by serological tests. Donor and recipient pairs should be of identical ABO blood group, and in addition should be matched as closely as possible.

histological The microscopic structure of tissue.

histology Science dealing with the microscopic identification of cells and tissue.

histoplasma capsulatum A microscopic fungus that causes the disease histoplasmosis.

histoplasmosis Fungal infection from breathing dust that contains fungus spores or through direct contact into an open skin wound. Fungus is found in the feces of birds and bats and in soil contaminated by feces. Although the acute disease is benign, other forms are very serious and may be fatal. *Synonym:* Darling's disease.

history of **present illness** A chronological description of the development of the patient's present illness from the first sign and/or symptom to the present.

histrionic personality disorder A personality disorder characterized by overly reactive and intensely expressed or overly dramatic behavior, proneness to exaggeration, emotional excitability, and disturbances in interpersonal relationships.

HIV Human Immunodeficiency Virus.

HIV antibody Presence of antibody is associated with having been infected by the virus known to cause AIDS (Acquired Immune Deficiency Syndrome).

HIVD Herniated intervertebral disc.

HKAFO Hip-Knee-Ankle-Foot Orthosis.

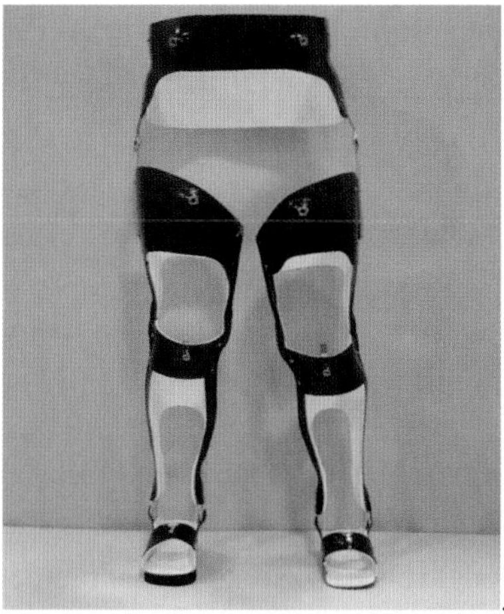

Hip-Knee-Ankle-Foot Orthosis

HKO Hip-Knee Orthosis (splint).

HLA type Antigens present on most cells of the body which are unique to the individual. It may be considered to be the individual's genetic fingerprint.

HMO Health Maintenance Organization.

HMO act The Health Maintenance Organization Act of 1973, also known as the HMO Act of 1973, provided grants and loans to provide, start, or expand a Health Maintenance Organization (HMO); removed certain state restrictions for federally qualified HMOs; and required employers with 25 or more employees to offer federally certified HMO options alongside traditional indemnity insurance upon request (the "dual choice provision"). HMOs were required to meet three basic requirements. These were to offer a specified list of benefits to all members, charge all members the same monthly premium, and be structured as a nonprofit organization. The Act solidified the term HMO and gave HMOs greater access to the employer-based market, providing for the rapid expansion of HMOs in later years.

HMO regulatory agency A state agency with the authority to grant or deny an HMO the right to do business in a state.

HMSA Health Manpower Shortage Area.

Hodgkin's disease Malignant tumor of the lymph glands characterized by progressive enlargement of the lymph nodes, loss of appetite, weight loss, fever, itching skin, night sweats and anemia. *Synonym:* Hodgkin's lymphoma.

Hodgson disease Uniform aneurysmal dilation of the aorta associated with insufficiency of the aortic valve, often accompanied by dilation or hypertrophy of the heart.

Hodgson procedure Anterior approach to C-1 and C-2 area for drainage of tuberculous abscess.

Hoffman apparatus An external fixation system for bone fractures.

Hofmeister operation Partial gastrectomy with anastomosis to the jejunum.

hold harmless A clause frequently found in managed care contracts, whereby the HMO and the physician agree not to hold each other liable for malpractice or corporate malfeasance if either of the parties is found to be liable. It may also refer to language that prohibits the provider from billing patients in the event a managed care company becomes insolvent.

Holter monitor A portable device for continuously monitoring various electrical activity of the central nervous system for at least 24 hours. The most common use is for monitoring the heart or ECG, but can also be used for monitoring EEG.

hom(o)- Denotes something as 'the same' as another or common.

Homan's sign Pain upon passive dorsiflexion of the foot as a positive sign for deep venous thrombus.

Home and Community-Based Services (HCBS) Programs which provide services in the home or at a convenient location in the community. Commonly these programs provide assistance with meals, transportation or homemaking.

home and community based waiver Medicaid waiver that provides a menu of community long term care services as an alternative to nursing home care. Limited to a specified number of slots in each state. The waiver generally provides a more liberal eligibility level than state plan Medicaid services.

home care In contrast with inpatient and ambulatory care, home care is medical care ordinarily administered in the house setting when a patient is not sufficiently ambulatory to make frequent office or hospital visits. With these patients, intravenous therapy for example is administered at the patient's residence, usually by a health care professional. Home care reduces the need for hospitalization and it's associated costs.

Home Health Agency (HHA) A public agency or private organization that is primarily engaged in providing the following services in the home; skilled nursing services, other therapeutic services (such as physical, occupational, or speech therapy), and home health aide services.

home health care Services given at home to aged, disabled, sick, or convalescent individuals not needing institutional care. The most common types of home care are visiting nurse services and speech, physical, occupational, and rehabilitation therapy. These services are provided by home health agencies, hospitals, or other community organizations.

Home Health Quality Initiative (HHQI) (HHA) Program administered by the Centers for Medicare and Medicaid Services (CMS) that aims to further improve the quality of care for Medicare beneficiaries who use home care through a combination of regulation and enforcement; improved consumer information; quality improvement programs; and collaboration and partnerships to leverage knowledge and resources.

home infusion therapy The intravenous administration of medication to patients in their own home.

home medical equipment Durable medical equipment prescribed by a physician for use by a patient at home. It is a means of continuing access to health care without remaining in the hospital. Such equipment may help the patient function more independently, it may assist recuperation, or it may be palliative. The equipment may be leased or purchased. These costs may be covered by a health plan.

home patients Medically-able individuals, who have their own dialysis equipment at home and after proper training, perform their own dialysis treatment alone or with the assistance of a helper.

home services Services provided to new and established patients in the patient's home.

home(o)- Similar.

homocysteine An amino acid found in the blood. High homocysteine levels are a risk factor for blood clots in the veins (DVT, PE) or arteries (heart attack, stroke), and hardening of the arteries (atherosclerosis).

homocystinuria A rare hereditary disease due to a deficiency of an enzyme needed to prevent the buildup of homocysteine in the blood.

homograft A transplant consisting of cells, tissues or organs sourced from a genetically non-identical donor.

homograft valves Replacement valves recovered from the hearts of humans who have died (cadavers).

homologous chromosomes Chromosomes that are paired during meiosis. Such chromosomes are alike with regard to size and also position of the centromere. They also have the same genes, but not necessarily the same alleles, at the same locus or location.

homozygous Having two abnormal genes. If you are homozygote for factor V Leiden, you inherited an abnormal gene from both parents.

Hoover test Similar to the thigh adduction test, the examiner differentiates true organic paralysis from hysterical, factitious or malingered paralysis by instructing the plaintiff to move the good leg while monitoring the involuntary movement of the paralyzed leg.

hordeolum An infection of the sebaceous gland of the eyelid. *Synonym:* stye.

Horizontal Plane divides the body into a superior (or upper) and an inferior (or lower) section. *Synonym:* transverse plane.

hormone antagonists Chemical substances which inhibit the function of the endocrine glands, the biosynthesis of their secreted hormones, or the action of hormones upon their specific sites.

hormones Chemical substances having a specific regulatory effect on the activity of a certain organ or organs. The term was originally applied to substances secreted by various endocrine glands and transported in the bloodstream to the target organs.

Horton syndrome Histaminic or cluster headache. (cephalalgia).

hospice A facility or program that is licensed, certified or otherwise authorized by law, which provides supportive care of the terminally ill.

hospice care Care that address the physical, spiritual, emotional, psychological, financial, and legal needs of the dying patient and the family; provided by an inter-disciplinary team of professionals and perhaps volunteers in a variety of settings, including hospitals, freestanding facilities, and at home.

hospital An institution whose primary function is to provide inpatient diagnostic and therapeutic services for a variety of medical conditions, both surgical and non-surgical. In addition, most hospitals provide some outpatient services, particularly emergency care. Hospitals may be classified by length of stay (short-term or long-term), as teaching or non-teaching, by major types of services (psychiatric, tuberculosis, general, and other specialties, such as maternity, pediatric, or ear, nose and throat), and by type of ownership or control (Federal, State, or local government; for-profit and non-profit).

hospital affiliation A contractual relationship between a health insurance plan and one or more hospitals whereby the hospital provides the inpatient benefits offered by the plan.

hospital alliance A group of hospitals that have joined together to improve competitive positions and reduce costs by sharing common services and developing group purchasing programs.

hospital assumptions These include differentials between hospital labor and non-labor indices compared with general economy labor and non-labor indices; rates of admission incidence; the trend toward treating less complicated cases in outpatient settings; and continued improvement in DRG coding.

hospital care Reimbursement for both inpatient and outpatient medical care expenses incurred in a hospital. Inpatient Benefits include; Charges for room and board, charges for necessary services and supplies sometimes referred to as 'hospital extras,' 'other hospital extras,' 'miscellaneous charges,' and 'ancillary charges. Outpatient Benefits include; surgical procedures, rehabilitation therapy, and physical therapy.

hospital coinsurance For the 61st through 90th day of hospitalization in a benefit period, a daily amount for which the beneficiary is responsible, equal to one-fourth of the inpatient hospital deductible; for lifetime reserve days, a daily amount for which the beneficiary is responsible, equal to one-half of the inpatient hospital deductible. *See* Lifetime reserve days.

hospital inpatient services Hospital inpatient services refer to hospital visits during the course of an inpatient hospital stay. The services may be provided by the patient's primary physician and/or other physicians in the event of multiple illnesses or injuries.

hospital input price index An alternate name for hospital market basket.

Hospital Insurance (HI) The Medicare program that covers specified inpatient hospital services, post-hospital skilled nursing care, home health services, and hospice care for aged and disabled individuals who meet the eligibility requirements. Also known as Medicare Part A.

Health Insurance Claim Number (HICN) The number assigned by the Social Security Administration to an individual identifying him/her as a Medicare beneficiary. This number is shown on the beneficiary's insurance card and is used in processing Medicare claims for that beneficiary.

hospital market basket The cost of the mix of goods and services (including personnel costs but excluding nonoperating costs) comprising routine, ancillary, and special care unit inpatient hospital services.

hospital observation services Occasionally a physician will watch or observe a patient in an area of an inpatient hospital designated as an observation area. This area is frequently located in or near the emergency room, and the observation typically after any acute care is rendered.

hospitalist A hospital-based internist who can be used to assume management of adult admissions from the primary care physician (PCP), freeing the PCP to do more office-based work. Hospitalists act as the hospital gatekeeper, to provide a valuable service by assessing the clinical needs of patients presenting to the emergency room and supervising inpatient care for those patients who are more critically ill, thereby reducing hospital inpatient costs.

hospital-surgical coverage A form of health insurance that offers coverage of certain costs related to hospitalization and surgical procedures. A hospital-surgical plan does not cover other types of medical services, such as physician office visits and outpatient prescription drugs.

Howard test A renal function test involving the catheterization of each ureter to determine and analyze the urinary output of each kidney.

Howell-Jolly bodies Spherical or ovoid nuclear fragments found in newly differentiated erythrocytes. Red blood cells with these bodies appear in greater numbers after a splenectomy.

HPSA Health professional shortage area.

HPV Human papillomavirus.

HPVD Hypertensive pulmonary vascular disease.

HQCB Health care quality certification board.

h-reflex study A diagnostic test that uses stimulation of a nerve and recording the reflex electrical discharge from a muscle in the limb.

HRSA Health Resources and Services Administration.

HRT Hormone replacement therapy.

HSA Health service area.

HSV Herpes simplex virus.

HTLV Human T-lymphotropic virus.

HTN Hypertension.

Hubbard tank A large, specially designed tank in which a patient may be immersed for various therapeutic underwater exercises.

Huhner's test An examination of seminal fluid obtained from the vaginal fornix and cervical canal after a specified interval following coitus; used in fertility studies to evaluate spermatozoal survival and activity in the female lower genital tract.

human chorionic gonadotropin Human chorionic gonadotropin (HCG) is a hormone produced when women are pregnant, and in some rare instances when certain tumors develop.

human herpes viruses A family of viruses including herpes simplex, varicella zoster, and Epstein-Barr.

human immunodeficiency virus A virus that can lead to acquired immunodeficiency syndrome (AIDS), a condition in humans in which the immune system begins to fail, leading to life-threatening opportunistic infections.

human papillomavirus A virus that infects the epidermis and mucous membranes of humans. Human papillomavirus can lead to cancers of the cervix, vulva, vagina, and anus in women and to cancers of the anus and penis in men.

human serum albumin A plasma protein very important in maintaining fluid balance in the blood. Important in maintaining blood pressure, regulating fatty acids, and hormone transport. Clinical uses include blood volume replacement during shock, serious burns and surgeries, as an adjunct during kidney dialysis and carrying drugs through the bloodstream.

humer(o)- of or pertaining to the shoulder (or [rarely] the upper arm).

humeral of or relating to the humerus.

humerus Bone extending from the shoulder to the elbow.

Hummelshein operation Transplant of a normal ocular rectus muscle to substitute for a paralyzed muscle.

humoral Relating to any fluid or semi fluid of the body.

Huntington's chorea Rare, abnormal, hereditary condition characterized by involuntary, purposeless, rapid movements of various body parts, as well as progressive mental deterioration. Symptoms often appear in the 40s with death occurring about 15 years later. *Synonym:* hereditary choreas.

Hurler disease (syndrome) A genetic disorder marked by progressive deterioration, hepato-splenomegaly, dwarfism and gargoyle-like faces. There is a progressive mental retardation, with death frequently occurring by the age of 10 years. *Synonym:* mucopolysaccharidosis type i, gargoylism.

HVD Hypertensive vascular disease.

hx History.

hybrid entity A covered entity whose covered functions are not its primary functions.

Hybrid-Model HMO A combination of at least two managed care organizational models that are molded into a single health plan. Since its features do not uniformly fit only one type of model, it is called a hybrid.

hydatidiform mole Disease occurring during early pregnancy resulting in death of the fetus and an overgrowth of tissue within the uterus.

hydr(o)- Water.

hydration The level of fluid in the body. The loss of fluid, or dehydration, occurs when the body loses more water or fluid than it takes in. The body cannot keep adequate blood pressure, get enough oxygen and nutrients to the cells, or get rid of wastes if it has too little fluid.

hydro Hydrotherapy.

hydrocele A painless swelling of the scrotum, caused by a collection of fluid around the testicle; commonly occurs in middle-aged men.

hydrocelectomy A surgical procedure to remove a hydrocele.

hydrocephalus Condition characterized by an excessive accumulation of fluid with the cranial vault.

hydrogen breath test A test used as a clinical medical diagnosis for people with irritable bowel syndrome, and common food intolerances. The test is simple, non-invasive, and is performed after a short period of fasting (typically 8-12 hours).

hydronephrosis Caused by an obstruction in the tube that carries urine from the kidney to the bladder (ureter). Because urine cannot flow past the obstruction, it backs up into the kidney causing distention or dilation. Prolonged hydronephrosis eventually results in loss of kidney function; surgery to remove the obstruction may be necessary.

hydrops Swelling from excessive accumulation of serous fluid in tissue.

hydrotherapy The use of water to revitalize, maintain, and restore health. Hydrotherapy treatments include saunas, steam baths, foot baths, sitz baths, and the application of cold and hot water compresses.

hygienist A dental auxiliary who cleans teeth, provides patient education, administers local anesthetic and nitrous oxide and performs periodontal scaling.

hygroma Accumulation of fluid in a sac, cyst, or bursa.

hymen A fold of mucous membrane which surrounds or partially covers the external vaginal opening.

hymenotomy Surgical removal of the hymen to enlarge the vaginal opening.

hyoid bone A U-shaped bone at the base of the tongue that supports the tongue muscles.

hyp(o)- Denotes something as 'below normal'.

hyper- Abnormally increased; excessive.

hyperactivity A physical state in which a person is abnormally and easily excitable or exuberant. Strong emotional reactions, impulsive behavior, and sometimes a short span of attention are also typical for a hyperactive person.

hyperacusis Abnormal acuteness of hearing due to increased irritability of the sensory neural mechanism; characterized by intolerance for ordinary sound levels.

hyperalimentation Supplying total nutritional needs of patients who are unable to eat normally by intravenous feeding or by tube through the nose into the stomach. Provides nutrients containing essential proteins, fats, carbohydrates and vitamins.

hyperbaric oxygen therapy The medical use of oxygen at a level higher than atmospheric pressure.

hypercalcemia Presence of excessive calcium in the blood.

May result from tumor of the parathyroid gland (due to overproduction of parathyroid hormone), Paget's disease, some cancers, multiple fractures or prolonged immobility. May also occur from excessive ingestion of calcium, such as overuse of antacids that contain calcium.

hyperchloremia Presence of excessive amounts of chloride in the blood. May result from severe dehydration, complete shutdown of kidneys and primary aldosteronism. *See* Aldosteronism, primary.

hypercholesterolemia The presence of high levels of cholesterol in the blood.

hypercoagulable This refers to an increased tendency to form blood clots, due to an inherited state or acquired disorder.

hyperemesis Severe and excessive vomiting.

hyperemesis gravidarum Extreme, persistent nausea and vomiting during pregnancy that may lead to dehydration.

hyperemia Increased blood in an organ or other body part.

hyperestrogenism Condition characterized by and caused by excessive secretion or intake of estrogen.

hyperfibrinogenemia Presence of excessive fibrinogen in the blood. *See* Fibrinogen. May indicate cancer of the stomach, breast or kidney or an inflammatory disorder.

hyperfunctioning tumor Any tumor that leads to higher than normal action of the chemicals (usually hormones) usually secreted by the tissue from which the tumor arises. For example, hyperfunctioning tumor of the thyroid gland leads to an increase in thyroid hormone released.

hyperhidrosis The condition characterized by abnormally increased perspiration, in excess of that required for regulation of body temperature.

hyperhomocysteinemia A condition where elevated homocysteine levels are present in the blood that may damage the lining of blood vessels and lead to the formation of blood clots.

hyperinsulinism Excessive secretion of insulin.

hyperkalemia Abnormally high blood potassium level. May be seen in people who have suffered severe burns, crushing injuries, diabetic ketoacidosis or myocardial infarction. *See* Myocardial infarction. Also seen in those who have Addison's disease or kidney failure. *See* Addison's disease.

hyperkeratosis Thickening of the outer layer of the skin.

hyperkinesis 1) A state of overactive restlessness in children. 2) A medical condition resulting in uncontrolled muscle movement, akin to spasms.

hyperkinetic syndrome of childhood A childhood or adolescent disorder characterized by excessive activity, emotional instability, significantly reduced attention span, and an absence of shyness and fear, and that occasionally develops in individuals with brain injury, mental defect, or epilepsy.

hyperlipidemia An elevation of lipids in the bloodstream. These lipids include cholesterol, cholesterol esters, phospholipids and triglycerides.

hyperlipoproteinemia Condition in which excessive lipoproteins (cholesterol and other fatty materials) accumulate in the blood.

hypermagnesemia Elevated levels of magnesium in the blood. Most commonly occurs in people with kidney failure. Can also result from Addison's disease. *See* Addison's disease.

hypermobility A condition in which the joints easily move beyond the normal range expected for a particular joint.

hypernatremia Excess of sodium in the blood, usually caused by excessive loss of water and electrolytes. Symptoms include mental confusion, seizures and eventually coma.

hyperopia A condition in which the eyeball is too short from front to back, or the eye's focusing mechanism is too weak, causing light rays to be focused behind, rather than on, the retina. *Synonym:* farsightedness, longsightedness.

hyperosmolarity Increase in the osmolality of the body fluids.

hyperostosis An excessive growth of bone.

hyperoxaluria Hereditary defect of metabolism, marked by excessive oxalate in the urine. May result in kidney stones, early onset of kidney failure (due to calcium deposits in the filtering system) and calcium-oxalate deposits in other areas of the body.

hyperparathyroidism Excessive amounts of parathyroid hormone circulating in the blood. Excess amounts increase blood levels of calcium (hypercalcemia) and decrease blood levels of phosphorus (hypophosphatemia).

hyperphosphatemia Abnormally high level of phosphates in the blood. May result from bone diseases, healing fractures, hypoparathyroidism, diabetic acidosis or kidney failure. *See* Hypoparathyroidism; diabetic ketoacidosis.

hyperpigmentation A skin condition in which there is excessive pigmentation, often seen as dark spots on the skin.

hyperplasia Excessive growth of normal cells of an organ.

hyperplasia of prostate A non-malignant enlargement of the prostate gland commonly occurring in men after the age of 50, and sometimes leading to compression of the urethra and obstruction of the flow of urine.

hyperploidy Condition of having one or more chromosomes in excess of the normal number. The result is unbalanced sets of chromosomes. One example of hyperploidy is Down's syndrome. *See* Down's syndrome.

hyperpotassemia Excessive amounts of potassium in the blood.

hyperprolactinemia The presence of abnormally-high levels of prolactin in the blood. May cause production and spontaneous flow of breast milk and disruptions in the normal menstrual period in women and hypogonadism, infertility and erectile dysfunction in men.

hyperprolinemia, type-a Disorder of amino acid metabolism.

hypersecretion Excessive secretion.

hypersensitivity Refers to damaging, discomfort-producing and sometimes fatal reactions produced by the normal immune system.

hypersomnia An inability to stay awake.

hypersplenism A disorder which causes the spleen to rapidly and prematurely destroy blood cells.

hypertelorism Abnormally increased distance between two organs or parts.

hypertension Increase in the force of blood against the arteries as blood circulates through them. Often has no symptoms. Essential or primary hypertension, the most common kind, has no single identifiable cause. Secondary hypertension is caused by an underlying disease. *Synonym:* high blood pressure.

hypertension table The Hypertension Table, found under the main term, Hypertension, in the Alphabetic Index of ICD-9-CM, contains a complete listing of all conditions due to or associated with hypertension and classifies them according to malignant, benign, and unspecified.

hypertensive chronic kidney disease Diseases of the kidney caused by high blood pressure.

hypertensive heart and chronic kidney disease Diseases of the heart and kidneys cause by high blood pressure.

hypertensive heart disease Heart disease caused by high blood pressure, especially localised high blood pressure.

hyperthyroidism Overactivity of the thyroid, an endocrine gland that regulates all body functions.

hypertonic Solution that contains substances that flow outward through a semipermeable membrane into a solution of lower concentration.

hypertonicity (Of muscular tissue) the state of being hypertonic.

hypertrichosis Refers to hair density or length beyond the accepted limits of normal for a particular age, race, or sex.

hypertrophic anal papilla Excessive growth of the papilla of the rectum. *See* Papilla.

hypertrophic and atrophic conditions of skin Are conditions that cause enlargement or wasting away of the skin.

hypertrophic scar A raised and red scar, similar to a keloid scar, but different in that it stays within the boundaries of the injury site.

hypertrophy Increase in the size of a cell or group of cells. Causes an increase in the size of an organ or part.

hypertropia A condition of misalignment of the eyes (strabismus), whereby the visual axis of one eye is higher than the fellow fixating eye.

hyperventilation Breathing so rapidly that carbon dioxide levels in the blood are decreased, upsetting normal blood chemistry. Can be caused by fever, heart disease, lung disease or severe injury. Can also be caused by anxiety. May be accompanied by numbness and tingling of mouth, hands and feet, weakness and faintness.

hypervitaminosis Any of various abnormal conditions in which the physiological effect of a vitamin is produced to a pathological degree by excessive intake of the vitamin.

hyphema Bleeding into the interior chamber of the eye.

hypnotherapy Hypnotherapy is a technique that uses the hypnotic state, which enables changes in perception and memory, a major increase in response to suggestion, and the potential for controlling many physiologic functions that are usually involuntary.

hypo Hypodermic injection.

hypoalbuminemia Abnormally low levels of albumin (protein) in the blood.

hypoalderostonism Deficiency of aldosterone secreted by the outer layer of the adrenal glands. May result from Addison's disease, salt-losing syndrome and toxemia of pregnancy. *See* Addison's disease; salt-losing syndrome; toxemia; eclampsia.

hypocalcemia Abnormally low level of calcium in the blood. May result from hypoparathyroidism or malabsorption of calcium. May be associated with Cushing's syndrome, kidney failure, pancreatitis or peritonitis.

hypochloremia Abnormally low levels of chloride in the blood. Low chloride levels can occur from prolonged vomiting, intestinal fistula, chronic kidney failure and Addison's disease. *See* Addison's disease; fistulas.

hypochondriasis Preoccupation with the fear of having, or the idea that one has, a serious disease based on the person's misinter-pretation of bodily symptoms.

hypochromic anemia *See* Anemia, hypochromic.

hypodermic Relating to or located below the epidermis; hypodermic needle.

hypodermis The innermost and thickest layer of the skin. The hypodermis is responsible for conserving the body's heat and protecting the vital inner organs.

hypofibrinogenemia Abnormally decreased level of fibrinogen in the blood. *See* Fibrinogen. May result from disseminated intravascular coagulation, fibrinolysis, severe liver disease and some cancers.

hypofunctioning tumor Tumor that causes the anatomical part it encroaches on to have less than normal function.

hypogammaglobulinemia Abnormally low levels of gammaglobulins in the blood, which results in an immunity deficiency. This makes you more susceptible to infectious diseases. You can be born with this condition or it can result from other diseases, such as nephrosis. *See* Nephrosis.

hypoglossal Supplies intrinsic muscles of the tongue and other tongue muscles.

hypoglycemia Abnormally low blood sugar level caused by abnormal function, not disease, of the pancreas. Excessive insulin produces symptoms of sweating, nervousness, weakness, nausea and rapid heartbeat. Excessive insulin may be caused by a tumor, called an insulinoma, that secretes too much insulin. Or it may result from a diabetic person injecting too much insulin. *See* Insulinoma. May also result from kidney failure, liver disease, alcoholism or decreased food intake. The brain must have glucose available at all times or brain cells are damaged. Hypoglycemia must be treated promptly.

hypoglycemic of or relating to hypoglycemia; hypoglycemic agents;.

hypoglycemic syndrome Condition caused by low blood sugar, characterized by cold sweat, low body temperature, headache, confusion, hallucinations and ultimately (if left untreated) convulsions, coma and death.

hypogonadism Decreased functional activity of gonads, with hindered growth and slowed sexual development.

hypogonadotropism Abnormal condition caused by decreased production of gonadotropins. *See* Gonadotropins.

hypokalemia Below normal level of potassium in the blood. May result from aldosteronism, Cushing's syndrome, excessive loss of body fluids and licorice addiction. *See* Aldosteronism; Cushing's syndrome.

hypolipoproteinemia Abnormally low levels of lipoproteins in blood.

hypomania An episode of illness that resembles mania, but is less intense and less disabling. Hypomania is characterized by a euphoric mood, unrealistic optimism, increased speech and activity, and a decreased need for sleep.

hyponatremia Less than normal concentration of sodium in the blood. Caused by excessive water in circulating blood or excessive loss of sodium from severe vomiting or diarrhea, or inadequate intake of sodium.

hypo-osmotic swelling test Determination of sperm viability by placing a sample in a hypo-osmotic solution, which causes swelling and curling of the tails of spermatozoa with normal plasma membranes.

hypooxaluria Decreased amount of oxalic acid in the urine.

hypoparathyroidism Decreased production of hormones by the parathyroid glands, causing low calcium blood level.

hypophosphatasia Inborn error of metabolism that causes difficulty building and healing bones.

hypophysectomy Surgical removal or destruction of the hypophysis, or pituitary gland.

hypophysis The pituitary gland.

hypopigmentation A skin condition in which there is a lack of pigmentation.

hypopituitarism Underactivity of the pituitary gland, resulting in inadequate hormone production.

hypoplasia Incomplete development or underdevelopment of an organ or tissue, usually from a decrease in the number of cells.

hypospadias repair Surgery to correct a birth defect in boys in which the urethra does not end at the tip of the penis.

hypostasis The suppression of a gene by the effect of an unrelated gene.

hypotension Abnormally low blood pressure.

hypotensive The accumulation of blood in an organ.

hypothalamic of or relating to the hypothalamus.

hypothenar Refers to a group of three muscles of the palm that control the motion of the little finger.

hypothermia A condition of characterized by low body temperature.

hypothermic of or relating to or affected by hypothermia.

hypothyroidism Underactive thyroid gland, which results in decreased metabolic rate. Early symptoms may include decreased tolerance for cold, fatigue, unexplained weight gain, constipation and forgetfulness. If left untreated, the disorder may progress to myxedema and eventually coma. Treatment includes thyroid replacement hormones.

hypothyroidism, primary Caused by dysfunction of the thyroid gland and may be due to surgical removal of the thyroid, radioactive iodine treatment, Hashimoto's thyroiditis or inflammatory conditions, such as sarcoidosis. *See* Hashimoto's thyroiditis; sarcoidosis.

hypothyroidism, secondary Caused outside the thyroid. It may result from decreased activity of the pituitary gland, which secretes thyroid stimulating hormone (TSH), dysfunction of the hypothalamus, which regulates TSH production, iodine deficiency in the diet or use of drugs that depress thyroid function.

hypotonic (Of living tissue) lacking normal tone or tension.

hypotony Low intraocular pressure (IOP) occasionally is associated with decreased vision.

hypotropia Downward deviation of the visual axis of one eye.

hypoventilation Abnormally slow and shallow respiration, resulting in an increased level of carbon dioxide in the blood.

hypovolemia An abnormally low volume of blood circulating through the body. It may result in hypovolemic shock.

hypoxemia Low oxygen levels in the blood.

hypoxia A condition in which the body as a whole or a region of the body is deprived of adequate oxygen supply.

hyster(o)- of or pertaining to the womb, the uterus.

hysterectomy Surgical removal of the uterus. Hysterectomy may be total (removing the body, fundus, and cervix of the uterus) or partial (removal of the uterine body but leaving the cervical stump, also called supracervical).

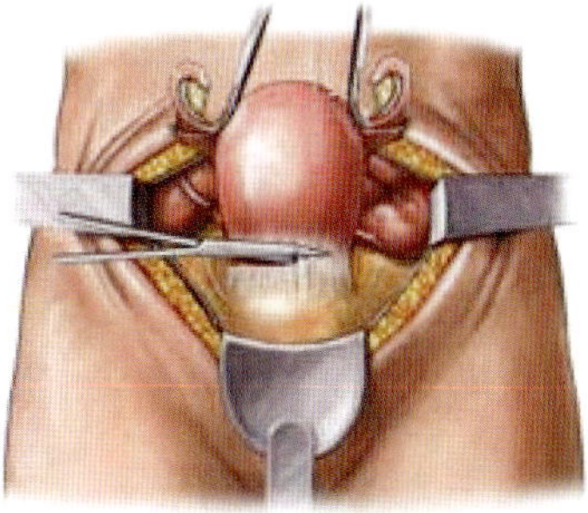

Abdominal Hysterectomy.

hysteresis The difference between the pulmonary pressure of inhalation and the pressure of exhalation.

hysteria Neurotic disorder characterized by violent emotional outbreaks and disturbances of sensory and motor functions.

hysterolysis Severing or separation of adhesions of the uterus.

hysteroplasty Plastic repair of the uterus.

hysterorrhaphy Suture repair of a lacerated uterus.

hysterosalpingography A procedure in which x-rays are taken of the female reproductive tract after injection of a dye. Purpose is to determine if the fallopian tubes are open, or if there are any apparent abnormalities or defects in the uterus.

hysterosalpingostomy Surgical restoration of a connection between the uterus and an occluded fallopian tube.

hysteroscopy Endoscopic examination, therapy or surgery of the interior of the uterus.

hysterosonography A noninvasive technique for evaluation of abnormalities of the uterus and endometrium that involves the slow infusion of sterile saline solution into the uterus during ultrasound imaging.

hysterotomy An incision in the uterus, performed through either the abdomen or the vagina.

hysterotrachelectomy Surgical removal of the uterine cervix.

I

I & D Incision and drainage.

-ia(sis) Condition.

iab Intra-aortic balloon.

iatr(o)- of or pertaining to medicine, or a physician [uncommon as a prefix; common as suffix, see -iatry].

iatrogenic Refers to adverse effects or complications caused by or resulting from medical treatment or advice.

-iatry Denotes a field in medicine of a certain body component.

IAV Intermittent assisted ventilation.

IBC Iron-binding capacity.

IBD Inflammatory bowel disease, irritable bowel disease.

IBID The same, in the same place.

IBS Irritable bowel syndrome.

-ic Pertaining to.

ICCU Intensive coronary care unit.

ICD-10 International Classification of Diseases, 10th Revision.

ICD-10-CM International Classification of Diseases, 10th Revision, Clinical Modification.

ICD-10-PCS International Classification of Diseases, 10th Revision, Procedure Coding System.

ICD-9 International Classification of Diseases - Ninth Revision.

ICD-9-CM International Classification of Diseases, Ninth Revision, Clinical Modification is the official system of assigning codes to diagnoses and procedures associated with hospital utilization in the United States. ICD-9-CM is based on the World Health Organization's Ninth Revision, International Classification of Diseases (ICD-9).

ICF Intermediate care facility.

ichthyosis Skin condition in which skin is dry, thickened and fissured, resembling fish scales. Usually appears at or shortly after birth; it may be associated with one of several rare syndromes. Treatment with bath oil or vitamin-A solution (retinoic acid) applied to the skin may help some types.

ichthyosis follicularis Skin disorder characterized by dryness, roughness and scaliness.

-icle Small.

-ics Organized knowledge, treatment.

ICU Intensive care unit.

ID The same.

idio- Self, one's own.

idiopathic Arising from an unknown cause.

idiopathic cold-agglutinin diseases Disease of unknown cause associated with laboratory findings of an agglutinin that acts only at relatively low temperatures.

idiopathic hypertrophic subaortic stenosis Chronic heart condition that produces an enlarged heart muscle, which restricts the amount of blood the heart pumps. Condition may be inherited, but cause is usually unknown. Symptoms may include chest pain, shortness of breath, fainting, heart rhythm irregularity, heart murmur, swollen feet and ankles, and enlarged, tender liver. Usually curable with medication or surgery.

idiopathic thrombocytopenic purpura Bleeding into the skin and other organs due to a deficiency of platelets.

ileitis *See* Crohn's disease.

ileo- Ileum.

ileocolostomy Surgical anastomosis of the ileum to the colon.

ileoileostomy Surgical anastomosis between two parts of the ileum.

ileoproctostomy Surgical construct-ion of an opening between the ileum and the rectum.

ileoscopy Use of a flexible instru-ment to examine the ileum.

ileostomy A stoma that has been constructed by bringing the end or loop of small intestine out onto the surface of the skin.

ileum The lowest part of the small intestine, located beyond the duodenum and jejunum, just before the colon.

ileus Blockage of the intestine (especially the ileum) that prevents the contents of the intestine from passing to the lower bowel.

iliac artery Either of two large arteries that conduct blood to the pelvis and the legs.

iliac bone A part of the pelvic bone that is above the hip joint and from which autogenous bone grafts are frequently obtained.

iliac crest The large, prominent portion of the pelvic bone at the belt line of the body.

iliac vein One of three veins drain-ing the pelvic area.

ilio of or referring to the ilium.

iliopsoas The great flexor muscle of the hip joint, divisible into two parts, the iliac and great psoas, - often regarded as distinct muscles.

ilium The uppermost and largest bone of the pelvis.

IM Intramuscular.

IME Independent Medical Evaluation.

immediate denture A denture constructed for immediate placement after removal of the remaining teeth.

immersion The placing of a body or a part thereof into a liquid.

immobilization test Detection of antibody based on its ability to inhibit the motility of a bacterial cell or protozoan.

immune Resistance or protection against infection by the body's natural defenses. A person may be immune to one kind of infection but not immune to another. Some infections, such as measles or chickenpox, cause permanent immunity to that infection.

immune globulins A medicine given by intramuscular injection that is used to prevent the immuno-logical condition known as Rhesus disease (or hemolytic disease of newborn).

immune serum globulin A sterile solution of globulins derived from pooled human blood that contains antibodies that are normally present in the blood of adults, used as a passive immunizing agent against rubella, measles, and hepatitis A and as treatment for hypogammaglobulinemia.

immunization The process of inducing immunity by administering an antigen to allow the immune system to prevent infection or illness.

immunization programs Preventive care programs designed to monitor and promote the administration of vaccines to guard against child-hood illnesses, such as chicken pox, mumps, and measles, and adult illnesses, such as pneumonia and influenza.

immunoassay Immunochemical assay or detection of a substance by serologic or immunologic methods. Usually the substance being studied serves as antigen both in antibody production and in measurement of antibody by the test substance.

immunodeficiency diseases Defects in the body's immune system. A healthy immune system protects the body against germs (bacteria, viruses, fungi), cancer (partial protection) and any foreign material that enters the body. When the system fails, the body becomes susceptible to infection and cancer. Can range from minor to very severe.

immunofluorescence A technique that uses antibodies linked to a fluorescent dye in order to study antigens in a sample of tissue.

immunoglobin alpha A type of immunoglobulin present in blood and body secretions which may aid in fighting infections.

immunoglobin-deficiency disease Illness caused by deficiency of a protein molecule with known antibody activity.

immunologic tests Diagnostic techniques involving the demon-stration or measurement of an immune response, including antibody production or assay, antigen-antibody reactions, serologic cross-reactivity, delayed hypersensitivity reactions, or heterogenetic responses.

immunology The study of the body's immune system.

immunomedicated disease Illness caused by medicines that decrease the efficiency of the immune system in preventing or decreasing severity of disease.

immunosuppressed A condition brought about by disease or chemotherapy where the individual is highly susceptible to infection.

immunosuppressive drugs Trans-plant drugs used to reduce the risk of rejecting a new organ after transplant. Transplant patients need to take these drugs for the rest of their lives.

immunosuppressive therapy Drugs used to prevent the body from forming a normal immune response. Therapy is used to treat diseases (especially when organs must be transplanted) when certain antibodies must be inactivated.

immunotherapy Therapy designed to produce immunity to a disease or to enhance resistance by the immune system.

impacted cerumen A collection of cerumen (ear-wax) in the external auditory canal.

impacted tooth Usually associated with a wisdom tooth, it is a tooth that is submerged under the gum tissue.

impaction A partial or completely unexposed tooth that is wedged against another tooth, bone, or soft tissue, precluding the eruption process.

impairment Any loss or abnormality of psychological, physiological, or anatomical structure or function from injury or disease. It represents a deviation from the person's usual biomedical state.

impaired risk An insurance applicant who has pre-existing poor health or is in substandard physical condition, is engaged in dangerous activities, or has a hazardous occupation.

imperforate Lacking a normal opening.

impetigo A contagious bacterial skin disease forming pustules and yellow crusty sores, chiefly on the face and hands.

Implant An artificial device that replaces the tooth root and may anchor an artificial tooth, bridge or denture.

implantation A surgical procedure that places something in the human body.

implantation intraocular lens Insertion of an artificial lens following removal of the crystalline lens, usually after cataract extraction.

implementation guide A document explaining the proper use of a standard for a specific business purpose. The X12N HIPAA igs are the primary reference documents used by those implementing the associated transactions, and are incorporated into the HIPAA regulations by reference.

implementation specification Under HIPAA, this is the specific instructions for implementing a standard.

impression An imprint in plastic material of the surfaces of the teeth and adjacent portions of the jaw from which a likeness may be produced in dentistry Incision A cut into a body tissue or organ.

improvement outcome (Home Health) An outcome measure that assesses whether a specific health status attribute (such as transferring or dyspnea) improves between two specified time points, as measured on the OASIS scale. An improvement measure can not be computed if the patient can not possibly improve (i.e., the patient's health status is optimal for the attribute of interest at start of care.

improvement plan A plan for measurable process or outcome improvement. The plan is usually developed cooperatively by a provider and the Network. The plan must address how and when its results will be measured.

impulse control disorders Disorders whose essential features are the failure to resist an impulse, drive, or temptation to perform an act that is harmful to the individual or to others.

in utero Within the uterus.

in vitro fertilization A process by which egg cells are fertilized by sperm outside the womb. Used as a major treatment in infertility when other methods have failed.

inappropriate utilization Utilization of services that are in excess of a beneficiary's medical needs and condition (over utilization) or receiving a capitated Medicare payment and failing to provide services to meet a beneficiary's medical needs and condition (underutilization).

incidence The frequency of new occurrences of a condition within a defined time interval. The incidence rate is the number of new cases of specific disease divided by the number of people in a population over a specified period of time, usually one year.

incidental findings Unanticipated information discovered in the course of testing or medical care. Used in discussions of information that may have social or psychological consequences.

incision The cutting of or into body tissues or organs.

incisional chest discomfort The pain or discomfort associated with a surgical incision or cut is called incisional discomfort.

incontinence Inability to control excretions. Urinary incontinence is the inability to keep urine in the bladder. Fecal incontinence is the inability to retain feces in the rectum.

incubators Insulated enclosures in which temperature, humidity, and other environmental conditions can be regulated at levels optimal for growth, hatching, reproduction, or metabolic reactions.

incurral date The date on which health care services are provided to a covered person. The incurral date, not the date on which the insurance company pays a health care claim, is the critical date in determining health insurance benefits. For example, a health insurance company will not pay a claim for health care services incurred prior to the effective date of the health insurance coverage.

incurred basis The costs based on when the service was performed rather than when the payment was made.

incurred but not reported (ibnr) claims Claims or benefits that occurred during a particular time period, but that have not yet been reported or submitted to an insurer or MCO, so they remain unpaid.

incurred claims A term that refers to the actual carrier liability for a specified period and includes all claims with dates of services within a specified period, usually called the experience period. Due to the time lag between dates of services and the dates claims payments are actually processed, adjustment must be made to any paid claims data to determine incurred claims.

indemnity benefits Benefits for which the insurance company payment is a fixed dollar amount.

indemnity health plan These are the types of plans that primarily existed before the rise of HMOs and ppos. With indemnity plans, the individual pays a predetermined percentage of the cost of health care services, and the health plan pays the other percent-age. For example, an individual might pay 20% for services and the insurance company pays 80%. The fees for services are defined by the health care providers and vary from physician to physician and hospital to hospital. *Synonym:* fee for service plan.

indemnity insurance Insurance providing a stipulated level of reimbursement for hospital/medical expenses, without regard to the actual expenses incurred during hospitalization.

indemnity plans An insurance policy in which beneficiaries are allowed total freedom to choose their health care providers. Those providers are reimbursed a set fee each time they deliver a service. Reimbursement is usually limited to a percentage of customary and reasonable charges (which may be less than the billed amount). Also see fee for service.

indemnity schedule *See* Schedule of Allowances.

indemnity wraparound policy An out-of-plan product that an HMO offers through an agreement with an insurance company.

independent agents Agents that represent the products of several health plans or insurers.

independent case management Comprehensive professional coordination of the health resources necessary to the support of the patient's diagnosis, treatment, and recovery, facilitating the ability of the patient to function with as much independence as possible through the convergence of physical, psychological, social, functional, and personal services. The case manager may organize services that are more cost-effective and appropriate to the needs of the patient that would not otherwise be covered under a beneficiary's health benefit.

independent clinic A location, not part of a hospital and not described by any other place of service code, that is organized and operated to provide preventive, diagnostic, therapeutic, rehabilitative, or palliative services to outpatients only.

independent laboratory A freestanding clinical laboratory meeting conditions for participation in the Medicare program and billing through a carrier. A laboratory certified to perform diagnostic and/or clinical tests independent of an institution or a physician's office.

Independent Medical Evaluation (IME) An examination carried out by an impartial health care provider, generally board certified, for the purpose of resolving a dispute related to the nature and extent of an illness or injury.

independent practice association An HMO that contracts with individual physicians to provide services to HMO members in a negotiated per capita or fee-for-service rate. Physicians maintain their own offices and can contract with other HMO's and see other fee-for-service patients.

index to external causes of **injuries & poisonings (E-codes)** This section contains the index to the codes that classify environmental events, circumstances, and other conditions as the cause of injury and other adverse effects.

indicator A key clinical value or quality characteristic used to measure, over time, the performance, processes, and outcomes of an organization or some component of health care delivery.

indicator dilution techniques Methods for assessing flow through a system by injection of a known quantity of an indicator, such as a dye, radionuclide, or chilled liquid, into the system and monitoring its concentration over time at a specific point in the system.

indigent medical Care Care given by health care providers to patients who are unable to pay for it.

indigestion Symptoms of poor digestion including heartburn, nausea, bloating and gas. *Synonym:* dyspepsia.

indirect pulp cap A procedure in which the nearly exposed pulp is covered with a protective dressing to protect the pulp from additional injury and to promote healing and repair via formation of secondary dentin.

individual health care account A method of financing health care by giving tax advantage to individuals who establish and maintain personal accounts for health care purposes; similar to an Individual Retirement Account for retirement purposes. Also referred to as medical savings account.

individual health insurance Health insurance coverage on an individual, not group, basis. The premium is usually higher for an individual health insurance plan than for a group policy, but you may not qualify for a group plan.

individual market A market segment composed of customers not eligible for Medicare or Medicaid who are covered under an individual contract for health coverage.

Individual Practice Association Model (IPA) The individual practice association contracts with independent physicians who work in their own private practices, and see fee-for-service patients as well as HMO enrollees. They are paid by capitation for the HMO patients and by conventional means for their fee-for-service patients. Physicians belonging to the IPA guarantee that the care needed by each patient for whom they are responsible will fall under a certain amount of money. They guarantee this by allowing the HMO to withhold an amount of their payments (i.e., usually 20% per year). If, by the end of the year, the physician's cost for treatment falls under the set amount, then the physician receives his entire "withhold fund". If the opposite is true, the HMO can then withhold any part of this amount, at its discretion, from the fund. Essentially, the physician is put "at risk" for keeping down the treatment cost. This is the key to the HMO's financial viability. Also called independent practice association.

individual stop-loss coverage A type of stop-loss insurance that provides benefits for claims on an individual that exceed a stated amount in a given period. *Synonym:* specific stop-loss coverage.

induction A method of artificially or prematurely stimulating labor.

indwelling catheter A catheter designed to be left within an organ or passage for an extended period of time.

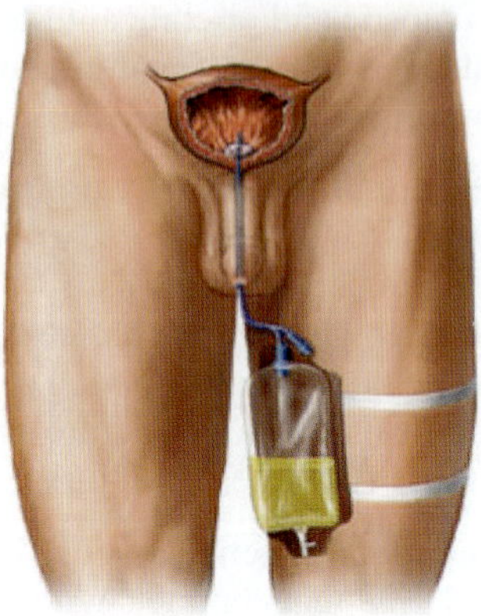

indwelling catheter

infant mortality rate Deaths in the first year of life per 1000 births. According to the U.S. General Accounting Office, 50% of these deaths are due to lifestyle factors, 20% due to environmental factors, 20% due to biological factors, and 10% due to inadequate health care.

infantile cerebral palsy The term used for a group of nonprogressive disorders of movement and posture caused by abnormal development of, or damage to, motor control centers of the brain. Cerebral palsy.

infarct Infarction.

infarction Tissue death due to the obstruction of blood to that tissue.

infect Infection, infectious.

infection The growth of a parasitic organism within the body.

infectious mononucleosis An acute disease characterized by fever and swollen lymph nodes and an abnormal increase of mononuclear leucocytes or monocytes in the bloodstream. *Synonym:* mono, glandular fever, kissing disease.

inferior Situated below or directed downward.

inferior vena cava Large vein that returns unoxygenated blood to the heart from parts of the body below the mid chest.

inferolateral Below and to one side.

inferoposterior Below and behind.

infestation The state of being invaded or overrun by parasites.

infiltration A local anesthetic procedure effective for upper teeth and soft tissue or the placement of anesthetic under the gum, allowing it to seep into bone.

inflammatory of or pertaining to inflammation.

inflammatory and toxic neuropathy Refers to pathology of the peripheral nerves caused by inflammation or toxins.

inflammatory bowel disease Characterized by fever, pain, abscess formation, severe diarrhea, bleeding and ulceration of the intestine's mucous membrane lining. Cause is unknown. Treatment includes fluids, cortisone drugs, antibiotics, diet change and sometimes surgery.

inflammatory disease A general term for infection of the uterus lining, fallopian tubes, or ovaries.

influenza A highly infectious respiratory disease. The disease is caused by certain strains of the influenza virus.

information Data to which meaning is assigned, according to context and assumed conventions.

information access control Formal, documented policies and procedures for granting different levels of access to health care information.

informed consent Informed consent is a legal term referring to the right of individuals to make informed medical treatment decisions. Under State law, informed consent typically includes the right to be told of one's medical condition and prognosis, the risks and benefits associated with a recommended procedure or course of treatment, and the risks and benefits of other available treatment options, including the option of refusing treatment. When a person becomes mentally incapacitated, his or her right to give or withhold informed consent typically passes to the person's legal representative, usually an agent or attorney-in-fact under a durable power of attorney, a court-appointed guardian, or a close family member.

infra- Prefix meaning below or under.

infracardiac Situated below the heart.

infraorbital Below the orbit.

infrapatellar Situated below the patella.

infrared light treatment The use of infrared light to promote healing.

infrarenal Situated or occurring below the kidneys.

infraspinatus muscle A muscle of the rotator cuff.

infratemporal fossa An irregularly shaped cavity, situated below and medial to the zygomatic arch.

infratentorial Beneath the tentorium of the cerebellum.

infraumbilical Inferior to the umbilicus.

infundibular Pertaining to any of the body's infundibula.

infusion pumps Pumps for giving fluid or medication into the vein at a specific rate or over a set amount of time.

infusions The administration of liquid medication, nutrient, or other fluid through some other route than the alimentary canal, usually over minutes or hours, either by gravity flow or often by infusion pumping.

inguinal Of, relating to, or situated in the region of the groin or in either of the lowest lateral regions of the abdomen.

inguinal hernia A protrusion of the abdominal viscera through the inguinal canal.

inguinofemoral hernia A bilocular or double hernia, both inguinal and femoral.

inhalation administration The administration of drugs by the respiratory route. It includes insufflation into the respiratory tract.

inhalation therapy The therapeutic use of gases or of aerosols by inhalation.

initial (claim) determination The first adjudication made by a carrier or fiscal intermediary (FI) (i.e., the affiliated contractor) following a request for Medicare payment or the first determination made by a PRO either in a prepayment or post payment context.

initial enrollment period The Initial Enrollment Period is the first chance a beneficiary has to enroll in Medicare Part B. Your Initial Enrollment Period starts three months before you first meet all the eligibility requirements for Medicare and lasts for seven months.

initial enrollment questionnaire A questionnaire sent to a patient to find out if that patient has other insurance that should pay his medical bills before Medicare. *See* Medicare Secondary Payer.

inlay A cast gold, porcelain, or composite custom-made filling cemented into the tooth that is used to replace part of a tooth.

inlier A patient whose length of stay or service cost resembles those of most other patients. Also see outlier..

in-network Providers or health care facilities which are part of a health plan's network of providers with which it has negotiated a discount. Insured individuals usually pay less when using an in-network provider, because those networks provide services at lower cost to the insurance companies with which they have contracts.

innominate artery An artery that arises from the arch of the aorta and divides into the right subclavian and right carotid arteries.

inoculation The introduction of an antigenic substance or vaccine into the body to produce immunity to a specific disease.

inpatient hospital A facility, other than psychiatric, which primarily provides diagnostic, therapeutic (both surgical and nonsurgical) and rehabilitation services by or under the supervision of physicians, to patients admitted for a variety of medical conditions.

inpatient hospital deductible An amount of money that is deducted from the amount payable by Medicare Part A for inpatient hospital services furnished to a beneficiary during a spell of illness.

inpatient hospital services These services include bed and board, nursing services, diagnostic or therapeutic services, and medical or surgical services.

inpatient psychiatric facility A facility that provides inpatient psychiatric services for the diagnosis and treatment of mental illness on a 24-hour basis, by or under the supervision of a physician.

inpatient services Items and services furnished to a patient staying overnight in a hospital including bed and board, nursing and related services, diagnostic and therapeutic services, and medical or surgical services.

INR International normalized ratio. This blood test result helps physicians monitor patients taking anticoagulant medications. It measures the blood's ability to clot based on the prothrombin time (PT), the time it takes for blood to clot in a test tube.

insemination, artificial Artificial introduction of semen into the vagina for the purpose of inducing conception.

insertion The point at which a muscle attaches to the skin, a bone, or another muscle. The insertion attaches to the structure that will be moved by the contraction of the muscle. Insertions are usually connections of muscle via tendon to bone.

insomnia Difficulty falling asleep or staying asleep when one has the opportunity to be sleeping.

instillation The administration of therapeutic agents drop by drop, as eye drops, ear drops, or nose drops. It is also administered into a body space or cavity through a catheter.

institutional care Usually refers to nursing home or hospital care.

Instrumental Activities of **Daily Living (IADL)** Normal day-to-day housekeeping activities such as cooking, cleaning, shopping, etc. with which functionally impaired individuals may need assistance. Also see activities of daily living.

instrumentation The use of instruments such as metal screws or braces during a surgical procedure to support bone as it heals.

insufflation The act of blowing a powder, vapor, gas, or air into a cavity such as the lungs.

insulin Hormone secreted by the isles of Langerhans in the pancreas; regulates storage of glycogen in the liver and accelerates oxidation of sugar in cells.

insulin-like growth factor i Insulin-like growth factor 1 (IGF-1) is mainly secreted by the liver as a result of stimulation by growth hormone (GH). Growth factors are proteins that bind to receptors on the cell surface, with the primary result of activating cellular proliferation and/or differentiation.

insulinoma Benign (nonmalignant) tumor of insulin secreting cells of the islets of Langerhans in the pancreas. It results in excessive insulin production and is one of the main causes of hypoglycemia. *See* Hypoglycemia. It is a rare disease and very difficult to diagnose because symptoms are often vague and mimic neurologic and psychiatric disorders. Treatment is usually surgical removal of the tumor. Frequent high carbohydrate meals or medication may also be used.

insulin-resistant states Severe insulin dependent diabetes mellitus that no longer responds to treatment with insulin.

Insurance Sharing the costs of the risk of incurring losses, whether for health expenses or property and casualty losses, across a base large enough to protect any one entity against the actual costs of an incurred loss. The costs of spreading the risk are assumed to be less than the costs of an actual loss. The insured group or insurance company is at financial risk for assuming the guarantee against loss for the specific instance.

insurance clerk A health care professional's employee who has been assigned the very important job of managing health insurance claims in the medical office.

insurance market reform The goal of most insurance market reform initiatives is to materially change the nature of competition in health insurance markets by prohibiting, or severely limiting, the marketing, rating, and underwriting practices that identify and select the most favorable risks while rejecting the least favorable. Requirements that often accompany insurance market reform proposals include prohibition of experience rating in favor of modified community rating, open enrollment, use of a standard benefit package and elimination of preexisting conditions exclusions. Imposition of such regulations would have the effect of reducing the rate differential among groups, and among competing insurers. However, while premium costs would fall for some groups, they would rise for others.

insurance reform Changing insurance companies' practices that prevent some consumers from obtaining health care coverage. Also see insurance market reform.

insured The person who represents the family unit in relation to the health insurance program. Usually the employee whose employment makes this coverage possible.

insurer An insurer of a GHP entity that, in exchange for payment of a premium, agrees to pay for GHP-covered services received by eligible individuals.

Insurer HMO An HMO whose primary purpose is to provide health insurance and who contracts with independent providers for the health care network.

integrated care An approach used to manage all aspects of health care including primary care, acute care and long term care.

integrated delivery system A provider organization that is fully integrated operationally and clinically to provide a full range of health care services, including physician services, hospital services, and ancillary services.

Integrated Provider Network (IPN) A group of hospitals, physicians and ancillary providers which have joined together to create a system which provides comprehensive health care services through a coordinated, client-centered continuum designed to improve health care services in specified geographic markets also known as an integrated delivery system (IDS) or an integrated delivery and financing system, especially when the organization offers an insurance plan. Also see community care network..

Integrated Services Network (ISN) *See* integrated provider network..

integration For provider organizations, the unification of two or more previously separate providers under common ownership or control, or the combination of the business operations of two or more providers that were previously carried out separately and independently.

integrity controls HIPAA security mechanism employed to ensure the validity of the information being electronically transmitted or stored.

integumentary system The organ system that protects the body from damage, comprising the skin and its appendages, including hair, scales, and nails.

intelligence test A set of problems or tasks posed to assess an individual's innate ability to judge, comprehend, and reason.

intensive care The provision of life support or organ support systems in patients who are critically ill and who usually require intensive monitoring.

Intensive Care Unit (ICU) Highly specialized care requiring sophisticated technologies given to patients who are in danger of disability or death.

inter- Between, among.

intercondylar Between condyles; as, the intercondylar fossa or notch of the femur.

intercostal Located or occurring between the ribs.

interferometry Measurement of distances or movements by means of the phenomena caused by the interference of two rays of light (optical interferometry) or of sound (acoustic interferometry).

intermediary A health insurance carrier, or data processing company, designed to receive and process Medicare or Medicaid claims on behalf of the government.

intermediate care A degree of nursing care evaluation that is less than that provided for skilled nursing care, but greater than that provided for custodial care. This level of care provides a planned, continuous program of nursing care that is preventive or rehabilitative in nature.

Intermediate Care Facility (ICF) A facility providing an inter-mediate level of care to individuals who do not require the degree of care and treatment that a hospital or skilled nursing facility is designed to provide, but who do require care above the level of room and board.

intermediate care facility for mentally retarded A facility which primarily provides health-related care and services above the level of custodial care to mentally retarded individuals but does not provide the level of care available in a hospital or skilled nursing facility.

intermediate entities Entities which contract between an MCO or one of its subcontractors, and a physician or physician group, other than physician groups themselves.

intermittent peritoneal dialysis An intermittent (periodic), supine regimen, which uses intermittent flow technique, automated assisted manual, or manual method in dialysis sessions two to four times weekly.

Intermittent Positive-Pressure-Breathing (IPPB) Form of treatment for disorders of the lungs using a sophisticated, expensive instrument that forces air into the lungs by controlled positive pressure. Treatment is usually given by a trained pulmonary therapist or technician.

internal audit The in-house review of the records of system activity (for example, logins, file accesses, security incidents) maintained by an organization.

internal controls Management systems and policies for reasonably documenting, monitoring, and correcting operational processes to prevent and detect waste and to ensure proper payment.

internal derangement of knee A term that describes internal damage to the knee joint, generally caused by trauma. It a nonspecific term that usually must be further refined by history, physical exam, x-rays, and frequently MRI studies.

internal fixation The immobilization of bone fragments or joints with implants in order to promote healing or fusion.

internal mammary arteries Vessels inside the chest wall that are commonly used to create an alternative pathway for blood to reach the heart muscle.

internal rotation A motion of the shoulder or hip that points the toes or the flexed forearm inwards (towards the midline). *Synonym:* medial rotation.

internal thoracic artery An artery on the inside of the chest wall used for bypass grafting.

International Classification of Diseases, 9th Revision, Clinical Modification Coding system maintained by the National Center for Health Statistics and the Center for Medicare and Medicaid Services (CMS). This coding system differentiates diagnostic conditions and is used by hospitals, governments, health insurance plans, and health care providers around the world.

internist A physician who finds and treats health problems in adults.

interocclusal The space between upper and lower teeth.

interpretation and report Refers to the process of reviewing the results of a diagnostic test, such as an EKG, x-ray, CT scan, etc., and preparing a written report.

interproximal The area between two adjacent teeth.

interscapular Between the shoulders or shoulder blades.

interscapular region Between the shoulders or shoulder blades.

intersex surgery Surgery performed for the purpose of changing a male to a female or vice versa.

interstitial Occupies space between tissues, such as interstitial fluid.

interstitial fibrosis Formation of fibrous tissue between normal tissues.

interstitial fluid The fluid in spaces between the tissue cells.

intervertebral disc disorders Result from a protrusion or herniation of one of the gel-like cushions (discs) that separate the vertebrae of the spine.

intervertebral disk chemolysis The dissolving of the nucleus pulposus of a displaced intervertebral disk, usually by the direct injection of a proteolytic enzyme, especially chymopapain, into the diseased disk.

intestinal of or relating to the intestines.

intestinal fistula Abnormal opening leading from the intestinal tract to another abdominal organ or to the skin.

intestinal malabsorption A state arising from abnormality in digestion or absorption of food nutrients across the gastrointestinal tract.

intestinal obstruction without mention of **hernia,** A blockage in the intestine which prevents the normal flow of waste down the length of the intestine.

intestine The section of the alimentary canal from the stomach to the anus. It includes the large intestine and small intestine.

intra- Within.

intra-abdominal Within the abdomen.

intra-aortic Within the aorta.

intra-arterial Within an artery.

intra-atrial Within the atrium.

intracavitary Within a cavity.

intracerebral hemorrhage A medical condition indicated by the rupturing of a blood vessel in the brain and the subsequent bleeding into the tissues of the brain.

intracoronal The area within the crown of a tooth.

intracranial Within the cranium , the bony dome that houses and protects the brain.

intracranial and intraspinal abscess An abcess occuring inside the cranium or the spinal column.

intracranial hemorrhage Bleeding in the brain caused by the breaking (rupture) of a blood vessel in the head.

intractable Unstoppable. For example, intractable diarrhea or intractable pain.

intracutaneous Within the skin.

intracutaneous test A skin test in which the antigen is injected intradermally. *Synonym:* intradermal test.

intradermal Within the dermis.

intradural Within or beneath the dura mater.

intraepithelial Within the layer of cells that forms the surface or lining of an organ.

intraepithelial neoplasia Small tumor or cancer in the epithelial layer of the skin.

intrafallopian Within the fallopian tube.

intrahepatic Within the liver.

intralesional Within a lesion.

intraluminal Within the lumen of a structure.

intramedullary The inside of a bone.

intramuscular Within a muscle.

intranasal Within the nose.

intranasal administration The administration of drugs through the nasal passage.

intranet An internal (private) computer network, built on Web-based technologies and standards, that is only available to members of the computer network.

intraocular Within the eye.

intraocular lens A man-made silicone or plastic lens used to replace the natural crystalline lens of the eye. Used in cataract surgery, lens (P-IOL) implantation, or refractive lens exchange.

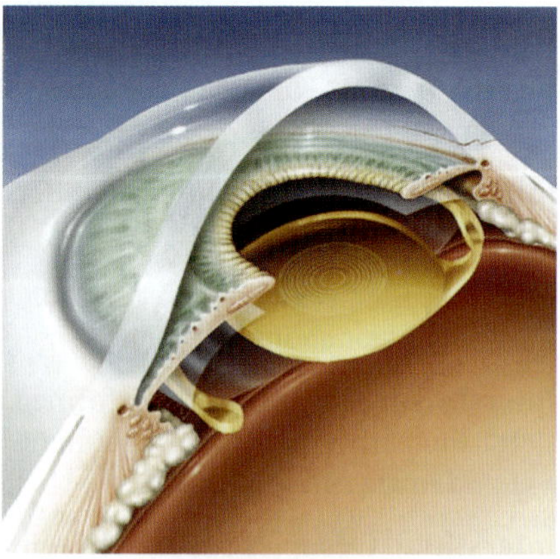

intraocular lens

intraocular pressure Pressure within the eye. High intraocular pressure is called glaucoma.

intraoperative The period of time during a surgical procedure.

intraoral Within the mouth.

intraosseous Within bone.

intrapelvic Within the pelvis.

intraperitoneal Within the peritoneum.

intrapleural Within the pleural cavity.

intrapulmonary Within the lungs.

intraretinal Within the retina.

intraspinal Within the spine.

intrastromal Within the stroma, especially of the cornea.

intrathecal Within the sheath of the spinal cord.

intrathoracic Within the thorax.

intrauterine Within the uterus.

intravaginal Within the vagina.

intravascular Within blood vessels or a blood vessel.

intravenous (IV) Into a vein.

intravenous pyelogram (IVP) A radiological procedure used to visualize abnormalities of the urinary system, including the kidneys, ureters, and bladder. *Synonym:* pyelography.

intravenously Through a vein.

intraventricular In the ventricle of the heart or brain.

intravesical Within the bladder.

intravitreal Within the eye, refers to a route of administration of a drug, or other substance, in which the substance is delivered via an eye.

intrinsic factor levels Substance secreted by the stomach lining that is necessary for vitamin B-12 to be absorbed by the intestine. A deficiency of intrinsic factor results in pernicious anemia. *See* Anemia, pernicious.

introduction The act of putting one thing into another. *Synonyms* cannulation, instillation, injection, perfusion, transfusion.

introitus Entrance or opening to a hollow organ or tube.

intubation Introduction of a tube into a hollow organ to restore or maintain patency if obstructed. It is differentiated from catheterization in that the insertion of a catheter is usually performed for the introducing or withdrawing of fluids from the body.

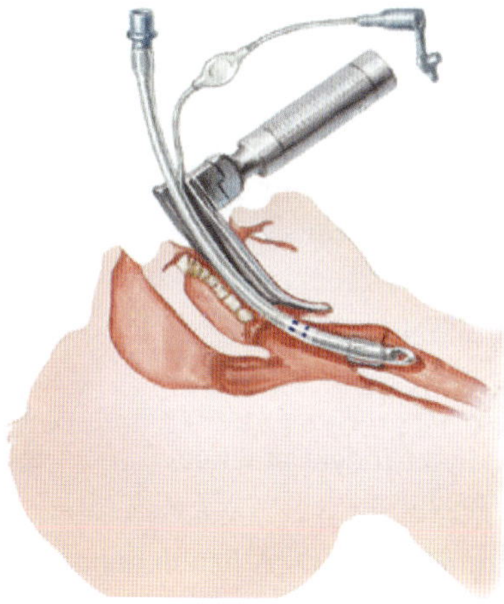

intubation

intussusception Intussusception is the enfolding of one segment of the intestine within another. It is characterized by and initially presents with recurring attacks of cramping abdominal pain that gradually become more painful.

invagination The infolding of one part within another part of a structure, as of the blastula during gastrulation.

inversion The movement of the sole towards the median plane (same as when an ankle is twisted).

IO Intraocular.

iodine-deficient goiter Enlarged thyroid gland due to too little iodine in the diet. Iodine is an essential trace element and is usually found in drinking water. Using small amounts of iodized table salt (if you live in an area with insufficient iodine in drinking water) prevents the occurrence of a goiter. A goiter causes a pronounced swelling in the front part of he neck.

IOL Intraocular lens.

iontophoresis Therapeutic introduction of ions of soluble salts into tissues by means of electric current.

IOP Intraocular pressure.

IP Inpatient.

IPA Independent practice association.

IPA model HMO A health maintenance organization which contracts with one or more associations of physicians in independent practice who agree to provide medical services to HMO members.

IPPB Intermittent positive pressure breathing.

IPPS Acute care hospital inpatient prospective payment system.

IPPV Intermittent positive-pressure ventilation.

IPR Independent professional review.

ipsilateral On or relating to the same side of the body.

IPSP Inhibitory postsynaptic potential.

IRDS Idiopathic respiratory distress syndrome.

IRF Inpatient Rehabilitation Facility.

irid(o)- Iris.

iridectomy Surgical removal of a section of the iris most frequently performed in the treatment of closed-angle glaucoma and iris melanoma[. *Synonym:* corectomy.

iridencleisis Confinement of a portion of the iris in a wound of the cornea as a surgical measure in treating glaucoma.

iridocapsulectomy Surgical procedure to remove a secondary membranous cataract. *Synonym:* iridocapsulotomy.

iridocyclitis An inflammation of the iris and of the ciliary body.

iridodialysis A localized separation or tearing away of the iris from its attachment to the ciliary body.

iridoplasty Surgery to alter the iris.

iridoschisis Splitting of the mesodermal stroma of the iris into two layers.

iridotasis Surgical stretching of the iris for glaucoma.

iridotomy A surgical incision into the iris.

iris Colored portion of the eye that expands or contracts to control the size of the pupil.

iritis Inflammation of tissues that support the iris (the ring of colored tissue around the pupil of the eye). Symptoms include eye pain, sensitivity to light and blurred vision. May be caused by infection that spreads to the eye from other body parts, injury to the eye or an autoimmune reaction. Often cause is unknown.

iron deficiency anemia A form of anemia due to lack of iron in the diet or to iron loss as a result of chronic bleeding.

iron overload Too much iron in blood, liver or other organs.

iron-deficiency anemia *See* Anemia, iron deficiency.

irradiated red blood cells Red blood cells treated with exposure to radiation in order to inactivate white blood cells which may cause graft-versus-host disease.

irradiation The treatment of disease by exposure to a radioactive substance.

irrigation The washing of a body cavity or surface by flowing solution which is inserted and then removed.

irritable bowel syndrome A functional bowel disorder characterized by chronic abdominal pain, discomfort, bloating, and alteration of bowel habits in the absence of any organic cause. *Synonym:* spastic colon.

IRV Inspiratory reserve volume.

ischemia Decreased blood supply to a body organ or part.

ischemic Condition in which there is decreased blood flow to a body organ or part.

ischemic bowel disease Intestinal problems caused by inadequate supply of blood to the cells of the intestines.

ischemic heart disease A disease characterized by reduced blood supply to the heart muscle, usually due to coronary artery disease (atherosclerosis of the coronary arteries).

ischemic preconditioning A technique in which tissue is rendered resistant to the deleterious effects of prolonged ischemia and reperfusion by prior exposure to brief, repeated periods of vascular occlusion.

ischiectomy Surgical removal of a segment of the hip bone including the ischium.

ischio- of or pertaining to the ischium, the hip-joint.

ischium One of the three sections of the hipbone; situated below the ilium.

Ishihara test Test for color blindness that utilizes plates upon which figures are formed from round dots of various colors.

islets of Langerhans The regions of the pancreas that contain its endocrine.

-ism Condition, disease.

-ismus Spasm, contraction.

iso- Denoting something as being 'equal'.

isochromosome Abnormal chromosome characterized by abnormal splitting of a chromosome during the process of duplicating itself. May cause inherited diseases or disorders.

isoenzyme One of many forms of a protein catalyst differing in characteristics (chemical, physical, immunological) but catalyzing the same reaction. For example, lactate dehydrogenase may exist in five different forms.

isola instrumentation Posterior fixation device.

isothermal infusion Injection with a fluid at the same temperature as the recipient.

IST Insulin shock therapy.

-ist One who specializes in.

isthmus A cord-like tissue connecting two larger parts of an anatomical structure.

isthmusectomy Standard surgical technique for removal of unilateral thyroid nodules.

IU International unit.

IUD Intrauterine device.

-ium Structure, tissue.

IUP Intrauterine pregnancy.

IV Intravenous.

IVAC Intravenous automated controller.

IVP Intravenous pyelogram.

IVU Intravenous urogram.

J

Jaboulay operation An operation to repair a hydrocele involving excision and eversion of the hydrocele sac. This procedure is typically performed as a day case under general or local anesthesia employing an incision through the scrotum.

Jacobs locking hook Thick, threaded rods for fixation of various spinal deformities.

Jaeger card Card with printed letters of varying sizes. Used to test vision.

Jakob-Creutzfeldt disease Spastic pseudoparalysis; a rare, usually fatal, transmissible spongiform encephalopathy characterized by progressive dementia, myoclonus and ataxia.

Jannetta procedure The most common surgical procedure for the treatment of trigeminal neuralgia. *Synonym:* microvascular decompression.

Jarcho-Levin syndrome Defects of the spine associated with a small, stiff thorax and pulmonary compromise.

Jatene procedure An open heart surgical procedure used to correct dextro-transposition of the great arteries.

jaundice Condition of yellow skin, yellow whites of the eyes, dark urine and light-colored stools. It is a symptom of diseases of the liver and blood caused by abnormally elevated amounts of bilirubin in the blood.

jaw fixation techniques The stable placement of surgically induced fractures of the mandible or maxilla through the use of elastics, wire ligatures, arch bars, or other splints. It is used often in the cosmetic surgery of retrognathism and prognathism.

jaw jerk reflex The mandible is tapped with a rubber hammer when the jaw is half open. If there is brain injury to the motor portion of the fifth cranial nerve, the jaw jerks closed. When the jaw jerk reflex is increased on the opposite side, a unilateral frontal lobe lesion may be suspected.

JCAH Joint Commission on Accreditation of Hospitals.

JCAHO Joint Commission on Accreditation of Health care Organizations.

J-codes A subset of the HCPCS Level II code set with a high-order value of J that has been used to identify certain drugs and other items. The final HIPAA transactions and code sets rule states that these J-codes will be dropped from the HCPCS, and that NDC codes will be used to identify the associated pharmaceuticals and supplies.

jejunoileal bypass A surgical procedure consisting of the anastomosis of the proximal part of the jejunum to the distal portion of the ileum, so as to bypass the nutrient-absorptive segment of the small intestine, to treat morbid obesity.

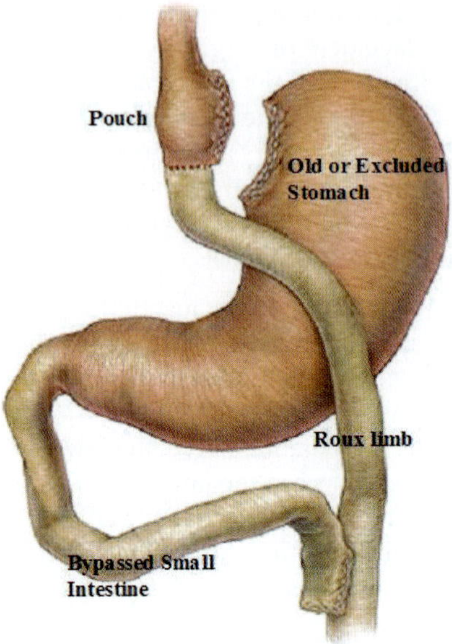

jejunoileal bypass.

jejunostomy Creation of an artificial opening between the jejunum and the anterior abdominal wall performed to allow feeding tube placement.

jejunum The part of the small intestine between the duodenum and the ileum.

joint aspiration The clinical procedure of using a syringe to collect synovial fluid from a joint capsule. Used in the diagnosis of gout, arthritis, and synovial infections. *Synonym:* arthrocentesis.

Joint Commission on Accreditation of Health care Organizations (JCAHO) Founded in 1951, the JCAHO evaluates and accredits health care organization in the U.S., including hospitals, health plans, and other care organizations that provide home care, mental health care, laboratory, ambulatory care and long-term services.

Jones procedure A procedure for correction of a clawed hallux.

Joplin procedure Correction of bunion with or without sesamoidectomy; with tendon transplants.

jugular vein Veins in the neck that return blood from the head.

justice or equity An ethical principle, which, when applied to managed care, states that managed care organizations and their providers allocate resources in a way that fairly distributes benefits and burdens among the members.

K

KAFO Knee-ankle-foot orthosis.

Kaneda device Anteriorly placed fixation device for spinal deformities.

Kaposi's sarcoma A cancer that causes patches of abnormal tissue to grow under the skin, in the lining of the mouth, nose, and throat or in other organs. Most often found in patients with acquired immunodeficiency syndrome (aids).

karyo- Nucleus.

karyotyping Determining the chromosome constitution of the nucleus of a cell. Useful in predicting abnormalities in a fetus before birth, using amniotic fluid to study cells.

Kasai procedure An operation to create an open duct so bile can drain.

Kawasaki syndrome Febrile mucocutaneous lymph node disease.

Keen operation Removal of sections of the posterior branches of the spinal nerves to the affected muscles, and of the spinal accessory nerve, as a cure for torticollis.

Kelikian procedure Surgical procedure for the repair of webbed toe(s).

Keller procedure Surgical procedure for hallux valgus.

keloid scar A type of scar that continues to grow beyond what is needed at the site of an injury. This type of scar is caused by too much collagen forming while the skin is being repaired. The tendency to develop keloid scars is genetic.

kerat(o)- Cornea (eye or skin).

keratectomy Surgical excision (removal) of any portion of the cornea.

keratitis Infection or inflammation of the cornea which can be caused by a variety of conditions, including infections, dry eyes, foreign objects, contact lenses, intense light, vitamin a deficiency or allergies.

keratoconjunctivitis Inflammation of the cornea and conjunctiva.

keratoconus A disorder that involves a thinning of the central cornea. The normally round shape of the cornea becomes distorted. A cone-like bulge develops, resulting in significant visual impairment.

keratoderma Any skin disorder consisting of a growth that appears horny.

keratolytic agents Agents that soften, separate, and cause desquamation of the cornified epithelium or horny layer of skin. They are used to expose mycelia of infecting fungi or to treat corns, warts, and certain other skin diseases.

keratomalacia Softening and drying and ulceration of the cornea resulting from vitamin A deficiency; symptom of cystic fibrosis or sprue.

keratometry The measurement of the curvature of the cornea.

keratomileusis A refractive surgical technique where a partial thickness circular flap of cornea is removed, frozen, reshaped on a lathe and replaced upon the cornea.

keratopathy Noninflammatory disease of the cornea.

keratophakia Keratoplasty in which corneal tissue from a donor is frozen, reshaped, and transplanted into the corneal stroma of the recipient to modify refractive error.

keratoplasty Plastic repair on the cornea.

keratoprosthesis A plastic replacement for an opacified inner part of a cornea.

keratosis A skin condition marked by an overgrowth of layers of horny skin.

keratosis follicularis Uncommon hereditary skin disorder characterized by small, horny growths that grow together to form brown or black, crusted, wart-like patches. They can spread rapidly, ulcerate and become covered with pus. Treatment includes large doses of vitamin-A by mouth, vitamin-A acid cream applied to lesions and sometimes steroids taken by mouth or applied to the skin.

keratotomy Surgical incision into the cornea.

kernicterus An abnormal accumulation of bile pigment in the brain and other nerve tissue; causes yellow staining and tissue damage.

Kernig's sign Flexion of hip and extension of leg while recumbent causes pain; a positive sign for meningitis.

ketoacidosis Serious disorder that results from a deficiency or inadequate use of carbohydrates. Characterized by fluid and electrolyte disorders, dehydration and mental confusion. If left untreated, coma and death may occur. It is usually a complication of diabetes mellitus but may also be seen in starvation and rarely in pregnancy if diet is inadequate.

ketone bodies Substances formed when the body rapidly breaks down fats to use for energy.

ketonuria Presence of ketone bodies in the urine. Usually seen in people with uncontrolled diabetes mellitus or as a result of starvation. *See* Diabetes mellitus.

ketsuekigata The study of personality analysis by blood type. It has become a nearly indispensable part of Japanese popular culture. Most of Japanese women and members of the younger generation believe that there is some correlation between blood type and personality.

Kidner procedure Relocation of tibialis posterior tendon insertion in the treatment of symptomatic accessory navicular.

kidney Either of two bean-shaped excretory organs that filter wastes (especially urea) from the blood and excrete them and water in urine.

kidney failure The sudden loss of the kidneys' ability to eliminate excess fluid and electrolytes as well as waste material from the blood.

kidney shut down Sudden failure of kidneys to function. Usually has a short, relatively severe course but is often curable. *Synonym:* kidney failure, renal failure.

kidney stones Hard, unyielding material produced by the kidney. May lodge in the kidney or pass through the ureter, the bladder and finally the urethra to the outside of the body.

Killian's operation Excision of the anterior wall of the frontal sinus.

kilo Kilogram.

kin(e)-, kin(o), kinesi(o)- Movement.

kineplasty An amputation of a limb in which tendons are arranged in the stump to permit their use in moving parts of the prosthetic appliance.

King's operation Surgical fixation of arytenoid cartilage or muscle. *Synonym:* arytenoidopexy.

Kirschner wire (apparatus) Steel wire used for skeletal fixation of, and obtaining skeletal traction in, fractures.

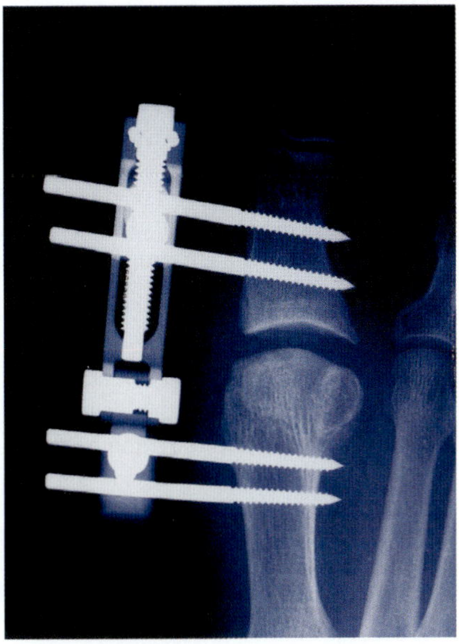

X-ray showing Kirschner wires.

Kleihauer-Betke procedure A procedure performed to diagnose fetomaternal hemorrhage.

Klinefelter's syndrome XXY syndrome; feminization of males due to extra X chromosomes combined with one Y chromosome, resulting in small testes and infertility.

Klippel-Feil syndrome Rare, congenital malformation of the neck due to fewer than normal vertebrae in the neck or because vertebrae are joined together. Results in limited neck movement and a low hairline. May require no treatment. It can cause pressure on nerves; if this occurs, traction or surgery may be necessary. *Synonym:* congenital short-neck syndrome.

knee jerk reflex This test is conducted by striking the Patellar tendons of the knee for reflex indications of a lesion in the L2, L3-L4 segments.

Knodt distraction rod Device used for distraction stabilization of the thoracic and lumbar spine.

Kocher operation A surgical procedure for the treatment of goiter.

Kock pouch Abdominovesical pouch one formed by reflection of the peritoneum from the abdominal wall to the anterior surface of the bladder.

Koenig syndrome Diarrhea alternating with constipation, seen with abdominal pain, meteorism and gurgling sounds on the right iliac fossa, symptomatic of cecal tuberculosis.

KOH Potassium hydroxide.

kojic acid A skin treatment product derived from a fungus that studies have shown is effective as a lightening agent and in inhibiting the production of melanin.

Kostmann's syndrome A rare inherited form of Severe Chronic Neutropenia usually detected soon after birth. *Synonym:* severe congenital neutropenia.

Kostuick-Harrington Anteriorly placed device for spinal deformity instrumentation correction.

Kraske's operation Removal of the coccyx and part of the sacrum for access to a rectal carcinoma.

Krebs cycle A basic metabolic mechanism involving the oxidation of acetic acid for energy stored in phosphate bonds. *Synonym:* citric acid cycle.

Kroenlein procedure Lateral orbital decompression to relieve forward pressure on the eye.

Krönlein's hernia A complicated hernia having a double sac, one part in the inguinal canal, the other projecting from the internal inguinal ring in the subperitoneal tissues.

Krukenberg procedure A surgical technique that converts a forearm stump into a pincer.

KUB Kidneys, ureters, bladder.

Kuhlmann test A modification of the Binet test of intelligence for use in infants.

Kussmal respirations Rapid, deep respiration due to diabetic ketoacidosis.

Kussmaul disease A vasculitis of medium-sized arteries, which become swollen and damaged from attack by rogue immune cells. *Synonym:* polyarteritis nodosa.

Kveim test A skin test used to detect sarcoidosis, where part of a spleen from a patient with known sarcoidosis is injected into the skin of a patient suspected to have the disease.

kwashiorkor A virulent form of childhood malnutrition characterized by edema, irritability, anorexia, ulcerating dermatoses, and an enlarged liver with fatty infiltrates.

kyph(o)- Humped.

kyphectomy Excision of kyphotic portion of lumbar spine combined with spinal fixation.

kyphoplasty Surgical procedure to restore vertebra bone height and reverse spine deformity.

kyphoscoliosis An abnormal curvature of the spine in both a coronal and sagittal plane.

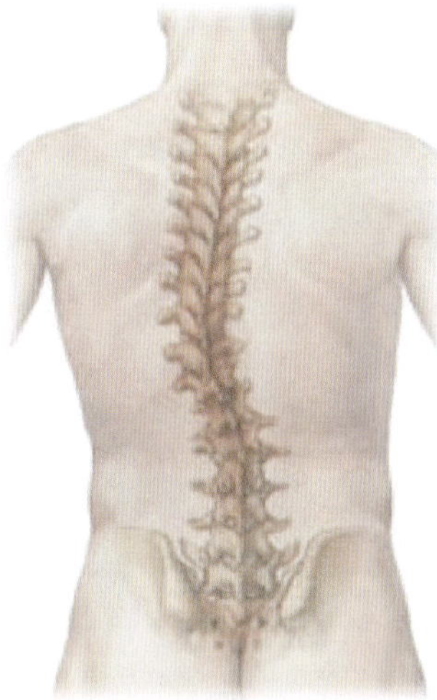

kyphoscoliosis

kyphosis Abnormal condition in which the upper spinal column (between the neck and midback) curves outward excessively. Sometimes occurs in adolescents. Usually causes no symptoms and requires no treatment. Can be caused by rickets or tuberculosis of the spine. If very severe, may be treated with a back brace; rarely surgery is needed. *Synonym:* hunchback.

L

lab Laboratory.

labi(o)- of or pertaining to the lip.

labia Any of the four lip-shaped folds of the female vulva.

labia majora The two outer rounded folds of adipose tissue that lie on either side of the vaginal opening and form the external lateral boundaries of the vulva.

labia minora The two folds of mucous membrane within the labia majora.

labial Of or pertaining to, or around, a lip.

labor Childbirth, the aptly-named experience of delivering the baby and placenta from the uterus to the vagina to the outside world. There are two stages of labor. During the first stage (called the stage of dilatation), the cervix dilates fully to a diameter.

labyrinthectomy Excision of the labyrinth of the ear.

labyrinthitis An inflammation of the inner ear.

labyrinthotomy Incision into the labyrinth of the ear.

laceration A jagged wound or cut.

Lachman test Test used to confirm anterior or posterior cruciate instability.

lacrim(o)- Tear.

lacrimal bone A thin scalelike bone, roughly resembling a fingernail in size and shape, at the anterior part of the medial wall of the orbit, articulating with the frontal and ethmoidal bones and the maxilla and inferior nasal concha.

lacrimal duct Any of several small ducts that carry tears from the lacrimal glands.

lacrimal punctum The minute circular opening of the lacrimal duct on the margin of each eyelid.

lacrimation Shedding tears.

lact(i)-, lact(o) Milk.

lactation The secretion of milk from the mammary glands.

lactic acidosis Increased acidity in body due to accumulation of excessive lactic acid production.

Ladd procedure Surgical division of Ladd's bands, widening of the small intestine's mesentery, performing an appendectomy and correctional placement of the cecum and colon.

Laënnec's cirrhosis Cirrhosis of the liver associated with alcohol abuse.

lagophthalmos The inability or difficulty in closing the eye. May be caused by Bell's Palsy, trauma, neurosurgery, bacterial infection, stroke, and cosmetic surgery. Common symptoms are severe dry eye and discomfort, corneal ulceration, decrease or loss of vision.

Lagrange's operation A combined iridectomy and sclerectomy that is performed in glaucoma for the purpose of forming a filtering cicatrix. *Synonym:* Sclerecto-iridectomy.

lamina An anatomical portion of a vertebra. For each vertebra, two lamina connect the pedicles to the spinous process as part of the neural arch.

laminaria A product made from a certain type of seaweed that is physically placed near the cervix to cause it to dilate.

laminate A thin plastic or porcelain veneer produced in a dental laboratory and then bonded to a tooth.

laminectomy An operation for removal of part or all of the lamina of a vertebra, commonly performed in order to be able to remove an intervertebral disc protrusion or to decompress a nerve root.

laminoplasty A surgical procedure for treating spinal stenosis by relieving pressure on the spinal cord.

laminotomy A neurosurgical procedure that removes part of a lamina of the vertebral arch in order to decompress the corresponding spinal cord and/or spinal nerve root.

Landry's syndrome Acute idiopathic polyneuritis.

Langerhans adenoma Islet cell adenoma of the pancreas; insulinoma.

language tests Tests designed to assess language behavior and abilities. They include tests of vocabulary, comprehension, grammar and functional use of language.

LAP Laparotomy.

lapar(o)- of or pertaining to the abdomen-wall, flank.

laparoscopic surgery Technique in which abdominal operations are performed through small incisions.

laparoscopy Direct visualization of the peritoneal cavity, ovaries, outside of the tubes and uterus by using a laparoscope.

laparotomy A surgical procedure involving an incision through the abdominal wall to gain access into the abdominal cavity.

Lapidus procedure Procedure for correction of metatarsus primus varus and hallux valgus.

large cell carcinoma A group of lung cancers in which the cells are large and look abnormal.

large group health plan A plan provided by an employer who employs 100 or more persons or a plan belonging to a multi-employer plan where at least one employer has 100 or more full or part time employees.

Laroyenne operation Puncture of Douglas pouch to evacuate the pus and to secure drainage in cases of pelvic suppuration.

laryng(o)- of or pertaining to the larynx.

laryngeal of or relating to the pharynx.

laryngectomy Total or partial excision of the larynx.

laryngitis Inflammation of the mucous membrane of the larynx, characterized by hoarseness or loss of voice and coughing.

laryngocele A congenital anomalous air sac communicating with the cavity of the larynx, which may bulge outward on the neck.

laryngofissure Surgical opening of the larynx that is usually made through the midline of the thyroid cartilage.

laryngography Radiography of the larynx.

laryngopharyngectomy Excision of the larynx and pharynx.

laryngopharyngitis Inflammation of the larynx and the pharynx.

laryngopharynx The portion of the pharynx below the upper edge of the epiglottis.

laryngoplasty Plastic repair of the larynx.

laryngoscopy Examination, therapy or surgery of the interior of the larynx performed with a specially designed endoscope.

laryngospasm Spasmotic closure of the larynx or voice box. When spasms occur, air cannot pass through the larynx properly. May occur with croup in infants, in tetany, caused by abnormally low calcium level in the blood, or in tetanus (lockjaw). Can be life-threatening if condition is severe.

laryngotomy Incision of the larynx.

laryngotracheitis Inflammation of the larynx and trachea.

larynx Part of the air passage connecting the throat with the trachea or windpipe.

Laseque's sign A limitation of straight leg raising usually associated with lumbar nerve root compression. Also, in sciatica, flexion of the hip is painful with the knee extended but painless when the knee is flexed.

LASER Light amplification by stimulated emission of radiation. The device that produces a focused beam of light at a defined wavelength that can vaporize tissue. In surgery, lasers can be used to operate on small areas without damaging delicate surrounding tissue.

laser coagulation The coagulation of tissues using lasers. These lasers produce light in the visible green wavelength that is selectively absorbed by hemoglobin, and thus it is possible to seal bleeding blood vessels.

laser surgery The use of a laser either to vaporize surface lesions or to make bloodless cuts in tissue. It does not include the coagulation of tissue by laser (laser coagulation).

laser-doppler flowmetry A method of non-invasive, continuous measurement of microcirculation. The technique is based on the values of the Doppler effect of low-power laser light scattered randomly by static structures and moving tissue particulates.

LASIK Laser-assisted in situ keratomileusis.

late effect A residual effect (condition produced) after the acute phase of an illness or injury has ended.

lateral Situated away from the midline of the body.

lateral sclerosis Degeneration of the lateral columns of the spinal cord.

latero- Lateral.

latex agglutination test A type of agglutination test in which antigen to a given antibody is adsorbed to latex particles and mixed with a test solution to observe for agglutination of the latex.

Latzko operation A method for the closure of small vesico-vaginal fistulas occurring in the vaginal dome after hysterectomy.

laughing gas Nitrous oxide; odorless inhalation agent that produces relative analgesic (sedation); reduces anxiety and creates a state of relaxation.

Laveen shunt Peritoneal-jugular shunt.

LBBB Left bundle branch block.

LBVP Luminal balloon valvuloplasty.

LBW Low birth weight.

LDH LDH is a material found in blood cells and liver cells. Breakdown of the blood cells as in heart disease or liver damage may increase values.

LDP Labor, delivery, and postpartum.

Leeds procedure Segmental wiring of a contoured square-ended Harrington rod for scoliosis.

LEEP procedure The loop electro-surgical excision procedure uses a thin, low-voltage electrified wire loop to cut out abnormal tissue.

Lefort's fracture Bilateral horizontal fracture of the maxilla.

Lefort's operation Uniting the anterior and posterior vaginal walls at the middle line to repair or prevent uterine prolapse.

left ventricle The main pumping chambers of the heart are the ventricles. The heart has a right side that pumps blood to the lungs, and a left side that pumps blood to the body. The left side of the heart, therefore, must work harder than the right.

legally induced abortion An abortion performed by medical professionals conforming to the legal guidelines of the state where the abortion is performed.

legend drug Drug that can only be obtained by prescription.

Legg-Calvé-Perthes disease Osteochondritis deformans juvenilis; necrosis of the upper end of the femur.

legionella The motile aerobic rod-shaped Gram-negative bacterium that thrives in central heating and air conditioning systems and can cause Legionnaires" disease.

lei(o)- Smooth.

leiomyoma Benign tumor of smooth muscle (usually in the uterus or digestive tract).

leiomyomata A benign smooth muscle neoplasm that is not premalignant.

leishmania Flagellate protozoan that causes leishmaniasis.

leishmaniasis A disease caused by protozoan parasites that belong to the genus leishmania and is transmitted by the bite of certain species of sand fly.

length of **stay** The number of days, counted from the day of admission to the day of discharge, that a plan member is confined to a hospital or other facility for each admission.

length-of-stay guidelines A utilization review resource that establishes an average inpatient length of stay based on a patient's diagnosis, the severity of the patient's condition, and the type of services and procedures prescribed for the patient's care.

lens A transparent double convex (outward curve on both sides) structure between the iris and the vitreous humor.

leprosy Chronic disease characterized by the production of fibrous connective-tissue lesions (granulomatous) of the skin, mucous membranes and peripheral nervous system (excluding the brain and spinal cord). It is not very contagious and requires prolonged, intimate contact to be transmitted to another person. The more serious form of leprosy may cause blindness and severe disfigurement. Treatment can result in improvement of skin lesions, but recovery of nerve damage is limited.

-lepsis, -lepsy Attack, seizure.

lept(o)- Light, slender.

leptomeningioma A slow-growing tumor of the meninges that is not cancerous. Symptoms are determined by the size and location of the tumor.

leptospira Important pathogens causing Weil's disease or canicola fever.

leptospirosis Also known as swamp fever, acute, infectious, febrile disease of both humans and animals, caused by spirochetes of the genus leptospira. *Synonym:* swamp fever.

lesion Injury or damage to an organ or tissue.

leuc(o)-, leuk(o)- Denoting a white color.

leucocoria A condition characterized by a whitish reflex within the pupil.

leucoma Eye disease consisting of an opaque white spot on the cornea.

leukemia Malignant neoplasm of blood-forming tissues; characterized by abnormal proliferation of leukocytes; one of the four major types of cancer.

leukemia, acute Malignant overgrowth of white blood cells in bone marrow or tissues that are part of the lymphatic system (lymph glands, spleen, liver). These excess cells accumulate and spill into the blood, eventually involving other tissues. Most common form of cancer in children.

leukemia, granulocytic Malignant blood disease of granulocytes, a form of white blood cell.

leukemia, lymphatic Cancer that primarily involves lymphatic cells. Affects children and adults.

leukemia, lymphocytic Very slow-growing cancer of blood-forming organs in older people. About 35% of all leukemia victims have this form of the disease. It is often discovered in a routine blood test for unrelated purposes.

leukemia, monocytic Malignancy of blood-forming tissues in which the predominant cells are monocytes (a type of white blood cell). The disease has an erratic course characterized by malaise, fatigue, fever, weight loss, enlarged spleen, bleeding gums, anemia and unresponsiveness to therapy. *See* Anemia.

leukemia, myeloblastic Malignancy of blood cells in which the predom-inant cells are myeloblasts (a form of white blood cell).

leukemia, myelogenous *See* Leukemia, myelocytic.

leukemia, myeloid Malignancy of white blood cells with polymorph-onuclear cells predominant.

leukemia, myelomonocytic Malig-nancy of blood cells in which the predominant cells are monocytes and myelocytes.

leukemia, myleocytic Disorder characterized by the unregulated, excessive production of myelocytes. *See* Myelocytes.

leukoagglutinins Antibodies directed against white blood cells.

leukocyte White blood cell.

leukocyte-reduced blood components Helps to prevent blood transfusion reactions caused by white cells contaminating red cell and platelet preparations and may reduce the likelihood of certain infections. A filtering process is used.

leukocytopenia A decrease in the number of white blood cells (leukocytes) found in the blood.

leukocytosis A condition character-ized by an abnormally high total number of circulating leukocytes.

leukodystrophy Refers to a group of disorders characterized by progres-sive degeneration of the white matter of the brain.

leukoencephalopathy The destruct-ion of the myelin sheaths that cover nerve fibers.

leukomalacia Softening of the white matter of the brain.

leukopenia A condition character-zed by an abnormally low total number of circulating leukocytes.

leukoplakia Adherent white plaques or patches on the mucous memb-ranes of the oral cavity, including the tongue.

leukoreduced Removal of white blood cells from products in order to prevent certain transfusion reactions such as fever, chills, and alloimmunization.

leukorrhea Discharge of white mucous material from the vagina; often an indication of infection.

Leveen shunt A tube that is surgically implanted to connect the peritoneal cavity and the superior vena cava to drain accumulated fluid from the peritoneal cavity.

Level II codes *See* HCPCS.

Level of Care (LOC) An assessment of the type of care necessary to meet the individual needs of the client. The assessment takes into consideration the client's needs in all aspects of develop-ment, level of functioning, and potential to benefit from a particular program.

Lhermitte sign Flexing the neck forward causes electric-shock-like pain in the extremities as a sign of multiple sclerosis or compression and other disorders of the cervical cord.

liability determination Determination based of whether the beneficiary and the provider did not and could not have been reasonably expected to know that payment would not be made for services.

licensed by the state as a risk-bearing entity An entity that is licensed or otherwise authorized by the state to assume risk for offering health insurance or health benefits coverage. The entity is authorized to accept prepaid capitation for providing, arranging, or paying for comprehensive health services under an M + C contract. Designation that an M + C organization has been reviewed and determined fully accredited by a CMS-approved accrediting organization for those standards within the deeming categories that the accrediting organization has the authority to deem.

Licensed Practical Nurse (LPN) Performs a variety of non-professional nursing care duties such as assisting in bathing patients, taking temperatures, blood pressure, pulse and respiration. Records results on charts. Observes patients for reactions to drugs, excessive respiratory rate or any other unusual conditions.

Licensed Social Worker (LSW) An individual who is licensed by the State to practice social work.

lichen Any of several eruptive skin diseases characterized by hard thick lesions grouped together and resembling lichens growing on rocks.

lifetime maximum benefit The maximum amount a health plan will pay in benefits to an insured individual during that individual's lifetime.

lifetime reserve days Under HI, each beneficiary has 60 lifetime reserve days that he or she may opt to use when regular inpatient hospital benefits are exhausted. The beneficiary pays one-half of the inpatient hospital deductible for each lifetime reserve day used.

ligament A band of flexible, fibrous connective tissue that is attached at the end of a bone near a joint. The main function of a ligament is to attach bones to one another, to provide stability of a joint, and to prevent or limit some joint motion.

ligation Tying a duct or blood vessel with a ligature (as to prevent bleeding during surgery).

light coagulation The coagulation of tissue by an intense beam of light, including laser (laser coagulation). In the eye it is used in the treatment of retinal detachments, retinal holes, aneurysms, hemorrhages, and malignant and benign neoplasms.

light therapy Or phototherapy, consists of exposure to daylight or to specific wavelengths of light using lasers, light-emitting diodes, fluorescent lamps, dichroic lamps or very bright, full-spectrum light, for a prescribed amount of time and, in some cases, at a specific time of day. Light therapy directed at the skin is used to treat acne vulgaris and neonatal jaundice.

lightwood's syndrome Renal tubular acidosis.

limb salvage An alternative to amputation in patients with neoplasms, ischemia, fractures, and other limb-threatening conditions. Generally, sophisticated surgical procedures such as vascular surgery and reconstruction are used to salvage diseased limbs.

limbus The visible borderline between the clear cornea and the white sclera of the eye. The conjunctival layer that covers the globe also joins at the limbus.

limitation of liability A provision designed to protect the beneficiary from liability under certain conditions when services he or she received are found not to be reasonable and necessary.

limitations A limit on the amount of benefits paid out for a particular covered expense.

limited license practitioner A professional licensed to perform certain health services in independent practice; for example, podiatrists, dentists, optometrists and chiropractors.

limited policy A policy that covers only specified accidents or sicknesses (e.g. a cancer policy).

limiting charge The maximum amount that a nonparticipating physician is permitted to charge a Medicare beneficiary for a service.

limulus test An extract of blood cells from the horseshoe crab is exposed to a blood sample from a patient; if gram-negative endotoxin is present in the sample, it will produce gelation of the extract of blood cells.

line item Service or item specific detail of claim.

lingu(a)-, lingu(o)- of or pertaining to the tongue.

lingual The area pertaining to, or around, the tongue.

liniments Heat-generating liquids that are thinner than ointments and are applied to the skin with friction.

liothyronine toxicosis Overactive thyroid function due to T3 poisoning.

lip augmentation A procedure done to improve deflated, drooping or sagging lips, correct their symmetry or to reduce fine lines and wrinkles around them. This is often done through injections or implants.

lip(o)- Fat.

lipectomy Removal of localized subcutaneous fat deposits by suction curettage or blunt cannulization in the cosmetic correction of obesity and other esthetic contour defects.

lipid panel A group of tests that are often ordered together to determine risk of coronary heart disease.

lipidoses A disorder of lipid metabolism, whether congenital or acquired.

lipids A generic term for fats and lipoids, the alcohol-ether-soluble constituents of protoplasm, which are insoluble in water.

lipodystrophy A medical condition characterized by abnormal or degenerative conditions of the body's adipose (fat) tissue.

lipoid An oily organic compound insoluble in water but soluble in organic solvents; essential structural component of living cells.

lipolysis The breakdown of fat stored in fat cells.

lipoma A benign tumor composed chiefly of fat cells.

lipoproteins Proteins combined with lipids that serve as carriers of cholesterol. The higher the value, the less likely that cholesterol deposits are in the blood stream and the less likely the chance of coronary heart disease. Cholesterol or HDL ratio measures the coronary risk factors.

liposuction A cosmetic procedure in which a special instrument called a cannula is used to break up and suck out fat from the body. *Synonym:* lipoplasty.

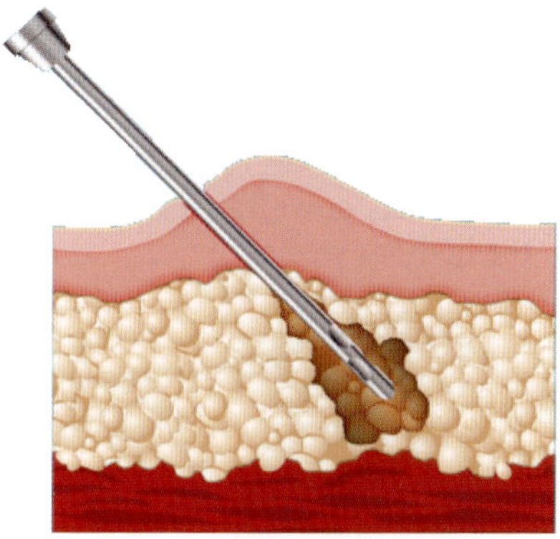

Liposuction with a cannula.

lips Aside from the lips of the mouth, there are two pairs of lips at the entrance to the vagina. They are the labia majora (the larger outside pair) and the labia minora (the smaller inside pair). Together they form part of the vulva.

listeriosis An infectious disease of animals and humans (especially newborn or immunosuppressed persons) caused by the bacterium Listeria monocytogenes; in sheep and cattle the infection frequently involves the central nervous system and causes various neurological symptoms.

lith(o)- Stone, calculus.

litholapaxy The procedure of crushing of a stone in the bladder and washing out the fragments through a catheter.

lithotripsy The destruction of a calculus of the kidney, ureter, bladder, or gallbladder by physical forces, including crushing with a lithotriptor through a catheter. Focused percutaneous ultrasound and focused hydraulic shock waves may be used without surgery.

liver An organ in the body that changes food into energy, removes alcohol and poisons from the blood, and makes bile, a substance that breaks down fats and helps rid the body of wastes.

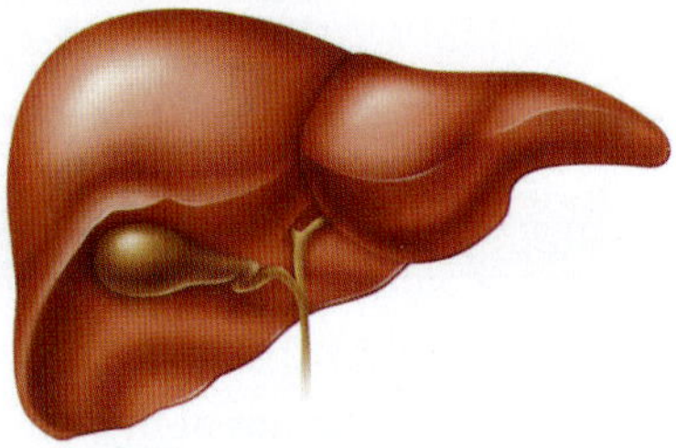

liver

liver enzymes Most often SGPT, SGOT; or alkaline phosphatase. Injury to the liver from infection or obstruction of bile flow causes damage to the cells; they leak various enzymes into the bloodstream; their detection in increased amounts most often means injury to the liver.

liver profile A panel of laboratory tests to determine liver function. Tests performed include Bilirubin, Protein, LDL, Alkaline Phosphatase, SGOT, SGPT, Albumin, and Globulin.

liver transplantation The transference of a part of or an entire liver from one human or animal to another.

living donor kidney transplant The surgical procedure of excising a kidney from a living donor and implanting it into a suitable recipient.

living wills A legal document that states a person's wishes regarding life-support or other medical treatment in certain circumstances, usually when death is imminent. *Synonym:* medical directive, advance medical directive.

LLE Left lower extremity.

LLP Limited license practitioner.

LLQ Left lower quadrant.

LMP Last menstrual period.

LMRP Local medical review policy.

lobe Part of an organ that appears to be separate in some way from the rest. A lobe may be demarcated from the rest of the organ by a fissure (crack), sulcus (groove), connective tissue or simply by its shape.

lobectomy Surgical removal of a lobe from any organ of the body (as the lung or brain).

lobotomy Surgical interruption of nerve tracts to and from the frontal lobe of the brain; often results in marked cognitive and personality changes.

Lobstein's syndrome Osteogenesis imperfecta.

LOC Level of Care.

local coverage determination A decision by a fiscal intermediary or carrier whether to cover a particular service on an intermediary-wide or carrier-wide basis. The difference between LMRPs and LCDs is that LCDs consist only of reasonable and necessary information, while LMRPs may also contain category or statutory provisions.

local lymph node assay The local lymph node assay (LLNA) is an alternative method for the identification of chemicals that have the ability to cause skin sensitization and allergic contact dermatitis.

Local Medical Review Policy (LMRP) An administrative and educational tool to assist providers, physicians and suppliers in submitting correct claims for payment. Local policies outline how contractors will review claims to ensure that they meet Medicare coverage requirements. CMS requires that LMRPs be consistent with national guidance (although they can be more detailed or specific), developed with scientific evidence and clinical practice, and are developed through certain specified federal guidelines. Contractor Medical Directors develop these policies. Reviewing Local Medical Review Policies assists in understanding why Medicare claims may be paid or denied.

localio procedure Method of partial excision of the sacrum for sacral tumors.

locality [Medicare] A geographic area for which a carrier calculates prevailing charges. Localities can be states, aggregations of counties, parts of counties, metropolitan zip code areas, or townships.

localization audiometry A technique for measuring the capacity to locate the source of a pure tone received binaurally in a sound field.

log(o)- Speech.

-logy Denotes the academic study or practice of a certain field.

LOINC Logical Observation Identifiers, Names, and Codes.

Lombard test The observation of fluctuations in the intensity of a patient's voice when a masking noise is increased or decreased; a test useful in assessing functional hearing loss.

Long Beach pedicle screw Posterolateral fusion screw and rod device.

Longmire operation Intrahepatic cholangiojejunostomy with partial hepatectomy for biliary obstruction.

long-term care A variety of services that help people with health or personal needs and activities of daily living over a period of time. Long-term care can be provided at home, in the community, or in various types of facilities, including nursing homes and assisted living facilities. Most long-term care is custodial care.

long-term care insurance A private insurance policy to help pay for some long-term medical and non-medical care, like help with activities of daily living. Because

Medicare generally does not pay for long-term care, this type of insurance policy may help provide coverage for long-term care that you may need in the future. Some long-term care insurance policies offer tax benefits; these are called Tax-Qualified Policies.

Long Term Care Ombudsman Program (LTCOP) Program that protects the health, welfare, safety, and rights of residents of long term care facilities. Trained and certified volunteers and professional staff visit long term care facilities, receive and investigate complaints, advocate for residents and mediate disputes.

long-term care policy Insurance policies that cover specified services for a specified period of time. Long-term care policies (and their prices) vary significantly. Covered services often include nursing care, home health care services, and custodial care.

long-term disability income insurance A provision to pay benefits to a covered disabled person as long as he or she remains disabled, up to a specified period.

long-term disability insurance Pays an insured a percentage of their monthly earnings if they become disabled.

loopogram An x-ray of an ileal or urinary conduit.

LOQ Lower outer quadrant.

lordosis Forward curvature of the lumbar spine (the small of the back).

Lorenz's operation An operation for congenital dislocation of the hip.

LOS Length of stay.

Loughheed and White procedure Coccygectomy and drainage from space procedure anterior to sacrum for drainage of lower abdominal abscesses.

louse-borne typhus Any of several forms of infectious disease caused by rickettsia, especially those transmitted by fleas, lice, or mites, and characterized generally by severe headache, sustained high fever, depression, delirium, and the eruption of red rashes on the skin. *Synonym:* prison fever, ship fever, typhus fever.

low molecular weight heparin An injectable form of heparin (a blood thinner) that is given underneath the skin. LMWH lasts longer, must be monitored differently and generally has fewer side effects than standard heparin. It is often used as an alternative to heparin or as bridging therapy for patients on warfarin, when dental work or surgery are needed or during pregnancy. Examples of brand names are Lovenox®, Fragmin®, and Innohep®.

low vision Visual loss that cannot be corrected with eyeglasses or contact lenses and interferes with daily living activities.

LRQ Lower right quadrant.

LS Lumbosacral.

LTC Long term care.

LTC-DRG Long-term care diagnosis-related group.

LTCH Long-term care hospital.

LUE Left upper extremity.

lumbago Backache affecting the lumbar region or lower back; can be caused by muscle strain or arthritis or vascular insufficiency or a ruptured intervertebral disc.

lumbar of or relating to or near the part of the back between the lower part of the rib cage and the hip bone.

lumbar puncture A procedure to collect cerebrospinal fluid surrounding the brain and spinal cord. *Synonym:* spinal tap.

lumbar stenosis Narrowing or stricture in the lower part of the back.

lumpectomy The surgical removal of a small tumor (lump) which may be benign or malignant, usually from the breast.

Lundh test A test for pancreatic function in which trypsin concentrations in the duodenum after a test meal are measured, with lowered levels of trypsin indicating low pancreatic secretion.

lung nodule A small growth in the lung.

lungs The lungs are a pair of breathing organs located with the chest which remove carbon dioxide from and bring oxygen to the blood. There is a right and left lung.

LUPA Low Utilization Payment Adjustment. An episode of 4 or less visits paid by national standardized per visit rates instead of case-mix groups.

lupus anticoagulant A type of antiphospholipid antibody associated with an increased risk for blood clots.

lupus band test An immunofluorescence test to determine the presence and extent of immunoglobulin and complement deposits at the dermal-epidermal junction of skin specimens from patients with systemic lupus erythematosus.

lupus erythematosus, systemic Inflammatory disease of connective tissue. Symptoms may include arthritis, swelling of the face and legs, anemia, mental changes, shortness of breath, hair loss and chest pain. Treatment usually requires immunosuppressive steroid and non-steroid antiinflammatory drugs. It is not inherited or cancerous.

LUQ Left upper quadrant.

Luque ISF Pedicle screw and plate device used for posterolateral fusion fixation.

luteinization Process by which a follicle in the ovary transforms into a luteum.

luteinized granulosa Thick, scarred, yellow lesion.

luteum Yellow-colored cyst.

LVAD Left ventricular assist device.

LVP Left ventricular pressure.

LVRS Lung volume reduction surgery.

Lyme Disease Recurrent multisystemic disorder caused by a tick-borne spirochete characterized by erythema chronicum migrans lesions, fever, malaise, headache and stiff neck, followed by arthritic pain in the large joints.

lymph Transparent, slightly yellow liquid found in lymph vessels throughout the body. Derived from tissue fluids.

lymph node Lymph nodes are small, bean-shaped structures that are laced throughout the body along the lymphatic routes.

lymph node excision Surgical excision of one or more lymph nodes. Its most common use is in cancer surgery.

lymph(o)- Lymph.

lymphadenectomy The surgical removal of one or more groups of lymph nodes, almost always performed as part of the surgical management of cancer.

lymphadenitis Inflammation of a lymph node. It is often a complication of a bacterial infection of a wound, although it can also be caused by viruses or other disease agents.

lymphadenopathy Chronic abnormal enlargement of the lymph nodes (usually associated with disease).

lymphangiogram A test of the lymphatic system using photographs taken with X-rays after injection of a special dye.

lymphangioma A lymphatic malformation, a benign proliferation of lymph vessels, forming a yellowish tumor on the skin, composed of a mass of dilated lymph vessels.

lymphangiotomy Incision of lymphatic vessels.

lymphangitis An infection of the lymph vessels, commonly resulting from an acute streptococcal or staphylococcal infection of the skin or an abscess in the skin or soft tissues. The infection causes the lymph vessels to become swollen and tender.

lymphatic Pertaining to lymph system of the body.

lymphatic leukemia *See* Leukemia, lymphatic.

lymphatic system Vast, complex network of vessels, valves, ducts, nodes and organs that help protect and maintain the internal fluid environment of the body. Responsible for transporting fats, proteins and other substances to the bloodstream. Lymph glands produce antibodies that help fight infections.

lymphedema A condition of localized fluid retention and tissue swelling caused by a compromised lymphatic system. Synonym: lymphatic obstruction.

lymphoblastic lymphoma Malignant tumor of lymph tissue. Lymphomas are classified according to the predominant cell type causing the disease. Lymphoblastic lymphoma's predominant cell is structured similarly to the lymphoblast. Treatment for lymphoma includes intensive radiotherapy and chemotherapy. *Synonym:* lymphoblastoma, lymphoblastic lymphosarcoma.

lymphocele A mass surrounded by an abnormal sac that contains lymph (fluid that is collected from tissues throughout the body) from diseased or injured lymphatic channels.

lymphocyte A small white blood cell (leukocyte) that plays a large role in defending the body against disease. Lymphocytes are responsible for immune responses.

lymphocytic proliferative disease Disease with an overproduction of lymphocytes, one form of white blood cells.

lymphocytopenia An abnormally small number of lymphocytes in the circulating blood.

lymphocytosis An abnormal increase in the number of lymphocytes in the circulating blood.

lymphogranuloma venereum A sexually transmitted disease (STD) or infection involving the lymph glands in the genital area. It is caused by a specific strain of Chlamydia.

lymphoid Referring to lymphocytes.

lymphoid leukemia A form of leukemia associated with hyperplasia and overactivity of the lymphoid tissue, with increased levels of circulating malignant lymphocytes or lymphoblasts.

lymphoma Disorders involving new, abnormal growth or tumor of lymph tissue. Usually malignant but may be benign. Usually afflicts men.

lymphoreticular malignancy Cancer of the reticuloendothelial cells of lymph nodes. *See* Reticuloendothelial system.

lymphosarcoma A type of cancer that originates in lymphocytes of the immune system. The diseases often originates in lymph nodes, presenting as an enlargement of the node (a tumor).

lymphs There are different kinds of white blood cells; Lymphocytes and Neutrophils are the major types. Neutrophils are the first to arrive on the scene when there is acute infection from bacteria. Lymphocytes accumulate when there is chronic injury or irritation. White blood cells help fight infections. White blood cells, especially lymphocytes, are the cells that attack bacteria in the blood.

lymphs (absolute) A test for the actual number for each of the 5 white blood cells. This is based on the percentage of white blood cells in the body.

Lynch procedure Transorbital frontal sinusotomy and ethmoidectomy.

lysis Dissolution or destruction of cells such as blood cells or bacteria.

-lysis Destruction.

lytes Electrolytes.

lytic therapy A clot-busting medication given in the hospital into the blood vessel to break up clots. The treatment has a risk of bleeding. Drug names are tpa, streptokinase, and urokinase.

M

M + C plan Health benefits coverage offered under a policy or contract offered by a Medicare + Choice Organization under which a specific set of health benefits are offered at a uniform premium and uniform level of cost-sharing to all Medicare beneficiaries residing in the service area of the M + C plan.

MAAC The Maximum Allowable Actual Charge is a limitation on billed charges for Medicare services provided by non-participating physicians. For physicians with charges exceeding 115 percent of the prevailing charge for non-participating physicians, MAACs limit increases in actual charges to 1 percent a year. For physicians whose charges are less than 115 percent of the prevailing, MAACs limit actual charge increases so they may not exceed 115 percent.

MABP Mean arterial blood pressure.

Maccarthy procedure Method of excision of the sacrum for sacral tumors.

Macewen's operation An operation for the radical cure of hernia by closing the internal ring with a pad made of the hernial sac.

macr(o)- Large, long.

macroamylaemia Excess of starch in the blood.

macrocheilia A condition of permanent swelling of the lip that results from greatly distended lymphatic spaces. This causes an abnormal largeness of the lips.

macrocytes Cells which are abnormally large, especially red blood cells.

macrocytic anemia *See* Anemia, macrocytic.

macrodactylia Condition characterized by enlargement of one or more digits.

macrodactyly An uncommon birth defect in which toes or fingers are abnormally large due to overgrowth of underlying bone and soft tissue.

macrogenia A large chin out of proportion to a person's facial features.

macroglobulinemia The presence of increased levels of macroglobulins in the circulating blood. The circulating macroglobulin produces symptoms of hyperviscosity syndrome weakness, fatigue, bleeding disorders, and visual disturbances.

macroglossia A congenital disorder characterized by an abnormally large tongue; often seen in cases of Down's syndrome.

macroscopic Large enough to be visible to the naked eye.

macrostomia Abnormal largeness of the mouth.

macula The small, sensitive area of the central retina; provides vision for fine work and reading.

macular degeneration A medical condition usually of older adults that results in a loss of vision in the center of the visual field.

macular disease Stain, spot or thickening of the cornea.

macular edema The collection of fluid in and under the macular portion of the retina causing swelling.

macular stain A small birthmark that is often nothing more than a small, mild, red blemish on the skin.

maculopathy Any pathological condition of the macula.

Magerl fusion Transarticular facet screw fusion for posterior C-1 on C-2 with the use of bilateral screws directed from inferior posterior lateral mass to anterior superior C-1.

magnesium An element absorbed in the intestine. Abnormal levels are found in pancreatitis, alcoholism and Addison's disease.

Magnetic Resonance Angiography (MRA) A group of techniques based on Magnetic Resonance Imaging to image blood vessels. Magnetic Resonance Angiography is used to generate images of the arteries in order to evaluate them for stenosis, occlusion or aneurysms. MRA is often used to evaluate the arteries of the neck and brain, the thoracic and abdominal aorta, the renal arteries, and the legs.

magnetic resonance imaging A test that uses a magnetic field and pulses of radio wave energy to provide pictures of organs and structures inside the body.

magnetoencephalography An imaging technique used to measure the magnetic fields produced by electrical activity in the brain.

Magnuson procedure A treatment for recurrent dislocation of the shoulder.

Magpi operation A simple surgical procedure that is designed to correct minor to moderate degrees of coronal or subcoronal hypospadias.

main term Refers to listings in the alphabetic index of the ICD-9-CM coding system appearing in boldface type.

major depressive disorder A major mood disorder characterized by one or more (recurrent) episodes of major depression, with or without full recovery between episodes. *Synonym:* clinical depression.

Major Diagnostic Category (MDC) A clinically coherent grouping of ICD-9-CM diagnoses by major organ system or etiology that is used as the first step in assignment of most diagnosis related groups (DRGs). MDCs are commonly used for aggregated DRG reporting.

major medical insurance Health insurance to finance the expense of major illnesses and injuries. Major medical policies usually include a substantial deductible clause. Above the initial deductible, major medical insurance is characterized by large benefit maximums.

major puerperal infection A bacterial infection following childbirth. *Synonym:* puerperal fever, postpartum fever.

malabsorption syndromes Poor absorption of nutrients from the intestinal tract into the blood.

-malacia Softening.

malaria An infective disease caused by sporozoan parasites that are transmitted through the bite of an infected anopheles mosquito; marked by paroxysms of chills and fever.

male infertility The biological inability of the male to contribute to conception.

male menopause Symptoms, such as depression, change in libido, impotence, in men at midlife. Many authorities claim no such condition exists.

malformation Abnormal or anomalous formation or structure.

malignancy Refers to cancerous cells that usually have the ability to spread, invade, and destroy tissue.

malignant Capable of causing destruction of normal tissue; may lead to death. Usually refers to cancer growth.

malignant neoplasm A tumor that tends to grow, invade, and metastasize. The tumor usually has an irregular shape and is composed of poorly differentiated cells. If untreated, it may result in death.

malleolus Either of the two rounded protuberances on each side of the ankle.

malleus The ossicle attached to the eardrum.

Mallory-Weiss syndrome A condition characterized by massive bleeding following a tear in the mucous membrane at the junction of the esophagus and stomach. Tear is usually caused from prolonged vomiting, most common in alcoholics or people who have an obstruction prevent-ing food from passing out of the stomach into the small intestine. Surgery is usually required to stop bleeding.

malnutrition A health problem caused by the lack (or too much) of needed nutrients.

malocclusion A condition in which the opposing teeth do not mesh normally.

malposition An abnormal position, as of an organ or a body part.

malpractice A dereliction from professional duty or a failure to exercise an accepted degree of professional skill or learning by one (as a physician) rendering professional services which results in injury, loss, or damage. Also an injurious, negligent, or improper practice.

malpractice expense refers to the relative value assigned to malpractice in the Medicare Physician Fee Schedule. .

malpractice insurance Insurance purchased by doctors and other providers to cover them against malpractice lawsuits.

malpresentation Abnormal position of the child at birth, making normal delivery difficult or impossible.

mamm(o)- of or pertaining to the breast.

mammaplasty Surgical reconstruction of the breast including both augmentation and reduction.

mammary dysplasia A common condition marked by benign (non-cancerous) changes in breast tissue. These changes may include irregular lumps or cysts, breast discomfort, sensitive nipples, and itching.

mammogram An X-ray of the breast with the breast in a device that compresses and flattens it. There are two basic mammogram tests; screening mammograms and diagnostic mammograms.

mammography The process of using low-dose X-rays to examine the human breast for diagnostic and screening purposes. The goal of mammography is the early detection of breast cancer.

mammoplasty Any reconstructive or cosmetic surgical procedure that alters the size or shape of the breast.

mammotomy *See* mastotomy.

managed behavioral health organization An organization that provides behavioral health services by implementing managed care techniques.

managed care Organized programs designed to control access to impatient and ambulatory health services, to ensure the medical necessity of the proposed service and the delivery of the service at the most efficient and cost effective level of care consistent with high quality. Managed care is essential to the structure of alternative delivery and financing systems, such as health maintenance organizations and preferred provider arrangements. The requirements can also be a component of traditional indemnity or fee-for-service health coverage.

Managed care may include pre-admission or pre-treatment certification, second surgical opinion programs, fee or price negotiation, pre-treatment protocol review, pre-admission testing, continued stay review, discharge planning, and individual/large case management. Failure to comply with managed care requirements or decisions usually reduces health benefit coverage for claims. The penalties may affect both the patient and the provider(s).

Managed Care Organization (MCO) Managed Care Organizations are entities that serve Medicare or Medicaid beneficiaries on a risk basis through a network of employed or affiliated providers. The term generally includes HMOs, PPOs, and Point of Service plans. In the Medicaid arena, other organizations may set up managed care programs to respond to Medicaid managed care. These organizations include Federally Qualified Health Centers, integrated delivery systems, and public health clinics. It is a health maintenance organization, an eligible organization with a contract under 11876 or a Medicare-Choice organization, a provider-sponsored organization, or any other private or public organization, which meets the requirements of 11902 (w) to provide comprehensive services.

managed care payment suspension Includes Health Maintenance Organizations (HMO), Competitive Medical Plans (CMP), and other plans that provide health services on a prepayment basis, based either on cost or risk, depending on the type of contract they have with Medicare. *See* also Medicare + Choice.

managed care system Integrates the financing and delivery of appropriate health care services to covered individuals by means of arrangements with selected providers to furnish a comprehensive set of health care services to members, explicit criteria for the selection of health care provides, and significant financial incentives for members to use providers and procedures associated with the plan. Managed care plans typically are labeled as HMOs (staff, group, IPA, and mixed models), ppos, or Point of Service plans. Managed care services are reimbursed via a variety of methods including capitation, fee for service, and a combination of the two.

managed competition A series of financial structures and methods used to manage the process by which individuals select health insurance coverage in a competitive market. The goal of managed competition is to encourage cost-conscious consumer choice when individuals select a plan. This, in turn, is intended to strengthen financial incentives for plans to deliver services in the most cost-effective manner. The basic structures of managed competition include a national board which would make decisions affecting benefit design and market rules, "sponsors" which manage the process of individual health insurance choice, and integrated health care delivery networks which provide and manage care. These structures have been termed as a National Health Board, Health Insurance Purchasing Cooperative (HIPCs), and Accountable Health Partnerships (AHPs) in several reform proposals.

managed health care plan One or more products which (1) integrate financing and management with the delivery of health care services to an enrolled population; (2) employ or contract with an organized provider network which delivers services; (3) between a network or individual provider shares financial risk or has some incentive to deliver quality, cost-effective services; and (4) use an information system capable of monitoring and evaluating patterns of enrollees' use of services and the cost of those services. *See* health maintenance organization, preferred provider organization, exclusive provider organization, prepaid health plan, and primary care case management.

managed indemnity plans Health insurance plans that are administered like traditional indemnity plans but which include managed care overlays such as precertification and other utilization review techniques.

management services organization An organization, owned by a hospital or a group of investors, that provides management and administrative support services to individual physicians or small group practices in order to relieve physicians of non-medical business functions so that they can concentrate on the clinical aspects of their practice.

mandated benefits Each state is responsible for the conduct of the insurance business within its boundaries rather than the Federal Government. Each state establishes its requirements for insurance company licensure. A state may establish minimum health insurance policy coverage provisions, such as a specified scope of services and covered providers. A state may require that all insured benefit plans include specific benefits, or both approaches may be used, depending upon the specific coverage under consideration. ERISA exempts self-insured employers from state mandates.

mandated services Services related to mandated consultation and/or related services (eg, third party payer, governmental, legislative or regulatory requirement) may be identified by adding the modifier '-32' to the basic procedure.

mandatory access control A means of restricting access to objects that are based on fixed security attributes assigned to users and to files and other objects. The controls are mandatory in the sense that they cannot be modified by users or their programs.

mandatory spending Outlays for entitlement programs (Medicare and Medicaid) that are not subject to the Federal appropriations process.

mandible The bone forming the lower jaw; the largest and strongest bone of the face, presenting a body and a pair of rami, which articulate with the skull at the temporomandibular joints.

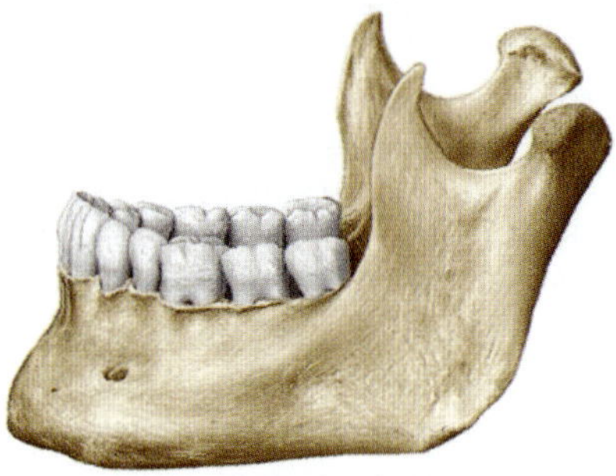

mandible

mandibular of or relating to the mandible.

mandibular advancement Moving a retruded mandible forward to a normal position. It is commonly performed for malocclusion and retrognathia.

mandibulectomy Surgical removal of the mandible (lower jaw bone).

manic depression A serious mental disorder that describes a category of mood disorders defined by the presence of one or more episodes of abnormally elevated mood clinically referred to as mania or, if milder, hypomania. *Synonym:* bipolar disorder.

manifestation Characteristic signs or symptoms of an illness.

manipulation refers to the process chiropractors use to apply to vertebrae that have abnormal movement patterns or fail to function normally. The objective of this chiropractic treatment is to reduce the subluxation, which results in an increased range of motion, reduced nerve irritability and improved function. *Synonym:* adjustment.

manometer A pressure gauge for comparing pressures of a gas.

manometry Measurement of the pressure or tension of liquids or gases with a manometer.

Mantoux test An intracutaneous tuberculin test.

manu- of or pertaining to the hand.

manual claim review Pre- or post-payment review of a health insurance claim by a person, instead of, or in addition to, a computer review.

manual rating A rating method under which a health plan uses the plan's average experience with all groups, and sometimes the experience of other health plans, rather than a particular group's experience to calculate the group's premium. .

MAOI Monoamine oxidase inhibitor.

maple-syrup urine disease Hereditary defect of metabolism. Usually diagnosed in infancy because it is recognized by the characteristic maple-syrup odor of urine. Other symptoms may include mental and physical retardation and feeding difficulties.

Marfan's syndrome This condition is an inherited disease affecting the bones, joints, and heart and great vessels. It can cause valves to become leaky and/or the aorta to become aneurysmal or to dissect.

Marie's sign Tremor of the extremities seen in Graves' Disease.

Marie-Bamberger disease Hypertrophic pulmonary osteoarthropathy; a disorder usually affecting the long bones of the arms and legs, often secondary to chronic pulmonary and heart disease.

Marie-Strümpell disease Chronic, inflammatory arthritis and autoimmune disease. It mainly affects joints in the spine and the sacroiliac in the pelvis, causing eventual fusion of the spine. *Synonym:* ankylosing spondylitis.

market-based reform Reliance on competition in the health care market to assure services of acceptable cost and quality to consumers without government mandates or involvement in rate-setting, financing, or administration. Can also refer to the reduction of barriers in the operation of a health care market.

market penetration The part of the total health care market that a managed care company has captured.

Marshall-Marchetti-Krantz proce-dure Surgery to relieve stress incontinence where the z operation anterior portion of the urethra, vesical neck, and bladder are sutured to the posterior surface of the pubic bone.

marsupialization The surgical technique of cutting a slit into a cyst and suturing the edges of the slit to form a continuous surface from the exterior to the interior of the cyst. Sutured in this fashion, the cyst remains open and can drain freely.

MAS Meconium aspiration syndrome.

MASER Microwave amplification by stimulated emission of radiation.

mass The mass of extra cells that forms a growth or tumor. Tumors can be benign or malignant.

mass immunization center A location where providers administer pneumococcal pneumonia and influenza virus vaccinations and submit these services as electronic media claims, paper claims, or using the roster billing method. This generally takes place in a mass immunization setting.

mass spectrometry The identification of chemicals in a substance by their molecular mass and charge.

massage therapy The practice of soft tissue manipulation with physical (anatomical), functional (physiological), and in some cases psychological purposes and goals.

mast cells Part of connective tissue.

mast(o)- of or pertaining to the breast.

mastectomy Surgical removal of part or all of the breast.

mastectomy, radical Removal of the breast, pectoral muscles, axillary lymph nodes, and assoc-iated skin and subcutaneous tissue.

mastectomy, segmental Removal of only enough breast tissue to ensure that the margins of the resected surgical specimen are free of tumor.

mastectomy, simple Removal of only the breast tissue and nipple and a small portion of the overlying skin.

mastectomy, subcutaneous Excision of breast tissue with preservation of overlying skin, nipple, and areola so that breast form may be reconstructed.

master two-step exercise test An early exercise test for coronary insufficiency in which electrocardiograms were recorded while and after the subject repeatedly ascended and descended two steps.

mastocytosis Overproduction of mast cells. May rarely infiltrate liver, spleen, bones, the gastrointestinal system and skin. May precede mast cell leukemia, which is a malignant disorder.

mastodynia Pain, tenderness, or pressure in the breast.

mastoid Process of the temporal bone behind the ear at the base of the skull.

mastoidectomy A surgical procedure that removes an infected portion of the mastoid bone.

mastoiditis An infection of the spaces within the mastoid bone. It is almost always associated with otitis media, an infection of the middle ear. In the most serious cases, the bone itself becomes infected.

mastoidotomy Surgical removal of some or all of the mastoid process.

mastopathy Any pathology of the breast.

mastopexy Plastic repair to lift or reshape the breasts.

mastotomy Surgical incision of a breast.

market-based reform Reliance on competition in the health care market to assure services of acceptable cost and quality to consumers without government mandates or involvement in rate-setting, financing, or administration. Can also refer to the reduction of barriers in the operation of a health care market.

market penetration The part of the total health care market that a managed care company has captured.

materials supplied by physician Materials such as surgical trays, irrigation sets, bandages, casting materials, etc. supplied by the physician.

maxilla A fusion of two bones along the palatal fissure that form the upper jaw.

maxillary of or relating to the maxilla.

maxillectomy Surgical removal of the maxilla.

maxillofacial prosthesis implantation Surgical insertion of an appliance for the replacement of areas of the maxilla, mandible, and face. When only portions of the mandible are replaced, it is referred to as mandibular prosthesis implantation.

maxillofacial surgery The specialty of treating problems of the mouth, jaw, neck and facial bones with surgery.

Maximum Allowable Charge (MAC) The largest dollar amount to which an insurance carrier will apply plan benefits.

maximum allowable costs list A list of prescription medications established by the health plan and distributed to pharmacies, which will be covered at a generic product level.

maximum out of pocket costs A limit on the total amount of co-payments, deductibles and co-insurance that a beneficiary is responsible for paying.

maximum defined data set Under HIPAA, this is all of the required data elements for a particular standard based on a specific implementation specification. An entity creating a transaction is free to include whatever data any receiver might want or need. The recipient is free to ignore any portion of the data that is not needed to conduct their part of the associated business transaction, unless the inessential data is needed for coordination of benefits.

maximum enrollee out-of-pocket costs The beneficiary's maximum dollar liability amount for a specified period.

maximum fee schedule A compensation arrangement in which a participating physician agrees to accept the Schedule of Allowances as his total fee for covered services.

maximum plan benefit coverage The maximum dollar amount per period that a plan will insure. This is only applicable for service categories where there are enhanced benefits being offered by the plan, because Medicare coverage does not allow a Maximum Plan Benefit Coverage expenditure limit.

maximums The top limit of the amount a carrier will pay for a specific benefit or policy during a specified time period.

Maydl operation Colostomy in two steps, used in cases of inoperable cancer of the rectum.

Mayo's operation An operation for the radical correction of umbilical hernia.

MBC Maximum (maximal) breathing capacity.

MBD Minimal brain dysfunction.

McAffee fusion Anterior retropharyngeal approach to upper cervical spine; often used for fusion, allowing excision of tumor.

McBride procedure A surgical procedure for the treatment of hallux valgus.

McBurney operation Radical surgery for the cure of inguinal hernia.

McBurney's point Spot on the abdomen overlying the normal position of the base of the appendix—this is a point of tenderness in acute appendicitis.

MCCA Medicare Catastrophic Coverage Act.

Mccannel procedure A suture technique for IOL fixation during cataract surgery.

Mccarran-Ferguson act A federal act that placed the primary responsibility for regulating health insurance companies and HMOs that service private sector (commercial) plan members at the state level.

MCCU Mobile coronary care unit.

McDonald's operation An operation for incompetent cervix, in which the cervical os is closed with a purse-string suture.

MCE Medicare code editor.

mcg Microgram.

Mcgill's operation Suprapubic transvesical prostatectomy.

MCH The mean corpuscular hemoglobin, or mean cell hemoglobin (MCH), is a measure of the mass of hemoglobin contained by a red blood cell. It is reported as part of a standard complete blood count. It is diminished in microcytic anemia's, and increased in macrocytic anemia's.

MCHC The mean corpuscular hemoglobin concentration, or MCHC, is reported as part of a standard complete blood count. It is used to assess the possibility of different kinds of anemia's.

Mcindoe procedure A procedure that corrects vaginal agenesis by creating a vagina with a skin graft.

McKissock operation A procedure for reduction mammoplasty.

MCM Medicare carrier manual.

McMurray's test As the patient lies supine with one knee fully flexed, the examiner rotates the patient's foot fully outward and the knee is slowly extended; a painful "click" indicates a tear of the medial meniscus of the knee joint; if the click occurs when the foot is rotated inward, the tear is in the lateral meniscus.

MCO Managed Care Organization.

MCO or PHP standards These are standards that states set for plan structure, operations, and the internal quality improvement or assurance system that each MCO or PHP must have in order to participate in the Medicaid program.

MCV The mean corpuscular volume, or MCV, is a measure of the average red blood cell volume (i.e. Size) that is reported as part of a standard complete blood count.

Mcvay's operation Surgical repair of femoral hernias by suture of the transverse muscle of the abdomen and its associated fasciae to the pectineal ligament.

MD Medical doctor.

MDC Major Diagnostic Category.

MDH Medicare-dependent small rural hospital.

measles A viral infection which causes an illness displaying a characteristic skin rash. Measles is also sometimes called rubeola, 5-day measles, or hard measles.

measurement The systematic process of data collection, repeated over time or at a single point in time.

meatoplasty Plastic repair of a meatus.

meatotomy A form of penile modification in which the underside of the glans is split.

meatus a small tubular opening.

mechanical valves Artificial valves made from metal, plastic, and/or pyrolytic carbon. They have excellent durability and most will last indefinitely.

Meckel's diverticulum Abnormal sac or pouch near the ileum due to remains of the embryonic sac.

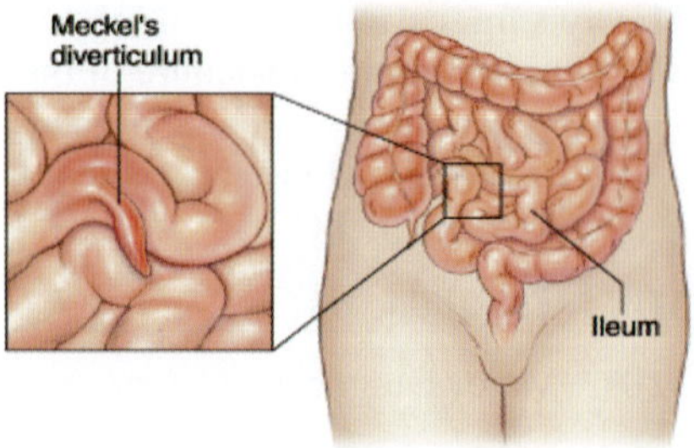

Meckel's diverticulum

meconium Thick, sticky, dark-green material that collects in the intestines of a fetus and forms the first stools of a newborn.

meconium ileus Obstruction of the small intestine in the newborn caused by a plug of meconium. *See* Meconium. Often the plug may be dislodged by giving enemas. Rarely, surgery is required. Condition may be an indication of cystic fibrosis. *See* Cystic fibrosis.

MECT Multiple electroconvulsive therapy.

medial Situated closer to the midline of the body.

median plane divides the body into right and left halves. *Synonym:* midsagittal plane.

median sternotomy The incision traditionally used to perform heart surgery in which the sternum or breastbone is divided down the middle from top to bottom.

mediastinitis Inflammation of the mediastinum.

mediastinoscope An instrument inserted through an incision above the sternum to visually examine the mediastinum (the part of the thoracic cavity between the lungs that contains the heart, aorta, esophagus, trachea and thymus).

mediastinoscopy A surgical procedure that enables visualization of the contents of the mediastinum, usually for the purpose of obtaining a biopsy.

mediastinotomy Surgical opening of the mediastinum.

mediastinum Central portion of the chest cavity that contains the heart and its large blood vessels, trachea (windpipe), esophagus, thymus gland and other structures and tissues. It separates the two lungs.

Medicaid (Title XIX) A joint Federal-State program that pays for medical and other services on behalf of certain groups of low-income persons.

Medicaid fiscal agent The organization responsible for administering claims for a state Medicaid program.

Medicaid management information system A CMS approved system that supports the operation of the Medicaid program. The MMIS includes the following types of sub-systems or files recipient eligibility, Medicaid provider, claims processing, pricing, SURS, MARS, and potentially encounter processing.

Medicaid MCO A Medicaid MCO provides comprehensive services to Medicaid beneficiaries, but not commercial or Medicare enrollees.

Medicaid state agency The state agency responsible for overseeing the state's Medicaid program.

medical aid unit A medical facility where ambulatory patients can be treated without an appointment, and receive immediate, non-emergency care. The medical aid units are not usually opened 24 hours a day; patients calling an HMO after hours with urgent, but not emergent, clinical problems, are often referred to these facilities. A similar facility is an Urgent Care Center or Unit, which may be opened 24 hours a day.

medical code sets Codes that characterize a medical condition or treatment. These code sets are usually maintained by professional societies and public health organizations. Examples of medical code sets include CPT, HCPCS, ICD-9-CM, DRG and CDT.

Medical Consumer Price Index An inflationary statistic that measures the cost of all purchased health care services.

medical decision making Refers to the complexity of establishing a diagnosis and/or selecting a management option. The level of complexity is determined by the number of diagnoses, and the amount or complexity of medical records and tests that must be reviewed, and the risk of significant complications, morbidity and/or mortality.

medical errors Errors or mistakes committed by health professionals which result in harm to the patient. They include errors in diagnosis (diagnostic errors), errors in the administration of drugs and other medications (medication errors), errors in the performance of surgical procedures.

Medical Foundations (MF) An organization through which physicians, hospitals and other providers can integrate the delivery of medical service. Usually an MF is an affiliate of a hospital through a common parent organization or is a subsidiary of a hospital. In most cases MFs are non-profit entities that own and manages facilities, equipment and supplies of a medical practice. They usually contract directly with patients and third party payers and employ non-professional personnel as well as physicians.

medical genetics The specialty of medicine that involves the diagnosis and management of hereditary disorders.

Medical Indigence Inability to pay for needed medical care, whether through insurance, savings, current income, or borrowing against future income.

medical insurance (Part B) Medicare medical insurance that helps pay for physicians services, outpatient hospital care, durable medical equipment, and some medical services that aren't covered by Part A.

medical necessity Medical information justifying that the service rendered or item provided is reasonable and appropriate for the diagnosis or treatment of a medical condition or illness.

medical nutrition therapy The assessment of nutritional status followed by nutritional therapy. The nutrition assessment includes review and analysis of 1) medical, nutrition and medication histories, 2) physical examination, 3) anthropometric measurements, and 4) laboratory test.

medical protocols Medical protocols are the guidelines that physicians in the future may be required to follow in order to have an acceptable clinical outcome. The protocol would provide the caregiver with specific treatment options or steps when faced with a particular set of clinical symptoms or signs or laboratory data. Medical protocols would be designed through an accumulated database of clinical outcomes.

medical records Institute An organization that promotes the development and acceptance of electronic health care record systems.

medical review The review of medical records or information as it relates to services rendered and billed by a provider or beneficiary for payment. This review is performed by the medical staff of physicians, registered nurses, licensed practical nurses, etc.

Medical Savings Account (MSA) A method of financing health care by giving a tax advantage to individuals who establish and maintain personal accounts for health care purposes; similar to an Individual Retirement Account for retirement purposes. Also referred to as individual health care account.

medical team conferences Medical team conferences involve in-person communication and consultation among health care professionals regarding health care services needed by the patient.

medical technology Includes drugs, devices, techniques, and procedures used in delivering medical care and the support systems for that care. There are no accurate estimates of how much new technology contributes to health spending.

medical transcriptionist A person who transcribes from dictating machine diagnostic work-ups, case histories, physicals, consultations, discharge summaries, and operations, using knowledge of medical terminology. .

medically appropriate services Diagnostic or treatment measures for which the expected health benefits exceed the expected risks by a margin wide enough to justify the measures.

medically necessary services Services or supplies as provided by a physician or other health care provider to identify and treat a member's illness or injury, which, as determined by the payer, are consistent with the symptoms, diagnosis, and treatment of the member's condition; in accordance with the standards of good medical practice; not solely for the convenience of the member, member's family, physician, or other health care provider; and furnished in the least intensive type of medical care setting required by the member's condition.

medically needy Optional component of the Medicaid program that allows states to offer Medicaid to persons who would otherwise be eligible, but whose incomes are too high. Such persons become eligible by spending a portion of their income each month on outstanding medical bills. *See* spend down, and categorically needy.

Medically Unnecessary Days (MUD) A term used to describe that part of a stay in a facility deemed to be excessive to diagnose and treat a medical condition because the stay was either too long, or more.

Medicare (Title XVIII) Federal program that provides basic health care and limited long term care for retirees and certain disabled individuals without regard to income level. Beneficiaries must pay premiums, deductibles and coinsurance. *See* beneficiary, cost sharing, medically necessary, and medigap.

Part A - Medicare hospital insurance that helps pay for medically necessary inpatient hospital care, and, after a hospital stay, and limited inpatient care in a skilled nursing facility, for limited home health care or hospice care.

Part B - Medicare medical insurance that helps pay for medically necessary physician services, outpatient hospital services and supplies that are not covered by the hospital insurance.

Part C - *See* Medicare + Choice.

Medicare + Choice An expanded set of options, established by the Balanced Budget Act of 1997, for the delivery of health care under Medicare. Most Medicare beneficiaries can choose to receive benefits through the original fee-for-service program or through one of the following Medicare + Choice plans; (1) coordinated care plans (such as health maintenance organizations, provider sponsored organizations, and preferred provider organizations); (2) Medical Savings Account (MSA) or High Deductible plans (through a demonstration available to up to 390,000 beneficiaries); or (3) private fee-for-service plans.

Medicare advantage The new name for Medicare + Choice Plans, such as HMOs, PPOs, Private Fee-for-Service Plans or Medicare Specialty Plans.

Medicare advantage drug plan Some Medicare Advantage Plans include coverage for a prescription drug plan.

Medicare benefits Health insurance available under Medicare Part A and Part B through the traditional fee-for service payment system.

Medicare benefits notice A notice sent to patients after the physician files a claim for Part A services in the Original Medicare Plan. The notice states what the provider billed for, the Medicare-approved amount, how much Medicare paid, and how much the patient must pay.

Medicare bonus payment An additional 10% payment to the physician above the allowed charge for services delivered to Medicare Beneficiaries in designated Health Professional Shortage Areas.

Medicare carrier A private company that contracts with Medicare to pay Part B bills.

Medicare Catastrophic Coverage Act of 1988 A law enacted enacted and repealed in 1989. Established ICD-9-CM coding requirements for all Medicare claims.

Medicare contractor A Medicare Part A Fiscal Intermediary (institutional), a Medicare Part B Carrier (professional), or a Medicare Durable Medical Equipment Regional Carrier (DMERC).

Medicare coordinated care plan A Medicare Advantage HMO or PPO Plan.

Medicare Cost HMO or Contract Prospective payment for acute and primary health care (monthly fee per patient with settlement annually based on actual costs). Primarily used in rural areas where full capitation is not feasible.

Medicare Cost Report (MCR) An annual report required of all institutions participating in the Medicare program. The MCR records each institution's total costs and charges associated with providing services to all patients, the portion of those costs and charges allocated to Medicare patients, and the Medicare payments received.

Medicare coverage Made up of two parts Hospital Insurance (Part A) and Medical Insurance (Part B). *See* Medicare Part A; Medicare Part B.

Medicare Economic Index (MEI) An index often used in the calculation of the increases in the prevailing charge levels that help to determine allowed charges for physician services. In 1992 and later, this index is considered in connection with the update factor for the physician fee schedule.

Medicare entitlement When an individual becomes entitled to Medicare, he or she receives a Health Insurance Claim card which shows his or her name, sex, Medicare number, and the effective dates of entitlement to hospital (Part A) benefits and medical (Part B) benefits. Entitlement begins the first day of the month of the individual's birth and ends the last day of the month, with the exception of death.

Medicare fee schedule The resource based fee schedule currently used by Medicare to pay for physicians' services. This method replaced the customary, prevailing and reasonable (CPR) payment method in the first quarter of 1992. This fee schedule is based on resource costs, and composed of factors representing physician work and practice costs.

Medicare handbook The Medicare Handbook provides information on such things as how to file a claim and what type of care is covered under the Medicare program. This handbook is given to all beneficiaries when first enrolled in the program.

Medicare Insured Group (MIG) Employer (or union) groups receiving a capitated rate from Medicare in exchange for integrating Medicare covered services into the employers own traditional retiree health plan.

Medicare managed care plan A type of Medicare Advantage Plan that is available in some areas of the country. In most managed care plans, you can only go to physicians, specialists, or hospitals on the plan's list. Plans must cover all Medicare Part A and Part B health care. Some managed care plans cover extras, like prescription drugs. Your costs may be lower than in the Original Medicare Plan.

Medicare medical savings account plans The Medicare + Choice delivery option that consists of a high-deductible catastrophic insurance policy and a tax-deferred medical savings account established for individual Medicare beneficiaries.

Medicare medical savings account plan A Medicare health plan option made up of two parts. One part is a Medicare MSA Health Insurance Policy with a high deductible. The other part is a special savings account where Medicare deposits money to help you pay your medical bills.

Medicare national coverage determinations manual (Formerly the Coverage Issues Manual). The National Coverage Determinations Manual contains implementing instructions for National Coverage Determinations. The manual includes information whether specific medical items, services, treatment procedures, or technologies are paid for under the Medicare program on a national level.

Medicare Part A The Medicare component that provides basic hospital insurance to cover the costs of inpatient hospital services, confinement in nursing facilities or other extended care facilities after hospitalization, home care services following hospitalization, and hospice care.

Medicare part a fiscal intermediary A Medicare contractor that administers the Medicare Part A (institutional) benefits for a given region.

Medicare Part B The Medicare component that provides benefits to cover the costs of physicians' professional services, whether the services are provided in a hospital, a physician's office, an extended-care facility, a nursing home, or an insured's home.

Medicare Part B carrier A Medicare contractor that administers the Medicare Part B (Professional) benefits for a given region.

Medicare Part B premium reduction amount Since CY 2003, MCOs are able to use their adjusted excess to reduce the Medicare Part B premium for beneficiaries. When offering this benefit, a plan cannot reduce its payment by more than 125 percent of the Medicare Part B premium. In order to calculate the Part B premium reduction amount, the PBP system must multiply the number entered in the indicate your MCO plan payment reduction amount, per member field by 80 percent. The resulting number is the Part B premium reduction amount for each member in that particular plan (rounded to the nearest multiple of 10 cents).

Medicare Part C The part of Medicare that expands the list of different types of entities allowed to offer health plans to Medicare beneficiaries. *Synonym:* Medicare + Choice.

Medicare Payment Advisory Commission (MedPAC) A non-partisan congressional advisory body charged with providing policy advice and technical assistance concerning the Medicare program and other aspects of the health system. It conducts independent research, analyzes legislation, and makes recommendations to Congress. The Physician Payment Review Commission (PPRC) has been merged with the Prospective Payment Assessment Commission (ProPAC) to create MedPAC.

Medicare preferred provider organization plan A type of Medicare Advantage Plan in which you use physicians, hospitals, and providers that belong to the network. You can use physicians, hospitals, and providers outside of the network for an additional cost.

Medicare premium collection center The contractor that handles all Medicare direct billing payments for direct billed beneficiaries. MPCC is located in Pittsburgh, Pennsylvania.

Medicare prescription drug plan A stand-alone drug plan, offered by insurers and other private companies to beneficiaries that receive their Medicare Part A and/or B benefits through Original Medicare; Medicare Private Fee-for-Service Plans that don't offer prescription drug coverage; and Medicare Cost Plans offering Medicare prescription drug coverage.

Medicare private fee-for-service plan A type of Medicare Advantage plan in which the patient may go to any Medicare-approved physician or hospital that accepts the plan's payment. The insurance plan, rather than the Medicare program, decides how much it will pay and what the patient must pay for the services provided.

Medicare Provider Analysis and Review File (MedPAR) A CMS data file that contains charge data and clinical characteristics, such as diagnoses and procedures, for every hospital inpatient bill submitted to Medicare for payment.

Medicare remittance advice remark codes A national administrative code set for providing either claim-level or service-level Medicare-related messages that cannot be expressed with a Claim

Adjustment Reason Code. This code set is used in the X12 835 Claim Payment & Remittance Advice transaction.

Medicare remittance notice A summarized statement for providers including payment information for one or more beneficiaries.

Medicare risk contract A contract between Medicare and an HMO or competitive medical plan under which the plan provides Medicare covered services for enrollees and receives monthly capitated payments from Medicare, thereby assuming health insurance risk for its enrollees.

Medicare savings program Medicaid programs that help pay some or all Medicare premiums and deductibles.

Medicare secondary payer Another insurance company that is primary to Medicare; the primary insurance company pays first and Medicare would be secondary payer for the service(s).

Medicare Select A form of Medigap insurance that allows insurers to experiment with the provision of supplemental benefits through a network of providers. Coverage is often limited to those services furnished by the participating network providers and emergency out-of-area care.

Medicare Self Referral Option A Medicare + Choice point of service option that allows enrollees in a Medicare risk HMO to go out of plan at a higher cost.

Medicare supplement A private medical expense insurance policy that provides reimbursement for out-of-pocket expenses, such as deductibles and coinsurance payments, or benefits for some medical expenses specifically excluded from Medicare coverage.

Medicare trust funds Treasury accounts established by the Social Security Act for the receipt of revenues, maintenance of reserves, and disbursement of payments for the HI and SMI programs.

Medicare-approved amount In the Original Medicare Plan, this is the Medicare payment amount for an item or service. This is the amount a physician or supplier is paid by Medicare and you for a service or supply. It may be less than the actual amount charged by a physician or supplier. The approved amount is sometimes called the approved charge.

medication therapy management services Describes in-person patient assessment and intervention as appropriate by a pharmacist. The purpose of MTMS is to maximize medication response and/or managed medication interactions or complications. MTMS includes review of history, medication profile, an.

Medigap A policy guaranteeing to pay a Medicare beneficiary's co-insurance, deductible and co-payments and will provide additional health plan or non-Medicare coverage for services up to a predefined benefit limit. In essence, the product pays for the portion of the cost of services not covered by Medicare.

Medigap open enrollment period A one-time-only six month period when you can buy any Medigap policy you want that is sold in your state. It starts in the first month that you are covered under Medicare Part B and you are age 65 or older. During this period, you can't be denied coverage or charged more due to past or present health problems.

Medigap policy A Medicare supplement insurance policy sold by private insurance companies to fill gaps in Original Medicare Plan coverage. Except in Massachusetts, Minnesota and Wisconsin, there are 10 standardized plans labeled Plan A through Plan J. Medigap policies only work with the Original Medicare Plan.

MedPAC Medicare payment advisory committee.

MedPAR Medicare Provider Analysis and Review.

MedPRO Medical education resources program.

medulla Lower or hindmost part of the brain; continuous with spinal cord.

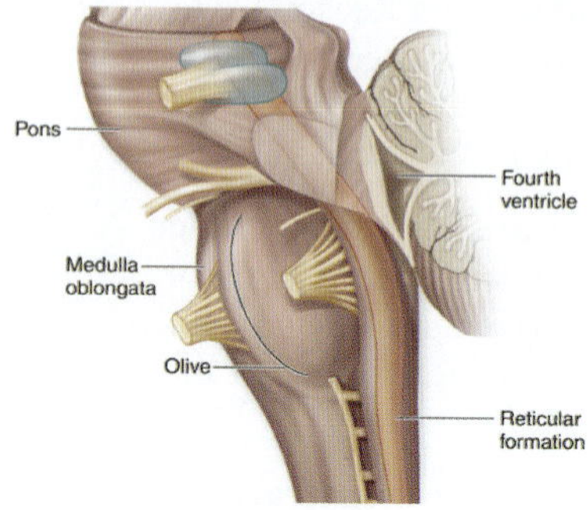

medulla

medullary of or referring to the medulla.

MEFR Maximum (maximal) Expiratory Flow Rate.

MEFV Maximum (maximal) Expiratory Flow Volume.

meg(a)-, megal(o)-, megaly Enlargement.

MEI Medicare economic index.

meibomian glands Large specialized sebaceous glands in the eyelid. There are about 50 glands on the upper lids and 25 glands on the lower lids. They create and distribute an oily substance called lipids. Meibomian gland secretions help keep the eye moist.

meibomitis A dysfunction of the meibomian glands that provide an oily film over natural tears to keep them from evaporating too quickly.

meiosis Cell division in specialized tissues of ovaries and testes which results in the production of sperm or ova. Meiosis involves two divisions and results in four daughter cells, each containing only half the original number of chromosomes--23 in the case of humans. These cells can develop into gametes.

melan(o)- Denoting a black color.

melanin Dark pigment of the skin, hair and iris of the eye.

melanocytes A pigment producing cell found in the skin, hair and eyes that gives them their color.

melanoma A malignant tumor of melanocytes which are found predominantly in skin but also in the bowel and the eye. It is one of the less common types of skin cancer but causes the majority of skin cancer related deaths.

melasma A condition in which pigmentation of the cheeks of the face darkens into tan or brown patches. This condition occurs in half of all women during pregnancy.

melioidosis An infectious disease caused by a gram-negative bacterium, burkholderia pseudomallei, found in soil and water. *Synonym:* Whitmore disease, Nightcliff gardener's disease.

member services The department responsible for helping members with any problems, handling member grievances and complaints, tracking and reporting patterns of problems encountered, and enhancing the relationship between members of the plan and the plan itself.

Meniere's syndrome (disease) Nausea, vomiting, tinnitus, vertigo and hearing loss caused by disease of the labyrinth.

mening(o)- Meninges.

meninges Thin membranes that cover the brain and spinal cord.

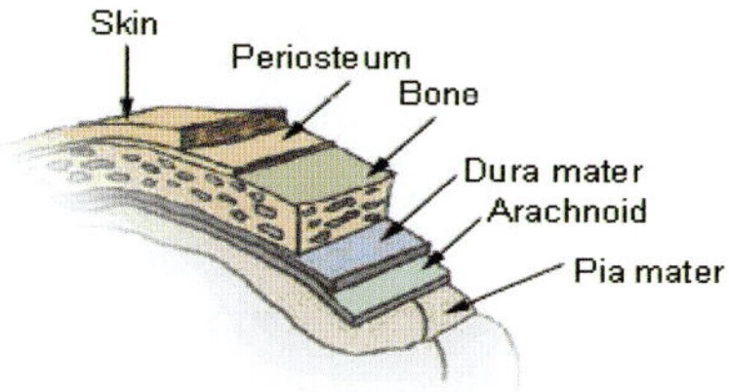

Meninges of the CNS.

meningioma Hard, usually vascular tumor of the membranes covering the brain and spinal cord. Usually grows slowly. May invade the skull causing bone erosion and pressure on brain tissues. Usually occurs in adults, in some cases following head injury.

meningitis Inflammation or infection of the meninges. It is contagious and may be caused by viruses, fungi or bacteria. Symptoms may include fever, headache, stiff neck, irritability, sensitivity of eyes to light, confusion, drowsiness or unconsciousness. Death or permanent brain damage may occur if treatment is delayed (especially in bacterial meningitis).

meningocele Protrusion of the membranes that cover the spine and part of the spinal cord through a bone defect in the vertebral column.

meningococcal infection An infection with the bacterium neisseria meningitidis. Neisseria was formerly called meningococcus but the term meningococcal is still common.

meningococcus A bacterium (Neisseria meningitidis) that causes cerebrospinal meningitis.

meningoencephalitis Inflammation of the brain and meninges.

meningomyelocele A saclike cyst containing brain tissue, cerebro-spinal fluid, and the meninges that protrudes through a congenital defect in the skull.

meniscectomy The surgical removal of all or part of a torn meniscus.

meniscus A disk of cartilage that serves as a cushion between the ends of bones that meet at a point.

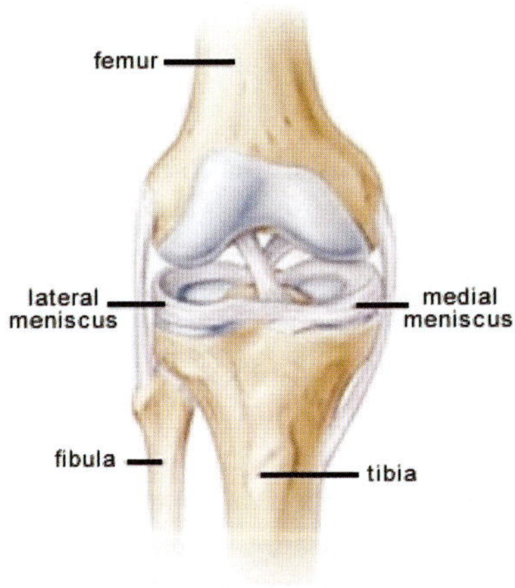

meniscus

Menke's kinky-hair syndrome Inherited disorder caused by a defect in intestinal absorption of copper. Characterized by the growth of sparse, kinky hair. Infants with syndrome suffer brain damage, retarded growth and early death.

menopausal and postmenopausal disorders Refer to disorders occuring during and after the menopausal period.

menopause Permanent cessation of menstruation. Occurs as early as age 35 or as late as age 55; usually spans 1 to 2 years. Menopause is only one event in the climacteric, a biological change in body tissue and body systems that occurs in both sexes between the mid-40s and mid-60s.

menorrhagia Abnormally heavy or prolonged menstruation; can be a symptom of uterine tumors and can lead to anemia if prolonged.

menstrual Pertaining to menstruation.

menstrual extraction A procedure for early termination of pregnancy by withdrawing the uterine lining and a fertilized egg if present by means of suction.

menstruating Normal discharge of blood and tissues through the vagina that come from the uterine lining. Lining builds up each month in preparation for a fertilized egg. If fertilization does not occur, lining is shed. This process is controlled by hormones and usually occurs about every 4 to 6 weeks.

mental health parity act A federal act which prohibits group health plans that offer mental health benefits from applying more restrictive limits on coverage for mental illness than for physical illness.

mental retardation A generalized disorder, characterized by sub average cognitive functioning and deficits in two or more adaptive behaviors with onset before the age of 18.

mes(o)- Middle.

mesenteric adenitis Lymph glands in mesentery become inflamed. Symptoms may mimic appendicitis, but the pain is usually more generalized and does not become more severe.

mesentery A double layer of peritoneum that attaches to the back wall of the abdominal cavity and supports the small intestines.

MESH The National Library of Medicine's controlled vocabulary thesaurus. It consists of sets of terms naming descriptors in a hierarchical structure that permits searching at various levels of specificity.

message [HIPAA] A digital representation of information.

message authentication [HIPAA] Insuring, typically with a message authentication code, that a message received (usually via a network) matches the message sent.

message authentication code [HIPAA] Data associated with an authenticated message that allows a receiver to verify the integrity of the message.

message integrity [HIPAA] The assurance of unaltered transmission and receipt of a message from the sender to the intended recipient.

messenger model A type of independent practice association (IPA) that simply negotiates contract terms with MCOs on behalf of member physicians, who then contract directly with MCOs using the terms negotiated by the IPA. This type of IPA is most often used with fee-for-service or discounted fee-for-service compensation arrangements.

meta- After, behind.

metabolic of or relating to metabolism.

metabolic alkalosis Too much base in the body due to loss of acid.

metabolism Sum of all the chemical and physical processes by which living substance is produced and maintained. Also includes the concept of the transformation by body cells by which energy is made available.

metabolites Any substance produced by metabolism. *See* Metabolism.

metacarpal Any bone of the hand between the wrist and fingers.

metachromatic leukodystrophy Inherited condition that causes blindness, mental retardation, rigidity and convulsions.

metamorphopsia Defective vision in which objects appear distorted. Sometimes results from disease of the retina.

metastases The spreading of a disease to another part of the body.

metastasis Process by which cancerous cells or infectious germs spread from their original location to other parts of the body.

metastatic Relating to or affected by metastasis.

metastatic cancer Cancerous cells that spread from their original location to other parts of the body.

metastatic disease Disease that has transferred from an organ or body part not directly connected to a new location, due to transfer of the germ. For example, tuberculosis is usually found in the lungs but can spread to bones and other organs. In this case, the lungs are the primary site of disease, and the bones or other organs are the site(s) of metastatic disease. *See* Tuberculosis.

metatarsal Refers to a group of five long bones in the foot located between the tarsal bones of the hind- and mid-foot and the phalanges of the toes.

metatarsals Any bone of the foot between the ankle and the toes.

metatarsectomy Excision or resection of a metatarsal bone.

-meter Measurement.

metr(o)- Pertaining to conditions or instruments of the uterus.

metroplasty Plastic repair on the uterus.

metrorrhagia Bleeding from the uterus that is not due to menstruation; usually indicative of disease (as cervical cancer).

-metry Process of measuring.

Meyer fusion Posterior fusion using vertical strut grafts and wires.

mg Milligram.

MGCRB Medicare Geographic Classification Review Board.

MGMA Medical group management association.

MI Myocardial infarction.

micro- Denoting something as small, or relating to smallness.

microaneurysms Microscopic aneurysms, characteristic of certain diseases. Capillary microaneurysms are often seen in the retina of the eye in diabetic retinopathy. *See* Aneurysms; diabetic retinopathy.

microbes Microorganism (small, living organism) capable of producing disease.

microcephalus An abnormally small head and underdeveloped brain.

microcytes Cells which are abnormally small, especially red blood cells.

microcytic anemia *See* Anemia, microcytic.

microdissection Dissection using a microscope.

microdosimetry A technique for measuring the microscopic distribution of energy, useful with different types of radiation.

microphthalmia Abnormally small size of eye.

micropigmentation A form of tattooing commonly used to apply permanent makeup by injecting iron oxide pigment into the middle layer of the skin (dermis).

microscopic angioscopy The noninvasive microscopic examination of the microcirculation, commonly done in the nailbed or conjunctiva. In addition to the capillaries themselves, observations can be made of passing blood cells or intravenously injected substances.

microsurgery The performance of surgical procedures with the aid of a microscope.

MICU Medical Intensive Care Unit.

mid level practitioner Group of health professionals with advanced health care training (including nurse practitioners and physician assistants) that can perform specialized health care tasks usually in support of, and under the supervision of, a physician.

midsagittal plane divides the body into right and left halves. *Synonym:* median plane.

middle ear The space between the eardrum and the inner ear that contains the three auditory ossicles, which convey vibrations through the oval window to the cochlea.

MIF test *See* migration inhibitory factor test.

MIFR Maximum (maximal) inspiratory flow rate.

migraine A severe, disabling headache, usually affecting only one side of the head, and often accompanied by nausea, vomiting, photophobia and visual disturbances.

migration inhibitory factor test An in vitro test for production of MIF by lymphocytes in response to specific antigens; used for evaluation of cell-mediated immunity. MIF production is absent in certain immunodeficiency diseases.

miliary tuberculosis Acute infection associated with the spread of tuberculosis throughout the body through the bloodstream. Tiny tubercles (small, rounded masses produced by infection with mycobacterium tuberculosis, the germ causing tuberculosis) are formed in a number of organs. If treatment is not delayed, the infection can usually be successfully treated with a combination of medications.

military health system A worldwide health care system operated by the U.S. Department of Defense that focuses its efforts on population health improvement by integrating the delivery of health care services for active-duty personnel, retirees, and the families of active-duty personnel and retirees.

military treatment facility A medical facility operated by one or more of the Uniformed Services. An MTF also refers to certain former U.S. Public Health Services (USPHS) facilities now designated as Uniformed Service Treatment Facilities (USTF).

Milk Teeth The deciduous (baby) teeth.

Millard-Gubler syndrome Gubler hemiplegia or paralysis; 6th and 7th nerve palsy with contralateral hemiplegia affecting limbs on one side of the body and the face on the other, together with paralysis of outward movement of the eye, caused by infarction of the pons.

Miller procedure A surgical procedure for the treatment of symptomatic mobile flat feet in adolescents.

Miller-Abbott intubation A treatment for obstruction of the small intestine using a double-channel intestinal tube with an inflatable balloon at its distal end.

Milroy's disease Congenital hereditary lymphedema.

MIM Medicare intermediary manual.

minimally invasive cardiac surgery Surgery on the heart that is performed either through a smaller than normal incision, or without the use of cardiopulmonary bypass (the heart-lung machine), or both.

Minimum Data Sets (MDS) Federal data collection system for assessing nursing home patients. The MDS for nursing facility residents is a comprehensive resident assessment instrument (RAI) that measures functional status, mental health status, and behavioral status to identify chronic care patient needs and formalize a care plan in response to 18 Resident Assessment Protocols (RAPs). Under Federal regulation, assessments are conducted at a time of admission into a nursing facility, upon return from a 72-hour hospital admission, whenever there is a significant change in status, quarterly, and annually, *See* resource utilization groups.

minimum scope of disclosure The principle that, to the extent practical, individually identifiable health information should only be disclosed to the extent needed to support the purpose of the disclosure.

Minnesota Multiphasic Personality Inventory (MMPI) One of the most frequently used personality tests in mental health. The test is used by trained professionals to assist in identifying personality structure and psychopathology.

miscarriage The spontaneous end of a pregnancy at a stage where the embryo or fetus incapable of surviving, generally defined in humans at prior to 20 weeks of gestation. Miscarriage the most common complication of early pregnancy. *Synonym:* spontaneous abortion.

miscellaneous and experimental services A section of the HCPCS coding system that provides codes and descriptions for medical services that are considered miscellaneous and/or experimental.

missed abortion Retention in the uterus of an fetus that has been dead for at least eight weeks.

Mitchell procedure A surgical procedure for the treatment of adolescent hallux valgus.

mitogen Substance that triggers mitosis.

mitosis Type of cell division in which the body produces new cells for growth and repair of injured tissues.

mitral of or relating to or located in or near the mitral valve.

mitral regurgitation Defective closure of the heart's mitral valve, which allows some of the blood to backflow or regurgitate. Normally, the mitral valve allows blood to flow from the top left chamber of the heart (atrium) to the bottom left chamber of the heart (ventricle), but prevents blood from flowing back into the left atrium. Although there are several causes, rheumatic heart disease is the single most common cause of this condition. Symptoms include fatigue and slight breathlessness. Eventually the condition may progress and result in severe congestion of lungs. Surgery to replace or repair the mitral valve is required in patients with severe symptoms.

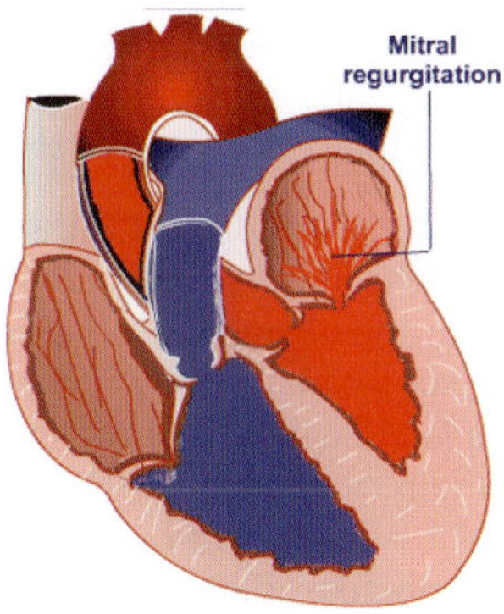

mitral regurgitation

mitral stenosis A narrowing of the mitral valve opening that increases resistance to blood flow from the left atrium to the left ventricle.

mitral valve The valve that separates the two chambers on the left side of the heart. The aortic vale is a valve between the left ventricle and the aorta; prevents blood from flowing from the aorta back into the heart.

mitral valve prolapse Condition in which the mitral valve becomes floppy, resulting in mitral regurgitation. *See* Mitral regurgitation.

mixed connective tissue disease Disease affecting the entire body characterized by the combined symptoms of various collagen diseases. Symptoms may include joint pain, inflammation of muscles, non-deforming arthritis and swollen hands. May also affect esophagus and lungs. Treatment often includes administration of corticosteroids.

Mixed Model HMO A health plan that includes more than one form of HMO within a single plan.

MMEFR Maximum (maximal) midexpiratory flow rate.

MMFR Maximum (maximal) midexpiratory flow rate.

MMIS Medicaid management information system.

MMPI The Minnesota Multiphasic Personality Inventory, a global test of personality used to detect pre-existing personality disorders.

MMR Measles, mumps, rubella.

mobile unit A facility or unit that moves from place-to-place equipped to provide preventive, screening, diagnostic, and/or treatment services.

modality Methods of treatment for kidney failure or ESRD. Modality types include transplant, hemodialysis, and peritoneal dialysis.

model fee schedule The sample fee schedule developed by CMS in 1990 from Phase I of the Harvard study.

moderate (conscious) sedation Moderate (conscious) sedation induces an altered state of consciousness that minimizes pain and discomfort through the use of pain relievers and sedatives.

modified community rating A separate rating of medical service usage in a given geographic area using age-sex data.

Modified Fee-For-Service A system in which providers are paid on a fee-for-service basis, with certain fee maximums for each procedure.

modifiers Two digit codes that indicate services or procedures have been altered by some specific circumstance. Modifiers do not change the definition of the reported procedure codes.

Mohs surgery A surgical technique used primarily in the treatment of skin neoplasms, especially basal cell or squamous cell carcinoma of the skin. This procedure is a microscopically controlled excision of cutaneous tumors either after fixation in vivo or after freezing. *Synonym:* chemosurgery.

molars The broad, multicuspid back teeth, used for grinding food that are considered the largest teeth in the mouth. In adults, there are a total of twelve molars (including the four wisdom teeth or third molars), three on each side of the upper and lower jaws.

molluscum contagiosum A viral infection of the skin caused by a poxvirus. The disease can affect any area of the skin but is most common on the body, arms and legs.

Moloney test One for detection of delayed hypersensitivity to diphtheria toxoid.

mon(o)- Single.

monaural Relating to or having or hearing with only one ear.

moniliasis An opportunistic fungal infection that develops after administering an antibiotic. Not uncommon in the mouth. Synonym: thrush.

monitoring A planned, systematic, and ongoing process to gather and organize data, and aggregate results in order to evaluate performance.

monitoring of MCO or PHP standards Activities related to the monitoring of standards that have been set for plan structure, operations, and quality improve-ment or assurance to determine that standards have been established, implemented, adhered to, etc.

mono Infectious mononucleosis.

mono spot This is the more quickly performed blood test for infectious mononucleosis.

monoamine oxidase inhibitors Drugs used in the treatment of clinical depression. These substances decrease depressive symptoms by stopping an enzyme that breaks down the mood stimulating chemicals in the brain.

monoclonal Forming or derived from a single clone.

monocytes A white blood cell that has a single nucleus and can take in foreign material. Monocytes play an important role in killing some bacteria, protozoa, and tumor cells, release substances that stimulate other cells of the immune system.

monocytes (absolute) The absolute count is the actual number for each of the 5 white blood cells in your test. This is based on the percentage of white blood cells in the body.

monocytic leukemia A type of leukemia characterized by the proliferation of monocytes and monoblasts in the blood.

mononeuritis The inflammation of a single nerve of a upper limb. There are many causes of mononeuritis including diabetes mellitus, carpal tunnel syndrome, rheumatoid arthritis and lyme disease.

mononucleosis An acute disease characterized by fever and swollen lymph nodes and an abnormal increase of mononuclear leucocytes or monocytes in the bloodstream; not highly contagious.

monoplegia Paralysis of a single limb, usually an arm.

monosomy Chromosomal abnormality characterized by the absence of one chromosome from the normally occurring pair of chromosomes. One example is Turner's syndrome. *See* Turner's syndrome.

Monteggia fracture A fracture of the ulna that affects the joint with the radius.

Montgomery glands Sweat glands located in the areola of the nipple.

mood disorders Those disorders that have a disturbance in mood as their predominant feature.

Moore's syndrome Abdominal epilepsy; producing paroxysmal abdominal pain as a sign of abnormal neuronal discharge from the brain.

morbidity A diseased state, often used in the context of a morbidity rate— the rate of disease or proportion of diseased people in a population. In common clinical usage, any disease state, including diagnosis and complications is referred to as morbidity.

morbidity rate The rate of illness in a population. The number of people ill during a time period divided by the number of people in the total population.

Moro reflex Startle reflex; contraction of the limb and neck muscles in infants when startled by a sudden noise, jolt or a short drop.

morph(o)- Form, shape.

morphology Refers to form, structure and configuration of an organism.

morphometry Measurement of the form or the body or its parts.

mortality rate The death rate often made explicit for a particular characteristic (e.g. Gender, sex, or specific cause of death). Mortality rate contains three essential elements the number of people in a population exposed to the risk of death (denominator), a time factor, and the number of deaths occurring in the exposed population during a certain time period (the numerator).

Morton's neuroma Benign tumor of the tissue that surrounds the digital nerve leading to the toes.

Morvan's syndrome A rare disorder characterized by neuromyotonia, hyperhidrosis, and central nervous system dysfunction.

mosaicplasty A surgical procedure used for treatment of cartilage damage.

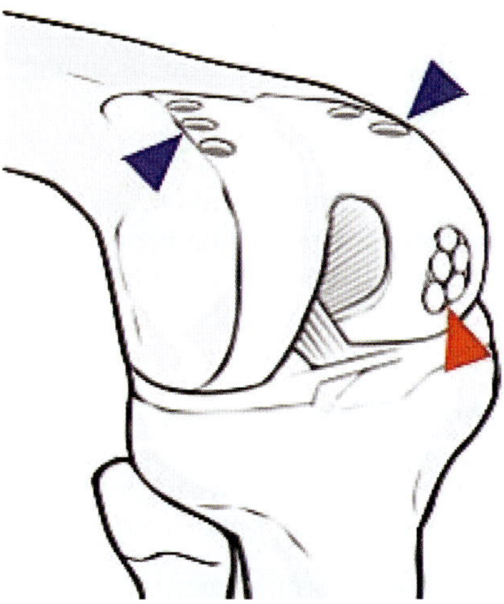

Mosaicplasty.

Moschcowitz operation Femoral herniorrhaphy via inguinal approach.

Mosenthal test An infrequently used test to evaluate renal concentrating ability by measuring the density of urine every two hours.

mosquito-borne viral encephalitis An inflammation of the brain, caused by a mosquito-borne virus.

Motais' operation Transplantation of a portion of the tendon of the superior rectus muscle of the eyeball into the upper lid, for ptosis.

motility disorders Any disorder or disease characterized by inability to remove intestinal waste contents efficiently.

motor In medicine, having to do with the movement of a part of the body. Something that produces motion or refers to motion. For example, a motor neuron is a nerve cell that conveys an impulse to a muscle causing it to contract.

Moynahan syndrome Progressive cardiomyopathic lentiginosis.

MPFS Medicare physician fee schedule.

MRA Magnetic resonance angiography.

MRI Magnetic resonance imaging.

MRSA Methicillin-resistant staphylococcus aureus.

MSA 1) medical savings accounts 2) metropolitan statistical area.

MSO Management services organization.

MSP Medicare secondary payer.

MUA Medically underserved area.

mucocele Dilation of a cavity with accumulated mucus secretion.

mucopolysaccharides Chemicals that contain hexosamine combined with proteins.

mucopolysaccharidosis Any of a group of genetic disorders caused by a defect in metabolism of mucopolysaccharides. Characterized by skeletal changes, mental retardation, clouding of the cornea and excessive mucopolysaccharides in urine.

mucopurulent Containing or composed of mucus and pus.

mucosal of or relating to mucous membranes.

mucosectomy Excision of the mucosa, usually of the rectum prior to ileoanal anastomosis for treatment of ulcerative colitis.

mucositis Inflammation and ulceration of the mucous membranes lining the digestive tract, usually as an adverse effect of chemotherapy and radiotherapy treatment for cancer.

Muller procedure A surgical procedure for the treatment of lower limb varices.

multi-employer group health plan A group health plan that is sponsored jointly by two or more employers or by employers and employee organizations.

multigravida Refers to a woman who has been pregnant more than one time.

multinodular goiter Enlarged thyroid gland causing a swelling in the front part of the neck. Swelling is very irregular (multinodular). Rarely toxic or malignant; may occur with chronic inflammatory thyroid disease.

multiple coding Refers to the need to use more than one ICD-9-CM code to fully identify coding a condition.

multiple employer plan A health plan sponsored by two or more employers. These are generally plans that are offered through membership in an association or a trade group.

multiple gestation A multiple birth occurs when more than one fetus is carried to term in a single pregnancy.

multiple myeloma Malignancy beginning in the plasma cells of the bone marrow. Plasma cells normally produce antibodies to help destroy germs and protect against infection. With myeloma, this function becomes impaired, and the body cannot deal effectively with infection.

multiple procedures More than one procedure, excluding E & M services, physical medicine or supplies, are performed at the same time by the same provider. Reported by adding CPT modifier -51 to the basic procedure code.

multiple-puncture test A skin test in which the material used (e.g., tuberculin) is introduced into the skin by pressure of several needles or pointed tines or prongs.

multiple option plan A health plan design that offers employees the option of electing to enroll under one of several types of coverage, usually from among an HMO, a

PPO, and a major medical indemnity plan.

multiple sclerosis Chronic disorder affecting many nervous system functions. Patches of white matter in the brain and spinal cord break down and cannot conduct normal nerve impulses. Usually begins in young adulthood. Early signs of the disease are often vague, including visual problems, abnormal skin sensations and muscle weakness or imbalance. Later, symptoms may include marked weakness, speech difficulty, loss of bladder or bowel control, and extreme mood swings. Currently not curable. Symptoms can be relieved or controlled with treatment. One-third of MS patients have a mild, nonprogressive disease. Another third worsen slowly. The rest worsen rapidly.

multiple-puncture test A skin test in which the material used (e.g., tuberculin) is introduced into the skin by pressure of several needles or pointed tines or prongs.

multispecialty group A group of doctors who represent various medical specialties and who work together in a group practice.

Mumford operation Arthroscopic resection of the shoulder joint.

mumps Mild, contagious, viral disease that causes painful swelling of the salivary glands. Other symptoms may include fever, headache and sore throat. Rarely, other organs may become involved, including testicles, ovaries, pancreas, breasts or brain. *Synonym:* parotitis.

Munchausen syndrome Repeated presentation to a physician and/or hospital with claims of an acute illness that is false, for the purpose of gaining medical attention.

muscle Muscle is the tissue of the body which primarily functions as a source of power. There are three types of muscle in the body. Muscle which is responsible for moving extremities and external areas of the body is called skeletal muscle. Cardiac muscle tissue forms the bulk of the wall of the heart. Smooth muscle tissue is located in the walls of hollow internal structures such as blood vessels, the stomach, intestines, and urinary bladder.

muscle relaxants A heterogeneous group of drugs used to produce muscle relaxation, excepting the neuromuscular blocking agents. They have their primary clinical and therapeutic uses in the treatment of muscle spasm and immobility associated with strains, sprains, and injuries.

muscle sparing incision A less invasive surgical procedure using a smaller incision(s) than a conventional surgical procedure. This incision does not require division of the chest muscles.

muscul(o)- Muscle.

muscular dystrophy A group of genetic, hereditary muscle diseases that weaken the muscles that move the human body. Muscular dystrophies are characterized by progressive skeletal muscle weakness, defects in muscle proteins, and the death of muscle cells and tissue.

musculoplasty Plastic repair of muscle(s).

musculoskeletal A general term which is defined as relating to muscles and the skeleton.

MVA Motor vehicle accident.

MVC Maximum (maximal) vital capacity.

MVP Mitral valve prolapse.

MVPS Medical volume performance standard.

my(o)- of or relating to muscle.

myasthenia gravis Disorder of muscles, especially the face and head, with increasing fatigue and weakness as muscles are used.

myc(o)- Fungus.

mycobacteria A bacteria that causes tuberculosis and leprosy.

mycoplasma A genus of bacteria which lack a cell wall. Several species cause disease in humans.

mycoplasma pneumonia Lung infection caused by germ mycoplasma.

mycosis An inflammatory condition caused by a fungus.

mycotoxin A toxin produced by a fungus.

mydriasis Reflex pupillary dilation as a muscle pulls the iris outward; occurs in response to a decrease in light or certain drugs.

myectomy Excision of a muscle.

myel(o)- of or relating to bone marrow.

myelitis Inflammation of the spinal cord.

myeloblastic leukemia *See* Leukemia, myeloblastic.

myelocele Saclike protrusion of the spinal cord through a congenital defect in the spinal column.

myelocytes Immature white blood cells normally found in bone marrow.

myelocytic leukemia *See* Leukemia, myelocytic.

myelogenous leukemia *See* Leukemia, myelocytic.

myelography X-ray of the spinal cord to detect possible lesions (usually after injection of a contrast medium into the subarachnoid space).

myeloid leukemia A type of leukemia affecting myeloid tissue (bone marrow).

myeloma A tumor of the bone marrow (usually malignant) composed of cells normally found in bone marrow.

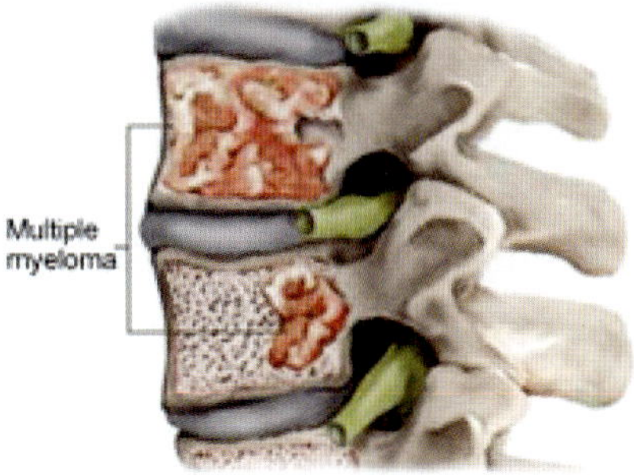

myeloma

myelomonocytic leukemia *See* Leukemia, myelomonocytic.

myelopathy Refers to pathology of the spinal cord.

myelophthisis A severe kind of anemia found in some people with diseases that affect the bone marrow.

myelosuppressive Inhibiting bone marrow activity, resulting in the decreased production of blood cells and platelets.

myelotomy Incision of the spinal cord.

myiasis Infestation of the body by the larvae of flies (usually through a wound or other opening) or any disease resulting from such infestation.

myocardial of or relating to the myocardium.

myocardial failure Condition that exists when the heart is no longer able to pump all the blood efficiently.

myocardial fibrosis Formation of fibrous material in the heart.

myocardial infarction Commonly known as a heart attack, occurs when the blood supply to part of the heart is interrupted causing some heart cells to die. *Synonym:* heart attack.

myocardial revascularization The restoration of blood supply to the myocardium.

myocarditis Inflammation of the heart muscle (myocardium) that usually occurs as a complication of underlying illness, hypersensitive immune reactions, injury or radiation therapy. Symptoms may include fatigue, shortness of breath, irregular heartbeat and fever.

myocarditis bacterial Inflammation of heart muscle (myocardium) caused by bacterial infection.

myocardium The middle layer of the heart, consisting of cardiac muscle.

myocutaneous flap A compound flap of skin and muscle with adequate vascularity to permit sufficient tissue to be transferred to the recipient site.

myofibroma A benign tumor that consists chiefly of fibrous connective tissue, with variable numbers of muscle cells forming portions of the tumor.

myoglobin Chemical stored in muscle that contains iron and oxygen.

myoglobinuria The presence of myoglobin in the urine.

myoma A benign tumor composed of muscle tissue.

myomectomy The surgical removal of uterine fibroids, also known as myomas.

myoneural of or relating to both muscles and nerves, especially to nerve endings in muscle tissue.

myoneural disorders Disorders affecting both muscles and nerves, especially to nerve endings in muscle tissue.

myopathy Any pathology of the muscles that is not attributable to nerve dysfunction.

myopia Eyesight abnormality resulting from the eye's faulty refractive ability; distant objects appear blurred.

myoplasty Plastic repair of muscular tissue.

myorrhaphy Suture of a muscle.

myositis Inflammation of muscle tissue.

myotomy Surgical incision or division of a muscle.

myotonia Abnormally long muscular contractions; slow relaxation of a muscle after a contraction.

myotonic of or relating to or caused by myotonia.

myring(o)- Eardrum.

myringitis An inflammatory contagious condition of the eardrum caused by viral or bacterial infection.

myringoplasty Surgical repair of a perforated eardrum with a tissue graft.

myringostomy Insertion of tympanostomy tubes for chronic serious otitis media resistant to medical therapy.

myringotomy A surgical procedure in which a tiny incision is created in the eardrum, so as to relieve pressure caused by the excessive buildup of fluid, or to drain pus. Myringotomy is often performed as a treatment for otitis media.

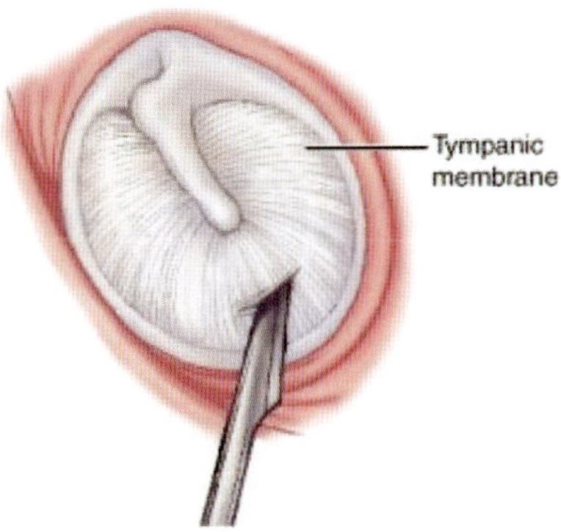

myringotomy

myx(o)- Mucus.

myxedema Condition of swollen lips, thickened nose, swelling of the skin and mental dullness caused by reduced function of the thyroid gland. *See* Hypoparathyroidism.

N

Naffziger syndrome A disorder characterized by pain and tingling in the forearm and hand similar to that occurring in cervical rib syndrome, caused by compression of the brachial plexus and subclavian artery against the first thoracic rib by a hypertonic anterior scalene muscle. Synonym: Scalenus anticus syndrome.

NAHC National Association for Home Care.

narcolepsy A sleep disorder characterized by sudden and uncontrollable episodes of deep sleep.

narcosynthesis A method of treating an acute traumatic neurosis by working with a patient while the patient is under the influence of a hypnotic drug.

narcotic antagonists Agents inhibiting the effect of narcotics on the central nervous system.

nas(o)- of or pertaining to the nose.

nasal bone small oblong bones that meet at the middle and superior part of the face. Their fusion forms the superior part of the bridge of the nose.

nasal polyps Are small, sac-like growths made up of inflamed tissue lining the nose (nasal mucosa).

nasal provocation tests Application of allergens to the nasal mucosa. Interpretation includes observation of nasal symptoms, rhinoscopy, and rhinomanometry. Nasal provocation tests are used in the diagnosis of nasal hypersensitivity, including hay fever.

nasoethmoid fracture Fracture of the naso-orbito-ethmoid complex typically caused by a forceful blow to the central aspect of the midface.

nasogastric Referring to the passage from the nose to the stomach.

nasogastric tube A tube that is passed through the nose and down through the nasopharynx and esophagus into the stomach.

nasolabial Pertaining to the nose and lip.

nasolacrimal duct The passage the lacrimal sac on each side of the nose, through which tears are conducted into the nasal cavity.

nasomaxillary Pertaining to the maxilla and the nasal cavity.

nasopharyngeal Pertaining to the pharynx and the nasal cavity.

nasopharyngitis Inflammation of the nasal passages and of the upper part of the pharynx.

nasopharyngoscopy A diagnostic procedure that examines the nasal passageways and pharynx with an instrument outfitted with an optical system.

nasopharynx The uppermost part of the pharynx. It extends from the base of the skull to the upper surface of the soft palate.

nasotracheal intubation Tracheal intubation through the nose.

National Center for Health Services Research (NCHSR) A division within the U.S. Department of Health and Human Services that supports analyses and evaluations of the health care system and its financing and underwrites the development and testing of new approaches to improve the distribution, use and cost-effectiveness of services.

National Center for Health Statistics (NCHS) The federal agency responsible for the collection and dissemination of the nation's vital and health statistics. Its mission is to provide statistical information that will guide actions and policies to improve the health of the American people.

National Claim History (NCH) A HCFA data reporting system that combines both Part A and Part B claims in a common file.

National Committee for Quality Assurance (NCQA) A non-profit organization created to improve patient care quality and health plan performance in partnership with managed care plans, purchasers, consumers, and the public sector.

National Coverage Determinations (NCD) A determination that sets forth the extent to which Medicare will cover specific services, procedures, or technologies on a national basis. Medicare contractors are required to follow ncds. If an NCD does not specifically exclude or limit an indication or circumstance, or if the item or service is not mentioned at all in an NCD or in a Medicare manual, it is up to the Medicare contractor to make the coverage decision (see LMRP). Prior to an NCD taking effect, CMS must first issue a Manual Transmittal, CMS ruling, or Federal Register Notice giving specific directions to our claims-processing contractors. That issuance, which includes an effective date and implementation date, is the NCD. If appropriate, the Agency must also change billing and claims processing systems and issue related instructions to allow for payment. The NCD will be published in the Medicare National Coverage Determinations Manual. An NCD becomes effective as of the date listed in the transmittal that announces the manual revision.

National Coverage Policy A policy developed by CMS that indicates whether and under what circumstances certain services are covered under the Medicare program. It is published in CMS regulations, published in the Federal Register as a final notice, contained in a CMS ruling, or issued as a program instruction.

National Drug Code (NDC) Numerical coding system for drug identification. NDC numbers are assigned by the Food and Drug Administration (FDA) and are typically used to bill payers for the drugs provided to health care beneficiaries.

national employer id A system for uniquely identifying all sponsors of health care benefits.

national health insurance Proposed Federal program that would use tax funds to finance the provision of comprehensive health benefits for the population. Scope of benefits, provider and beneficiary eligibility, financing, and ownership and control of resources, among other issues, must be defined.

national improvement projects Health care quality improvement projects developed by a group consisting of representatives of some or all of the following groups; CMS, Public Health Service, Networks, renal provider, and consumer communities. The object is to use statistical analysis to identify better patterns of care and outcomes, and to feed the results of the analysis back into the provider community to improve the quality of care provided to renal Medicare beneficiaries.

national median charge The national median charge is the exact middle amount of the amounts charged for the same service. This means that half of the hospitals and community mental health centers charged more than this amount and the other half charged less than this amount for the same service.

National Institute of **Health** The primary Federal agency for conducting and supporting medical research. Helping to lead the way toward important medical discoveries that improve people's health and save lives, NIH scientists investigate ways to prevent disease as well as the causes, treatments, and even cures for common and rare diseases.

national patient id A system for uniquely identifying all recipients of health care services. This is sometimes referred to as the National Individual Identifier (NII), or as the Health care ID.

national payer id A system for uniquely identifying all organizations that pay for health care services. *Synonym:* health plan ID.

national practitioner data bank A database maintained by the federal government that contains information on physicians and other medical practitioners against whom medical malpractice claims have been settled or other disciplinary actions have been taken.

national provider identifier A unique standardized identifier for a providers and suppliers of health care services, as required under the Administrative Simplification are of the Health Insurance Portability and Accountability Act (HIPAA). The NPI consists of an eight digit alphanumeric identifier plus a two digit alphanumeric location identifier to indicate the provider's practice location. Npis are good for life and only the location identifier may change. NPI has not yet been implemented.

national standard per visit rates National rates for each six home health disciplines based on historical claims data. Used in payment of lupus and calculation of outliers.

National Uniform Billing Committee (NUBC) An organization, chaired and hosted by the American Hospital Association, that maintains the UB-92 hardcopy institutional billing form and the data element specifications for both the hardcopy form and the 192-byte UB-92 flat file EMC format. The NUBC has a formal consultative role under HIPAA for all transactions affecting institutional health care services.

national uniform claim committee An organization, chaired and hosted by the American Medical Association, that maintains the HCFA-1500 claim form and a set of data element specifications for professional claims submission via the HCFA-1500 claim form, the Professional EMC NSF, and the X12 837. The NUCC also maintains the Provider Taxonomy Codes and has a formal consultative role under HIPAA for all transactions affecting non-dental non-institutional professional health care services.

navicular The largest wrist bone on the thumb side.

NCHS National Center for Health Statistics. The federal agency responsible for the collection and dissemination of the nation's vital and health statistics. Its mission is to provide statistical information that will guide actions and policies to improve the health of the American people.

NCVHS National Committee on Vital and Health Statistics.

NDC National drug code.

nearsightedness Common term for myopia.

nebulizer A device used to administer medication to people in the form of a mist inhaled into the lungs. It is commonly used in treating cystic fibrosis, asthma, and other respiratory diseases.

NEC Not Elsewhere Classified. Used with ill-defined terms to alert the coder that a specified form of the condition is classified differently. The category number for the term including NEC is to be used only when the coder lacks the information necessary to code the term to a more specific category.

necatoriasis Hookworm disease caused by species of Necator.

neck The part of the body joining the head to the shoulders. Also, any narrow or constricted part of a bone or organ that joins its parts as, for example, the neck of the femur bone.

neck dissection Dissection in the neck to remove all disease tissues including cervical lymph nodes and to leave an adequate margin of normal tissue. This type of surgery is usually used in tumors or cervical metastases in the head and neck.

necr(o)- Death.

necrolysis Disintegration and dissolution of dead tissue.

necropsy An examination and dissection of a dead body to determine cause of death or the changes produced by disease.

necrosis Localized death of tissue that occurs in groups of cells in response to disease or injury.

needle biopsy Biopsy sample obtained via a needle.

negotiated fee schedule Fees set through an organized bargaining process usually used to help determine a global budget. Also called negotiated payment schedule.

neisseria meningitides Bacteria that is often the cause of meningitis.

neo- New.

neo-adjuvant therapy Therapy given before the primary therapy; for example, neo-adjuvant chemotherapy, which is chemotherapy given prior to surgery.

neonatal Relating to or affecting the infant during the first month after birth.

neonatal isoimmune thrombocytopenia An alloimmune disorder characterized by low platelets at birth which can be accompanied by severe bleeding.

neoplasm A tumor. An abnormal growth of tissue.

neoplasm table A table in the Alphabetical Index of ICD-9-CM that includes a list of code numbers for neoplasms by anatomical site. For each site there are six possible code numbers according to whether the neoplasm in question is malignant, benign, in situ, of uncertain behavior, or of unspecified nature.

neoplastic diseases Disease characterized by abnormal growth of new tissue. Cell multiplication is uncontrolled and progressive. Can be benign or malignant.

neostigmine test On injection of neostigmine methylsulfate mixed with atropine sulfate, lessening of myasthenic symptoms indicates myasthenia gravis.

NEP Negative expiratory pressure.

nephelometry A technique used in immunology to determine levels of igm, igg, and iga. It is performed by shining light on a sample, and measuring the amount of light scattered.

nephr(o)- of or pertaining to the kidney.

nephrectomy The surgical removal of a kidney.

nephritis Any one of a large group of diseases of the kidney characterized by inflammation and abnormal function.

nephrocutaneous fistula A fistula between the kidney and the skin, mostly secondary to trauma, including surgery.

nephrogenic Arising in the kidneys.

nephrolith A kidney stone.

nephrolithiasis The presence of kidney stones (calculi) in the kidney.

nephrolithotomy The surgical removal of a kidney stone.

nephrologist A physician who has been trained in the diagnosis and management of kidney disease.

nephron Anatomical and functional unit of the kidney consisting of tubules and blood vessels.

nephropathy A disease affecting the kidneys.

nephropexy The surgical fixation of a floating or mobile kidney (nephroptosis).

nephroplasty Plastic repair of the kidney.

nephroptosis An abnormal condition in which the kidney drops down into the pelvis when the patient stands up. *Synonym:* floating kidney, renal ptosis.

nephropyeloplasty Plastic repair of the kidney and renal pelvis.

nephrorrhaphy Suture of the kidney.

nephrosclerosis Involves small arteries and kidney's filtering system. Caused by hypertension. *See* Hypertension. If the condition is severe and left untreated, kidney failure and heart failure result. *Synonym:* nephroangiosclerosis.

nephroscopy Visualization of the kidney by using a nephroscope.

nephrosis Form of chronic kidney disease beginning in early childhood. Characterized by protein in the urine, swelling of skin and organs, and low protein and high cholesterol blood levels. *Synonym:* nephrotic syndrome.

nephrosonephritis Renal disease with nephrotic and nephritic components.

nephrostogram A radiograph of the kidney after a contrast agent has been administered through a nephrostomy tube.

nephrostolithotomy A percutaneous procedure used to break up small kidney stones.

nephrostomy The insertion of a catheter through the skin and body wall into the kidney pelvis, mainly to provide urine drainage where the ureter is not functional. It is used also to remove or dissolve renal calculi and to diagnose ureteral obstruction.

nephrostomy tube Flexible plastic tube passed into an opening made in the kidney that leads outside the body.

nephrotic syndrome A collection of symptoms which occur because the glomeruli (tiny blood vessels) in the kidney become leaky. This allows protein, normally never passed out in the urine, to leave the body in large amounts.

nephrotomogram A series of x-rays of the kidneys.

nephrotomy Incision into a kidney (usually to remove a kidney stone).

nerv- of or pertaining to nerves and the nervous system [uncommon as a root neuro- mostly always used].

nerve A bundle of fibers that uses chemical and electrical signals to transmit sensory and motor information from one body part to another.

nerve root The bony arch of the posterior aspect of a vertebra that surrounds the spinal cord, also referred to as the vertebral arch.

nerve (root) canal The internal chamber of a tooth (dental pulp).

nerve transfer Surgical reinnervation of a denervated peripheral target using a healthy donor nerve and/or its proximal stump.

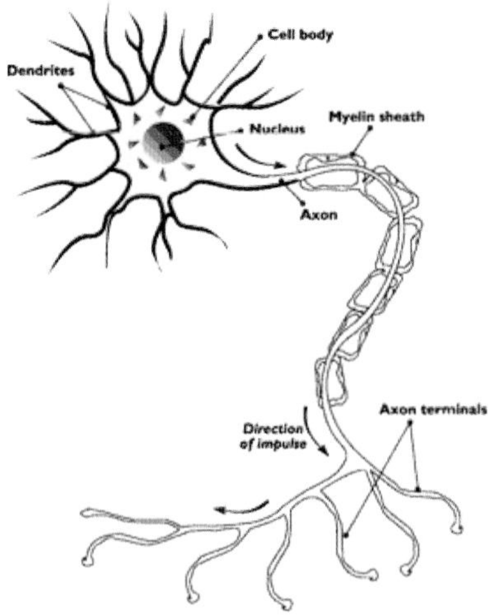

illustration of a nerve

nervous system The system of cells, tissues, and organs that regulates the body's responses to internal and external stimuli. It consists of the brain, spinal cord, nerves, ganglia, and parts of the receptor and effector organs.

network A group of physicians, hospitals and other health care providers contracted to provide services to insurance companies customers for less than their usual fees. Provider networks can cover a large geographic market or a wide range of health care services. Insured individuals typically pay less for using a network provider.

network model HMO An HMO that contracts with more than one group practice of physicians or specialty groups.

network provider Physicians, hospitals or other providers of medical services that have agreed to participate in a network, to offer their services at negotiated rates, and to meet other negotiated contractual provisions. *Synonym:* participating provider.

neur(i)-, neur(o)- of or pertaining to nerves and the nervous system.

neurasthenia A psycho-pathological term describing a condition with symptoms of fatigue, anxiety, headache, impotence, neuralgia and depressed mood.

neuraxial analgesia Pertains to local anesthetics placed around the nerves of the central nervous system. *Synonym:* epidural.

neurectomy The surgical removal of a nerve or a section of a nerve.

neurinoma Tumor of the nerve covering. Usually benign, but may undergo malignant change.

neuritis Inflammation of a nerve. Can cause pain, numbness, paralysis or sensitivity of the affected area.

neuro Neurologic.

neuroblastoma Highly malignant tumor that usually originates in the adrenal glands of young children. Tumor metastasizes early and widely to lymph nodes, liver, lung and bone. Prior to metastasis, treatment is often successful.

neurocognitive Memory, thinking skills.

neuroendocrine tumor A tumor derived from cells that release a hormone in response to a signal from the nervous system. Examples of neuroendocrine tumors include carcinoid tumors islet cell tumors, medullary thyroid carcinoma, and pheochromocytoma.

neuroendoscopy The use of an endoscope to gain access to the brain, spine and peripheral nervous system. Used in the management of hydrocephalus, cystic lesions of the brain and spinal cord, tumors, vascular lesions, degenerative spine disease and nerve entrapments.

neurofibroma Fibrous tumor of nerve tissue.

neurofibromatosis Genetic disorders of the nervous system that primarily affect the development and growth of neural (nerve) cell tissues. These disorders cause tumors to grow on nerves and produce other abnormalities such as skin changes and bone deformities.

neurogenic 1) Forming nervous tissue or stimulating nervous energy. 2) Originating in the nervous system.

neuroleptic Tranquilizer used to treat psychotic conditions when a calming effect is desired.

neurologic Refers to the brain, spinal cord, and nerves.

neurological Having to do with the nerves or the nervous system.

neurology Refers to the study and treatment of the nervous system. Neurology services are usually performed in conjunction with a medical consultation.

neurolysis Destruction of nerve tissue.

neuroma A growth or tumor of nerve tissue.

neuromuscular agents Drugs used for their actions on skeletal muscle.

neuromyelitis optica An auto-immune, inflammatory disorder in which a person's own immune system attacks the optic nerves and spinal cord. This produces an inflammation of the optic nerve (optic neuritis) and the spinal cord (myelitis). *Synonym:* devic's disease.

neuropathies Any pathology of the peripheral nerves.

neuropathy Refers to disorders of the nerves of the peripheral nervous system.

neuroplasty Plastic repair of a nerve.

neuroprotective agents Drugs intended to prevent damage to the brain or spinal cord from ischemia, stroke, convulsions, or trauma.

neuropsychological tests Tests designed to assess neurological function associated with certain behaviors. They are used in diagnosing brain dysfunction or damage and central nervous system disorders or injury.

neurorrhaphy Suture of a divided nerve.

neurosis A mental or personality disturbance not attributable to any known neurological or organic dysfunction.

neurostimulation The stimulation of the spinal cord by tiny electrical impulses. These impulses block the transmission of pain messages to the brain.

neurosurgeon A physician trained in surgery of the nervous system and who specializes in surgery on the brain and other parts of the nervous system. Sometimes called a brain surgeon.

neurosurgery The specialty of treating the central nervous system, including the brain and spinal cord, with surgery.

neurosurgical procedures Surgery performed on the nervous system or its parts.

neurosyphilis The slowly progressive degeneration of the spinal cord that occurs in the late (tertiary) phase of syphilis a decade or more after contracting the infection. *Synonym:* tabes dorsalis.

neurotic disorders Disorders in which the symptoms are distressing to the individual and recognized by him or her as being unacceptable. Social relationships may be greatly affected but usually remain within acceptable limits.

neurotomy The surgical severing of a nerve.

neurotransmitters and neurotransmitter agents A collective grouping for neurotransmitters and substances that act on the neurotransmitter system.

neurotrophic factor Generic term for any of a family of substances with roles in maintenance and survival of neurons.

neurovascular of or pertaining to nerves and blood vessels.

neutralization test One for the neutralization power of an antiserum or other substance by testing its action on the pathogenic properties of a microorganism, toxin, virus, bacteriophage, or toxic substance.

neutropenia Leukopenia in which the decrease is primarily in number of neutrophils.

neutrophils Neutrophils are a type of white blood cell that is responsible for much of the body's protection against infection. Neutrophils are produced in the bone marrow and released into the bloodstream to travel to wherever they are needed. Large numbers of immature forms of neutrophils, called neutrophilic band cells, are produced by the bone marrow when the demand is high.

neutrophils (absolute) The absolute count is the actual number for each of the 5 white blood cells in your test. This is based on the percentage of White blood cells in the body. For example, let's say your total WBC is 5.4; this would mean there was a total of 5, 400 white blood cells in your body for every 1,000 millimeters of blood collected.

nevus A blemish on the skin formed before birth.

new patient A patient who has not received any professional services from the physician or another physician of the same specialty who belongs to the same group practice within the past three years.

newborn care services Services provided to newborns (birth through the first 28 days) in several different settings.

Newborns' And Mothers' Health Protection Act A law which specifies that group health plans or group health care insurers cannot mandate that hospital stays following childbirth be shorter than 48 hours for normal deliveries or 96 hours for cesarean births.

Newman fusion C-1 to C-2 posterior fusion without fixation.

NICU Neonatal intensive care unit.

Niemann-Pick disease Autosomal-recessive inherited lipid histiocytosis with accumulation of phospholipid (sphingomyelin) in histiocytes in the liver, spleen, lymph nodes and bone marrow. *Synonym:* sphingolipidosis.

night guard A plastic mouthpiece for the prevention of damage caused by grinding teeth at night.

NIH National Institute of Health is the primary Federal agency for conducting and supporting medical research. Helping to lead the way toward important medical discoveries that improve people's health and save lives, NIH scientists investigate ways to prevent disease as well as the causes, treatments, and even cures for common and rare diseases.

Nissen operation A surgical procedure to treat gastroesophageal reflux disease (GERD) and hiatus hernia. *Synonym:* fundoplication.

nitrous oxide A controlled mixture of nitrogen and oxygen gases (N2O) that is inhaled by the patient in order to decrease anxiety. *Synonym:* laughing gas.

NMES Neuromuscular electrical stimulation.

no balance billing provision A provider contract clause which states that the provider agrees to accept the amount the plan pays for medical services as payment in full and not to bill plan members for additional amounts (except for co-payments, coinsurance, and deductibles).

NOC Not otherwise classified.

nocturia Excessive urination at night; especially common in older men.

nocturnal penile tumescence test Monitoring of erections occurring during sleep; used in the differential diagnosis of psychogenic and organic impotence.

no-fault insurance No-fault insurance is insurance that pays for health care services resulting from injury or damage to property regardless of who is at fault for causing the accident.

non-arthropod-borne viral diseases Diseases caused by a virus that is not carried by insects, spiders, crustaceans, centipedes or millipedes.

non-assigned claim A claim for which the suppliers do not agree to accept Medicare's allowed charges; the supplier bills the beneficiary for all charges, and then submits claim as non-assigned; Medicare sends any payment to the beneficiary.

non-covered service A service that a) does not meet the requirements of a Medicare benefit category, or b) is statutorily excluded from coverage, or c) is not reasonable and necessary.

non-entity assets Assets that are held by an entity but are not available to the entity. These are also amounts that, when collected, cannot be spent by the reporting entity.

non-formulary drugs Drugs not on a plan-approved list.

non-group market A market segment that consists of customers who are covered under an individual contract for health coverage or enrolled in a government program.

non-hemolytic Refers to transfusion reactions where the red blood cell is not destroyed.

non-Hodgkin's lymphoma Malignant tumor of the lymph glands, which is more common than Hodgkin's disease. Cause is unknown, but viral infection may be a factor. Symptoms may include swollen, rubbery, non-tender lymph glands anywhere in the body, weight loss, malaise, anemia, jaundice and bleeding from the digestive tract. *Synonym:* lymphosarcoma.

non-invasive vascular diagnostic studies Refers to diagnostic procedures performed to determine blood flow and/or the condition of arteries and/or veins.

non-maleficence An ethical principle which, when applied to managed care, states that managed care organizations and their providers are obligated not to harm their members.

non-operating room procedure A procedure classification of the DRG system, which defines procedures which would not usually require the use of an operating room.

non-participating physician (Medicare) A physician who does not sign a Medicare participation agreement, and therefore is not obligated to accept assignment on all claims. Frequently defined as nonpar.

non-renewable An insurance policy that cannot be renewed or continued after its expiration date.

non-residential substance abuse treatment facility A location which provides treatment for substance (alcohol and drug) abuse on an ambulatory basis. Services include individual and group therapy and counseling, family counseling, laboratory tests, drugs and supplies, and psychological testing.

non-small cell lung cancer A lung cancer in the form of squamous cell carcinoma, adenocarcinoma, or large cell carcinoma. Non-small cell lung cancer is a disease in which malignant (cancer) cells form in the tissues of the lung.

non-specific code Refers to CPT codes with descriptions that include the term specify instructing the coder to include additional information such as the quadrant, the nerve, the muscle, the level of spine, the number of joints, the type of study, the method of dosimetry, the hormone, the receptor, etc.

non-specific liver disease Poor liver function in the absence of a known cause.

non-spherocytic hemolytic anemia *See* Anemia, non-spherocytic hemolytic.

non-stress test The monitoring of the response of the fetal heart rate to fetal movements by cardiotocography.

non-toxic nodular goiter A type of simple goiter with enlargement caused by nodules, or lumps, on the thyroid.

nontreponemal antigen test Any of various tests detecting serum antibodies to reagin (cardiolipin and lecithin) derived from host tissues in the diagnosis of the Treponema pallidum infection of syphilis.

non-union Failure of the fragments of a fractured bone to heal or to obtain bony fusion following an arthrodesis.

nootropic agents Drugs used to specifically facilitate learning or memory, particularly to prevent the cognitive deficits associated with dementias. These drugs act by a variety of mechanisms.

no-rap LUPAs A billing scenario in which only a claim, not a RAP, is submitted for an episode by an HHA because the HHA is aware from the outset that the episode will be four visits or less.

norepinephrine A hormone that regulates blood pressure by causing blood vessels to narrow and the heart to beat faster. It also has a role in regulating mood.

NOS Not Otherwise Specified. Equivalent to Unspecified. This abbreviation refers to a lack of sufficient detail in the statement of diagnosis to be able to assign it to a more specific sub division within the classification.

novocain A generic name for the many kinds of anesthetics used in the dental injection, such as Xylocaine, Lidocaine, or Novocain. See local anesthetic. The older brand name for a local anesthetic, currently replaced by safer, more effective agents.

NPDR Nonproliferative diabetic retinopathy.

NPI National provider identifier.

NPI registry A publicly available, Internet-based real-time query database that displays publicly available health care provider data from the NPPES in response to a user's query.

NSAID A non-steroidal anti-inflammatory drug.

NSR Normal sinus rhythm.

NUBC National uniform billing committee.

NUCC National uniform claim committee.

nuclear imaging A method of producing images by detecting radiation from different parts of the body after a radioactive tracer material is administered. The images are recorded on computer and on film.

nuclear medicine A specialty of medicine and medical imaging that uses radioactive isotopes (radio-nuclides) in the diagnosis and treatment of disease.

nuclear sclerosis Commonly known as cataracts. Nuclear sclerosis is an opacity or clouding of the natural crystalline lens that may prevent a clear image from forming on the retina. Cataracts occur naturally and can be induced by trauma.

nucleus pulposus The semi-gelatinous tissue in the center of an intervertebral disc. It is surrounded and contained by the annulus fibrosus which prevents this material from protruding outside the disc space.

nurse practitioner A nurse who has 2 or more years of advanced training and has passed a special exam. A nurse practitioner often works with a physician and can do some of the same things a physician does.

nursing facility A facility which primarily provides skilled nursing care and related services for the rehabilitation of injured, disabled, or sick persons, or on a regular basis, health related care services above the level of custodial care to other than mentally retarded individuals.

nursing home A residence that provides a room, meals, and help with activities of daily living and recreation. Generally, nursing home residents have physical or mental problems that keep them from living on their own. They usually require daily assistance.

nutrition therapy Improving health status of an individual by adjusting the quantities, qualities, and methods of nutrient intake.

nutritional deficiencies A disease caused by a deficiency of a particular nutrient such as minerals, vitamins, carbohydrates, fats and proteins.

nutritional marasmus Extreme malnutrition and emaciation, especially in children; resulting from inadequate intake of food.

nystagmus Involuntary movements of the eyeballs; the presence or absence of nystagmus is used to diagnose a variety of neurological and visual disorders.

O

O_2 Oxygen.

OASIS Outcome Assessment Information Set. The Home Health assessment instrument required by CMS.

OB/GYN Obstetrics and gynecology.

Ober and Barr procedure A surgical method for treating weak biceps muscles by transfer of the brachioradialis muscle.

OBG Obstetrics and gynecology.

obliteration To cause to disappear by surgical methods.

OBRA Omnibus Budget Reconciliation Act of 1993.

OBS Organic brain syndrome.

obsessive-compulsive disorder An anxiety disorder characterized by recurrent, persistent obsessions or compulsions. Obsessions are the intrusive ideas, thoughts, or images that are experienced as senseless or repugnant.

obstetrical pulmonary embolism A blood clot that lodges in the lungs and blocks the lung arteries during pregnancy so the flow of blood to the lungs and heart is reduced.

obstetrics The specialty of treating women before, during and after childbirth which may include surgery such as a C-section.

obstructed labor A labor in which delivery is prevented by mechanical factors; delivery often requires cesarean section.

obstructive jaundice Interruption in the flow of bile through any part of the biliary tract. Causes can occur in or outside the liver. Causes outside the liver may be a gallstone, tumor in the common bile duct or cancer of the pancreas. *Synonym:* cholestasis.

obturator neurectomy Surgical removal of all or part of the obturator nerve.

obturator prosthesis A prosthesis used to restore speech after maxillectomy and other surgical procedures.

occipital Pertaining to the occiput, the back of head.

occipital bone a single trapezoid-shaped bone situated at the posterior and inferior part of the cranium.

occlusal surface The chewing surface of the back teeth.

occlusal x-ray An intraoral x-ray taken with the film held between the teeth in biting position.

occlusion 1. Closing or obstruction. Usually describes a blockage in blood vessels. 2. Any contact between biting or chewing surfaces of upper and lower teeth.

occult blood Chemical, spectroscopic, or microscopic detection of extremely small amounts of blood.

occupational therapy Services given to help you return to usual activities (such as bathing, preparing meals, housekeeping) after illness.

occupancy rate A measure of inpatient health facility use, determined by dividing available bed days by patient days. It measures the average percentage of facilities' beds occupied.

Occupational Safety and Health Administration (OSHA) A Federal agency within the U.S. Department of Labor that is responsible for setting standards to promote and enforce employee safety in the workplace.

Occupational Therapist (OT) Occupational therapists assess functioning in activities of everyday living, including dressing, bathing, grooming, meal preparation, writing, and driving, which are essential for independent living. In making treatment recommendations, the OT addresses (1) fatigue management, (2) upper body strength, movement, and coordination, (3) adaptations to the home and work environment, including both structural changes and specialized equipment for particular activities, and (4) compensatory strategies for impairments in thinking, sensation, or vision.

OCD Obsessive-compulsive disorder.

OCE Outpatient Code Editor (system).

OCG Oral cholecystogram.

ocul(o)- of or pertaining to the eye.

ocular adnexa The adjacent structures of the eye such as the lacrimal apparatus, the extraocular muscles and the eyelids, eyelashes, eyebrows and the conjunctiva.

oculoelectromyography Electromyogram of the eye.

oculography A method of recording eye position and eye movements.

oculomotor nerve The third of twelve paired cranial nerves. It controls most of the eye's movement, constriction of the pupil, and maintains an open eyelid.

odont(o)- of or pertaining to teeth.

odontoclasia A type of dental decay that ravages the teeth of very young children.

odontogenic 1) Of or pertaining to the formation and development of teeth. 2) Originating in the tissues of the teeth.

odontoid process A small, tooth like, upward projection from the second vertebra of the neck around which the first vertebra rotates.

odyn(o)- Pain.

offset The recovery by Medicare of a debt by reducing present or future Medicare payments and applying the amount withheld to the indebtedness.

OHD Organic heart disease.

-oid Resemblance to.

ole- Small or little.

olecranon process Process of the ulna that forms the outer bump of the elbow and fits into the fossa of the humerus when the arm is extended.

olfactory of or relating to olfaction (smell).

olig(o)- Denoting something as 'having little, having few'.

oligohydramnios A condition in pregnancy characterized by a deficiency of amniotic fluid.

oliguria Abnormally small production of urine; can be a symptom of kidney disease or obstruction of the urinary tract or edema or an imbalance of fluids and electrolytes in the body.

om(o)- of or pertaining to the shoulder.

-oma (singular), -omata (plural) Tumor.

ombudsman An individual who assists enrollees in resolving problems they may have with their MCO or PHP. An ombudsman is a neutral party who works with the enrollee, the MCO or PHP, and the provider (as appropriate) to resolve individual enrollee problem.

omentectomy Surgical removal of the omentum.

omentopexy A surgical procedure whereby the greater omentum is sutured to a nearby organ.

omentum A fold of peritoneum supporting the viscera.

Omnibus Budget Reconciliation Act A federal act which established the Medicare SELECT program, a Medicare supplement that uses a preferred provider organization to supplement Medicare Part B coverage.

omphal(o)- of or pertaining to the navel, the umbilicus.

omphalectomy Excision of the umbilicus.

omphalitis Infection of the umbilical cord stump in the neonatal newborn period.

omphalocele Protrusion of the intestine and omentum through a hernia in the abdominal wall near the navel; usually self correcting after birth.

OMT Osteopathic manipulative treatment.

onchocerciasis A disease caused by Onchocerca volvulus, a nematode that can live for up to fifteen years in the human body. It is transmitted to humans through the bite of a black fly. Onchocerciasis is the world's third leading cause of blindness. *Synonym:* river blindness.

onco- Tumor, bulk, volume.

oncologic and oncology Terms referring ot the study of cancer.

oncology The specialty of treating cancer with surgery.

onlay A cast, usually made of gold, attached to the occlusal surface of a tooth.

on-line electronic medical evaluation Consists of assessment and management services provided by a health care professional to a patient via the internet in response to an on-line inquiry.

on-site reviews Reviews performed on-site at the MCO or PHP health care delivery system sites to assess the physical resources and operational practices in place to deliver health care.

onych(o)- of or pertaining to the nail (of a finger or toe).

onychectomy Surgical removal of a toenail or fingernail.

onychia An inflammation of the matrix (surrounding tissue) of the nail with formation of pus and shedding of the nail. Onychia results from the introduction of microscopic pathogens through small wounds.

oo- of or pertaining to the an egg, a woman's egg, the ovum.

oophor(o)- of or pertaining to the woman's ovary.

oophorectomy The surgical removal of an ovary or ovaries.

oophoritis Inflammation of one or both ovaries.

oophorocystectomy Excision of an ovarian cyst.

OP Outpatient.

opacified Impervious to light rays or X-rays.

open access A provision that specifies that plan members may self-refer to a specialist, either in-network or out-of-network, at full benefit or at a reduced benefit, without first obtaining a referral from a primary care provider.

open enrollment A period each year during which employees have an opportunity to change their employer-provided health care coverage. They usually can choose among various plans from different health insurance providers.

open formulary The provision that drugs on the preferred list and those not on the preferred list will both be covered by a PBM or MCO.

open treatment Refers to the treatment of (compound) fractures involving wounds that communicate with the fracture and may expose bone to contamination. Open injuries carry an elevated risk of infection; they require antibiotic treatment and usually urgent surgical treatment.

open-ended HMO An HMO which allows enrolled individuals to use out-of-plan providers and still receive partial or full coverage and payment for the professional's services under a traditional indemnity plan.

open-panel HMO An HMO in which any physician who meets the HMO's standards of care may contract with the HMO as a provider. These physicians typically operate out of their own offices and see other patients as well as HMO members.

operating microscope Binocular microscope used in surgery to provide a clear view of small and inaccessible parts of the body (as in microsurgery).

operating room procedure A procedure classification of the DRG system, which defines procedures which usually require the use of an operating room.

operation A surgical procedure performed for the repair of damage or the restoration of health that usually involves incision, excision, or suturing.

operative dentistry Refers to dentistry involving restoration of parts of the teeth that are defective through disease, trauma, or abnormal development.

operculectomy The surgical removal of the mucosal flap partially or completely covering an unerupted tooth.

OPG Oculoplethysmography.

ophthalm(o)- of or pertaining to the eye.

ophthalmic of or relating to the eye.

ophthalmodynamometry Measurement of the blood pressure of the retinal vessels. It is used also for the determination of the near point of convergence.

ophthalmologic surgical procedures Surgery performed on the eye or any of its parts.

ophthalmologist A medical physician specializing in the treatment of diseases of the eye.

ophthalmology The study and treatment of diseases of the eye.

ophthalmopathy Any eye disease.

ophthalmoplegia Paralysis of the one or more extraocular muscles which are responsible for eye movements.

ophthalmoscopy Examination of the internal structures of the eye using an illumination and magnification system.

OPPS Outpatient Prospective Payment System.

optic atrophy Degeneration of the optic nerve.

optic cup The white, cup-like area in the center of the optic disc.

optic disk The circular area (disc) where the optic nerve connects to the retina. Also know as the optic nerve head.

optic nerve A nerve that transmits visual information from retina to brain.

optic neuritis Inflammation of the nerve that conducts vision impulses from the eye to the brain.

optic(o)- of or relating to chemical properties of the eye.

optometrist A person skilled in testing for defects of vision in order to prescribe corrective glasses.

OPV Oral poliovirus vaccine.

or(o)- of or pertaining to the mouth.

oral administration The giving of drugs, chemicals, or other substances by mouth.

oral and maxillofacial surgeon A dental specialist who manages the diagnosis and surgical treatment of diseases, injuries and deformities of the mouth and supporting structures.

oral cavity The mouth.

oral diagnosis Examination of the mouth and teeth toward the identification and diagnosis of intraoral disease or manifestation of non-oral conditions.

oral hygiene The process of maintaining cleanliness of the teeth and related structures.

oral medicine A branch of dentistry dealing with diseases of the oral and paraoral structures and the oral management of systemic diseases.

oral surgery A dental specialty concerned with the diagnosis and surgical treatment of disease, injuries, and defects of the human oral and maxillofacial region.

oral surgical procedures Procedures used to treat disease, injuries, and defects of the oral and maxillofacial region.

orbit The structural area of the facial skeleton into which the eye is set. *Synonym:* globe.

orbit evisceration The surgical removal of the contents of the orbit. This includes the eyeball, blood vessels, muscles, fat, nerve supply, and periosteum.

orbitotomy An incision into the orbit.

orchi(o)-, orchido- Testis.

orchidopexy Surgery to move an undescended testicle into the scrotum and permanently fix it there.

orchidoplasty Plastic repair of the testis.

orchiectomy Surgical removal of one or both testes.

orchiopexy Surgery to move an undescended testicle into the scrotum and permanently fix it there.

orchioplasty Plastic repair of the testis.

orchitis The inflammation and swelling of the testes as a result of infection or physical injury. Epididymitis is an inflammation of the epididymis which is located along the posterior aspect of the testicle.

ordering physician The physician who orders an item or service.

organ or disease oriented panels CPT codes for organ or disease oriented panels were included in cpt due to the increased use of general screening programs by physicians, clinics, hospitals, and other health care facilities.

organ procurement The administrative procedures involved with acquiring organs for transplantation through various programs, systems, or organizations. It includes obtaining consent and arranging for transportation of donor organs, after tissue harvesting, to the hospital.

organ procurement organization An organization that performs or coordinates the retrieval, preservation, and transportation of organs and maintains a system of locating prospective recipients for available organs.

organ transplantation Transference of an organ between individuals of the same species or between individuals of different species.

organic sleep disorders Are sleep disorders that are the result of an anatomic or physiologic abnormality or disease process.

organized delivery system A comprehensive, integrated network of providers who manage and deliver many levels of care in comprehensive set of health services.

orientation in space tests Holding objects in space and describing how to get from one point to another (the doctors office to home), are orientation in space tests used to locate dominant hemisphere parieto-occipital lesions.

ornithosis An atypical pneumonia caused by a rickettsia microorganism and transmitted to humans from infected birds.

orth(o)- Denoting something as straight or correct.

ortho Orthopedics.

orthodontics A dental specialty concerned with the prevention and correction of dental and oral anomalies (malocclusion).

orthokeratology A non-surgical procedure using contact lenses to alter the shape of the cornea to effect a change in the refractive error.

orthopantogram An x-ray that provides a panoramic view of the mouth, giving information on the teeth and the bones of the upper and lower jaw.

orthopedic procedures Procedures used to treat and correct deformities, diseases, and injuries to the musculoskeletal system, its articulations, and associated structures.

orthopedic surgery The specialty of treating problems of the bones, joints, ligaments and tendons with surgery.

orthopnea Shortness of breath (or dyspnea) which occurs when lying flat.

orthoptics The study and treatment of defects in binocular vision resulting from defects in the optic musculature or of faulty visual habits. It involves a technique of eye exercises designed to correct the visual axes of eyes not properly coordinated for binocular vision.

orthoroentgenogram A method of determining leg length discrepancy by placing a radio-opaque ruler beneath the limb and moving the x-ray tube to obtain separate exposures of the hip, knee and ankle.

orthosis A device applied to a human limb to control or enhance movement or to prevent bone movement or deformity, for example, a splint or an arch support.

orthostatic Pertaining to an upright standing posture.

orthotic training Training in the use of an orthosis.

orthotics An allied health care profession concerned with the design, development, fitting and manufacturing of orthoses, which are devices that support or correct musculoskeletal deformities and/or abnormalities of the human body.

oscillometry Measurement of oscillations of any kind. In medicine it is used in studying cardiovascular and respiratory physiology.

Osgood-Schlatter disease Osteochondrosis of the tibial tuberosity as seen in adolescents.

OSHA Occupational Safety and Health Administration.

-osis A condition, disease or increase.

Osler disease Polycythemia vera or erythremia; chronic disease characterized by bone marrow hyperplasia, increase in blood volume as well as in number of red cells, redness of the skin, and splenomegaly.

osmotic fragility test Heparinized or defibrinated blood is placed in sodium chloride solutions of varying concentrations; increased fragility, measured as hemolysis, indicates spherocytosis.

osseo- Bony.

osseous Composed of or containing bone.

ossi- Bone.

ossification The process of forming bone in the body.

ost(e)-, oste(o)- Bone.

ostectomy Surgical removal of a bone or part of a bone.

osteitis Inflammation of a bone as a consequence of infection or trauma or degeneration.

osteitis deformans A disease of bone occurring in the middle aged and elderly; excessive bone destruction sometimes leading to bone pain and fractures and skeletal deformities. *Synonym:* Paget's disease.

osteoarthritis Degeneration of cartilage at a joint and growth of bone spurs that inflame surrounding tissue. Can be caused by stress on the joint due to activity and aging or from an injury to the joint lining. Symptoms include stiffness and pain of the affected joint. Cold, damp weather often increases pain. *Synonym:* degenerative arthritis, degenerative joint disease.

osteoarthropathy Any disease of the bones and joints.

osteoarthrosis A chronic degenerative non-inflammatory condition of the joint characterized by structural changes of the joint surfaces.

osteochondritis A painful condition where the cartilage and bone in a joint is inflamed.

osteochondritis dissecans Inflammation of bone and cartilage, which results in pieces of cartilage splitting off into the affected joint.

osteochondroma A benign tumor that contains both bone and cartilage and usually occurs near the end of a long bone.

osteochondromatosis Occurrence of multiple osteochondromas.

osteochondropathies Diseases involving both bone and cartilage.

osteochondropathy A condition affecting both bone and cartilage.

osteochondrosis A condition of defective bone formation in the epiphysis or growing part of the skeleton.

osteodystrophy Any defective bone formation.

osteogenesis imperfecta A genetic disorder characterized by bones that break easily without a specific cause. *Synonym:* brittle bone disease.

osteolysis Lysis of bone caused by disease or infection or inadequate blood supply.

osteoma A slow growing benign tumor of consisting of bone tissue; usually on the skull or mandible.

osteomalacia Abnormal condition resulting in softening of bone. Accompanied by weakness, fracture, pain and weight loss. May be caused by a diet lacking in phosphorus, calcium or vitamin D, lack of exposure to sunlight or malabsorption.

osteomyelitis Infection of the bone and bone marrow caused by bacteria, usually staphylococcus. Bacteria are usually introduced directly by trauma or surgery, but may travel through the bloodstream from an infected organ or tissue, such as from a middle ear infection or pneumonia. Usually curable with prompt, aggressive treatment. Requires hospitalization for observation and administration of intravenous antibiotics.

osteopathic manipulative treatment A form of manual treatment applied by a physician to eliminate or alleviate somatic dysfunction and related disorders. This treatment may be accomplished by a variety of techniques.

osteopathic medicine A system of therapy based on the theory that the body is capable of making its own remedies against disease and other toxic conditions when it is in normal structural relationship and has favorable environmental conditions and adequate nutrition.

osteophytectomy Surgical removal of bone spurs.

osteoplasty Surgical repair or alteration of bone.

osteoporosis Loss of normal bone density, mass and strength, leading to increased porousness and vulnerability to fracture. Usually occurs in women after menopause. Treatment includes a well-balanced, nourishing diet, specific vitamin-mineral supplements, exercise and sometimes estrogen replacement. Treatment can halt, and may reverse, bone deterioration.

osteotomy A surgical operation whereby a bone is cut to shorten, lengthen, or change its alignment.

ostomy Surgical construction of an artificial opening (stoma) for external fistulization of a duct or vessel by insertion of a tube with or without a supportive stent.

ot(o)- of or pertaining to the ear.

otalgia An ache localized in the middle or inner ear.

OTC Over-the-counter.

other managed care arrangement Used if the plan is not considered either a PCCM, PHP, Comprehensive MCO, Medicaid-only MCO, or HIO.

other unlisted facility Other service facilities not previously identified.

otitis Inflammation of the ear.

otitis externa An inflammation of the outer ear and ear canal.

otitis media An inflammation of the outer ear and ear canal.

otogenic of or originating within the ear.

otolaryngology The specialty of treating problems of the ears, nose and throat with surgery.

otologic surgical procedures Surgery performed on the external, middle, or internal ear.

-otomy Act of cutting, incision.

otoplasty A surgical procedure done to correct misshaped or protruding ears.

otorhinolaryngologic surgical procedures Surgery performed on the ear and its parts, the nose and nasal cavity, or the throat, including surgery of the adenoids, tonsils, pharynx, and trachea.

otorhinolaryngology The study and treatment of diseases of the head and neck, including the ears, nose and throat.

otorrhea A discharge from the ear.

otosclerosis A hereditary disorder in which ossification of the labyrinth of the inner ear causes tinnitus and eventual deafness.

otoscopy Examination of the ear by means of an otoscope.

-ous Pertaining to.

out of **area** Services provided to enrollees by providers that have no contractual or other relationship with M + C organizations.

out of network benefit Generally, an out-of-network benefit provides a beneficiary with the option to access plan services outside of the plan's contracted network of providers. In some cases, a beneficiary's out-of-pocket costs may be higher for an out-of-network benefit.

out-of-pocket expenses or costs The share of health services payments paid by the enrollee.

out-of-pocket maximum or cap An annual limit on how much in deductibles and co-payments the patient is required to pay. Also called "stop-loss" provision.

outcome The result of performance (or nonperformance) of a function or process. The consequences of a medical intervention on a group of patients.

outcome audit A type of patient or medical care evaluation study in which criteria are designed to focus upon desired patient outcome or results of treatment, as distinguished from a process audit in which criteria focus upon the components of appropriate clinical intervention.

outcome data Data that measure the health status of people enrolled in managed care resulting from specific medical and health interventions (for example, the incident of measles among plan enrollees during the calendar year).

outcome indicator An indicator that assesses what happens or does not happen to a patient following a process; agreed upon desired patient characteristics to be achieved; undesired patient conditions to be avoided.

outcome measures Assessments to gauge the results of treatment for a particular disease or condition. Outcome measures include the patient's perception of restoration of function, quality of life and functional status, as well as objective measures of mortality, morbidity and health status.

Outcomes and Assessment Information Set (OASIS) Federal monitoring system for Home Health Agencies. A group of data elements that represent core items of a comprehensive assessment for an adult home care patient and form the basis for measuring patient outcomes for purposes of outcome-based quality improvement (OBQI). This assessment is performed on every patient receiving services of Home Health agencies that are approved to participate in the Medicare and/or Medicaid programs.

outlier A comparative term describing a patient whose stay in the hospital is unusually long or whose costs for hospital care are unusually high compared to other patients with the same diagnosis or condition. The Medicare program uses DRGs as categories to identify outliers. Under Medicare, additional payments are made for outliers meeting certain conditions.

out-of-network Health care services received outside the HMO or PPO network.

out-of-plan This phrase usually refers to physicians, hospitals or other health care providers who are considered non-participants in an insurance plan (usually an HMO or PPO). Depending on an individual's health insurance plan, expenses incurred by services provided by out-of-plan health professionals may not be covered, or covered at a reduced benefit level.

out-of-pocket costs Insured health care costs for which one is responsible, because of the application of deductibles, coinsurance and co-payments.

out-of-pocket maximum Total dollar amount an insured will be required to pay for covered medical services during a specified period, such as one year. The out-of-pocket maximum may also be called the stop-loss limit or catastrophic expense limit.

outpatient An individual (patient) who receives health care services (such as surgery) on an outpatient basis, meaning they do not stay overnight in a hospital or inpatient facility. Many insurance companies have identified a list of tests and procedures (including surgery) that will not be covered (paid for) unless they are performed on an outpatient basis. The term outpatient is also used synonymously with ambulatory to describe health care facilities where procedures are performed.

outpatient care Treatment that is provided to a patient who is able to return home after care without an overnight stay in a hospital or other inpatient facility.

outpatient hospital A portion of a hospital which provides diagnostic, therapeutic (both surgical and nonsurgical), and rehabilitation services to sick or injured persons who do not require hospitalization or institutionalization. Part of the Hospital providing services covered by SMI, including services in an emergency room or outpatient clinic, ambulatory surgical procedures, medical supplies such as splints, laboratory tests billed by the hospital, etc.

outpatient hospital services (Medicare) Medicare or surgical care that Medicare Part B helps pay for and does not include an overnight hospital stay, including blood transfusions; certain drugs; hospital billed laboratory tests; mental health care; medical supplies such as splints and casts; emergency room or outpatient clinic, including same day surgery; and emergency room or outpatient clinic, including same day surgery; and x-rays and other radiation services.

Outpatient Prospective Payment System (OPPS) The way that Medicare pays for most outpatient services at hospitals or community mental health centers under Medicare Part B.

outside referral Referral to a consultant provider not on the managed care company's staff or within its network of providers.

ov Office visit.

ovari(o)- of or pertaining to the ovaries.

ovarian of or referring to the ovaries.

ovarian agenesis Congenital absence of ovaries resulting in sterility.

ovarian cyst Any collection of fluid, surrounded by a very thin wall, within an ovary.

ovarian dysfunction Improper functioning of the ovaries.

ovarian pregnancy An abnormal pregnancy that takes place within the ovary itself due to the development of a fertilized ovum still lodged within an ovarian follicle.

ovaries The pair of female reproductive glands in which the ova, or eggs, are formed. The ovaries are located in the pelvis, one on each side of the uterus.

over the counter drugs A drug that does not require a prescription.

overbite A vertical overlap of the front teeth.

overdenture A denture that fits over residual roots or dental implants.

overjet A horizontal overlap of the front teeth.

overhydration Too much fluid in tissues.

overpayment assessment A decision that an incorrect amount of money has been paid for Medicare services and a determination of what that amount is.

Overton fusion Dowel graft that is applied across facet joints.

overvalued procedure A procedure for which the payment rate has been reduced because it was identified as "overvalued" under the customary, prevailing, and reasonable payment system.

oviduct Either of a pair of tubes conducting the egg from the ovary to the uterus.

oviducts A tube through which the ova pass from the ovary to the uterus or to the outside.

ovo-, ovi-, ov- of or pertaining to the eggs, the ovum.

oxo- Addition of oxygen.

oxy- Sharp, acid, acute, oxygen.

oxytocin challenge test A contraction stress test in which the uterine contractions are stimulated by intravenous infusion of oxytocin.

P

pacemaker A small device that's placed under the skin of the chest or abdomen to help control abnormal heart rhythms. This device uses electrical pulses to prompt the heart to beat at a normal rate.

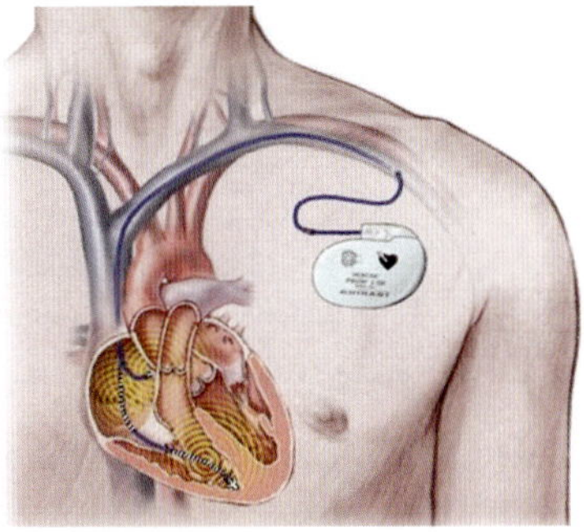

pacemaker

pachy- Thick.

pachymetry Measurement of the thickness of the cornea with a pachymeter. It is useful in monitoring the progression of certain disorders that cause the cornea to become thickened (or filled with water), resulting in a loss of vision. Pachymetry is also performed to determine whether the cornea is strong enough for procedures such as lasik.

PAD Peripheral artery disease.

Paget's disease Gradual, progressive bone disease, characterized by bones breaking down and regenerating excessively. New bone is fragile and weak. It is not cancerous. *Synonym:* osteitis deformans.

paid claims The amount paid to providers to satisfy the contractual liability of the carrier or plan sponsor. These amounts do not include any member liability for ineligible charges, deductibles, or co-payments.

pain An unpleasant sensation that can range from mild, localized discomfort to agony. Pain has both physical and emotional components. The physical part of pain results from nerve stimulation.

palate The upper surface of the mouth that separates the oral and nasal cavities.

palatine bone one of two irregularly shaped bones (L-shaped) forming the posterior part of the hard palate, the lateral wall of the nasal fossa between the medial pterygoid plate and the maxilla, and the posterior part of the floor of the orbit. The posterior part of the hard palate, which separates the nasal cavity from the oral cavity, is formed by the horizontal plates.

palatopharyngoplasty Surgical resection of unnecessary palatal and oropharyngeal tissue to open the airway; intended to cure extreme cases of snoring.

palatoplasty Plastic repair of the palate.

palatoschisis Cleft palate.

palliative vare Care which is provided to relieve pain rather than provide a cure. Also called "comfort care."

Palmer reflex The Palmar grasp reflex appears at birth and persists until five or six months of age. When an object is placed in the infant's hand and strokes their palm, the fingers will close and they will grasp it.

palpation A method of examination in which the examiner feels the size or shape or firmness or location of body parts.

palpebr- of or pertaining to the eyelid [uncommon as a root].

palpitations An abnormal awareness of the beating of the heart, whether it is too slow, too fast, irregular, or at its normal frequency. It can be caused by ectopic beat, which is a more specific diagnosis. Palpitations may be brought on by overexertion, adrenaline, alcohol, nicotine, caffeine, cocaine, amphetamines, and other drugs, disease (such as hyperthyroidism and pheochromocytoma) or as a symptom of panic disorder.

palsy Paralysis of a body part, often accompanied by loss of sensation and by uncontrolled body movements, such as shaking.

pan-, pant(o)- Denoting something as 'complete' or containing 'everything'.

Pancoast's tumor Adenocarcinoma of the lung involving pain in the shoulder and arm due to 8th cervical and 1st thoracic nerve involvement.

pancreas A gland organ in the digestive and endocrine system. It is both an endocrine gland producing several important hormones, including insulin, glucagon, and somatostatin, as well as an exocrine gland, secreting pancreatic juice containing digestive enzymes that pass to the small intestine. These enzymes help in the further breakdown of the carbohydrates, protein, and fat.

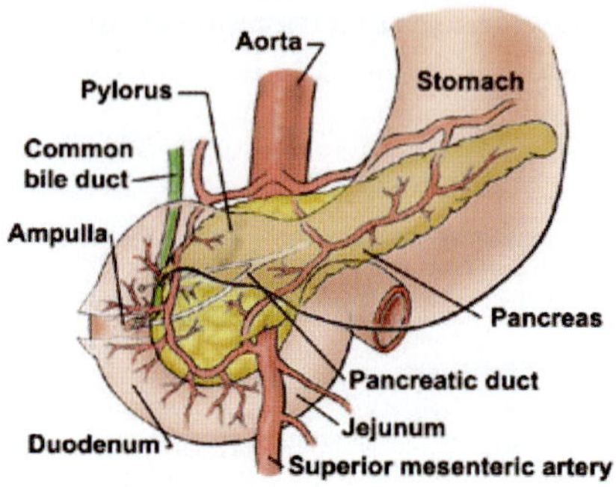

the pancreas

pancreatectomy Surgical removal of the pancreas.

pancreatic disease Any disease of the pancreas.

pancreaticoduodenectomy The excision of the head of the pancreas and the encircling loop of the duodenum to which it is connected. *Synonym:* Whipple procedure.

pancreaticojejunostomy Surgical anastomosis of the pancreatic duct, or the divided end of the transected pancreas, with the jejunum.

pancreatitis Inflammation of the pancreas. Chronic pancreatitis usually follows recurrent attacks of acute pancreatitis. Pancreas gradually becomes unable to supply digestive juices and hormones necessary for good health.

pancreatography Radiography of the pancreas.

pancreatojejunostomy The surgical formation of an artificial opening between the jejunum and a pancreatic duct, cyst, or fistula.

pancreatorrhaphy Suturing of the pancreas.

pancreatotomy Incision of the pancreas.

panel size The number of patients served by a physician or physician group. If the panel size is greater than 25,000 patients, then the physician group is not considered to be at substantial financial risk because the risk is spread over the large number of patients. Stop loss and beneficiary surveys would not be required.

panencephalitis Encephalitis that affects both gray and white matter of the brain, resulting in progressive loss of mental and motor functions.

panhypopituitarism Complex syndrome marked by deficiency of hormones secreted by the pituitary gland. It is very rare. Most often caused by a tumor of the pituitary gland. In children, it results in dwarfism and is characterized by dysfunction of metabolism, sexual immaturity and growth retardation.

panic disorder A type of anxiety disorder characterized by unexpected panic attacks that last minutes or, rarely, hours. Panic attacks begin with intense apprehension, fear or terror and, often, a feeling of impending doom.

panniculectomy Surgery to remove an apron of excess skin and underlying fat from the lower abdomen.

panniculitis Inflammation of subcutaneous adipose tissue. Symptoms include tender skin nodules, and systemic signs such as weight loss and fatigue.

pannus A hanging flap of tissue. When involving the abdomen, it is called a panniculus and consists of skin, fat, and sometimes contents of the internal abdomen as part of a hernia. A pannus can be the result of loose hanging tissues after pregnancy or weight loss. It can also be the result of obesity.

panophthalmitis Inflammation of all the eye structures or tissues.

panorex A full mouth x-ray (180 degree view) of the teeth, upper and lower jaws on one film.

PAOD Peripheral artery occlusive disease.

PAP Papanicolaou (smear, stain, test).

Papanicolaou test An exfoliative cytological staining procedure for detection and diagnosis of various conditions, particularly malignant and premalignant conditions of the female genital tract; also used in evaluating endocrine function and in the diagnosis of malignancies.

papill- of or pertaining to the nipple (of the chest or breast).

papilla Small nipple-like projection or elevation.

papillectomy Surgical removal of any papilla.

papilledema Swelling of the optic disk caused by increased intracranial pressure. Sometimes seen with serious conditions, such as a brain tumor, hemorrhage in the brain or swelling of the brain after head trauma.

papillitis Inflammation of the optic disk. Inflammation of a renal papilla.

papilloma Benign tumor of the skin.

papillotomy Incision into the major duodenal papilla.

papul(o)- Indicates papulosity, a small elevation or swelling in the skin, a pimple, swelling.

PAR Participating Physician and Supplier Program.

para A woman who has given birth. Number of pregnancies producing viable offspring para-0, para-i, para-ii, etc.

para- Alongside of, abnormal.

paracentesis A medical procedure involving needle drainage of fluid from a body cavity, most commonly the abdomen.

paralysis Loss of voluntary movement (motor function). Paralysis that affects only one muscle or limb is partial paralysis, also known as palsy; paralysis of all muscles is total paralysis, as may occur in cases of botulism.

paralytic syndromes Other forms of paralysis resulting in the complete loss of muscle function for one or more muscle groups.

parametritis Inflammation of the parametrium.

paranasal Adjacent to the nasal cavities.

paranasal sinus Any of the paired cavities, designated frontal, sphenoidal, maxillary, and ethmoidal, located in the bones of the face and lined by a mucous membrane continuous with that of the nasal cavity.

paranasal-sinus disease Any disease or disorder of one of the sinuses in the skull adjacent to the nose structure. There are eight paranasal sinuses.

paranoid disorders Chronic mental disorders in which there has been an insidious development of a permanent and unshakeable delusional system (persecutory delusions or delusions of jealousy), accompanied by preservation of clear and orderly thinking.

parapatellar synovitis Inflammation of the synovial membrane close to the kneecap.

paraplegia An impairment in motor and/or sensory function of the lower extremities. It is usually the result of spinal cord injury or a congenital condition such as spina bifida which affects the neural elements of the spinal canal.

paraproteinemias Disorder characterized by paraproteins in the blood including those for multiple myeloma, cryoglobulins and others. *See* Multiple myeloma; cryoglobulins.

parasites Organisms that live within, upon or at, the expense of another living organism. Human parasites include disease-causing agents, such as amoebas or worms, that infect the digestive system or fungi that live on skin.

parasitic disease Any one of many diseases caused by a parasite. *See* Parasites.

parasomnias Are a group of behavioral disorders during sleep that are associated with brief or partial arousals but not with marked sleep disruption or impaired daytime alertness. The presenting complaint is usually related to the behavior itself.

parasthesia A partial loss of sensation; may be temporary or permanent.

parathyroid gland Small endocrine glands in the neck that produce parathyroid hormone. Humans have four parathyroid glands, which are usually located behind the thyroid gland. Parathyroid glands control the amount of calcium in the blood and within the bones.

parathyroidectomy Excision of one or both of the parathyroid glands.

parathyroids Small glands that control calcium levels in the blood and bones. Located within or next to the thyroid gland in the lower neck, next to the trachea.

parenchyma The essential or functional tissue of an organ, as distinguished from its connective tissue, blood vessels, etc.

paresis A condition typified by partial loss of movement, or impaired movement.

-paresis Slight paralysis.

paresthesias Abnormal sensation of the skin, such as numbness, prickling and tingling, that occurs without apparent cause.

parietal bones one of the two quadrilateral bones on either side of the cranium forming part of the superior and lateral surfaces of the skull, and joining each other in the midline at the sagittal suture. The parietal bones form the greater portion of the sides and roof of the cranial cavity.

paring The act of removing the outer covering or skin.

Parkinson's disease Disease of the central nervous system in older adults characterized by gradual, progressive muscle rigidity, tremors and clumsiness. Cause is usually unknown, although medications, brain injury, tumor or infection may cause it. Currently incurable, but treatment can control or relieve symptoms.

paronychia Infection in the tissues adjacent to a nail on a finger or toe.

parotid gland The largest of the salivary glands. It is found wrapped around the mandibular ramus, and it secretes saliva through Stensen's duct into the oral cavity, to facilitate mastication and swallowing.

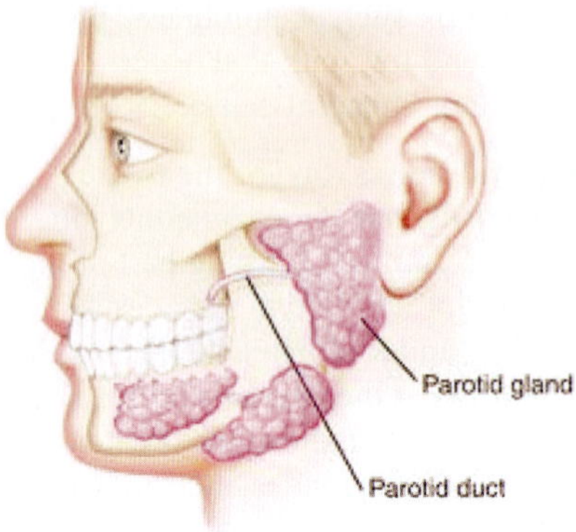

parotid gland and duct

parotidectomy Surgical removal of parotid gland.

parotitis A viral disease of the human species, caused by the mumps virus. It is an acute contagious viral disease characterized by fever and by swelling of the parotid glands. *Synonym:* mumps.

paroxysmal atrial tachycardia (PAT) Bouts of rapid, regular heart beating that originate in the upper chamber (atrium) of the heart due to abnormalities in the atrioventricular (AV) node that lead to rapid firing of electrical impulses from the atrium that bypass the AV node. PAT tends to occur under certain conditions, including excess alcohol consumption, stress, caffeine use, overactive thyroid or excessive thyroid hormone intake, and use of certain drugs.

paroxysmal nocturnal hemoglobinuria Disorder characterized by the destruction of red blood cells resulting in hemoglobin being excreted in the urine. It occurs in irregular episodes for several days in a row, especially at night. Usually afflicts adults between 25 and 45 years of age and is accompanied by abdominal pain, back pain and headache.

paroxysmal ventricular tachycardia (PSVT) A period of very rapid and regular heart beats that begins and ends abruptly. The heart rate is usually between 160 and 200 beats per minute. This condition is also known as paroxysmal supraventricular tachycardia.

Part A The Medicare Hospital Insurance program which covers hospital and related post-hospital services. As an entitlement program, it is available without payment of a premium. Beneficiaries are responsible for an initial deductible per spell of illness and coinsurance for some services.

Part A premium A monthly premium paid by or on behalf of individuals who wish for and are entitled to voluntary enrollment in the Medicare Hospital Insurance (HI) program. These individuals are those who are aged 65 and older, are uninsured for social security or railroad retirement, and do not otherwise meet the requiremints for entitlement to Part A. Disabled individuals who have exhausted other entitlement are also qualified.

Part B The Medicare Supplementary Medical Insurance program (SMI), which covers the costs of physician services, outpatient lab, x-ray, DME and certain other services. As a voluntary program, Part B requires payment of a monthly premium. Beneficiaries are responsible for a deductible and coinsurance payment for most covered services.

partial capitation An insurance arrangement where the payment made to a health plan is a combination of a capitated premium and payment based on actual use of services; the proportions specified for these components determine the insurance risk faced by the plan.

partial denture A removable appliance used to replace one or more lost teeth.

partial hospitalization A structured program of active treatment for psychiatric care that is more intense than care provided in the physician's or therapist's office.

partially capitated A stipulated dollar amount established for certain health care services while other services are reimbursed on a cost or fee-for-service basis.

participating An eligible provider or supplier who has entered into an agreement to accept assignment for all services rendered to Medicare patients, and to accept the Medicare approved amount as payment in full for all services rendered. A participating provider or supplier may not collect from the beneficiary more than the applicable deductible and coinsurance for covered services.

participating hospitals Those hospitals that participate in the Medicare program.

participating physician A physician who signs a participation agreement, agreeing to accept assignment on all Medicare claims for a period of one year. Frequently referred to as PAR.

participating physician and supplier program A program which provides financial and administrative incentives for physicians and suppliers to agree in advance to accept assignment on all Medicare claims for a period of one year.

participating provider A health care provider who has been contracted to render medical services or supplies to insured persons at a pre-negotiated fee. Providers include hospitals, physicians, and other medical facilities that are part of a PPO or HMO network.

Partsch's operation A technique for marsupialization of a dental cyst.

passive cutaneous anaphylaxis An evanescent cutaneous reaction occurring when antibody is injected into a local area on the skin and antigen is subsequently injected intravenously along with a dye.

passive-aggressive personality disorder A long-term (chronic) condition in which a person seems to actively comply with the desires and needs of others, but actually passively resists them. In the process, the person becomes increasingly hostile and angry.

PAT Paroxysmal atrial tachycardia.

Patau syndrome A chromosomal abnormality in which an extra chromosome 13 causes defects of the central nervous system, mental retardation, with cleft palate, polydactyly and cardiac problems, among others.

patch tests Skin tests in which the sensitizer is applied to a patch of cotton cloth or gauze held in place for approximately 48-72 hours. It is used for the elicitation of a contact hypersensitivity reaction.

patella a thick, circular-triangular bone which articulates with the femur and covers and protects the knee joint. It is the largest sesamoid bone in the human body. Synonym: knee cap.

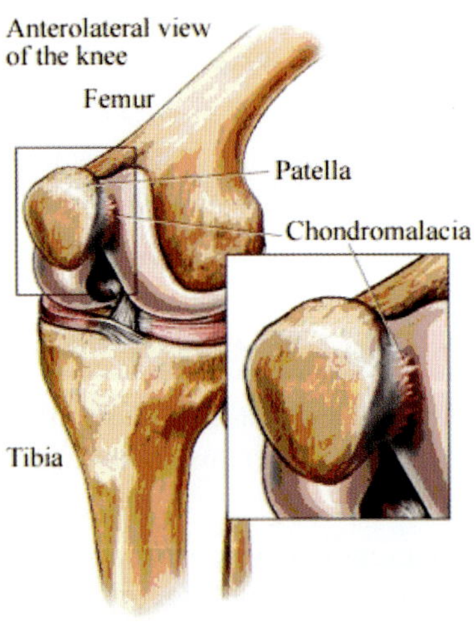

patella

patellar Near or relating to the patella or kneecap.

patellar reflex A deep tendon reflex and is a myotatic reflex. Striking the patellar ligament with a tendon hammer just below the patella stretches the quadriceps muscles in the thigh. The absence or decrease of patellar reflex may indicate the presence of nerve damage or disease, brain lesions or interruption of nerve impulse transmission. Synonym: knee jerk.

patellectomy Surgical removal of the knee bone.

Patey's operation Modified radical mastectomy.

path(o)- Disease.

pathology Pathology is that discipline of the practice of medicine that deals with the causes and nature of disease.

pathology laboratory Lab where tissues, blood, urine, feces and other parts of the human body are studied to determine cause of disease.

-pathy Denotes (with a negative sense) a disease, or disorder.

patient A person under treatment or care, as by a physician or surgeon, or in a facility.

patient advocate Serves as a liaison between patient and hospital staff. Assists patients in interpreting hospital policies, procedures, and services and to obtaining solutions to problems and concerns. Assists staff in gaining awareness of patients' perceptions of the hospital experience.

patient bill of rights Refers to the Consumer Bill of Rights and Responsibilities, a report prepared by the President's Advisory Commission on Consumer Protection and Quality in the Health Care

Industry in an effort to ensure the security of patient information, promote health care quality, and improve the availability of health care treatment and services. The report lists a number rights, subdivided into eight general areas, that all health care consumers should be guaranteed and describes responsibilities that consumers need to accept for the sake of their own health.

patient eligibility Requirements entitling individuals to Medicare benefits.

patient lifts Equipment to move a patient from a bed or wheelchair using your strength or a motor.

patient perception A type of outcomes measure related to whether the patient feels completely better after treatment or feels improved compared to how he or she felt prior to receiving treatment.

Patient Self-Determination Act A Federal law that requires health care facilities to determine if new patients have a living will and/or durable power of attorney for health care and take patients' wishes into consideration in developing their treatment plans.

patient status code A code in the Patient Discharge Status field on institutional claims which describes patient status at discharge or end of period.

Patrick's test With the patient supine, the thigh and knee are flexed. The external malleolus rests on the patella of the opposite leg and the knee is depressed. Production of pain indicates arthritis of the hip. Also called the Fabere sign after the initial letters for Flexion, abduction, External Rotation and Extension. *Synonym:* Fabere sign.

pattern analysis The clinical and statistical analysis of data sets. Frequently used ESRD data sets include the PMMIS, USRDS, the core indicators, Network files, or CMS analytic files.

Paul-Bunnell test Determination of the highest dilution of the patient's serum that will agglutinate sheep erythrocytes; used to detect serum heterophile antibodies in the diagnosis of infectious mononucleosis.

Paul-Bunnell-Davidsohn test a modification of the Paul-Bunnell test that differentiates among three types of heterophile sheep agglutinins those associated with infectious mononucleosis and serum sickness, and natural antibodies against Forssman antigen.

payer In health care, an entity that assumes the risk of paying for medical treatments. This can be an uninsured patient, a self-insured employer, a health plan, or an HMO.

payment rate The total amount paid for each unit of service rendered by a health care provider, including both the amount covered by the insurer and the consumer’s cost sharing.

payment safeguards Activities to prevent and recover inappropriate Medicare benefit payments including MSP, MR or UR, provider audits, and fraud and abuse detection.

PBI Protein-bound iodine.

PCG Phonocardiogram.

PCL Posterior cruciate ligament.

PDA Patent ductus arteriosus.

PDR Physician's desk reference.

PDT Photodynamic therapy.

Pean's operation A surgical procedure for the treatment of gastric ulcers.

pectoral reflex The anterior, (frontal) fold of the axilla, (armpit) that contains the pectoral muscle is tapped with a reflex hammer. In cortical spinal lesions above C5, there is a brisk and sometimes excessive contraction.

ped-, -ped-, -pes of or pertaining to the foot; -footed.

pediatric Pertaining to children.

pediatrics The branch of medical care that deals with the medical care of infants, children, and adolescents. The upper age limit ranges from age 12 to 21, depending on the country.

pediatric surgery The specialty of treating health problems of children with surgery.

pedicle The part of each side of the neural arch of a vertebra. It connects the lamina with the vertebral body.

pedicle flap A surgical flap sustained by a blood-carrying stem from the donor site during transfer.

pediculosis An infestation with lice (pediculus humanus) or true lice or crab lice (phthirius) resulting in severe itching.

peds Pediatrics.

pedunculotomy Total or partial surgical section of the cerebral peduncle.

PEEP Positive end-expiratory pressure.

peer review An examination by practicing physicians or other health professionals of the medical necessity, appropriateness, and quality of the health care services ordered or provided by other physicians or other health professionals. The efficiency and effectiveness of the patient care services are also reviewed. It may be conducted while the patient is in the hospital (concurrent review) or after discharge (retrospective review).

peer review committee The MCO committee that reviews cases of health care services delivery in which the quality of care is questionable or problematic.

Peer Review Organization (PRO) An entity established by the Tax Equity and Fiscal Responsibility Act of 1982 (TEFRA) to review quality of care and appropriateness of admissions, readmissions and discharges for Medicare and Medicaid. These organizations are held responsible for maintaining and lowering admission rates, and reducing lengths of stay while insuring against inadequate treatment.

PEFR Peak expiratory flow rate.

PEFV Partial expiratory flow volume.

Pel-Epstein fever Cyclic fever common with Hodgkin disease featuring intermittent febrile episodes lasting for several days.

pelv(i)-, pelv(o)- Hip bone.

pelvic adhesions Refer to scarring or tissue repair that occurs anywhere in the pelvis. They form as the first step in the healing process after any surgery, trauma, infection, or inflammation.

pelvic exam An exam to check if internal female organs are normal by feeling their shape and size.

pelvic exenteration Removal of all of the organs and adjacent structures of the pelvis. It is usually performed to surgically remove cancer involving the bladder, uterine cervix, or rectum.

pelvic inflammatory disease Infection of female reproductive organs. May be contagious if the infecting germ is sexually transmitted.

pelvic obliquity Deviation of the pelvis from the horizontal in the frontal plane. Fixed pelvic obliquities can be attributed to contractures either above or below the pelvis.

pelvimetry Measurement of the dimensions and capacity of the pelvis. It includes cephalo-pelvimetry (measurement of fetal head size in relation to maternal pelvic capacity), a prognostic guide to the management of labor, obstetric associated with disproportion.

pelviolithotomy Operative removal of a calculus from the kidney through an incision in the renal pelvis.

pelvis The part of the trunk inferoposterior (below-behind) to the abdomen in the transition area between the trunk and the lower limbs.

Pemberton osteotomy A surgical procedure used in the treatment of developmental dysplasia of the hip.

pemphigus A rare autoimmune blistering disorder of the skin.

PEN Parenteral and enteral nutrition.

pended A claims term that refers to a situation in which it is not known whether an authorization has or will be issued for delivery of a health care service, and the case has been set aside for review.

penectomy Surgical removal of the penis.

PENG Photoelectric nystagmography.

-penia Deficiency.

penile of or relating to the penis.

penile implantation Surgical insertion of cylindrical hydraulic devices for the treatment of organic impotence.

penis External male reproductive organ.

PEP Partial Episode Payment (adjustment). A reduced episode payment that may be made based on the number of service days in an episode (always less than 60 days, employed in cases of transfers or discharges with readmissions).

Pepper syndrome Neuroblastoma of the adrenal gland with metastases in the liver.

-pepsia Denotes something relating to digestion, or the digestive tract.

peptic ulcer Lesion of the mucous membrane lining of the stomach, duodenum or of any part of the digestive tract exposed to stomach acids. *See* Ulcers. Acute peptic ulcers are often shallow and cause no scars or symptoms. Chronic peptic ulcers are often deep, cause scarring of the tissue and are persistent. Symptoms may include a gnawing pain, vomiting, loss of appetite and weight loss. Serious complications include bleeding, perforation and malignant change. Treatment may include antacids, medication that blocks the formation of stomach acid and diet changes.

per- Through.

per case payment A set rate of payment for a hospital admission, including all ancillary services excluding separately billed physician services.

per diem rate A set price for one day of hospital care, including all ancillary services, excluding separately billed physician services.

Per Member Per Month (PMPM) The amount of money paid or received on a monthly basis for each individual enrolled in a managed care plan, often referred to as capitation.

percent of premium A predetermined percentage of premium is shared between the payer and provider to pay for the costs of medical services provided to the covered population.

percentile A number that corresponds to one of the equal divisions of the range of a variable in a given sample and that characterizes a value of the variable as not exceeded by a specified percentage of all the values in the sample. .

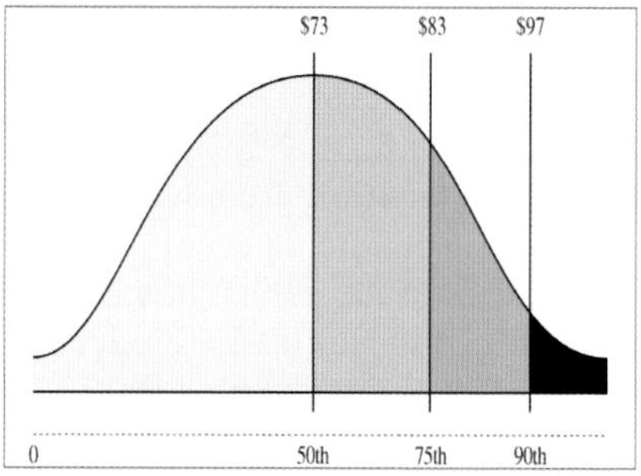

Bell curve illustrating the percentile distribution of fees for CPT code 99213

percutaneous Performed through the skin. In some procedures, a needle is passed through the skin to a space below the skin to obtain fluid or to inject a fluid, dye or medication.

percutaneous skeletal fixation Defines fracture treatment which is neither open or closed. Prior to fixation a closed reduction may be performed if necessary for alignment of the broken bones. Pins or screws are then put through the skin and bone above and below the fracture.

Pereyra procedure A type of surgical procedure to suspend the bladder neck for relief of urinary incontinence.

performance The way in which an individual, group, or organization carries out or accomplishes its important functions or processes.

performance assessment Involves the analysis and interpretation of performance measurement data to transform it into useful information for purposes of continuous performance improvement.

performance improvement projects Projects that examine and seek to achieve improvement in major areas of clinical and non-clinical services. These projects are usually based on information such as enrollee characteristics, standardized measures, utilization, diagnosis and outcome information, data from surveys, and grievance and appeals processes. They measure performance at two periods of time to ascertain if improvement has occurred. These projects are required by the state and can be of the MCO or PHPs choosing or prescribed by the state.

performance measures A gauge used to assess the performance of a process or function of any organization. Quantitative or qualitative measures of the care and services delivered to enrollees (process) or the end result of that care and services (outcomes). Performance measures can be used to assess other aspects of an individual or organization's performance such as access and availability of care, utilization of care, health plan stability, beneficiary characteristics, and other structural and operational aspects of health care services.

performance standards Standards an individual provider is expected to meet, especially with respect to quality of care. The standards may define volume of care delivered per time period.

perfusion To supply nutrients and oxygen to the organs and tissues by way of blood flow through the vessels or the process of mechanically pumping blood through the body's blood vessels.

perfusion, regional Neoplasm drug therapy involving an extracorporeal circuit with temporary exclusion of the tumor-bearing area from the general circulation during which high concentrations of the drug are perfused to the isolated part.

peri- Denoting something with a position 'surrounding' or 'around' another.

periapical The area that surrounds the root tip of a tooth.

pericardial effusion Escape of fluid. Into the pericardium.

pericardial window techniques Surgical construction of an opening or window in the pericardium. It is often called subxiphoid pericardial window technique.

pericardiectomy Surgical excision (total or partial) of a portion of the pericardium.

pericardiocentesis A procedure where fluid is aspirated from the pericardium (the sac enveloping the heart).

pericardioscopy A diagnostic procedure to visualize macroscopically alterations in both the epicardium and pericardium.

pericardiostomy Creation of an opening into the pericardium, usually for the drainage of effusions.

pericardiotomy Surgical incision of the pericardium.

pericarditis Inflammation of the sac that covers the heart. Symptoms may include chest pain that worsens with movement, rapid breathing, cough, fever and chills, weakness and anxiety. Cause may be unknown. Sometimes caused by infection or as a complication of an illness or chest injury.

pericardium Thin, membranous, double-layered covering of the heart.

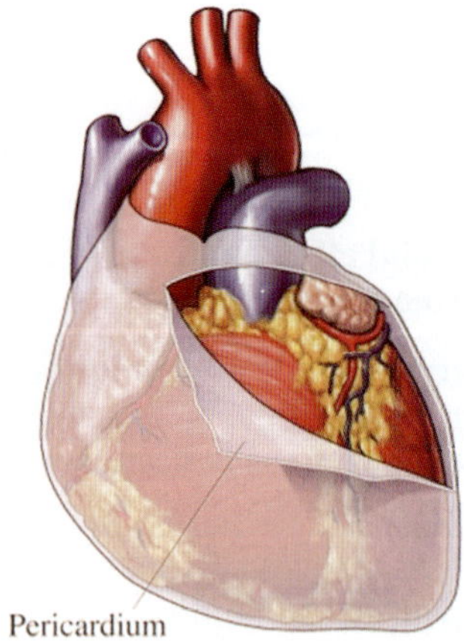

pericardium

perichondritis An infection of the skin and tissue surrounding the cartilage of the outer ear.

perineal of or referring to the perineum.

perineogram X-ray of the perineum.

perineoplasty Plastic repair on the perineum.

perineorrhaphy Suture of the perineum.

perineum The area between the vagina and the rectum.

periodontal of or relating to or involving or practicing periodontics; periodontal disease.

periodontal chart A record measuring the depth of gum pockets around the teeth.

periodontal disease Inflammation and infection of the gums, causing loss of supporting bone. Can result in tooth loss. *Synonym:* periodontitis.

periodontal pocket An abnormal deepening of the gingival crevice. It is caused when disease and infection destroy the ligament that attaches the gum to the tooth and the underlying bone.

periodontal surgery A surgical procedure involving the gums and jawbone.

periodontics A dental specialty concerned with the histology, physiology, and pathology of the tissues that support, attach, and surround the teeth, and of the treatment and prevention of disease affecting these tissues.

periodontitis Inflammation and infection of the ligaments and bones that support the teeth.

periodontosis A degenerative disease of the periodontal ligament and tooth sockets.

periods of care (hospice) A set period of time that you can get hospice care after your physician says that you are eligible and still need hospice care.

perionychia An inflammation of the folds of tissue surrounding the nail.

perioperative The period of time extending from the time of hospitalization for surgery through to the time of discharge from the hospital.

perioperative autologous transfusions The recovery, washing and reinfusion of a patient's own blood, which has been lost, during and after surgery in order to reduce the need for transfusions.

periorbital Situated around the orbit of the eye.

periosteum A fibrous membrane that covers the surface of bone except at the end of the bones where it is covered with cartilage as part of a joint. In children, periosteum is involved in forming new bone and molding the configuration of bone; and in the adult, the periosteum forms new bone secondary to injury or infection.

periostitis A medical condition caused by inflammation of the periosteum, a layer of connective tissue that surrounds bone.

peripheral On or near an edge or constituting an outer boundary.

peripheral circulation Network of arteries, veins and lymphatic channels supplying the head, arms and legs.

peripheral enthesopathies and allied syndromes Any pathological condition of the enthesis (teno-osseous junction), for example tennis elbow, and jumper's knee.

peripheral nervous system agents Drugs that act principally at one or more sites within the peripheral neuroeffector systems, the autonomic system, and motor nerve-skeletal system.

peripheral neuropathy Damage to nerves of the peripheral nervous system which may be caused either by diseases of the nerve or from the side-effects of systemic illness.

peripheral stem cell collection and processing The removal, separation and freezing of peripheral blood or marrow, which contain stem cells, for later reinfusion to restore a patient's blood manufacturing capability after radiation or chemotherapy.

peripheral vascular disease A term that includes all diseases caused by the obstruction of large arteries in the arms and legs. *Synonym:* peripheral artery disease, peripheral artery occlusive disease.

peripheral vessels *See* Peripheral circulation.

peripheral vision The ability to see objects and movement outside of the direct line of vision.

peripheral-artery disease Any abnormal condition that affects the arteries outside the heart. Signs and symptoms may include numbness, pain and paleness of the involved area(s) and hypertension. Causes include obesity, cigarette smoking, stress, inactive lifestyle, various metabolic disorders and emboli.

periradicular The area which surrounds a portion of the root of the tooth.

peritoneal of or referring to the peritoneum.

peritoneal cavity The space within the abdomen that contains the intestines, the stomach, and the liver.

peritoneal dialysis A procedure that introduces dialysate into the abdominal cavity to remove waste products through the peritoneum (a membrane which surrounds the intestines and other organs in the abdominal cavity). It functions in a manner similar to that of the artificial semi permeable membrane in the hemodialysis machine. Three forms of peritoneal dialysis are continuous ambulatory peritoneal dialysis, continuous cycling peritoneal dialysis, and intermittent peritoneal dialysis.

peritoneal lavage Washing out of the peritoneal cavity. The procedure is a diagnostic as well as a therapeutic technique following abdominal trauma or inflammation.

peritoneocentesis Paracentesis of the abdominal cavity.

peritoneogram Radiological study of the peritoneum.

peritoneoscopy Internal examination of the peritoneum with a peritoneoscope passed through an incision in the abdominal wall.

peritoneum Covering of the intestinal tract and lining of the walls of the abdominal and pelvic cavities.

peritonitis Serious infection or inflammation of part or all of the peritoneum. May be fatal if not treated promptly.

peritonsillar abscess An abscess forming in acute tonsillitis around one or both tonsils.

permanent teeth The 32 adult teeth that replace the baby or primary teeth; also known as secondary teeth.

pernicious anemia *See* Anemia, pernicious.

personal care Nonskilled, personal care, such as help with activities of daily living like bathing, dressing, eating, getting in and out of bed or chair, moving around, and using the bathroom. It may also include care that most people do themselves, like using eye drops. The Medicare home health benefit does pay for personal care services.

personal emergency response system A device, carried or worn, that can be activated in an emergency to alert a central location through the phone system. Family, friends, or emergency services are then contacted to check on the nature of the emergency.

personality disorder A class of personality types which deviate from the contemporary expectations of a society. Common types of personality disorders include paranoia, schizoid tendencies, antisocial behavior, narcissism, and obsessive-compulsive disorders. *Synonym:* (formerly) character disorders.

personality tests Standardized objective tests designed to facilitate the evaluation of personality.

pertussis A disease of the respiratory mucous membrane.

pes planus A medical condition in which the arch of the foot collapses. *Synonym:* flat foot.

pessary A small plastic or silicone medical device which is inserted into the vagina or rectum and held in place by the pelvic floor musculature. A pessary is most commonly used to treat prolapse of the uterus. It is also used to treat stress urinary incontinence, a retroverted uterus, cystocele and rectocele.

PET Positron Emission Tomography.

PET scan Advances in the fields of computerized tomography and in the production and detection of short lived radioactive isotopes has enabled the construction of scanners which monitor the course of radioactive labeled biological molecules. A variety of tracers can be administered which provide detailed images of cerebral functions such as metabolism, blood flow, and receptor distribution. The normal brain may be examined at rest as well as following activation can be observed. A variety of different pathological states have also been examined.

petechiae Tiny purple or red spots that appear on the skin as a result of very minute hemorrhages.

petit mal A form of epilepsy with very brief, unannounced lapses in consciousness. A petit mal seizure involves a brief loss of awareness, which can be accompanied by blinking or mouth twitching.

petrositis An inflammation of the temporal bone.

-pexy Fixation.

Peyronie's disease The development of abnormal scar tissue, or plaques, in tissues inside the penis.

PGH Pituitary growth hormone.

ph Symbol expressing the acidity of alkalinity of a solution on a scale of 0 to 14. Ph 7 is neutral. Above 7 is alkaline. Below 7 is acid.

phaco- Lens-shaped.

phacoemulsification A cataract surgical procedure which uses an ultrasonic vibration to shatter and break up a cataractous lens, making it easier to remove.

phacofragmentation Rupture and aspiration of the lens.

-phage, -phagia Forms terms denoting conditions relating to eating or ingestion.

-phagist Forms nouns that denote a person who 'feeds on' the first element or part of the word.

phago- Eating, devouring.

phagocytosis The process by which a cell engulfs particles such as bacteria, other microorganisms, aged red blood cells, foreign matter, etc. The principal phagocytes (cells that can engage in phagocytosis) include the neutrophils and monocytes (types of white blood cells).

-phagy Forms nouns that denotes 'feeding on' the first element or part of the word.

phalangeal of or pertaining to a phalanx.

phalangectomy Excision of one or more phalanges of the hand or foot.

phalanges The bones that form the fingers and toes.

Phalen's sign Procedure to assess for possible carpal tunnel syndrome wrists are flexed and held for one minute, if positive, there will be numbness in the fingers.

phallo- Phallus.

pharmaceutical cards Identification cards issued by a pharmacy benefit management plan to plan members. These cards assist pbms in processing and tracking pharmaceutical claims. *Synonym:* drug cards, prescription cards.

Pharmaceutical Care A strategy that attempts to utilize drug therapy more efficiently to achieve definite outcomes that improve a patient's quality of life. A pharmaceutical care system requires a reorientation of physicians, pharmacists, and nurses toward effective drug therapy outcomes. It is a set of relationships and decisions through which pharmacists, physicians, nurses, and patients work together to design, implement, and monitor a therapeutic plan that will produce specific therapeutic outcomes.

Pharmacist A health care professional who compounds and dispenses medications and other pharmaceutical supplies, using standard physical and chemical procedures to fill written prescriptions issued by physicians. Maintains records on all unit dose for each nursing unit and also IV additive program. Maintains inventory of supplies.

pharmaco- Drug, medication.

pharmacy benefit management plan A type of managed care specialty service organization that seeks to contain the costs, while promoting safer and more efficient use, of prescription drugs or pharmaceuticals. *Synonym:* prescription benefit management plan.

pharyng(o)- of or pertaining to the pharynx, the upper throat cavity.

pharyngeal of or referring to the pharynx.

pharyngectomy Surgical removal of a part of the pharynx.

pharyngitis Throat inflammation and infection that can be caused by a variety of germs (bacteria, viruses, fungi). Symptoms include sore throat, difficulty swallowing, fever, body aches and sometimes swollen glands in the neck. Treat-ment varies depending on the type of germ causing the pharyngitis. *Synonym:* sore throat.

pharyngoplasty Plastic repair of the pharynx.

pharyngorrhaphy Suture of the pharynx.

pharyngostomy External surgical fistulization of the pharynx for feeding.

pharyngotomy Incision of the pharynx.

pharynx The section of the aliment-ary canal that extends from the mouth and nasal cavities to the larynx.

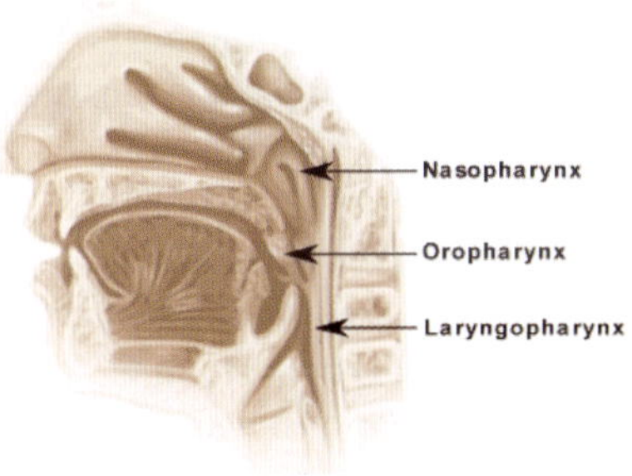

pharynx

phenylketonuria Inherited disorder marked by the inability of phenyl-alanine (an amino acid) to metab-olize appropriately. Results in an accumulation of phenyl-alanine, which is toxic to brain tissue. If left untreated, results in progressive mental retardation. Most states require a PKU screening test for all newborns. Treatment consists of a diet free of phenylalanine.

pheochromocytoma Tumor of the core (medulla) of the adrenal glands. Tumor is usually benign and does not spread to other organs. *See* Adrenal medulla tumors.

pheresis A procedure in which blood is collected, part of the blood such as platelets or white blood cells is taken out, and the rest of the blood is returned to the donor.

PHI Personal health information.

-phil(ia) Attraction for.

phleb(o)- of or pertaining to the (blood) veins, a vein.

phlebectasia Dilation of the veins.

phlebectomy A minimally invasive procedure used to remove varicose veins on the surface of the leg. This is usually done in a physician's office using local anesthesia.

phlebitis Inflammation of a vein.

phlebophlebostomy The surgical formation of an anastomosis between two veins. *Synonym:* venovenostomy.

phleborheography A procedure to measure venous volume changes in response to respiration and foot or calf compression. To perform the procedure, a plethysphygmograph with cuffs is applied to the abdomen, thigh, calf, and foot.

phleborrhaphy The surgical suturing of a vein.

phlebothrombosis Thrombosis of a vein without inflammation.

phlebotomy To puncture a vein for the purpose of withdrawing blood;

having to do with blood transfusion, diagnosis, or experiment, and treatment.

PHO Physician-hospital organization.

phob(o)- Exaggerated fear, sensitivity.

phobia An uncontrollable, irrational and persistent fear of a specific object, situation or activity.

phobic disorders Anxiety disorders in which the essential feature is persistent and irrational fear of a specific object, activity, or situation that the individual feels compelled to avoid. The individual recognizes the fear as excessive or unreasonable.

phon(o)- Sound.

phonophoresis Use of ultrasound to increase the percutaneous adsorption of drugs.

phosphorous Related to bone activity and usually follows exact opposite of calcium.

phot(o)- of or pertaining to light.

photo-aging The changes that occur to the skin due to exposure to the sun. This includes wrinkles and age spots.

photochemotherapy Therapy used to destroy cancer cells by the action of bright light and oxygen.

photocoagulation The coagulation (clotting) of tissue using a laser.

photodensitometry Measurement of the degree of darkening of X-ray film by means of a photocell which measures light transmission through the film.

photodynamic therapy A two-part treatment for esophageal cancer, gastric cancer, and lung cancer using a photosensitizing drug activated by red, non-thermal laser light.

photopheresis A form of apheresis in which blood is treated with photoactivable drugs which are then activated with ultraviolet light.

photophobia Sensitivity to light.

photoradiation Treatment of cancer by intravenous injection of a photosensitizing agent, followed by exposure to visible light by a fiberoptic probe.

photosensitizing agents Drugs that are pharmacologically inactive but when exposed to ultraviolet radiation or sunlight are converted to their active metabolite to produce a beneficial reaction affecting the diseased tissue.

phototherapy Treatment of a disease by exposure to light, especially variously concentrated light rays.

PHP Prepaid health plan.

phren(i)-, phren(o)-, phrenico Diaphragm.

phrenic nerve Motor nerve fibers that produce contractions of the diaphragm.

PHS Public health service.

physical access controls (limited access) Those formal, documented policies and procedures to be followed to limit physical access to an entity while ensuring that properly authorized access is allowed.

physical medicine The diagnosis, treatment, and prevention of disease with the aid of physical agents such as light, heat, cold, water, electricity or with mechanical devices. Physical medicine services may be provided by physicians or physical therapists.

physical safeguards Protection of physical computer systems and related buildings and equipment from fire and other natural and environmental hazards, as well as from intrusion. Also covers the use of locks, keys, and administrative measures used to control access to computer systems and facilities.

physical therapy Treatment consisting of exercising or treating specific parts of the body such as the legs, arms, hands or neck, in an effort to strengthen, regain range of motion, relearn movement and/or rehabilitate the musculoskeletal system to improve function.

Physician Assistant (PA) A medically trained professional who can provide many of the health care services traditionally performed by a physician, such as taking medical histories and doing physical examinations, making diagnoses, prescribing and administering therapies.

physician dispensing A physician gives the patient his or her initial doses of a commonly prescribed drug during an office visit. The prescription is usually refilled at the pharmacy and not the physician's office. Doctors who dispense medications usually stock 20 to 30 drugs (antibiotics, anti-inflammatories, etc.). Pharmacists see this as a reduction in their market share, whereas physicians see this as both an extra service and convenience to their patients.

physician group A partnership, association, corporation, individual practice association (IPA), or other group that distributes income from the practice among members. An IPA is considered to be a physician group only if it is composed of individual physicians and has no subcontracts with other physician groups.

Physician Hospital Organization (PHO) A separate legal entity owned by a hospital and participating physicians which can contract with health insurance companies, HMOs or self-insured employers for the provision of medical services.

physician incentive plan Any compensation arrangement at any contracting level between an MCO and a physician or physician group that may directly or indirectly have the effect of reducing or limiting services furnished to Medicare or Medicaid enrollees in the MCO. Mcos must disclose physician incentive plans between the MCO itself and individual physicians and groups and, also, between groups or intermediate entities (for example, certain IPAs or Physician-Hospital Organizations) and individual physicians and groups.

Physician Payment Review Commission (PPRC) A bipartisan congressional advisory group established in 1986 to advise Congress on setting Medicare and Medicaid reimbursement. In 1990, PPRCs responsibilities were expanded to include other payment policy issues.

physician practice management company A company, owned by a group of investors, that purchases physicians' practice assets, provides practice management services, and, in most cases, gives physicians a long-term contract to continue working in their practice and sometimes an equity (ownership) position in the company.

physician profiling In the context of a pharmacy benefit plan, the process of compiling data on physician prescribing patterns and comparing physicians' actual prescribing patterns to expected patterns within select drug categories.

physician services Services provided by an individual licensed under state law to practice medicine or osteopathy. Physician services given while in the hospital that appear on the hospital bill are not included.

physician standby services Refers to services requiring prolonged physician attendance, for example, standby for surgery, frozen section, cesarean section or monitoring, etc.

physician-hospital organization A joint venture between a hospital and many or all of its admitting physicians whose primary purpose is contract negotiations with MCOs and marketing.

physicians practice cost and income survey A survey sponsored by CMS of a national sample of physicians regarding practice characteristics, costs and reimbursement, conducted by the National Opinion Research Center in 1984 with a follow-up in 1987.

physiology The science of the functioning of living organisms, and of their component systems or parts.

pica The persistent eating of nonnutritive substances for a period of at least one month.

Pick's adenoma A neoplasm of the ovary, arising from the ovarian stroma, mimicking to a greater or lesser extent derivatives of the sex cord mesenchyme of the testis, and sometimes causing defeminization and virilization. Synonym: Androblastoma.

Pickwickian syndrome Name derived from the overweight boy in Charles Dickens' Pickwick Papers; obesity, somnolence and hypoxia with carbon dioxide retention.

PICU Pediatric intensive care unit.

PID Pelvic inflammatory disease.

PIFR Peak inspiratory flow rate.

pilonidal cyst A special kind of abscess that occurs in the cleft between the buttocks. Forms frequently in adolescence after long trips that involve sitting.

PIN Provider identification number.

pinguecula A a common, non-cancerous growth of the mucus membrane lining the eyeball and underside of the eyelids (conjunctiva).

pinta A human skin disease endemic to Mexico, Central America, and South America caused by infection with a spirochete, treponema pallidum carateum, which is morphologically and serologically indistinguishable from the organism that causes syphilis.

pit A recessed area found on the surface of a tooth, usually where the grooves of the tooth meet.

pituitary diabetes insipidus Metabolic disorder due to injury of the pituitary gland causing a deficient production of anti-diuretic hormone. Patients have great thirst and pass copious amounts of urine.

pituitary gland The master gland of the endocrine system; located at the base of the brain.

pituitectomy Total excision of the pituitary gland.

pityriasis Any of several skin disorders characterized by shedding dry flakes of skin.

PKD Polycystic kidney disease.

PKU Phenylketonuria.

place of service Where a service was performed, for example, inpatient hospital, outpatient hospital, physician's office, etc.

placement To position or implant an object such as a catheter or stent.

placenta The organ that connects the developing fetus to the uterine wall. The placenta supplies the fetus with oxygen and food, and allows fetal waste to be disposed of via the maternal kidneys.

placenta previa Bleeding late in pregnancy caused by placenta attaching too low in the uterus, covering the cervix completely or partially. (The cervix contains the opening into the birth canal). This can be life-threatening to the unborn child and to the mother. The most common sign is sudden, painless bleeding, usually in the last trimester. With prompt care, mothers and most infants survive without complications. In some cases, delivery is necessary before the fetus is mature enough to survive.

placental function tests Methods used for the assessment of placental function.

placental sulfatase deficiency Deficiency of sulfatase in the placenta.

plagiocephaly A condition characterized by an asymmetrical distortion (flattening of one side) of the skull.

plague A deadly infectious disease caused by the enterobacteria yersinia pestis (pasteurella pestis).

plan administration Supervising the details and routine activities of installing and running a health plan, such as answering questions, enrolling individuals, billing and collecting premiums, and similar duties.

plan funding The method that an employer or other payer or purchaser uses to pay medical benefit costs and administrative expenses.

planned change Change that is deliberate, controlled, collaborative, and proactive.

plantar fasciitis Inflammation of the band of tissue that runs from the heel along the arch of the foot.

plantar reflex Dorsiflexion of the big toe on stimulation of the plantar surface (sole), occurring in lesions of the pyramidal tract (nerve fibers arising in the brain and passing down through the spinal cord). *Synonym:* Babinski's toe sign.

plantar flexion Flexion of the entire foot inferiorly, as if pressing an automobile pedal. Occurs at ankle.

plaque 1) Deposits of fat, cholesterol, calcium and other cellular sludge from one's blood. 2) A film of sticky material containing saliva, food particles and bacteria that attaches to the tooth surface, both above and below the gum line. When left on the tooth, it can promote gum disease and tooth decay.

-plasia Formation, development.

plasma The non-cellular liquid component of un-clotted whole blood. Plasma is the liquid medium in which the formed elements of blood are suspended and comprises the major portion of whole blood. Plasma is used to treat clotting disorders, burn victims and shock.

plasma purpura *See* Purpura.

plasmapheresis blood is withdrawn from a vein in the arm and passed through a cell separator to remove cells from the plasma. The blood cells are then transfused back into the individual. TPE is used to treat immune disorders. *Synonym:* therapeutic plasma exchange.

plasmin Active portion of the chemical system that causes blood clots to dissolve.

plasminogen A substance naturally produced by the body that helps break down blood clots.

plasminogen-activator system System that stimulates the conversion of chemical substances to plasmin. *See* Plasmin.

plastic surgery The specialty of improving the appearance for cosmetic reasons, or to correct defects for a more appealing appearance.

-plasty Surgical repair, reconstruction.

platelet A type of blood cell that helps prevent bleeding by causing blood clots to form.

platelet transfusion refractoriness The inability of platelet transfusions to adequately increase the platelet count.

plateletpheresis An apheresis procedure where platelets are collected.

platelets Cytoplasmic fragments of megakaryocytes (bone marrow cells). Platelets contain cytoplasmic granules; however, they lack nuclei and are part of the formed elements of blood. They are colorless cells whose main function is to control bleeding. Platelets are essential to normal blood clotting. They can be destroyed during treatment for cancer, leukemia, aplastic anemia and other diseases.

play or pay mandate Employers are required to provide at least a minimum standard benefits package for their employees or pay a payroll tax. Employees in firms that choose to pay the tax will be "pooled" together for the purchase of health insurance either into a single public program like Medicare or a program in which enrollees choose from competing private health plans. Payroll tax revenues, individual premiums (with subsidies provided for low-income persons) and other general tax revenues would finance the health benefit costs.

-plegia Paralysis.

pleoptic training The use of eye exercises for eye movement and fixation training.

plethysmography Recording of change in the size of a part as modified by the circulation in it.

pleur(o)-, pleur(a) of or pertaining to the ribs.

pleura Thin tissue lining of the lungs and chest cavity.

pleural of or relating to the pleura or the walls of the thorax.

pleural cavity The body cavity that surrounds the lungs.

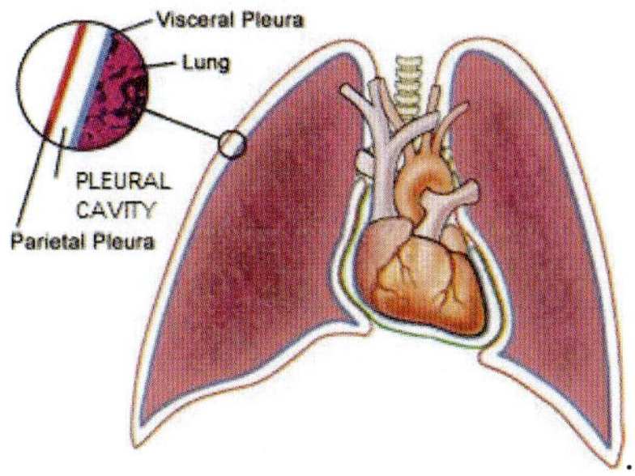

pleural cavity

pleurectomy Surgical procedure to remove the parietal pleura, the outermost lining around the lungs. This procedure is performed for a variety of disorders including pleural effusion, malignant pleural mesothelioma, and trauma.

pleurisy An inflammation of the membrane that surrounds and protects the lungs (the pleura). Inflammation occurs when an infection or damaging agent irritates the pleural surface.

pleuritis An inflammation of the pleura.

pleurocentesis *See* thoracentesis. *Synonym:* thoracentesis.

pleurodesis The adherence of the outer surface of a lung to the membrane surrounding that lung, which is performed to treat the buildup of fluid around the lung.

pleurosclerosis Intentional scarring of the lungs with a sclerosing agent (a type of drug that induces scarring).

plexectomy Surgical excision of a plexus.

PMB Postmenopausal bleeding.

PMS Postmenopausal syndrome.

PMT Premenstrual tension.

pneum(o)- of or pertaining to the lungs.

pneumat(o)- Air, lung.

pneumatosis cystoides intestinalis Disease characterized by the presence of air or gas in abnormal pockets in the intestinal tract. Usually associated with an infection.

pneumocentesis A procedure in which a lung is punctured to drain fluid contents.

pneumococcus Bacterium causing pneumonia.

pneumoconiosis Fibrosis and scarring of the lungs as a result of repeated inhalation of occupationally associated dust, such as silica, asbestos, and coal dust.

pneumocystosis An infection of the lungs caused by the microorganism Pneumocystis carinii.

pneumogram A radiograph of an organ inflated with air.

pneumohemothorax The presence of air or gas and blood in the lung cavity.

pneumolysis Surgical separation of the lung and costal pleura from the endothoracic fascia; formerly used in collapse therapy for tuberculosis.

pneumomediastinum Deliberate introduction of air or gas into the mediastinum as an aid to examination and diagnosis.

pneumonectomy The surgical removal of a lung.

pneumonia Inflammation of the lung(s) resulting in tiny air sacs in the lung becoming plugged with exudate. Can be caused by bacteria, viruses or fungi.

pneumonitis Inflammation of lung tissue that may be caused by a virus or it may be an allergic response to chemicals, dust or mold. A dry cough is a common sign. Treatment depends on the cause, but often includes the administration of corticosteroids to reduce inflammation.

pneumonology The branch of medicine that deals with diseases of the respiratory system.

pneumonolysis The separation of an adherent lung from the pleura, to permit collapse of the lung.

pneumonopathy Any disease or disorder involving the lungs.

pneumonostomy Surgical formation of an artificial opening (as for drainage of an abscess) into a lung.

pneumonotomy Incision of the lung.

pneumoperitoneum Deliberate introduction of air into the peritoneal cavity.

pneumoplethysmography A test used to measure the functional residual capacity (FRC) of the lungs and total lung capacity.

pneumothorax Collapse of all or part of a lung caused by pressure from free air in the chest between the two layers of the pleura. *See* Pleura.

pod-, -pod-, -pus of or pertaining to the foot, -footed.

podiatry The specialty of treating problems of the feet with surgery.

-poiesis Production.

point of purchase plan A benefit plan that expands enrollee options to choose providers. It usually consists of two or more delivery and financing options including an alternative delivery system, such as an HMO or PPO, and another plan such as traditional fee-for-service coverage. The participant is not locked-in but may change coverage options each time care is obtained. The scope of benefits and payment provisions are structured to provide incentives for greater use of the alternative delivery system option.

point-of-service plan A managed care plan that combines features of both prepaid and fee-for-service health insurance. Health plan enrollees decide whether to use network or non-network providers at the time care is needed and usually are charged sizable copayments for selecting the latter.

policy The insurance agreement or contract.

policy holder Under a group plan, the group is the policyholder; under an individual plan, the individual is the policyholder. The policyholder is the one who has the contract or agreement with the insurer.

policy year The twelve month period beginning with the effective date or renewal date of the policy.

policy or guidelines on work station use Documented instructions and procedures delineating the proper functions to be performed at an employees workstation, the manner in which those functions are to be performed, and the physical attributes of the surroundings, of a specific computer terminal site or type of site, dependant upon the sensitivity of the information accessed from that site.

polio A contagious viral illness that in its most severe form causes paralysis, difficulty breathing and sometimes death.

polio- Denoting a grey color.

poliomyelitis A highly infectious viral disease that may attack the central nervous system and is characterized by symptoms that range from a mild nonparalytic infection to total paralysis in a matter of hours. *Synonym:* polio, infantile paralysis.

poliovirus The virus causing poliomyelitis.

poly- Denotes a 'plurality' of something.

polyarteritis Inflammation of several arteries.

polyarteritis nodosa A progressive disease of connective tissue that is characterized by nodules along arteries; nodules may block the artery and result in inadequate circulation to the particular area.

polyarthropathy Inflammation of several joints simultaneously.

polycystic Containing many cysts.

polycystic ovaries Ovary enlargement from many small cysts. Ovary surface becomes too thick to allow ovulation. Women with this problem cannot become pregnant without treatment. *Synonym:* Stein-Leventhal syndrome.

polycystic ovary syndrome An endocrine disorder with principle features of obesity, anovulation and excessive amounts of androgenic hormones. *Synonym:* functional ovarian hyperandrogenism.

polycythemia Increase in red blood cells in the body. The disease has three forms. Polycythemia vera involves overproduction of red blood cells, white blood cells and platelets. Secondary polycythemia is a complication of diseases or factors other than blood cell disorders. Stress polycythemia involves decreased blood plasma.

polycythemia vera Overproduction of red blood cells, white blood cells and platelets. Cause is unknown. Treatment may include withdrawing blood at certain intervals, radio-isotope therapy and drug therapy. Treatment is needed to prevent blood clots from forming that could cause a stroke, heart attack or blockage in a vein or artery.

polydactyly Birth defect characterized by the presence of more than the normal number of fingers or toes.

polydipsia Excessive thirst (as in cases of diabetes or kidney dysfunction).

polyglandular dysfunction and related disorders Dysfunctional disorders involving multiple glands.

polyhydramnios A condition that exists when there is too much amniotic fluid in the uterus.

polymyalgia rheumatica A rheumatic disorder that is associated with moderate to severe muscle pain and stiffness in the neck, shoulder and hip areas.

polymyositis Inflammation of many muscles at one time. Usually accompanied by muscle weakness, deformity, swelling, pain, sweating and tension. Sometimes associated with malignant conditions.

polyneuritis Inflammation of many nerves simultaneously. In acute infectious polyneuritis (Guillain-Barre syndrome), inflammation of nerves and muscles progresses, rapidly causing weakness, loss of sensation and sometimes paralysis for weeks or months. Cause is unknown, but it sometimes follows an infection, immunization or minor surgery. May be an autoimmune disorder.

polyneuropathy Disease of multiple nerves.

polyp An abnormal growth of tissue projecting from a mucous membrane.

polypectomy Surgical removal of a polyp.

polyposis Formation of numerous polyps. Familial polyposis is an inherited condition in which the intestinal lining contains many polyps, some of which are highly likely to become malignant.

polyps Growths. Often on a stalk arising from dry mucous membranes, such as in the nose, cervix or colon.

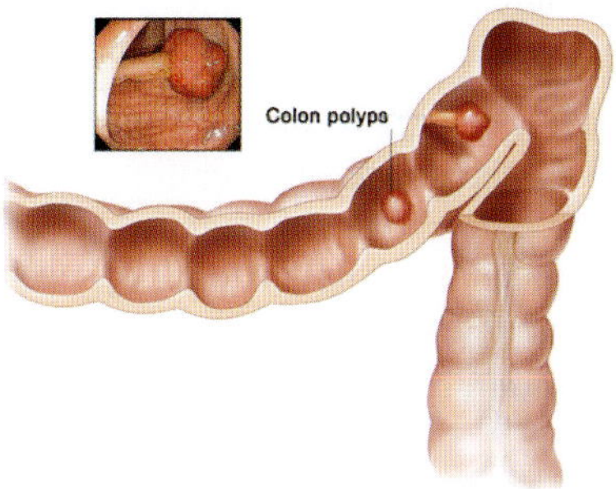

polyps

polysomnography A multi-parametric test used in the study of sleep and as a diagnostic tool in sleep medicine. *Synonym:* sleep study.

polytomography Body section radiography using a machine designed to effect complex motion; images a thinner tissue plane compared to simple linear or circular tomography.

polyuria Renal disorder characterized by the production of large volumes of pale dilute urine; often associated with diabetes.

Pomeroy's operation Excision of a ligated portion of the fallopian tubes.

POMR Problem-oriented medical record.

pontic An artificial tooth used in a bridge to replace a missing tooth.

pooling The mixing together, in a vat, of the blood plasma that has been separated from the whole blood donated by thousands to tens of thousands of blood donors for purposes of facilitating further treatment and ease of management of resources.

popliteal Refers to anatomical structures located in the back of the knee.

porcelain crown An all porcelain restoration covering the coronal portion of tooth (above the gum line).

Porcelain Fused to Metal (PFM) crown A restoration containing metal coping for strength covered by porcelain for appearance.

porcelain inlay/onlay A tooth-colored restoration made of porcelain and cemented or bonded in place.

porcelain veneers A thin layer of porcelain, fabricated by a laboratory and bonded to a natural tooth to replace lost tooth structure, close spaces, straighten teeth, or change color and/or shape.

por(o)- Pore, porous.

porphyr(o)- Denotes a purple color.

porphyria Excretion of porphyrins into the urine. *See* Porphyrins.

porphyria, cutanea tarda Type of porphyria usually associated with chronic alcoholism marked by skin lesions and enlarged liver. *See* Porphyria, acute intermittent.

porphyria, acute intermittent Rare inherited disorder characterized by excessive formation and excretion of porphyrins. Symptoms include recurrent abdominal pain often accompanied by nausea, vomiting, constipation and dark urine.

porphyrins Any of a group of pyrrole derivatives found in cytoplasm. These combine with iron and magnesium to form other substances.

portability The ability for an individual to transfer from one health insurer to another health insurer with regard to pre-existing conditions or other risk factors.

portacaval shunt Connection of the portal vein with the vena cava to release backed-up pressure in the veins that drain the intestinal tract.

portal hypertension Higher than normal blood pressure in the large vein that collects nourishment from intestinal absorption then drains into the liver.

portal vein thrombosis A form of venous thrombus is affecting the hepatic portal vein, which can lead to portal hypertension and reduction in the blood supply to the liver.

portoenterostomy Operation for biliary atresia by anastomosis of the bile ducts into the jejunum or duodenum.

portography A radiography of the portal vein after injection of radiopaque contrast material.

port-wine stain A type of hemangioma characterized by a mark on the skin that resembles the rich red color of port wine. Port-wine stains are caused by an abnormal concentration of capillaries. *Synonym:* nevus flammeus.

Posadas-Wernicke disease A systemic mycosis caused by of dust particles containing arthroconidia of Coccidioides immitis.

positron emission tomography A specialized imaging technique that uses radioactive substances to produce three-dimensional colored images of those substances functioning within the body. *Synonym:* PET scan.

post- Denotes something as 'after' or 'behind' another.

post and core Post and build-up to replace lost tooth structure and retain crown.

postcoital test Determination of the number and condition of spermatozoa in mucus aspirated from the cervical canal soon after intercourse.

post-core A post and buildup to replace lost tooth structure and retain crowns.

post-crown A single structure that combines post-core and crown.

posterior Located behind a structure, such as relating to the back side of the human body. *Synonym:* dorsal.

posterior chamber The space between the back of the iris and the front face of the vitreous; filled with aqueous fluid.

posterior optical segment The part of the eye behind to the crystalline lens, including the vitreous, choroid, retina, and optic nerve.

posterior vitreous detachment The separation of the vitreous body from the retinal surface due to shrinkage from degenerative or inflammatory conditions or trauma. Often an age-related condition.

posterolateral thoracotomy An incision through that extends from the back to the side of the chest, usually between the 5th to 7th rib space. This is the surgical route usually chosen for access to the lung, esophagus or descending aorta.

postnatal Occurring immediately after birth.

post-op Postoperative.

postoperative The period of time after a surgical operation.

postoperative management only Refers to a situation where postoperative management is performed by a different physician than the one performing the surgery. This reported by adding CPT modifier -55 to the procedure code.

postpartum care Encompasses management of the mother, newborn, and infant during the postpartum period. This period usually is considered to be the first few days after delivery, but technically it includes the six-week period after childbirth up to the mother's postpartum checkup.

postpartum hemorrhage Bleeding after delivery.

post payment review The review of a claim after a determination and payment has been made to the provider or beneficiary.

post-phlebitic or post-thrombotic syndrome Long-term, recurring leg symptoms that affect some patients as a result of permanent injury to veins and their valves from DVT.

post-streptococcal glomerulonephritis Inflammatory disease of kidney occurring about 3 weeks following a strep infection elsewhere in the body. Probably related to an effect on body's immune system.

post-traumatic stress disorder A debilitating condition that is related to a past terrifying physical or emotional experience causing the person who survived the event to have persistent, frightening thoughts and memories or flashbacks, of the ordeal. People with PTSD often feel chronically emotionally numb.

posterior Located behind a structure, such as relating to the back side of the human body.

posturography A general term that covers all the techniques used to quantify postural control in upright stance in either static or dynamic conditions.

potassium A body salt or electrolyte found mostly inside of cells. Water pills may lower potassium and increase kidney damage.

potassium channel blockers A class of drugs that act by inhibition of potassium efflux through cell membranes. Blockade of potassium channels prolongs the duration of action potentials. They are used as anti-arrhythmia agents and vasodilator agents.

potassium, serum Potassium is another blood electrolyte and is involved with the functioning of nervous tissue and in heart and muscle contraction. Abnormal levels may indicate diseases of the gastrointestinal tract, kidney and adrenal gland.

potential payments The maximum anticipated total payments (based on the most recent year's utilization and experience and any current or anticipated factors that may affect payment amounts) that could be received if use or costs of referral services were low enough. These payments include amounts paid for services furnished or referred by the physician or group, plus amounts paid for administrative costs. The only payments not included in potential payments are bonuses or other compensation not based on referrals (for example, bonuses based on patient satisfaction or other quality of care factors).

Pott's disease Rare, grave form of tuberculosis that is located in the spinal column. Segments of the spine may actually collapse. Symptoms include stiffness and painfulness of the spine. Abscesses may form and put pressure on the spinal cord, resulting in areas of paralysis. *Synonym:* tuberculous spondylitis.

Pott's fracture Fracture of the lower fibula and injury of the lower tibial articulation, producing outward displacement of the foot.

Potts-Smith procedure Descending aorta-left pulmonary artery anastomosis.

power of attorney A medical power of attorney is a document that lets you appoint someone you trust to make decisions about your medical care. This type of advance directive also may be called a health care proxy, appointment of health care agent or a durable power of attorney for health care.

poxvirus infections A group of viruses that produce spreading vesicular lesions, including smallpox, vaccinia, and molluscum contagiosum.

PPA Preferred provider arrangement.

PPB Positive-pressure breathing.

PPD Purified protein derivative (tuberculin).

PPO Preferred provider organization.

PPRC Physician payment review commission.

PPS Prospective payment system.

PPT Partial prothrombin time.

practice expense The cost of non-physician resources incurred by the physician to provide services. Examples include salaries and benefits for employees, the expenses associated with the purchase and use of medical equipment and supplies.

practice guidelines A statement of what is known about the benefits, risks and costs of particular courses of medical treatment to achieve the best possible patient outcome.

practice parameters Strategies for patient management developed to assist physicians in clinical decision-making. Parameters improve quality and assure appropriate utilization of health services.

PRC Peer review committee.

pre- Denotes something as 'before' another (in [physical] position or time).

pre-admission certification Review and approval process completed before hospital admission to ensure the medical necessity for the acute level of care and for the proposed services and procedures, to avoid a weekend admission, and to forecast the expected length of stay. The review process may include an assessment of the physician's proposed treatment protocol and fees. Compliance with changes in the treatment plan recommended by the reviewing entity may be a condition of receiving full coverage under the health benefit. The benefit level may be reduced or services not covered at all if the patient fails to comply with plan requirements. The pre-admission review process may also include an administrative confirmation of the patient's eligibility for benefits, covered services and restrictions, and the determination of applicable deductibles, co-payments, and maximums.

pre-admission notification Similar to pre-admission certification, a condition of receiving full benefits. Failure to notify the reviewing agency within the time limitations may result in a reduced level or denial of benefits. Differs from certification programs since the counseling offered by the notification agency is not binding upon the patient.

pre-admission review A review of an individual's health care status or condition, prior to an individual being admitted to a hospital or inpatient health care facility. Pre-admission reviews are often conducted by case managers or insurance company representatives (usually nurses) in cooperation with the individual, his or her physician or health care provider, and hospitals.

preadmission testing Medical tests that are completed for an individual prior to being admitted to a hospital or inpatient health care facility.

pre-authorization Similar to pre-admission certificate, a condition of receiving health benefits. Review and approval process that must be completed before services are provided, when an inpatient or ambulatory site is proposed for care. The review process may include an assessment of the physician's proposed protocol and fees. Compliance with changes in the proposed treatment plan recommended by reviewing entity may be a condition of receiving full coverage under the health benefit.

precertification The process of obtaining permission to perform a service from the health insurance carrier before the service is performed. *Synonym:* pre-authorization.

precipitin test Any serologic test based on a precipitin reaction.

predetermination A procedure where a provider submits a treatment plan to the health insurer before treatment begins. The insurer reviews the treatment plan and notifies the provider of one or more of the following patient's eligibility, covered services, amounts payable, co-payment and deductibles and plan maximums.

pre-eclampsia Serious disturbance in blood pressure, kidney function and the central nervous system that may occur from the 20th week of pregnancy until 7 days after delivery. Not accompanied by seizures. *Synonym:* toxemia of pregnancy.

pre-existing conditions When a physical or mental condition of a newly insured individual is present prior to the insurance of the new insurance policy. Normally, these exclusions last from 6 to 12 months, however, more severe conditions may be considered as lifetime exclusions.

pre-existing condition exclusion Practices of some health insurers to deny coverage to individuals for a certain period, for health conditions that already exist when coverage is initiated.

Preferred Provider Organization (PPO) A managed care health plan that contracts with networks or panels of providers to furnish services and be paid on a negotiated fee schedule. Enrollees are offered a financial incentive to use providers on the preferred list, but may use non-network providers as well.

preferred providers Physicians, hospitals, and other health care providers who contract to provide health services to persons covered by a particular health plan.

pregnancy care Federal maternity legislation, enacted in 1978, requires that employers engaged in interstate commerce who have 15 or more employees provide the same benefits for pregnancy, childbirth, and related medical conditions as for any other sickness or injury.

pregnancy-induced hypertension A rise in blood pressure, without proteinuria, during the second half of pregnancy. *Synonym:* pre-eclampsia.

preimplantation diagnosis Determination of the nature of a pathological condition or disease in the ovum, zygote, or blastocyst prior to implantation. Cytogenetic analysis is performed to determine the presence or absence of genetic disease.

premature atrial contractions The normal heart rhythm is set by the sinoatrial node, an area of specialized tissue in the atrium. Occasionally an early or premature beat or contraction originates from the atrium.

premium Prospectively determined rate for insurance coverage for specific health benefits. Generally, a health insurance plan will have different premium rates for single subscribers, married subscribers and for subscribers with dependants.

premium, community-rated Premiums based upon the claims experience of all those insured by the carrier and not dependent upon the claims experience of each policyholder. *See* community rating.

premium, cost sharing The sharing of the cost of the health plan premium between the employer or other group sponsors and the enrollees.

premium, experience-rated Premium based on the projected utilization and claims experience of a specific group. *See* experience rating.

prenatal Occurring or existing before birth.

prenatal care Services to pregnant women designed to insure that both expectant mother and the newborn are in the best health. A lack of prenatal care early in the pregnancy is associated with low birth weight and infant mortality.

prenatal diagnosis Determination of the nature of a pathological condition or disease in the postimplantation embryo, fetus, or pregnant female before birth.

pre-op Preoperative.

preoperative The period of time before surgery.

preoperative management only Refers to a situation where one physician provides preoperative care and another physician performs the surgery. Reported by adding CPT modifier -56 to the procedure code.

prep Preparation, prepare.

prepaid care Health care services provided to an HMO member in exchange for a fixed, monthly premium paid in advance of the delivery of medical care.

Prepaid Health Plan (PHP) In Medicaid terminology, a PHP is not the same as an HMO even though the terms are often used inter-changeably in commercial managed care business. PHPs can contract on a capitated basis for a non-comprehensive set of services (which is often called partial capitation) or on a cost basis. Federally qualified health centers (FQHCs) can also be designated as PHPs if they meet certain conditions.

prepayment review The review of claims prior to determination and payment.

prepuce A retractable piece of skin which covers part of the genitals. On a male, it covers the head of the penis. On a female, it surrounds and protects the head of the clitoris. *Synonym:* foreskin.

presby(o)- Old age.

presbycusis The loss of hearing that gradually occurs in most individuals as they grow older.

presbyopia A condition in which the lens of the eye loses its ability to focus, making it difficult to see objects up close.

prescription benefit management plan Pharmacy benefit management plan.

prescription cards *See* pharmaceutical cards.

prescription drug plan Medicare prescription drug plan benefit, will provide insurance coverage for prescription drugs. Like other insurance, if you enroll you will pay a monthly premium.

presenting problem A disease, condition, illness, injury, symptom, sign, finding, complaint, or other reason for the encounter, with or without a diagnosis being made at the time of the encounter.

pre-service review Pre-service review programs examine the medical necessity and appropriateness of proposed services to be provided in the ambulatory or inpatient setting that may require frequent treatment, extended courses of treatment, or require the use of expensive technologies. Dental and vision benefits may require predetermination for certain services or charges.

prevailing charge One of the factors determining a physician's payment for service under Medicare. Currently set at the 75th percentile of customary charges for all physicians in a locality.

prevalence The number of existing cases of a disease or condition in a given population at a specific time.

preventive care An approach to health care which emphasizes preventive measures and health screenings such as routine physicals, well-baby care, immunizations, diagnostic lab and x-ray tests, pap smears, mammograms and other early detection testing. The purpose of offering coverage for preventive care is to diagnose a problem early, when it is less costly to treat, rather than late in the stage of a disease when it is much more expensive, or too late to treat.

preventive dentistry The branch of dentistry concerned with the prevention of disease and the maintenance and promotion of oral health.

preventive medicine services Refers to the routine evaluation and management of adults and children in the absence of patient complaints or counseling and/or risk factor reduction intervention services to healthy individuals.

priapism Condition in which the penis is continually erect; usually painful and seldom with sexual arousal.

PRICER Software modules in Medicare claims processing systems, specific to certain benefits, used in pricing claims, most often under prospective payment systems.

pricing The process of deciding the premium to charge for a health plan or a given set of benefits.

prim- Denotes something as 'first' or 'most-important'.

primary biliary cirrhosis Disease of the liver caused from chronic bile retention. Cause is unknown. *See* Cirrhosis.

primary care General medical care that is provided directly to a patient without referral from another physician. It is focused on preventative care and the treatment of routine injuries and illnesses.

primary care case management A program where the state contracts directly with primary care providers who agree to be responsible for the provision and/or coordination of medical services to Medicaid recipients under their care. Currently, most PCCM programs pay the primary care physician a monthly case management fee in addition to reimbursing services on a fee-for-service basis.

primary care case management provider A provider (usually a physician, physician group practice, or an entity employing or having other arrangements with such physicians, but sometimes also including nurse practitioners, nurse midwives, or physician assistants) who contracts to locate, coordinate, and monitor covered primary care (and sometimes additional services).

Primary Care Network (PCN) A plan similar to an HMO which provides health services for a fixed price, relying on participating primary care physicians to serve as "gatekeepers" to control patient access to institutional services and specialty care. The primary care physician determines the patient's need for specialty care and any resulting referrals.

primary care physician Under a health maintenance organization (HMO) plan, the primary care physician is usually an insured person's first contact for health care. This is often a family physician, internist, or pediatrician. A primary care physician monitors patient health, treats most patient health problems, and refers patients, if necessary, to specialists.

primary care provider A physician or other medical professional who serves as a group member's first contact with a plan's health care system. Also known as a primary care physician, personal care physician, or personal care provider. *Synonym:* primary care physician, personal care physician, person care provider.

primary carrier The health insurance carrier which has first responsibility under Coordination of Benefits.

primary code The ICD-9-CM code that defines the main reason for the current encounter.

primary coverage That coverage which pays first when an individual is covered under two or more insurance plans.

primary hypothyroidism Overabundance of aldosterone, a hormone produced and secreted by the adrenal gland.

primary lymphedema Chronic swelling of a part due to the accumulation of fluid (lymph) caused by obstruction of lymph vessels. Primary lymphedema may be congenital or caused by abnormal increase in number of cells of lymph vessels.

primary payer An insurance policy, plan, or program that pays first on a claim for medical care. This could be Medicare or other health insurance.

primary source verification A process through which an organization validates credentialing information from the organization that originally conferred or issued the credentialing element to the practitioner.

primary teeth The first set of teeth that humans get, lasting until the permanent teeth come in; also referred to as deciduous teeth or baby teeth.

prinzmetal angina Angina pectoris in which attacks occur during rest and for longer duration, accompanied by an ST segment elevation.

principal diagnosis The principal diagnosis is defined in the Uniform Hospital Discharge Data Set (UHDDS) as that condition established after study to be chiefly responsible for occasioning the admission of the patient to the hospital for care.

prion A protein molecule that lacks nucleic acid, that is, no DNA or RNA, often considered to be the cause of various infectious diseases of the nervous system (such as Creutzfeldt-Jakob disease and scrapie.) Very resilient, not easy to kill.

prior approval An authorization for the delivery of services that must be obtained prior to the delivery of those services. Commonly used in the Medicaid program and managed care plans.

prior authorization Review of need for health care items or services before services are rendered or products are provided. This refers to a decision made by the health plan to cover or not cover the charges before the services are provided.

prison-correctional facility A prison, jail, reformatory, work farm, detention center, or any other similar facility maintained by either federal, state or local authorities for the purpose of confinement or rehabilitation of adult or juvenile criminal offenders.

private fee-for-service plan A type of Medicare Advantage Plan in which a patient may go to any Medicare-approved physician or hospital that accepts the plan's payment. The insurance plan, rather than the Medicare program, decides how much it will pay and what the patient pays for the services provided.

private review Review of patient care episodes to ensure the medical necessity and appropriateness of services and charges, usually for services financed through institutional purchaser health benefit programs. Private review services are offered by many entities, including insurance companies and their subsidiary companies specializing in managed care services, hospitals, and foundations for medical care. Peer review organizations (PRO), Federally authorized agencies, sell review services to private sector purchasers of health care. There are currently no licensure or certification standards for private review programs.

Private review is usually implemented through a contractual relationship between the purchaser and the reviewing entity; it may also be financed on a fee per review, an annual fee based upon the number of covered individuals, or percentage of the annual premium or expenditure, or some combination, and may include a performance incentive bonus relating the costs of conducting the review services, the projected health plan expenditures, and actual savings.

prn As needed.

PRO Peer review organization.

pro time Prothrombin time.

procedure code A CPT or HCPCS code used by a physician or provider of services to describe the procedure or service rendered to the patient.

procedure for emergency access Documented instructions for obtaining necessary information during a crisis.

procedures for verifying access authorizations prior to physical access Formal, documented policies and instructions for validating the access privileges of an entity prior to granting those privileges.

process audit A type of patient/medical care evaluation study in which the criteria are designed to focus on the components of appropriate clinical intervention.

procidentia A sinking or prolapse of an organ or part, for example rectal procidentia and uterine procidentia.

proct(o)- Anus, rectum.

proctectasis Dilation of the anus or rectum.

proctectomy Surgical resection of the rectum. *Synonym:* rectectomy.

proctitis Inflammation of the rectum and tissues around the anus. Can be caused by sexually transmitted infections, other infections, cancer of the rectum, food allergies or chronic constipation. Usually curable with appropriate treatment specific to the cause.

proctocele Prolapse of the rectum. *Synonym:* rectocele.

proctopexy Surgical fixation of a prolapsed rectum.

proctoplasty Reconstructive surgery of the anus or rectum.

proctorrhaphy Repair by suture of a lacerated rectum or anus.

proctosigmoidoscopy Examination of the lower colon using a sigmoid-oscope, inserted into the rectum.

proctotomy Incision into the rectum. *Synonym:* rectotomy.

professional component The part of the relative value or fee for a procedure that represents physician work. Reported by adding CPT modifier -26 to the main procedure code.

professional liability insurance The health insurance physicians must purchase to help protect themselves from the financial risks associated with malpractice claims and awards.

Professional Review Organization (PRO) An organization that reviews the activities and records of a health care provider, institution, or group. The reviewer is generally a physician if a physician is the subject of the review; a group of administrators, physicians, and allied health care personnel if a hospital is the subject of the review; etc. The PRO can be state-sponsored or independent.

profile Most hospital and commercial laboratories offer blood tests collected together in packages (sometimes called profiles). The number of tests in each package and the cost varies between laboratories. On your bill, a sum is usually quoted for the entire package of tests, without breaking out the charge for each test. In the lab report, the result and name of each test are clearly marked. Some common profiles include coronary risk profile, electrolyte package, hepatitis profile, liver profile, thyroid profile and chemical profile.

profiles Data segregated by specific time period (quarterly, annually) and target area (facility, state) for the purpose of identifying patterns.

profiling Expressing a pattern of practice as a rate (costs or services) or outcome (morbidity, mortality) collected over time for a defined population of patients to compare with other practice patterns.

progesterone A hormone produced by the ovaries and adrenal glands; essential for healthy functioning of the female reproductive system.

prognosis A prediction of the probable outcome of a disease based on a individual's condition and the usual course of the disease as seen in similar situations.

program management and medical information system An automated system of records that contains records primarily of current Medicare-eligible ESRD patients, but also maintains historical information on people no longer classified as ESRD patients because of death or successful transplantation or recovery of renal function. The PMMIS contains medical information on patients and the services that they received during the course of their therapy. In addition, it contains information on ESRD facilities and facility payment.

program of all-inclusive care for the elderly A combination Medicare Waiver or Medicaid Waiver that provides day health center-based comprehensive community and medical services. PACE capitates primary, acute and long term care services exclusively for frail dual eligibles at risk of institutionalization.

projective test Any of various tests in which an individual interprets ambiguous stimulus situations according to their own unconscious dispositions, yielding information about their personality and possible psychopathology.

prolonged activated partial thromboplastin time Longer-than-normal time required for clotting to take place in the activated thromboplastin time test.

prolonged services When a physician provides service involving direct (face-to-face) patient contact that is beyond the usual service in either the inpatient or outpatient setting.

PROM Passive range of motion.

pronation A rotation of the forearm that moves the palm from an anterior-facing position to a posterior-facing position, or palm facing down. This is not medial rotation as this must be performed when the arm is half flexed.

proof of eligibility Evidence of eligibility for health insurance benefits.

ProPAC Prospective payment assessment committee.

proprietary hospital An investor-owned hospital operated for the purpose of making a profit for its owner.

prophylactic Preventative.

prophylactic vaccination A vaccination performed to prevent infectious diseases. Suspension of attenuated or killed viruses or bacteria or parts thereof that is capable of producing a protective immune response to such infectious agents.

prophylaxis Cleaning of the teeth for the prevention of periodontal disease and tooth decay.

prospective authorization Authorization to deliver health care service that is issued before any service is rendered. *Synonym:* precertification.

Prospective Payment Assessment Commission (PPAC) A Federal commission established under the Social Security Act amendments of 1983 to advise and assist Congress and the DHHS in maintaining and updating the Medicare prospective payment system.

Prospective Payment System (PPS) A method of reimburse-ment in which Medicare payment is made based on a predetermined, fixed amount. The payment amount for a particular service is derived based on the classification system of that service (for example, drgs for inpatient hospital services).

prospective pricing Method of third party payment by which prices for services are established in advance for a specified period of time. These prices are firm regardless of the actual costs incurred in a specific episode of care.

prospective review The review and possible authorization of proposed treatment plans for a patient before the treatment is implemented.

prostate Gland surrounding the neck of the bladder and urethra in men.

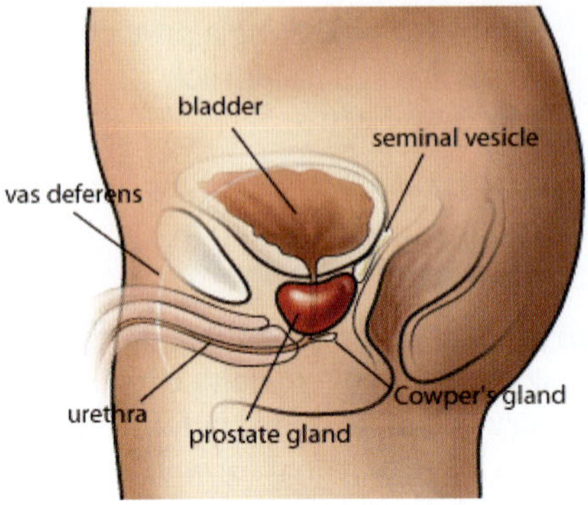

prostate

prostatectomy Surgical removal of part or all of the prostate.

prostate-specific ag, serum Prostate-specific antigen (PSA) is a protein produced by the cells of the prostate gland. The PSA test measures the level of PSA in the blood. It is normal for men to have low levels in their blood; however, prostate cancer or benign (not cancerous) conditions can increase PSA levels.

prostatic hypertrophy Enlargement of the prostate. May obstruct the flow of urine from the bladder. Not cancerous. Symptoms may include urinary urgency and frequency, burning on urination, weak urinary stream, a feeling that the bladder cannot be emptied and sometimes impotence. Curable with surgery.

prostatitis Inflammation or infection of the prostate. Symptoms may include urinary urgency and frequency, burning on urination, difficulty starting urination and emptying bladder completely, fever, chills, pain in scrotum, anus or lower back, and muscle or joint aches. Usually curable with treatment, which includes antibiotics.

prostatotomy Surgical incision of the prostate.

prosthesis An artificial body part such as an artificial leg or arm. The term prosthesis is also used to describe some of the implants used in the body such as a hip or knee replacement device.

prosthesis fitting The fitting and adjusting of artificial parts of the body.

prosthesis implantation Surgical insertion of a prosthesis.

prosthodontics A dental specialty concerned with the restoration and maintenance of oral function by the replacement of missing teeth and structures by artificial devices or prostheses.

prosthodontist A dental specialist skilled in restoring or replacing teeth with fixed or removable prosthesis (appliances) in order to maintain proper occlusion. May also treat facial deformities with artificial prostheses.

prot(o)- Denotes something as 'first' or 'most-important'.

Protected Health Information (PHI) Individually identifiable health information transmitted or maintained in any form or medium, which is held by a covered entity or its business associate. Identifies the individual or offers a reasonable basis for identification. Is created or received by a covered entity or an employer Relates to a past, present, or future physical or mental condition, provision of health care or payment for health care.

protein c deficiency Protein C deficiency is an uncommon clotting disorder.

protein electrophoresis A blood test to determine the levels of the immune proteins (globulins, or antibodies), and albumin.

protein metabolism Process by which protein foods are used by the body to make tissue proteins, together with breaking down tissue proteins to produce energy. Food proteins are first broken down into amino acids then absorbed into the blood and finally used in body cells to form new proteins. Diseases affecting protein metabolism include liver disease, maple-sugar urine disease and phenylketonuria. *See* Maple-sugar urine disease; phenylketonuria.

protein s deficiency Protein S deficiency is an uncommon clotting disorder.

protein, total, serum Protein tests measure the amounts and types of protein in the blood. Proteins are constituents of muscle, enzymes, hormones, transport proteins, hemoglobin, and other functional and structural elements of the body.

proteinuria The presence of excessive protein (chiefly albumin but also globulin) in the urine; usually a symptom of kidney disorder.

proteus infections Bacteria normally found in feces, water and soil. May cause urinary tract infections, kidney infections, wound infections, diarrhea and bacteremia. *See* Bacteremia.

prothrombin A protein in blood plasma that is the inactive precursor of thrombin.

protime A test of the blood clotting system and a general test of the liver's capacity to synthesize needed blood proteins. *Synonym:* prothrombin time.

protozoa A single-cell organism that can only divide within a host organism.

protozoal intestinal diseases Diseases of the intestinal system caused by protozoa, which are single-cell organisms that can only divide within a host organism. Malaria ,giardia and toxoplasmosis are examples of diseases caused by protozoa.

protraction Anterior movement of the arms at the shoulders.

protrusion The anterior movement of an object. This term is often applied to the jaw.

provider Generically, a professional engaged in the delivery of health services, including physicians, dentists, nurses, podiatrists, optometrists, clinical psychologists, etc. Hospitals and long term care facilities are also providers. The Medicare program uses the term "provider" more narrowly, to mean participating institutions hospitals, skilled nursing facilities, home health agencies, etc.

provider identification number An identification number assigned to providers by the carrier; required for any provider, regardless of participation status, who wishes to submit claims to Medicare for reimbursement.

provider network The providers with which an M + C Organization contracts or makes arrangements to furnish covered health care services to Medicare enrollees under an M + C coordinated care or network MSA plan.

provider profiling The collection and analysis of information about the practice patterns of individual providers.

Provider Reimbursement Review Board A Federal board responsible for making decisions regarding provider appeals on Medicare reimbursement issues.

provider sponsored organization A group of physicians, hospitals, and other health care providers that agree to give health care to Medicare beneficiaries for a set amount of money from Medicare every month. This type of managed care plan is run by the physicians and providers themselves, and not by an insurance company.

provider survey data Data collected through a survey or focus group of providers who participate in the Medicaid program and have provided services to enrolled Medicaid beneficiaries. The state or a contractor of the state may conduct the survey.

provider taxonomy codes An administrative code set for identifying the provider type and area of specialization for all health care providers. A given provider can have several Provider Taxonomy Codes. This code set is used in the X12 278 Referral Certification and Authorization and the X12 837 Claim transactions, and is maintained by the NUCC.

provider-sponsored organization A health care organization established, organized, or operated, by a health care provider or a group of affiliated health care providers to arrange for the delivery, financing, and administration of health care that meets requirements established by the Balanced Budget Act of 1997 and has the authority to contract directly with Medicare.

proximal Nearest the center of the body.

PRRB Provider reimbursement review board.

pruritus The medical term for itching. Pruritus can result from drug reaction, food allergy, kidney or liver disease, cancers, parasites, aging or dry skin, contact skin reaction, such as poison ivy, and for unknown reasons.

PSA Prostate specific antigen. Abnormal levels in the serum are associated with clinical abnormalities of the prostate, including prostate cancer. Because PSA is found in normal, malignant and benign prostatic tissue, clinical discrimination is based upon its serum level.

pseudoarthrosis A form of a non–union in which there is the formation of a false joint with some cartilage covering the ends of the bones and a cavity containing fluid that resembles a normal joint.

pseudocysts Abnormal or dilated space resembling a cyst but without a membrane lining. Condition commonly occurs after pancreatitis. *See* Pancreatitis. Surgery may be required to drain pseudocysts.

pseudogout Arthritic condition marked by attacks of gout-like symptoms, usually affecting a single joint (particularly the knee). Inflammation and pain may be relieved by hydrocortisone injections into the affected joint or by taking antiinflammatory medications.

pseudohypoparathyroidism Hereditary condition that resembles hypoparathyroidism. In hypoparathyroidism, there is a deficiency of parathyroid hormone. In pseudohypoparathyroidism, there is no deficiency of hormone, but the body fails to respond normally to the parathyroid hormone. Symptoms may include short stature, crossed eyes, calcium deposits in muscle and brain tissue, and mental retardation.

pseudomembranous enterocolitis Acute inflammatory bowel disorder that usually occurs in premature or low-birth-weight newborns. Cause is unknown. Characterized by death of tissue of the intestinal walls, which may lead to perforation and peritonitis. *See* Peritonitis. Early symptoms may include low body temperature, poor feeding, vomiting and blood in stools. *Synonym:* necrotizing enterocolitis.

pseudo-precocious puberty Premature sexual development; of unknown cause.

pseudotumors False or phantom tumor.

psoriasis Chronic, scaly skin disorder characterized by frequent remissions and recurrences. Affected skin areas are raised, have red borders and are covered with large, silver-white scales. Areas may crack and become painful. Treatment can control symptoms, but there is no cure.

PSRO Professional standards review organization.

psych Psychiatry, psychology.

psych(e)-, psych(o) of or pertaining to the mind.

psychiatric Relating to or used in or engaged in the practice of psychiatry.

psychiatric facility (partial hospitalization) A facility for the diagnosis and treatment of mental illness on a 24-hour basis by, or under, the supervision of a physician.

psychiatric residential treatment center A facility or distinct part of a facility for psychiatric care which provides a total 24-hour therapeutically planned and professionally staffed group living and learning environment.

psychiatry The study, treatment and prevention of mental disorders. Psychiatric services include diagnostic and therapeutic services in the hospital, office, or other outpatient setting.

psychodynamic therapy A branch of psychotherapy that deals with the psychology of mental or emotional forces or processes developed in early childhood and their effects on behavior and mental states.

psychogenic Mental or emotional rather than physiological in origin.

psychological test Any test to measure a subject's development, achievement, personality, intelligence, thought processes, etc.

psychologist A specialist in the study of the structure and function of the brain and related behaviors or mental processes. A psychologist may provide psychological evaluation, assessment, testing, and treatment, but may not prescribe medications.

psychometrics Assessment of psychological variables by the application of mathematical procedures.

psychomotor test A test that assesses the subject's ability to perceive instructions and perform motor responses.

psychopathology A term which refers to either the study of mental illness or mental distress, or the manifestation of behaviors and experiences which may be indicative of mental illness or psychological impairment, such as abnormal, maladaptive behavior or mental activity.

psychosis Any severe mental disorder in which contact with reality is lost or highly distorted.

psychosurgery Treatment of chronic, severe and intractable psychiatric disorders by surgical removal or interruption of certain areas or pathways in the brain, especially in the prefrontal lobes.

psychotherapy The treatment of mental or emotional problems by psychological means.

psychotic Suffering from psychosis.

psychotic disorders Disorders in which there is a loss of ego boundaries or a gross impairment in reality testing with delusions or prominent hallucinations.

psychotropic drugs A loosely defined grouping of drugs that have effects on psychological function. Here the psychotropic agents include the antidepressive agents, hallucinogens, and tranquilizing agents (including the antipsychotics and anti-anxiety agents).

PT Physical therapy.

pt (prothrombin time test) The prothrombin time test, also called PT, helps measure how well blood is able to clot. The test provides a control for long-term anticoagulant therapy that usually involves the use of warfarin. It is also known as INR or Protime.

PTCA Percutaneous Transluminal Coronary Angioplasty.

pterygium A thickened triangular layer of conjunctiva extending from the nasal edge of the eye to the cornea; pterygia arise from irritation of the pinguecula.

ptosis The drooping of a body part, especially the eyelids or the breasts.

-ptosis Falling, downward placement, prolapse.

PTSD Post-traumatic stress disorder.

PTT Partial thromboplastin time. A blood test that measures the length of time (in seconds) that it takes for clotting to occur when certain substances are added to the liquid portion of blood in a test tube. It is used to detect clotting factor deficiencies and to monitor heparin's effectiveness.

ptyalectasis Surgical dilation of a salivary duct.

ptygeria A growth of scar tissue on the cornea. These lesions like pinguecula are caused by an ultraviolet burn to the surface layer or epithelium.

-ptysis (A spitting), spitting, hemoptysis, the spitting of blood derived from the lungs or bronchial tubes.

pubic Relating or near the pubis.

pubic symphysis The joint located between the two bones of the pelvis.

pubis One of the three sections of the hipbone; together the two pubic bones form the front of the pelvis.

public health clinic A facility maintained by either state or local health departments that provide ambulatory primary medical care under the general direction of a physician.

Public Health Service A Federal agency responsible for public health services and programs including biomedical research.

public use file Non-identifiable data that is within the public domain.

PUD Peptic ulcer disease.

pudendal nerve A somatic nerve in the pelvic region that innervates the external genitalia of both sexes, as well as sphincters for the bladder and the rectum.

puerperal Relating to or connected with or occurring at the time of childbirth or shortly following, or to the woman who has just given birth.

puerperium The time period after childbirth (about 6 weeks) during which a woman's body returns to its normal physical state.

pulmon-, pulmo- of or relating to the lungs.

pulmonary Lungs.

pulmonary angiogram The most definitive test to diagnose PE, this is an invasive test requiring injection of a dye through a catheter (IV line) into the body.

pulmonary artery An artery that carries de-oxygenated blood from the right ventricle of the heart to the lungs.

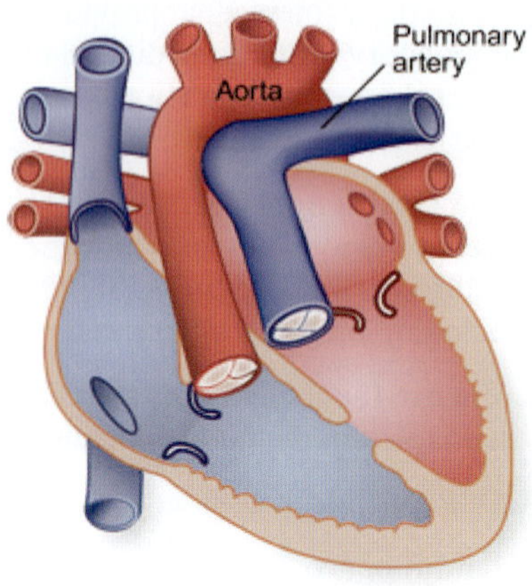

pulmonary artery

pulmonary autograft valves A new approach for replacement of a diseased aortic valve involves moving the patients own pulmonary valve (the valve on the right side of the heart that leads to the pulmonary artery and the lungs just as the aortic valve leads to the aorta and the body).

pulmonary circulation The circulation of blood through the lungs for the purpose of oxygenation and the release of carbon dioxide. *Synonym:* lesser circulation.

pulmonary congestion and hypostasis Excess fluid or blood in the lungs.

pulmonary disease Lung disease.

pulmonary edema Accumulation of fluid in the lungs. Caused by a failing heart.

pulmonary embolism blood clot or fat cells (rarely) in one of the arteries carrying blood to the lungs. blood clot begins in a deep vein of the leg or pelvis. Fat embolus usually begins at a fracture site. Embolus moves through the blood, passing through the heart and lodging in the branch of an artery that nourishes the lungs. This blockage decreases breathing ability and sometimes destroys lung tissue.

pulmonary fibrosis Fibrous tissue in the lungs causing scarring of tissue from one of many disease processes, such as emphysema.

pulmonary function test A series of tests that measure lung function.

pulmonary heart disease The enlargement and eventual failure of the right ventricle of the heart due to disorders of the lungs or their blood vessels or chest wall abnormalities.

pulmonary infarction The death of a small area of lung resulting from pulmonary embolism. It occurs in a small, dead-end pulmonary artery and often causes pain in the back or chest.

pulmonary insufficiency Subnormal function of the lungs.

pulmonary sequestration A condition where a piece of tissue that develops into lung tissue is not attached to the pulmonary blood supply and does not communicate with the other lung tissue. *Synonym:* cystic lung lesion.

pulmonary valve Separates the right bottom chamber of the heart (ventricle) from the pulmonary artery (the large artery that goes from the heart to the lungs).

pulmonary-valve stenosis Narrowing of the pulmonary valve. Impairs heart function. Usually there are no symptoms at first. As the condition worsens, chest pain, dizziness, faintness upon exertion and congestive heart failure symptoms develop. When symptoms become severe, surgery is recommended to stretch the defective pulmonary valve. *See* Congestive heart failure.

pulmonology The medical specialty that deals with diseases of the lungs and the respiratory tract.

pulp The hollow chamber inside the crown of the tooth that contains its nerves and blood vessels.

pulp cap A medicated covering over a small area of exposed pulp tissue.

pulp chamber The center or innermost portion of the tooth containing the pulp.

pulpectomy Removal of the entire pulp from the canals in the root.

pulpitis Inflammation of the pulp, which is common cause of toothache.

pulpotomy The removal of a portion of the tooth's pulp.

pulse generator A device that produces an electrical discharge at regular intervals, which can be modified as needed, as in an electronic pacemaker.

pulse oximetry A noninvasive (no blood needed) method used to monitor the percentage of hemoglobin that is saturated with oxygen.

punctal occlusion Closing off the punctum, either with plugs, cauterization, or other natural or artificial methods.

punctum A point or small area.

pupil Appears as a small black dot in the center of the iris. The pupil changes its diameter in response to changes in ambient lighting. The pupil varies the amount of light reaching the retina and the depth of focus of the eye.

pupillary reflex Contraction of the pupil after application of light, loud noise or other stimulus.

purchased diagnostic tests Refers to tests such as x-rays, ultrasound, laboratory tests, etc., purchased from an outside supplier for which a physician bills, but does not personally perform or supervise.

pure tone audiometry Audiometry utilizing pure tones that are relatively free of noise and overtones.

purines Any of a large group of nitrogen compounds. End products after digestion of certain proteins; also made by the body. Present in many medications and in some foods.

purpura Are purple-colored spots and patches that occur on the skin, organs, and in mucus membranes, including the lining of the mouth.

purulent Infected.

PUVA A Psoralen + UVA treatment for eczema, psoriasis and vitiligo, and mycosis fungoides. The Psoralen is applied or taken orally to sensitize the skin, then the skin is exposed to UVA.

PUVD Pulsed ultrasonic (blood) velocity detector.

PVB Premature ventricular beat.

PVC Premature ventricular contraction.

PVD Peripheral vascular disease.

pyel(o)- Pelvis.

pyelitis Acute inflammation of the pelvis of the kidney, caused by bacterial infection.

pyelocutaneous fistula A fistula between the kidney and the skin. Most are secondary to trauma, including surgery, chronic granulomatous disease or foreign bodies.

pyelography X-ray photography of the kidneys, renal pelvises, ureters, and urinary bladder after injection with a radiopaque dye.

pyelolithotomy Incision of the renal pelvis for removal of calculi.

pyelonephritis Noncontagious bacterial infection of the kidneys. Infection may begin in the bladder and ascend to the kidneys. May be acute or chronic. Acute infections come on rapidly and are often characterized by fever, chills, nausea, flank pain and urinary frequency and burning. Antibiotic therapy usually cures the infection in 10 to 14 days. Chronic infections develop slowly and last for months or years. They lead to scarring and eventual loss of kidney function. If chronic kidney failure develops in both kidneys, kidney transplant or kidney dialysis can be life saving. *Synonym:* kidney infection.

pyeloplasty The surgical reconstruction or revision of the renal pelvis to drain and decompress the kidney.

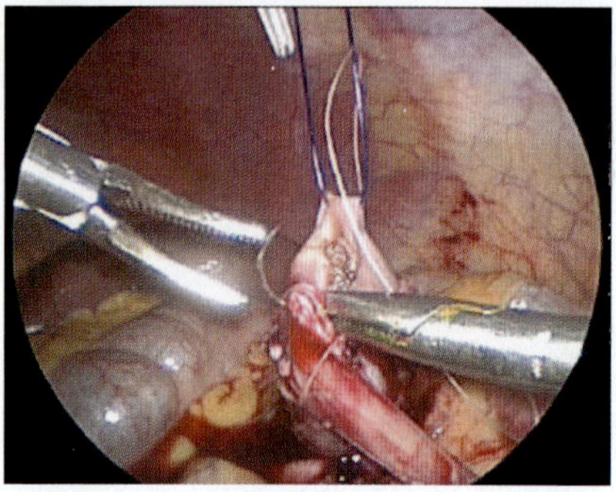

pyeloplasty

pyeloscopy Fluoroscopic observation of the pelvis and the calices of the kidney following injection of a contrast medium through the ureter.

pyelostolithotomy Surgical removal of a calculus (stone) through an incision into the renal pelvis.

pyelostomy Surgical formation of an opening into the renal pelvis.

pyelotomy Incision into the pelvis of the kidney. *Synonym:* pelviotomy.

pyeloureteritis Inflammation of a ureter and the renal pelvis.

pyeloureteroplasty Plastic repair of the kidney(s) and ureter(s).

pyemia Septicemia caused by pus-forming bacteria released from an abscess.

pyemic of or relating to pyemia.

pyloric stenosis Condition in infancy in which encircling muscles enlarge and cause obstruction. It occurs in infants, usually beginning at 2 to 5 weeks. Causes projectile vomiting after feedings.

pyloromyotomy A surgical procedure in which an incision is made in the longitudinal and circular muscles of the pylorus. It is used to treat hypertrophic pyloric stenosis.

pyloroplasty A surgical procedure performed to widen the opening between the stomach and the small intestine.

pyo- Pus.

pyoderma Any purulent skin disease.

pyogenic Producing pus.

pyrexia A rise in the temperature of the body; frequently a symptom of infection. *Synonym:* fever.

pyridoxine-responsive anemia *See* Anemia, pyridoxine-responsive.

pyro- Fever.

pyrosis A technical term for what is popularly called heartburn, a burning sensation in the upper abdomen.

Q

QRS Principle deflection in ECG.

quadr(i)- Four.

quadrant The dental term for the division of the jaws into four parts, beginning at the midline of the arch and extending towards the last tooth in the back of the mouth. There are four quadrants in the mouth; each quadrant generally contains five to eight teeth.

quadrantectomy Quadrantectomy is a surgical procedure in which a quadrant (approximately one-fourth) of the breast, including tissue surrounding a cancerous tumor, is removed. *Synonym:* segmental mastectomy.

quadriceps A muscle of the thigh that extends the leg.

quadricepsplasty A corrective surgical procedure on the quadriceps femoris muscle and tendon to release adhesions and improve mobility, with the goal of improving the range of flexion of the knee.

quadriplegia Paralysis of both arms and both legs.

qualified beneficiary Generally, qualified beneficiaries include covered employees, their spouses and their dependent children who are covered under the group health plan. In certain cases, retired employees, their spouses and dependent children may be qualified beneficiaries.

Qualified Medicare Beneficiary (QMB) A person whose income falls below 100% of Federal poverty guidelines and whose resources do not exceed twice the resource limit of the SSI program, for whom the state must pay the Medicare Part B premiums, deductibles and co-payments.

qualifying circumstances for anesthesia CPT codes that define circumstances such as age, condition, technique and other circumstances affecting the provision of anesthesia.

qualifying event An occurrence (such as death, termination of employment, divorce, etc.) That changes an employee's eligibility status under a group health plan. The term is most frequently used in reference to COBRA eligibility.

qualitative Refers to tests that identify the components of a mixture.

quality Defined by the Institute of Medicine as the degree to which health services for individuals and populations increase the likelihood of desired outcomes and are consistent with current professional knowledge.

quality assessment An ongoing process to monitor and evaluate aspects of patient/medical care against pre-established criteria and standards to determine the medical necessity, appropriateness, and effectiveness of the services provided.

quality assurance An interactive management process designed to objectively ensure the appropriateness and effectiveness of patient care. It includes identifying deficiencies, implementing corrective action(s) to improve performance, and monitoring the corrective actions to ensure that quality of care has been enhanced. In the broadest sense, this ongoing process should involve the medical and professional staff, the administration, and the governing body of the health care facility.

quality improvement A continuous process that identifies problems in health care delivery, examines solutions to those problems, and regularly monitors the solutions for improvement.

Quality Improvement Organization (QIO) Organization under contract with HCFA to review quality and cost issues for Medicare. Required to oversee Medicare HMOs. Formerly known as a peer review organization. Can also be used in a more general sense to refer to any independent quality review organization. Also see quality assurance.

quality management An organization-wide process of measuring and improving the quality of the health care provided by an MCO.

quality of care The degree or grade of excellence with respect to medical services received by patients, administered by providers or programs, in terms of technical competence, need, appropriateness, acceptability, humanity and structure.

quality-of-life measures An assessment of patient's perceptions of how they deal with their disease or with their everyday life when suffering from a particular condition. It is subjective in the sense that the kinds of information cannot be measured objectively; however, it has been in health care literature for at least 20 years. It has been tapped in the area of pharmaceuticals most recently in the last five or six years. Through statistical means, the indices that have been developed to measure various aspects of quality of life have been validated over time, and we know that these measures are reliable and reproducible.

quality program An organization-wide initiative to measure and improve the service and care provided by an MCO.

quant Quantitative.

quantitative Refers to tests that measure some quantity or number.

Quick's test 1) A test for liver function based on excretion of hippuric acid after administration of sodium benzoate. 2) Prothrombin time.

R

r/o Rule out.

ra latex A blood test for rheumatoid factor. Positive in juvenile rheumatoid arthritis.

rabies A viral disease that causes acute encephalitis in warm-blooded animals and people, characterised by abnormal behaviour such as excitement, aggressiveness, and dementia, followed by paralysis and death.

rachi(o)- Spine.

rachicentesis Lumbar puncture.

radial keratotomy A surgical procedure that permanently alters the shape of the cornea by placing microscopically thin relaxing incisions in the peripheral cornea. The incisions cause the central portion of the cornea to flatten, thereby reducing the power of the cornea.

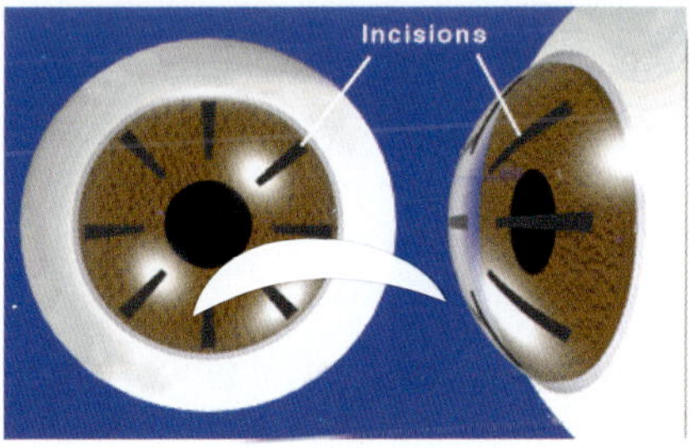

radial keratotomy

radiation dosimetry The calculation of the absorbed dose in matter and tissue resulting from the exposure to indirectly and directly ionizing radiation.

radiation oncology The use of ionizing radiation as part of cancer treatment to control malignant cells. Radiation therapy may be used for curative or adjuvant cancer treatment. It is used as palliative treatment or as therapeutic treatment. *Synonym:* radiotherapy.

radiation therapy Use of high-energy waves, generated by special X-ray machines, cobalt machines and other devices, to treat some forms of cancer. Radiation destroys cancerous tissue, but does little harm to healthy tissue. *Synonym:* radiotherapy.

radicular Pain caused by the root of a nerve.

radiculitis Inflammation of the radicle of a nerve.

radioallergosorbent test (rast) A radioimmunoassay test for the measurement of specific ige antibody in serum, using allergen extract antigens fixed in a solid-phase matrix and radiolabeled anti–human ige.

radiogrammetry A method of bone mineral analysis in which measurements are derived from radiographs, most commonly through determination of the metacarpal index.

radiograph A photographic image produced on a radiosensitive surface by radiation other than visible light (especially by X-rays or gamma rays).

radiographic Relating to or produced by radiography.

radiography Making X-ray films of internal structures of the body by exposure of film specially. sensitized to X-rays or gamma rays.

radioimmunoassay Classic quantitative assay for detection of antigen-antibody reactions using a radioactively labeled substance (radioligand) either directly or indirectly to measure the binding of the unlabeled substance to a specific antibody or other receptor system.

radioimmunosorbent test A radioimmunoassay technique for measuring serum ige concentration, using radiolabeled ige and anti–human ige bound to an insoluble matrix.

radioisotope Radioactive form of chemical normally present in the body. Chemical elements that give off radiation. A radioisotope of a chemical element normally present in the body, such as carbon, will mix with non-isotopes when it is injected into the body.

radioisotope scan Radioisotope is given orally or intravenously and becomes concentrated in organs, such as the heart, lungs or brain. Instruments measure the radiation given off by the radioisotopes and create a photographic image of the organ being studied. *See* Radioisotope.

radiologic examination A test that uses radiation or other imaging procedures to find signs of cancer or other abnormalities.

radiologic guidance The use of fluoroscopy, computed tomography, magnetic resonance or other forms of radiologic guidance for device placement or removal, needle placement, localization and breast biopsy.

radiology The branch of medical science dealing with the medical use of X-rays or other penetrating radiation.

radiometry The measurement of radiation by photography, as in x-ray film and film badge, by Geiger-Mueller tube, and by scintillation counting.

radiopaque Not transparent to X-rays or other forms of radiation.

radiosurgery A procedure that allows non-invasive treatment of benign and malignant tumors. *Synonym:* stereotactic radiotherapy, stereotactic body radiotherapy.

radiotherapy The use of ionizing radiation to treat malignant neoplasms and other benign conditions. The most common forms of ionizing radiation used as therapy are x-rays, gamma rays, and electrons.

radioulnar joint Any of three joints connecting the radius and ulna at their proximal and distal ends and along their shafts.

radius The outer and slightly shorter of the two bones of the human forearm.

railroad retirement A federal insurance program similar to Social Security designed for workers in the railroad industry. The provisions of the Railroad Retirement Act provide for a system of coordination and financial interchange between the Railroad Retirement program and the Social Security program.

Ramstedt operation A surgical procedure on the pylorus in order to relax a stenotic or closed-by-spasm sphincter. *Synonym:* pyloromyotomy.

random change Haphazard change.

random sample A random sample is a group selected for study, which is drawn at random from the universe of cases by a statistically valid method.

range of motion Refers to the distance and direction a joint can move to its full potential. Each specific joint has a normal range of motion that is expressed in degrees after being measured with a goniometer.

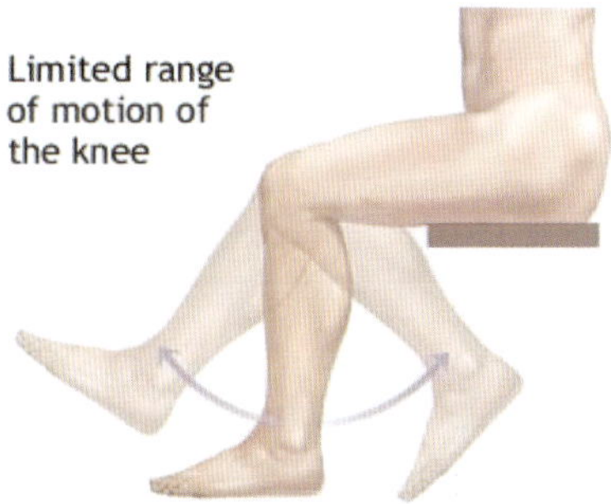

range of motion knee

RAP Request for Anticipated Payment. First of two transactions at opening and closing of Home Health PPS episode to receive one of two split percentage payments.

rapid plasma reagin test A screening flocculation test for syphilis, using a modified VDRL antigen.

Rapoport test A test used to evaluate suspected renovascular hypertension.

Raskind procedure Balloon atrial septostomy.

rat-bite fever An acute, febrile human illness caused by bacteria transmitted by rodents, rats in most cases, which is passed from rodent to human via the rodent's urine or mucous secretions. Two types of gram-negative facultative anaerobic bacteria can cause the infection.

rate setting An approach to cost containment where the government establishes payment rates for all payers for various categories of health services.

Raynaud's disease Primary disorder of the circulatory system that affects blood circulation to fingers and occasionally toes. Occurs mostly in people who smoke.

Raynaud's phenomenon Circulation system disorder affect-ing fingers and toes. A compli-cation of an underlying disease or emotional disturbance.

RBBB Right bundle branch block.

RBC Red blood cell.

RBRVS Resource Based Relative Value Scale. A government mandated relative value system, based on a study conducted at Harvard University, that is to be used for calculating national fee schedules for services provided to Medicare patients.

RDS Respiratory distress syndrome.

RDW The red blood cell distribution width, or RDW, is a measure of the variation of red blood cell width that is reported as part of a standard complete blood count. Usually red blood cells are a standard size of about 6-8 M. Certain disorders, however, cause a significant variation in cell size. Higher RDW values indicate greater variation in size. Normal range in human red blood cells is 11-15%.

re- Again, backward.

reactive change Change that is controlled, but rarely planned, and that can lead to positive, negative, or even unintended results.

realignment To restore a body part to its proper position.

reality therapy Method of psychotherapeutic treatment based on assumption of the patient's personal responsibility for their own behavior. The therapist actively guides patients to accurate self-perception for fulfillment of needs of self-worth and respect for others.

reasonable and customary Fee A reasonable charge is a charge that, in the context of the community is fair. A customary charge is a charge or fee that falls within the customary range of charges or fees prevailing in a specific geographic area for the provision of a similar service, procedure, or supply.

reasonable charge The amount Medicare will pay for a covered service. This is usually the lowest of the actual, customary and prevailing charges.

reasonable cost Fis and carriers use CMS guidelines to determine reasonable costs incurred by individual providers in furnishing covered services to enrollees. Reasonable cost is based on the actual cost of providing such services, including direct and indirect cost of providers and excluding any costs that are unnecessary in the efficient delivery of services covered by the program.

reasonable-cost basis The calculation to determine the reasonable cost incurred by individual providers when furnishing covered services to beneficiaries. The reasonable cost is based on the actual cost of providing such services, including direct and indirect costs of providers, and excluding any costs that are unnecessary in the efficient delivery of services covered by a health insurance program.

receded gums A condition characterized by the abnormal loss of gum tissue due to infection or bone loss.

rebate A reduction in the price of a particular pharmaceutical obtained by a PBM from the pharmaceutical manufacturer.

rebound stimulation Response is reversed when stimulus is withdrawn.

rebundling A comprehensive standardized package of computerized edits to identify and prevent improper reporting on a national level.

receivership A situation in which the state insurance commissioner, acting for a state court, takes control of and administers an HMO's assets and liabilities.

recidivism The frequency of the same patient returning to a provider with the same presenting problems. Usually refers to recurring inpatient hospital services.

recipient A person who receives a Medicaid service while eligible for the Medicaid program. Individuals may be Medicaid eligible without being Medicaid recipients. Also see Medicaid.

reciprocity The right of an enrollee in a health plan who is temporarily away from home to receive necessary medical care under the arrangements of a health plan in the area in which the enrollee receives medical care.

reconsideration Review of an adverse coverage determination that may be requested by the patient or representative, the attending physician, or the hospital. Reconsideration is performed by the original reviewing body, not by an independent appeals panel.

reconstruction A surgical procedure used to reconstruct, restore, or improve defective, damaged, or missing structures.

recoupment The recovery by Medicare of any Medicare debt by reducing present or future Medicare payments and applying the amount withheld to the indebtedness.

rect(o)- Rectum.

rectal of or involving the rectum.

rectal administration The insertion of drugs into the rectum, usually for confused or incompetent patients, like children, infants, and the very old or comatose.

rectocele A hernial protrusion of the rectum into the vagina.

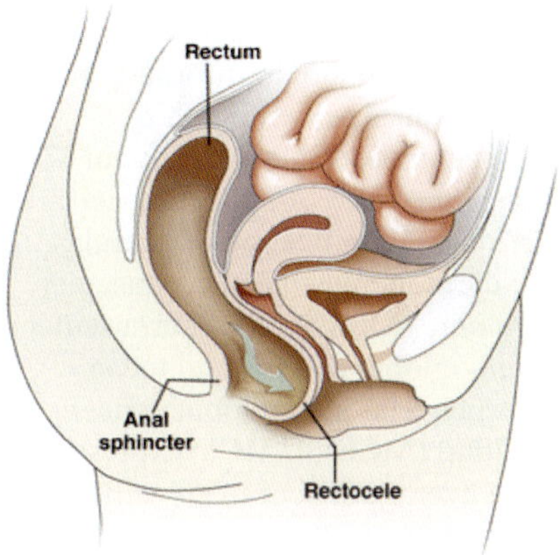

rectocele

rectopexy A procedure in which sutures are used to secure the rectum in its proper position using key-hole surgery.

rectoplasty Reconstructive surgery of the anus or rectum.

rectorrhaphy Repair by suture of a lacerated rectum or anus.

rectum The terminal section of the alimentary canal; from the sigmoid flexure to the anus.

rectus Any of various straight muscles.

rectus abdominis A large muscle in the front of the abdomen that assists in the regular breathing movement and supports the muscles of the spine while lifting and keeping abdominal organs such as the intestines in place.

recurrence The return of a sign, symptom or disease after a remission. The reappearance of cancer cells at the same site or in another location is, unfortunately, a familiar form of recurrence.

red cell indices Blood test that provides important information about the size, hemoglobin concentration and hemoglobin weight of an average blood cell. Aids in classification of anemias. Indices include mean corpuscular volume (MCV), mean corpuscular hemoglobin (MCH) and mean corpuscular hemoglobin concentration (MCHC). MCV expresses the average size of many cells and indicates whether most red blood cells are undersized (microcytic), oversized (macrocytic) or normal sized (normocytic). MCH is the hemoglobin-to-red-blood-cell ratio and gives the weight (concentration) of hemoglobin in an average red blood cell. MCHC defines the volume of hemoglobin in an average red cell and helps distinguish normally colored (normochromic) red blood cells from pale (hypochromic) red cells.

red cells Blood cells (erythrocytes) which appear as biconcave disks, lack nuclei and comprise the largest number of cells of the formed elements of whole blood. Red cells transport oxygen to body cells and remove carbon dioxide. Red cells contain iron in the hemoglobin.

red measles Serious viral disease of childhood. Uncommon today because immunizations have controlled this problem to a great extent in North America and Europe. *Synonym:* rubeola.

redlining An insurance practice used to exclude entire occupations, businesses, geographic areas, and age groups from health insurance coverage to limit loss.

reduced services Under certain circumstances a service or procedure is partially reduced or eliminated at the physician's discretion. This is reported by adding the CPT modifier -52 to the procedure code.

reduction The replacement or realignment of a body part in normal position or restoration of a bodily condition to normal.

reduction mammaplasty Plastic repair on the breast to reduce its size and often to improve its shape and position.

redundant prepuce A condition where the foreskin of the penis more than covers the glans when not erect and does not automatically fully retract upon erection. Phimosis a constriction of the foreskin of the penis resulting in the inability to retract the prepuce over the glans.

reference (outside) laboratory When laboratory procedures are performed by a party other than the treating or reporting physician, the procedure may be identified by adding the modifier '-90' to the usual procedure number.

referral The transfer of the total care or specific portion of care of a from one physician to another. A referral is not a request for consultation.

referral services Any specialty, inpatient, outpatient or laboratory services that are ordered or arranged, but not furnished directly. Certain situations may exist that should be considered referral services for purposes of determining if a physician or group is at substantial financial risk. For example, an MCO may require a physician group or physician to authorize retroactive referrals for emergency care received outside the MCO's network. If the physician group or physician's payment from the MCO can be affected by the utilization of emergency care, such as a bonus if emergency referrals are low, then these emergency services are considered referral services and need to be included in the calculation of substantial financial risk. Also, if a physician group contracts with an individual physician or another group to provide services that the initial group cannot provide itself, any services referred to the contracted physician group or physician should be considered referral services.

referring physician A physician who requests an item or service for the beneficiary for which payment may be made under the Medicare program.

Refined Diagnosis Related Group (RDRG) An expanded list of diagnosis related groups to take into account a patient's severity of illness.

reflux esophagitis Irritation of the esophagus from stomach acid splashing upward into the esophagus.

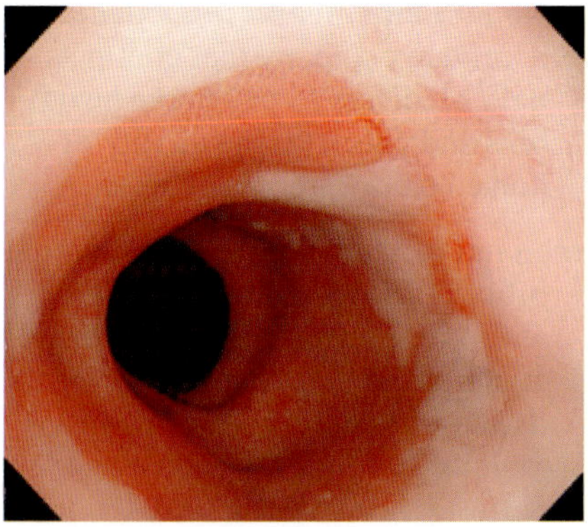

reflux esophagitis

refraction The ability of the eye to bend light so that an image is focused on the retina. Accommodation the automatic adjustment in focal length of the natural lens of the eye.

refractive surgery Any surgical procedure which permanently alters the focusing power of the eye in order to change refractive errors.

refractometry The method of measuring the refractive index of a substance to assess composition or purity.

refractory Not yielding to treatment.

Regenstrief institute A research foundation for improving health care by optimizing the capture, analysis, content, and delivery of health care information. Regenstrief maintains the LOINC coding system that is being considered for use as part of the HIPAA claim attachments standard.

regional enteritis Inflammation of the intestinal tract, especially of the small intestine.

regional home health intermediary A private company that contracts with Medicare to pay home health bills and check on the quality of home health care.

regional office CMS has ten regional offices that work closely together with Medicare contractors in their assigned geographical areas on a day-to-day basis. Four of these ros monitor network contractor performance, negotiate contractor budgets, distribute administrative monies to contractors, work with contractors when corrective actions are needed, and provide a variety of other liaison services to the contractors in their respective regions.

Registered Nurse (RN) An individual who provides nursing services after completing a course of study that results in a baccalaureate degree and who has been legally authorized or registered to practice as an RN and use the RN designation after passing examination by a state board of nurse examiners or similar state authority.

Registered Respiratory Therapist (RPT) Aids in the treatment of patients with serious respiratory problems and heart and lung disorders. The therapist assists with long term ventilation procedures, administers breathing treatments and maintains respiratory equipment.

regurgitation When a valve leaks it is said to be regurgitant, or to exhibit regurgitation.

rehab Rehabilitation.

rehabilitation To restore health following an accident, injury or illness.

rehabilitation, acute Early rehabilitation phase as soon as medically stable. Primary emphasis is to provide intensive physical and cognitive restorative services in the early months following injury. Typical stay 3-4 months (short term). Based in medical facility.

rehabilitation, long term May be called Extended Rehabilitation. Have full range of rehabilitation services available. Frequently after initial year of rehabilitation when progress is slower. Generally not permanent placement. May be facility or community based.

rehabilitation, sub acute Post-acute phase of rehabilitation. Capacity to treat for 6-24 months. Need not be hospital based. Stay based on demonstrated improvement.

rehabilitation, transitional To prepare for community re-entry. Non-medically based. Emphasis on functional skills for maximum independence. May be in group home or part of a continuum of rehabilitation center. Typical stay 4-8 months. Greater focus on compensation vs. restoration.

rehabilitative (restorative) care Skilled care provided by a trained medical person (physical therapist, R.M., speech therapist).

rehabilitation centers Facilities which provide programs for rehabilitating the mentally or physically disabled individuals.

Reichstein's substances One of several steroids.

reimplantation The insertion and temporary fixation of partially or completely avulsed teeth resulting from traumatic injury.

Reiter's syndrome (disease) An autoimmune condition that develops in response to an infection in another part of the body. The symptoms often include a combination of an inflammatory arthritis of large joints, inflammation of the eyes, and urethritis. *Synonym:* reactive arthritis.

reject status The encounter data did not pass the front-end edit process. M + C organization needs to correct the data and resubmit.

relapsing fever An infection caused by certain bacteria in the genus borrelia. It is a vector-borne disease that is transmitted through louse or soft-bodied tick bites. *Synonym:* typhinia.

relative value A value that reflects a comparison with an arbitrary standard.

Relative Value Scale (RVS) An index that assigns specific numeric values to medical services. Multiplying the relative value by a conversion factor results in a fee.

release of information The patient's signature indicating consent to the release of information necessary for settlement of his or her health insurance claim.

REM Rapid eye movement (sleep).

remission A return to the asymptomatic state, usually accompanied by a return to the usual level of functioning.

ren(o)- of or pertaining to the kidney.

renal of or pertaining to the kidney.

renal agents Drugs used for their effects on the kidneys regulation of body fluid composition and volume. The most commonly used are the diuretics.

renal disease Any of several diseases affecting the kidneys.

renal failure Severe malfunction of the kidneys, producing uremia and the resulting constitutional symptoms. *Synonym:* kidney failure.

renal plasma flow Rate of blood flow through the kidney.

renal replacement therapy Procedures which temporarily or permanently remedy insufficient cleansing of body fluids by the kidneys.

renal sclerosis A sclerosis or hardening of the kidney due to renovascular disease.

renal transplant center A hospital unit that is approved to furnish transplantation and other medical and surgical specialty services directly for the care of ESRD transplant patients, including inpatient dialysis furnished directly or under arrangement.

renal tubular acidosis Loss of base or accumulation of acid in the body due to disease of the kidney tubules.

renal tubular disease Disease of the kidney tubules.

Rendu-Osler-Weber syndrome Hereditary hemorrhagic telangiectasia.

renewal A continuation of an insurance policy on revised terms, such as adjusted health insurance rates.

renovascular hypertension Abnormally high blood pressure within the vessels of portal circulation. Caused by compression or obstruction of a blood vessel(s) decreasing blood flow in this area. The portal circulation system is a network of veins that carries blood from abdominal organs to the liver. Portal hypertension is frequently associated with alcoholic cirrhosis, but also results from blood clots in the hepatic (liver) or portal vein, constrictive pericarditis or a defective tricuspid valve in the heart. Portal hypertension results in an enlarged spleen and ascites, and in severe cases, generalized high blood pressure and esophageal varices. *See* Cirrhosis; hypertension; ascites; esophageal varices. *Synonym:* portal hypertension.

reopening An action taken, after all appeal rights are exhausted, to reexamine or question the correctness of a determination, a decision, or cost report otherwise final.

reoperation A repeat operation for the same condition in the same patient due to disease progression or recurrence, or as followup to failed previous surgery.

reperfusion Restoration of blood supply to tissue which is ischemic due to decrease in normal blood supply. The decrease may result from any source including atherosclerotic obstruction, narrowing of the artery, or surgical clamping.

replantation Restoration of an organ or other structure to its original site.

reproductive control agents Substances used either in the prevention or facilitation of pregnancy.

reproductive health services Health care services related to human reproduction and diseases of the reproductive system.

Request for Anticipated Payment (RAP) A payment request submitted by Home Health agencies at the beginning of every 60-day episode once verbal orders have been obtained and the first Medicare billable service has been provided.

resection Surgical removal of part of an organ.

reserves Estimates of money that an insurer needs to pay future business obligations.

resident 1) A physician in training after medical school graduation. In the modern era, specialties require at least three years of residency training. Many specialties require four years or more, and it is not uncommon for physicians to undertake fellowships for further specialty training after a residency. 2) An individual in a nursing home, assisted living or other residential facility.

Resident Assessment Protocols (RAPs) Process used to assess nursing home residents who have problems (such as incontinence, or dementia) that have an especially significant impact on their care. Also see minimum data set, or resource utilization groups.

residential care facilities Long-term care facilities which provide supervision and assistance in activities of daily living with medical and nursing services when required.

residential substance abuse treatment facility A facility which provides treatment for substance (alcohol and drug) abuse to live-in residents who do not require acute medical care. Services include individual and group therapy and counseling, family counseling, laboratory tests, drugs and supplies, psychological testing, and room and board.

residual The long-term condition(s) resulting from a previous acute illness or injury.

residual factors Factors other than price, including volume of services, intensity of services, and age or sex changes.

resistance Opposition to something, or the ability to withstand it. For example, some forms of staphylococcus are resistant to treatment with antibiotics.

resorption The removal of bone tissue by normal physiological process or as part of a pathological process such as an infection.

resource costs The costs of the inputs used by an efficient physician to provide a service or procedure, including both the costs of the physician's own time and effort and the costs of nonphysician inputs. The apparently redundant use of resource with costs is a convention used to indicate the average costs of an efficient physician, as distinguished from cost-based reimbursement such as that used for hospitals prior to the prospective payment system.

resource-based relative value scale A scale of national uniform relative values for all physicians' services. The relative value of each service must be the sum of relative value units representing physicians' work, practice expenses net of malpractice expenses, and the cost of professional liability insurance.

Resource Utilization Groups (RUGS III) Patient classification system for nursing home patients used by the Federal government and some states to determine reimbursement levels for nursing home care. Also see minimum data set.

respirator A breathing device for administering long-term artificial respiration.

respiratory distress syndrome A type of lung failure in newborns that may result from any disease that causes large amounts of fluid to collect in the lungs.

respiratory function tests Measurement of the various processes involved in the act of respiration inspiration, expiration, oxygen and carbon dioxide exchange, lung volume and compliance, etc.

respiratory syncytial virus A virus that causes infections of the lungs and respiratory tract.

respiratory therapy Care of patients with deficiencies and abnormalities associated with the cardiopulmonary system. It includes the therapeutic use of medical gases and their administrative apparatus, environmental control systems, humidification, aerosols, ventilatory support.

respite care Short term care which is needed in order to maintain health or safety and provides temporary relief from care-giving duties to a member of the immediate family (or any other unpaid, primary caregiver). Respite care can include such services as home care, home health care, adult day care and institutional care.

restoration The replacement of a portion of a damaged tooth.

restraints Physical restraints are any manual method or physical or mechanical device, material, or equipment attached to or adjacent to the resident's body that the individual cannot remove easily which restricts freedom of movement or normal access to ones body. Chemical restraints are any drug used for discipline or convenience and not required to treat medical symptoms.

restrictive pericarditis Pressure develops when an increasing amount of fluid restricts the pumping action of the heart. Caused by development of fluid between the heart and the sac covering the heart. Treatment may include medication, aspiration of fluid from the sac using a needle or surgery to remove fluid from the sac. *See* Pericarditis.

resuscitation Act of reviving a person and returning them to consciousness.

retained placenta A placenta that remains inside the womb after the birth of the baby.

retained root The partial root structure remaining in the jaw after extraction or fracture of a natural tooth.

retainer A removable dental appliance, usually used in orthodontics, that maintains space between teeth or holds teeth in a fixed position until the bone solidifies around them.

retardation Lack of normal development of intellectual capacities.

reticulocyte An immature red blood cell containing a network of filaments or granules.

reticulocytosis Excess amount of reticulocytes in the blood.

reticuloendothelial system Body system involved primarily in defense against infection and in disposal of products of the breakdown of cells. Made up of cells that are able to surround, engulf and digest microorganisms and cell debris (macrophages) and special cells in the liver, lungs, bone marrow, spleen and lymph nodes.

reticuloendotheliosis Proliferation of the reticuloendothelium in any organ or tissue. *Synonym:* hairy cell leukemia.

reticulosarcoma A malignant lymphoma, histiocytic or undifferentiated.

retina The light-sensitive membrane covering the back wall of the eyeball; it is continuous with the optic nerve.

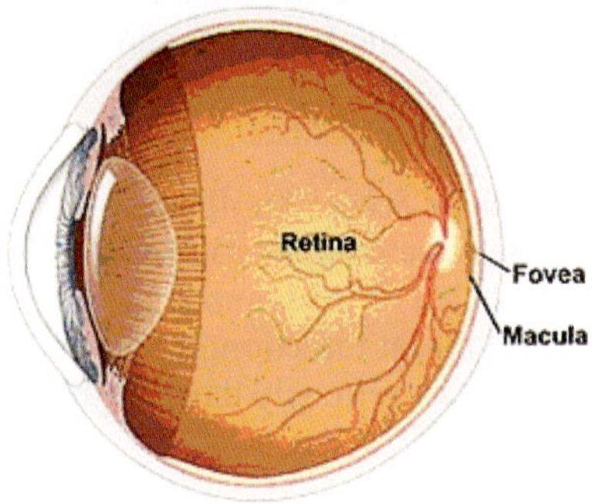

retina

retinal In or relating to the retina of the eye.

retinal detachment A disorder of the eye in which the retina peels away from its underlying layer of support tissue.

retinitis Inflammation of the retina.

retinitis pigmentosa Hereditary disease marked by progressive loss of retinal response, leading to partial or total blindness.

retinochoroiditis Inflammation of the retina and choroid.

retinopathy Any non-inflammatory disease of the retina. Associated with various conditions. It is most frequently seen in people with untreated hypertension or with diabetes mellitus.

retinopexy Surgical correction of a detachment of the retina.

retinoschisis A genetic eye disease that affects the retinal cells in the macula.

retraction Posterior movement of the arms at the shoulders.

retreatment The therapy of the same disease in a patient, with the same agent or procedure repeated after initial treatment, or with an additional or alternate measure or follow-up.

retro- Backward, behind.

retrograde Motion in the reverse of the normal direction of flow. For example, gastric reflux.

retrograde filling A method of sealing the root canal by preparing and filling it from the root tip, generally done at the completion of an apicoectomy.

retroperitoneal Pertaining to organs closely attached to the abdominal wall, behind the peritoneum.

retroperitoneal thrombosis Clotting of blood in the retroperitoneal space.

retrospective authorization Authorization to deliver health care service that is granted after service has been rendered.

retrospective review A type of utilization review that occurs after treatment is completed in order to authorize payment and medical necessity and appropriateness of care.

retrovirus Any of a group of viruses that contain two single-strand linear RNA molecules per virion and reverse transcriptase (RNA to DNA).

retrusion The opposite of protrusion, moving a part posteriorly.

Rett syndrome Cerebroatrophic hyperammonemia.

revascularization Reestablishment of blood supply to a part or organ.

revenue code Four position payment codes for services or items placed in the Revenue Codes field on UB-04 institutional claim formats.

revenues The amounts earned from a company's sales of products and services to its customers.

review of claims Using information on a claim or other information requested to support the services billed, to make a determination.

Reye's syndrome Disease in children and adolescents that involves brain and other major organs. Can cause permanent brain damage, coma or death due to pressure on brain. With treatment, most children survive and recover completely. Aspirin has been linked to influenza and various viral diseases as a possible cause.

Reynaud's phenomenon Intermittent ischemia of the fingers or toes marked by severe pallor and often accompanied by paralysis or pain, precipitated by exposure to the cold.

rf Radiofrequency.

rh The Rh factor is an inherited blood group on red blood cells like the ABO blood types. About 85% of the people in this country have it. Those who have it are Rh-positive, those who do not are Rh-negative.

rhabd(o)- Rod shaped, striated.

rheum Rheumatic.

rheumatic chorea A disease characterized by rapid, uncoordinated jerking movements affecting primarily the face, feet and hands. *Synonym:* Sydenham's chorea, Saint Vitus' dance.

rheumatic fever An illness which arises as a complication of untreated or inadequately treated strep throat infection. Rheumatic fever can seriously damage the valves of the heart.

rheumatic heart disease A thickening and stenosis of one or more of the heart valves and often requires surgery to repair or replace the involved valve(s).

rheumatism 1) Any painful disorder of the joints or muscles or connective tissues 2) A chronic autoimmune disease with inflammation of the joints and marked deformities; something (possibly a virus) triggers an attack on the synovium by the immune system, which releases cytokines that stimulate an inflammatory reaction that can lead to the destruction of all components of the joint.

rheumatoid of or pertaining to arthritis.

rheumatoid arthritis Illness characterized by joint disease that involves muscles, cartilage and membrane linings of the joints. Symptoms include red, warm, painful joints. Sometimes accompanied by weakness and fatigue. If disease is severe, permanent deformity and crippling may result.

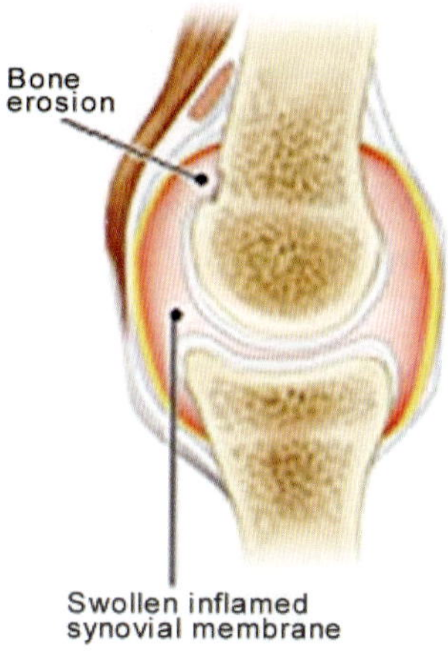

rheumatoid arthritis

rheumatoid factor test A laboratory test for rheumatoid factor used to diagnose rheumatoid arthritis.

RHF Right heart failure.

rh-factor Symbol for rhesus factor. Antigens present on the surface of red blood cells.

RHHI Regional Home Health Intermediary. Four fis nationally designated to process Medicare home health and hospice claims.

rhin(o)- of or pertaining to the nose.

rhinectomy The surgical removal of a nose. If only part of the nose is removed it is called a partial rhinectomy, while entire nose removal is called a total rhinectomy. Often, a nose prosthesis is required for rehabilitation.

rhinomanometry Technique for measuring air pressure and the rate of airflow in the nasal cavity during respiration.

rhinometry Diagnostic measurement of the nose and its cavity through acoustic reflections. Used to measure nasal anatomical landmarks, nasal septal deviation, and nasal airway changes in response to allergen provocation tests (nasal provocation tests).

rhinophototherapy A medical therapy for the treatment of allergic rhinitis and other nasal conditions using a device that emits a combination of ultraviolet A, ultraviolet B, and visible lights.

rhinophyma A descriptive term for a large, bulbous, ruddy appearance of the nose caused by granulomatous infiltration, commonly due to untreated rosacea.

rhinoplasty A plastic surgical operation on the nose, either reconstructive, restorative, or cosmetic.

rhinorrhea Persistent watery mucus discharge from the nose (as in the common cold).

rhinoscleroma A chronic granulomatous bacterial disease of the nose that can sometimes infect the upper respiratory tract.

rhinoscopy Examination of the nasal passages by means of a speculum or similar instrument.

rhinotomy Surgical procedure in which an incision is made in the nose to drain accumulated pus.

rhinovirus Any of a group of picornaviruses that are responsible for many upper respiratory infections.

rh-isoimmunization Development of agglutination against Rh-blood group antigens in an Rh-negative person in response to Rh-positive blood. It may lead to serious or fatal reactions to blood transfusion or development of erythroblastosis fetalis in the fetus of a subsequent pregnancy. *See* Agglutination; erythroblastosis fetalis.

rhizotomy Surgical procedure in which spinal nerve roots are cut; done (anterior roots) to relieve intractable pain or (posterior roots) to stop severe muscle spasms.

rhod(o)- Denoting a rose-red color.

rhytidectomy Plastic repair to remove wrinkles and other signs of aging from your face; an incision is made near the hair line and skin is pulled back and excess tissue is excised.

rhytidoplasty Plastic repair performed, usually by excision of skin, for the elimination of wrinkles from the skin.

RIA Radioimmunoassay.

Richardson hysterectomy Total abdominal hysterectomy.

rickets Condition caused by insufficient intake or absorption of vitamin D coupled with too little exposure to sunlight. Seen primarily in infants and small children. Characterized by abnormal bone formation. Symptoms include soft, pliable bones, enlarged skull, muscle pain and profuse sweating.

rickettsia A genus of bacteria carried as parasites by many ticks, fleas, and lice, and cause diseases such as typhus, rickettsialpox, Boutonneuse fever, African Tick Bite Fever, Rocky Mountain spotted fever, Australian Tick Typhus, Flinders Island Spotted Fever and Queensland Tick Typhus in human beings.

rickettsial disease Any disease caused by rickettsial micro-organisms. Transmitted to humans by bites from infected lice, fleas, ticks and mites. Rickettsial diseases have been responsible for some of the worst epidemics in history.

rickettsial-collagen disease Connective tissue disease caused by rickettsial germs.

rickettsiosis A disease caused by intracellular bacteria. Examples of rickettsioses include typhus, rocky mountain spotted fever, and rickettsialpox.

Ridell operation A rarely used surgical procedure for frontal sinus disease in which the entire anterior and inferior walls of the frontal sinus are removed.

rider An attachment, amendment or endorsement to an insurance policy.

righting reflex The assumption of an optimal body position after the patient has been moved from it.

rights of individuals Rights provided to individuals under HIPAA legislation include the right to; see and get a copy of health records, have corrections added to health information, receive a notice that explains how health information may be used and shared, grant permission before health information can be used or shared for certain purposes, get a report on when and why health information was shared for certain purposes, and the right to file complaints with providers, health insurers and/or the U.S. government.

Riley fusion Extensive anterior approach for fusion of C-1 to C-3 or lower.

ring-chromosome formation Chromosome in which both ends have been lost; broken ends have reunited to form a ring-shaped figure.

Rinne test A hearing test for conductive hearing loss that compares perception of sounds, as transmitted by air or by bone conduction through the mastoid.

Ripstein operation An operation used to treat rectal prolapse.

risk-adjustment The statistical adjustment of outcomes measures to account for risk factors that are independent of the quality of care provided and beyond the control of the plan or provider, such as the patient's gender and age, the seriousness of the patient's illness.

risk agreement Term used in the disability community to refer to a signed document by both an individual and a services provider that details the tasks that will be the responsibility of each party. In particular it refers to those services that the consumer does not choose to accept even though the service provider believes they are necessary.

risk-based health maintenance organization or competitive medical plan A type of managed care organization. After any applicable deductible or co-payment, all of an enrollee or member's medical care costs are paid for in return for a monthly premium. However, due to the lock-in provision, all of the enrollee or member's services (except for out-of-area emergency services) must be arranged for by the risk-HMO. Should the Medicare enrollee or member choose to obtain service not arranged for by the plan, he or she will be liable for the costs. Neither the HMO nor the Medicare program will pay for services from providers that are not part of the HMO's health care system or network.

risk contract A legal agreement between a payer and provider to share in either the net revenues after expenses or financial losses incurred as a result of providing health care services within a defined delivery system, such as an

HMO or PPO. A percentage of provider or professional payments that are withheld by the payer to satisfy the risk provisions at the end of the fiscal period.

risk factors Conditions that influence a person's health status and are capable of causing illness or injury, including genetic or biological risk factors, life style, or environmental conditions.

risk pool A distinct population group, such as employees of a company, insured against costs of their potential use of health care resources. Premium projections are based on variables such as the age of the covered population, health status, sex, occupation, group size, and location. Structure can provide positive incentives to the participants, such as sharing savings when expenses are below projections; sharing losses when actual expenses exceed budgeted expenses, or a combination of these. May also describe a financial arrangement among providers and payers to safeguard against unexpectedly high expenses or utilization.

Risser jacket A molded jacket used for the treatment of scoliosis or thoracolumbar fractures.

RIST Radioimmunosorbent test.

Ritter's disease A disease usually seen in infants where large areas of skin peel off, as in a second-degree burn, as a result of upper respiratory staphylococcal infection. *Synonym:* staphylococcal scalded skin syndrome, pemphigus neonatorum.

RLE Right lower extremity.

RLQ Right lower quadrant.

RLS Restless legs syndrome.

RNA Ribonucleic acid.

Roaf, Kirkaldy-Willis and Cattero procedure Drainage of a thoracic spinal abscess through dorsolateral approach.

rocky mountain spotted fever An infectious disease caused by bacteria carried by ticks. Symptoms include high fever, headache, body aches and skin rash. The tongue is covered with a thick, white coating that turns brown as the fever persists and rises.

rod cells One type of specialized light sensitive cells (photoreceptors) in the retina that provide side vision and the ability to see objects in dim light (night vision).

roentgenography Photography with the use of x-rays.

Rogozinki instrumentation Combined anteroposterior device used in correction of spinal deformities.

rollover test Comparison of the blood pressure of a pregnant woman lying on her back versus on her side; an excessive increase when she rolls to the supine position indicates increased risk of preeclampsia.

ROM Range of motion.

Romanowsky-type stains Blood smear dyes having modified mixtures of eosin and methylene blue. Wright's and Giemsa's stains are examples of these types of blood smear stains.

Romberg's sign Swaying of the body or falling when the eyes are closed with the feet placed close together.

root The part of the tooth below the crown, normally encased in the jawbone. It is made up of dentin, includes the root canal, and is covered by cementum.

root canal The hollow part of the tooth's root; it runs from the tip of the root into the pulp.

root canal Therapy The process of removing the pulp of a tooth and filling it with an inert material.

root planing The process of scaling and planing exposed root surfaces to remove all calculus, plaque, and infected tissue.

root resection The removal of a portion of diseased root structure, but retaining the remaining natural tooth.

Rorschach test An association technique for personality testing based on the patient's response to a series of inkblot designs.

rosacea A skin disease of unknown causes that causes an array of symptoms, including redness and puffiness on several areas of the face, including the cheeks and nose.

Ross procedure A type of specialized aortic valve surgery where the patient's diseased aortic valve is replaced with his or her own pulmonary valve.

roster billing Simplified billing process used when a provider accepts assignment and bills for mass immunizations.

rotator cuff The group of muscles and their tendons that act to stabilize the shoulder.

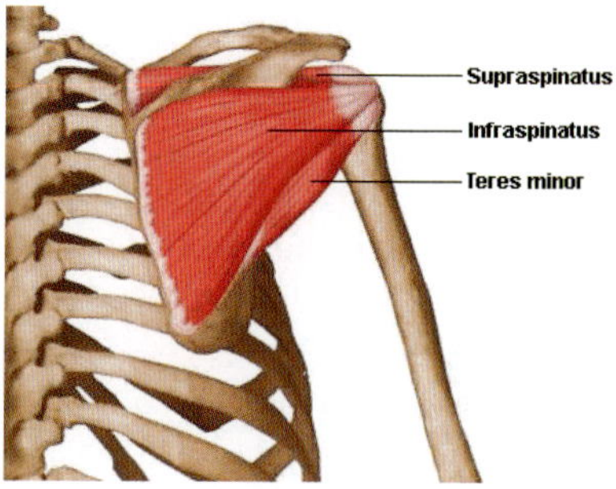

rotator cuff

rotavirus A virus that is the leading single cause of severe diarrhea among infants and young children, and is one of several viruses that cause infections commonly known as stomach flu.

Roux-en-y anastomosis Y-shaped anastomosis which includes the small intestine.

Roy-Camille fusion Posterior bone graft with wire and parallel vertical screw plate fixation from occiput to C-3.

Roy-Camille instrumentation Posterior pedicle screw and plate device for spinal stabilization.

-rrhage Burst forth.

-rrhagia Rapid flow of blood.

-rrhaphy Surgical suturing.

-rrhea Flowing, discharge.

-rrhexis Rupture.

RSV Respiratory syncytial virus.

rubella A highly contagious viral disease. The symptoms include swollen glands, joint pain, low fever, and a fine red rash. *Synonym:* german measles.

rubeola An acute and highly contagious viral disease marked by distinct red spots followed by a rash; occurs primarily in children. *Synonym:* measles.

Rubin's test A test for patency of the uterine tubes, performed by transuterine inflation with carbon dioxide gas.

rubr(o)- of or pertaining to the red nucleus of the brain.

RUG Resource utilization group.

rule out Refers to a method used to indicate that a condition is probable, suspected or questionable but unconfirmed.

rupture State of being torn or burst open.

RUQ Right upper quadrant.

rural health clinic An outpatient facility that is primarily engaged in furnishing physicians' and other medical and health services and that meets other requirements designated to ensure the health and safety of individuals served by the clinic. The clinic must be located in a medically under-served area that is not urbanized as defined by the U.S. Bureau of Census.

rural health services Health services, public or private, in rural areas. The services include the promotion of health and the delivery of health care.

RVU Relative value unit.

RW Relative weight.

RX Prescription.

S

s/p Status post.

Sabin vaccine Live oral attenuated poliovirus vaccine.

SACH Solid ankle, cushion heel (foot prosthesis).

sacral of or relating to or near the sacrum.

sacroiliac joint The joint between the sacrum, at the base of the spine and the ilium of the pelvis, which are joined by ligaments.

sacroiliitis An inflammation of the sacroiliac joint.

sacrospinous Pertaining to the sacrum and the spine of the ischium.

sacrum Wedge-shaped bone consisting of five fused vertebrae forming the posterior part of the pelvis; its base connects with the lowest lumbar vertebra and its tip with the coccyx.

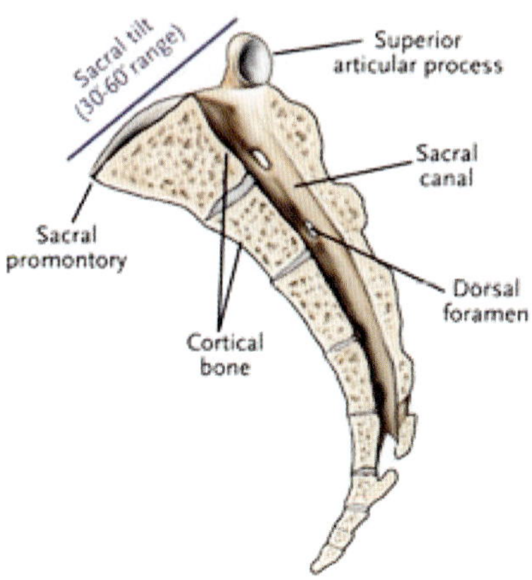

sacrum

SAD Seasonal affective disorder.

SADMERC Statistical analysis durable medical equipment regional carrier.

SAECG Signal-averaged electrocardiogram.

Saemisch's operation Transfixion of the cornea and of the base of the ulcer for cure of hypopyon.

sagittal Refers to a lengthwise cut that divides the body into right and left portions.

SAID Sexually acquired immunodeficiency syndrome.

salabrasion A technique in which salt or a salt solution is used to abrade the skin, for example to remove the pigment from a tattoo or permanent makeup.

saline A solution comprised primarily of salt water.

saline infusion The intravenous infusion of a sterile solution of sodium chloride (salt) in water.

saliva A clear lubricating fluid in the mouth containing water, enzymes, bacteria, mucus, viruses, blood cells and undigested food particles.

saliva ejector A suction tube placed in the mouth to remove saliva.

salivary duct Tube through which saliva is carried from the salivary gland to the mouth.

salivary gland A gland that secretes saliva, especially any of three pairs of large glands, the parotid, submaxillary, and sublingual, whose secretions enter the mouth and mingle in saliva.

salivary-gland disease Disease of the salivary glands, which secrete saliva.

Salk vaccine Original poliovirus vaccine containing inactivated strains of the poliomyelitis virus.

sallowness A term used to describe a yellowish color of the skin.

salmonella Thousands of kinds of salmonella bacteria cause many diseases, including typhoid fever, paratyphoid fever and some forms of gastroenteritis (inflammation of the stomach and intestines).

salmonellosis An infection with salmonella bacteria. Most persons infected with salmonella develop diarrhea, fever, vomiting, and abdominal cramps.

salping(o)- of or pertaining to the fallopian tubes.

salpingectomy The removal of one or both of the fallopian tubes.

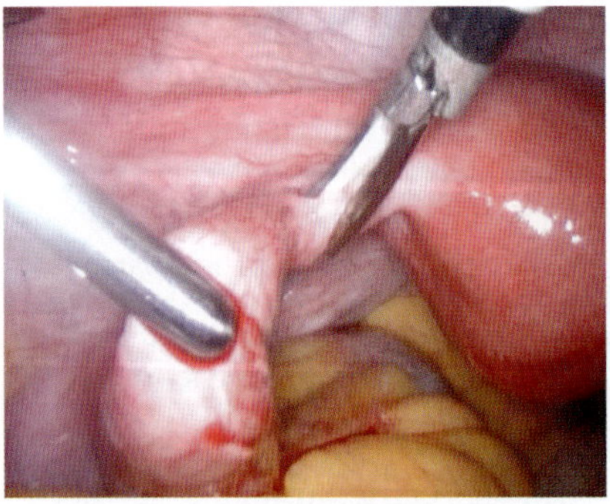

salpingectomy

salpingitis Inflammation of a Fallopian tube (usually the result of infection spreading from the vagina or uterus) or of a Eustachian tube.

salpingolysis Surgical separation of adhesions involving the Fallopian tubes.

salpingo-oophorectomy Removal of the fallopian tubes and ovaries.

salpingostomy Formation of an artificial opening in a fallopian tube.

salplingoplasty Plastic repair of a Fallopian tube.

salter osteotomy A procedure for the treatment of developmental dysplasia of the hip in children.

salt-losing syndrome Condition characterized by vomiting, dehydration, abnormally low blood pressure and even sudden death due to very large sodium losses from the body. Can occur due to large sodium loss from the gastrointestinal tract or from excessive sodium loss into the urine (as in congenital adrenal hyperplasia or adrenocortical insufficiency). *See* Adrenal hyperplasia.

sanctions Administrative remedies and actions (exclusion or civil monetary penalties) available to the Office of the Inspector General (OIG) to deal with questionable, improper, or abusive behaviors of providers under the Medicare, Medicaid, or any state health programs.

Sandhoff's disease Variant of Tay-Sachs disease that has a progressive, more rapid course. Found in the general population. Tay-Sachs disease usually only affects Ashkenazic Jewish infants. *See* Tay-Sachs disease.

sangui-, sanguine- of or pertaining to blood.

saphenous vein Vein on the inside of the leg running from the ankle to the groin can be used to make bypasses from the aorta to the coronary arteries.

sarco- Muscular, flesh like.

sarcoidosis A disease of unknown origin that causes small lumps (granulomas) due to chronic inflammation to develop in a great range of body tissues. Sarcoidosis can appear in almost any body organ, but most often starts in the lungs or lymph nodes.

sarcoma Tumor derived from connective tissue.

SARS Severe acute respiratory syndrome.

saucerization Excavation of tissue to form a shallow depression, performed in wound treatment to facilitate drainage from infected areas. *Synonym:* craterization.

Saundby's test A test for blood in the stool.

SBO Small bowel obstruction.

scabies A contagious ectoparasite skin infection characterized by superficial burrows and intense pruritus (itching). It is caused by the mite sarcoptes scabiei.

scalenotomy Surgical division or section of the anterior scalene muscle.

scaling Removing plaque, calculus, and stain from teeth.

scalp The skin that covers the top of the head.

scan The data or image obtained from the examination of organs or regions of the body by gathering information with a sensing device.

scanogram A radiographic technique for showing true dimensions by moving a beam of x-rays along the length of the structure being measured, fro example, the lower extremities.

scaphoid bone The largest wrist bone on the thumb side.

scapula Either of two flat triangular bones one on each side of the shoulder in human beings.

scapular Relating to or near the shoulder blade.

scapulopexy Surgical fixation of the scapula.

scarlatina Childhood disorder characterized by a bright-red rash. Scarlet fever is preceded by a streptococcal throat infection. Both are very contagious. *Synonym:* scarlet fever.

scarlet fever *See* scarlatina.

Schanz operation Osteotomy of the proximal femur.

Schauta operation Total removal of the uterus and the adnexa using a vaginal approach.

Schede procedure Surgical removal of part of the ribs to cause the collapse of a diseased lung. *Synonym:* thoracoplasty.

schedule of allowances A list of specific amounts which the carrier will pay toward the cost of medical services provided.

schedule of benefits and exclusions A health insurance listing of the benefits which are covered under the policy guidelines as well as services which are not provided under the policy.

Scheie procedure Surgical procedure for the treatment of aphakic glaucoma.

Scheuermann's disease Inflammation of the anterior cartilage of the thoracic and lumbar spine.

sciatica A lay term indicating pain along the course of a sciatic nerve, especially noted in the back of the thigh and below the knee.

Schick test An intradermal test for determination of susceptibility to diphtheria.

Schiller's test A test for early squamous cell carcinoma of the cervix, performed by painting the uterine cervix with a solution of iodine and potassium iodide, diseased areas being revealed by a failure to take the stain.

Schilling test A diagnostic test in which vitamin B12 is tagged with radioactive cobalt, taken orally, and gastrointestinal absorption is determined via measurement of the amount of radioactivity in a 24-hour urine collection.

Schirmer's test A test of tear production in keratoconjunctivitis sicca, performed by measuring the area of moisture on a piece of filter paper inserted over the conjunctival sac of the lower lid, with the end of the paper hanging down on the outside.

schist(o)- Split, cleft.

schistosomiasis A parasitic disease caused by several species of fluke of the genus schistosoma. Schistosomiasis often is a chronic illness that can damage internal organs and, in children, impair growth and cognitive development. *Synonym:* bilharzia, bilharziasis, snail fever.

schiz(o)- Denoting something 'split' or 'double-sided'.

schizoid personality disorder A personality disorder manifested by a profound defect in the ability to form social relationships, no desire for social involvement, and an indifference to praise or criticism.

schizophrenia A severe emotional disorder of psychotic depth characteristically marked by a retreat from reality with delusion formation, hallucinations, emotional disharmony, and regressive behavior.

schizophrenic of or relating to or characteristic of schizophrenia.

Schlatter's operation Gastrectomy with end-to-side oesophagus jejunostomy.

Schlemm's canal The passageway for the aqueous fluid to leave the eye.

Schlicter test A test that measures the activity of the patient's serum against an infecting pathogen.

Schmorl's nodes Protrusions of the cartilage of the intervertebral disc through the vertebral body endplate and into the adjacent vertebra.

Schocket procedure Anterior chamber tube shunt to an encircling band for treatment of refractory glaucoma.

Scholiner costoplasty Multiple rib partial excisions for rib deformity.

SCHP State child health plan.

Schwabach's test A hearing test made, with the opposite ear masked, placing the stems of vibrating tuning forks on the mastoid process first of the patient and then of the examiner.

sciatic nerve The longest nerve in the body, arising from the sacral plexus and passing about halfway down the thigh where it divides into the common peroneal and tibial nerves.

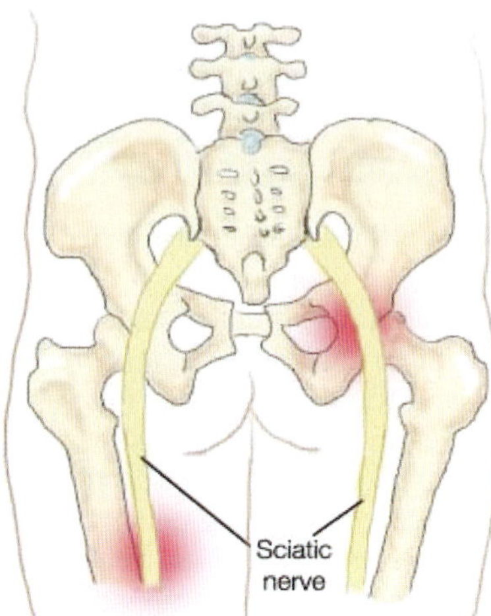

sciatic nerves

sciatica Neuralgia along the sciatic nerve.

scintigraphy A diagnostic test in which a two-dimensional picture of a body radiation source is obtained through the use of radioisotopes.

scler(o)- Hardness.

sclera Whitish fibrous membrane (albuginea) that with the cornea forms the outer covering of the eyeball.

scleral buckling An operation for retinal detachment which reduces the size of the globe by indenting the sclera so that it approximates the retina.

sclerectoiridectomy Excision of a portion of the sclera and the iris in the treatment of glaucoma.

sclerectomy Excision of part of the sclera.

scleritis Inflammation of the sclera.

scleroderma Widespread connective tissue disease in which skin and other body parts gradually degenerate, thicken and become stiff.

scleroplasty Plastic repair of the sclera. This procedure is used frequently to prevent blindness and poor vision in children with myopia.

sclerosing agent Chemical agents injected into veins to cause localized thrombosis and eventual fibrosis and obliteration of the vessels. They are used in the treatment of varicose veins, hemorrhoids, gastric and esophageal varices, and peptic ulcer hemorrhage.

sclerosing cholangitis Scarring and inflammation of a bile duct.

sclerosis Localized hardening of skin.

sclerotherapy A medical procedure used to eliminate varicose veins and spider veins. During the procedure, an injection of a solution (generally sodium chloride) in placed directly into the vein.

sclerotomy Surgical incision of the sclerotic coat of the eye.

scoli(o)- Twisted.

scoliosis Abnormal curving of the spine, especially in a lateral direction. *Synonym:* curvature of the spine.

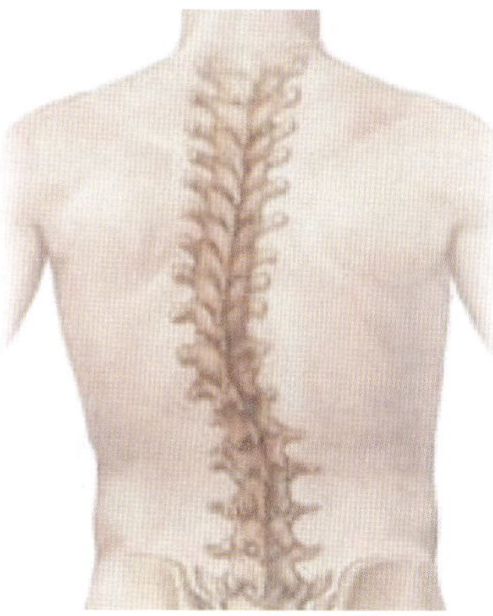

scoliosis

-scope Instrument for viewing.

Scope of **Benefits or Coverage** Refers to the range of services, providers, and settings covered by a health benefit plan.

-scopy Use of instrument for viewing.

scotoma Area of depressed or decreased vision in the visual field that is surrounded by an area of normal (or less depressed) vision.

Scott procedure Use of cross-wire fixation transverse process to inferior pedicle in stabilization of spondylolysis fusion.

scratch test A skin test in which the antigen is applied to a superficial scratch.

screening Screening is the testing for disease or disease precursors in seemingly well individuals so that early detection and treatment can be provided for those who test positive for the disease.

screening tests blood tests used to try to detect a disease when there is little or no evidence of a suspected disease.

Scribner cannulization Insertion of a cannula for prolonged hemodialysis.

scrotal of or referring to the scrotum.

scrotoplasty Reparative or plastic repair of the scrotum. *Synonym:* oscheoplasty.

scrotum The external pouch that contains the testes.

SCU Special care unit.

scurvy Illness caused by inadequate intake of vitamin C. Symptoms in children may include tender, swollen legs, bleeding and bruising under the skin, bleeding gums, fever and anemia. Adults may have swollen, bleeding gums, tooth loss, bleeding or bruising under the skin or bleeding into joints, weakness and mental changes. *Synonym:* Vitamin C deficiency.

sealants Thin resin material bonded in the pits and fissures of back teeth for the prevention of decay.

sebaceous cyst A common cyst of the skin; filled with fatty matter (sebum) secreted by a sebaceous gland that has been blocked.

sebaceous glands Are microscopic glands in the skin which secrete an oily matter (sebum) in the hair follicles to lubricate the skin and hair.

seborrhea A condition in which overactivity of the sebaceous glands causes the skin to become oily.

seborrheic dermatitis Skin condition characterized by greasy or dry, white scales. Dandruff and cradle cap are both forms of seborrheic dermatitis. Not contagious.

second degree burn A burn that manifests as erythema with superficial blistering of the skin, which may involve more or less pain depending on the level of nerve involvement. Second-degree burns involve the superficial (papillary) dermis and may also involve the deep (reticular) dermis layer.

second opinion A medical opinion provided by a second physician or medical expert, when one physician provides a diagnosis or recommends surgery to an individ-ual. Individuals are encouraged to obtain second opinions whenever a physician recommends surgery or presents an individual with a serious medical diagnosis.

second opinion program Voluntary or mandatory medical or surgical review program established by a health benefit program to ensure the medical necessity of proposed services or procedures. The second opinion is paid for by the plan and provided by a physician other than the professional recommending the treatment. Payment for care is usually assured under the benefit program regardless of the second opinion recommendation if the patient obtains the second opinion in accordance with the health benefit requirements. Coverage limitations may be imposed upon beneficiaries not complying with mandatory programs. Second opinion programs may be required for inpatient and for ambulatory services and procedures. These programs may be considered a cost containment mechanism as well as a means to help ensure the medical necessity of proposed services.

second-look surgery A followup operation to examine the outcome of the previous surgery and other treatments, such as chemotherapy or radiation therapy.

secondary carrier The health insurance carrier which is second in responsibility under Coordination of Benefits.

secondary care Services provided by medical specialists, such as cardiologists, urologists and dermatologists, who generally do not have first contact with patients.

secondary code ICD-9-CM code(s) listed after the primary code that further indicate the cause(s) for the current encounter or define the need for higher levels of care.

secondary coverage The plan that has the responsibility for payment of any eligible charges not covered by the primary coverage.

secondary diagnosis ICD-9-CM code(s) that define(s) illnesses, injuries or ill-defined conditions that are secondary to the patient's primary diagnosis.

secondary hypertension A type of hypertension caused by an identifiable underlying secondary cause.

secondary hypothyroidism Low thyroid function from drugs or other cause.

secondary lymphedema Swelling of a body part due to the accumulation of fluid caused by inflammation, obstruction or removal of lymph vessels. May follow mastectomy surgery when breast tissue and lymph vessels are removed. Obstruction of lymph vessels may be caused by malignant tumors or infestation with adult filarial parasites. *See* Filariasis.

secondary payer An insurance policy, plan, or program that pays second on a claim for medical care. This could be Medicare, Medicaid, or other insurance depending on the situation.

secondary syphilis Second stage of syphilis, characterized by skin rash, fever, swollen glands and headache. *See* Syphilis.

section The process of cutting, or dividing into parts.

sections Refers to portions of the Tabular List of ICD-9-CM that are organized in groups of three-digit code numbers. For example, Malignant Neoplasm of Lip, Oral Cavity and Pharynx (140-149).

security [HIPAA] Security encompasses all of the safeguards in an information system, including hardware, software, personnel policies, information practice policies, disaster preparedness, and the oversight of all these areas. The purpose of security is to protect both the system and the information it contains from unauthorized access from without and from misuse from within. Through various security measures, a health information system can shield confidential information from unauthorized access, disclosure and misuse, thus protecting privacy of the individuals who are the subjects of the stored data.

sed rate (Erythrocyte) sedimentation rate.

sedation 1) A state of reduced excitement or anxiety that is induced by the administrative of a sedative agent 2) The administration of a sedative agent or drug.

sedative A drug that reduces excitability and calms a person.

Seddon procedure Drainage of thoracic spinal abscess through anterolateral approach with partial resection of rib.

Seddon-Brookes procedure Tenoplasty with muscle transfer elbow to shoulder.

sedimentation rate A nonspecific measure of inflammatory response anywhere in the body; this test is elevated (above the normal range) in infections and a wide variety of so-called inflammatory diseases. *Synonym:* sed rate.

SEG Sonoencephalogram, sono-encephalography.

segment Under HIPAA, this is a group of related data elements in a transaction.

segmentectomy A surgical procedure to remove part of an organ or gland. It may also be used to remove a tumor and normal tissue around it. In lung cancer surgery, segmental resection refers to removing a section of a lobe of the lung. *Synonym:* segmental resection.

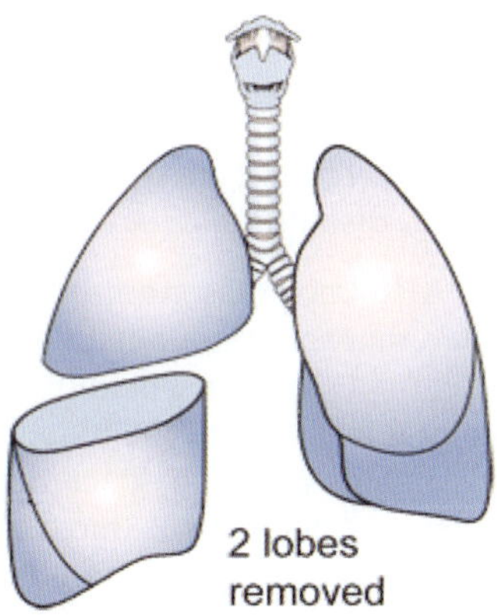

segmentectomy with removal of two lobes

Seidlitz powder test A diagnostic procedure for diaphragmatic hernia.

seizure Uncontrolled electrical activity in the brain, which may produce a physical convulsion, minor physical signs, thought disturbances, or a combination of symptoms.

seizure disorders One of a great many medical conditions that are characterized by episodes of uncontrolled electrical activity in the brain (seizures). Some seizure disorders are hereditary, but others are caused by birth defects or environmental hazards, such as lead poisoning.

self-administered plan Health benefit plan administered by the employer or health and welfare fund rather than through an insurance carrier or third party administrator.

self dialysis Dialysis performed with little or no professional assistance (except in emergency situations) by an ESRD patient who has completed an appropriate course of training, in a dialysis facility or at home.

self-funding Often confused with self-insurance, a self-funded health care plan is funded entirely by the employer. A self-funded plan may be self-administered, or the employer may contract with an outside administrator for an administrative services only arrangement. Self-funded plans obtain stop-loss insurance to cover catastrophic illnesses.

self-insured Employers who assume direct responsibility or risk for paying for employees' health care without purchasing health insurance. They usually contract with an outside firm to handle claims payment and/or utilization review.

self referral Arrangements for care beyond primary care made by the patient rather than the provider. HMOs generally specify to which in-house departments or services a patient may self refer. Physicians self-referral is when providers refer patients to a facility in which they have a vested interest.

sella turcica Depression in the floor of the skull that contains the pituitary gland.

semi- One-half, partly.

seminal vesicles A pair of simple tubular glands posteroinferior to the urinary bladder of males. The seminal vesicles secrete a significant proportion of the fluid that ultimately becomes semen.

Sengstaaken tamponade Esophagogastric tamponade with balloon.

senile Mentally or physically infirm with age.

senile aortic calcification As some individuals get older, calcium may accumulate on the leaflets of the aortic valve. The normal functioning of the valve requires that the leaflets open and close completely. When this calcium accumulates, the leaflets can no longer function normally.

senile dementia A progressive, abnormally accelerated deterioration of mental faculties and emotional stability in old age.

senility A progressive decline in mental functioning that is a part of the aging process.

sensorineural deafness Loss of hearing due to a lesion in the acoustic nerve (the eighth cranial nerve).

sentinel event An adverse health event that may have been avoided through appropriate care or alternative interventions. Providers are required to alert JCAHO and often state licensing authorities of all sentinel events, including a review of risk factors, preventative measures and case analysis.

SEP Sensory evoked potential.

separate procedure A procedure or service that is normally performed as an integral component of a total service or procedure. CPT codes identified as separate procedure codes should not be coded in addition to the basic procedure code.

separation The process of disconnecting, disuniting, or severing.

sepsis Also known as gram-negative bacteremia and gram-positive bacteremia. An overwhelming bacterial infection of the blood and body organs caused by bacteria that has entered body tissue, most often through a wound or incision, that leads to the formation of pus, and/or to the spread of the bacteria throughout the blood stream.

septal of or relating to a septum.

septal defects Abnormal, usually congenital, defect in the wall separating two chambers of the heart.

septectomy Surgical excision of a septum or part of a septum, especially the nasal or atrial septum.

septic Containing or resulting from disease-causing organisms.

septic arterial embolism A sudden interruption in arterial blood flow to an organ or body extremity. The blockage is caused by a bacterial infection in the bloodstream.

septic arthritis Infection in any joint in the body. *See* Arthritis.

septicemia A systemic illness with toxicity due to invasion of the bloodstream by virulent bacteria coming from a local seat of infect- ion. The symptoms of chills, fever and exhaustion are caused by the bacteria and substances they produce. *Synonym:* blood poisoning.

septoplasty A corrective surgical procedure done to straighten the nasal septum.

septostomy Surgical creation of an opening in a septum.

septum A dividing partition between two tissues or cavities.

sequencing The process of listing procedure and/or diagnosis codes in the proper order on the health insurance claim form.

sequestrectomy Excision of a sequestrum, a piece of dead bone separated from sound bone.

serial tonometry Multiple determinations of intraocular pressure over an extended period of time.

serialography Serial radiography.

sero Serology.

serologic tests Diagnostic procedures involving immunoglobulin reactions.

seroma A pocket of clear serous fluid that sometimes develops in the body after surgery.

serous of or producing or containing serum.

serum Liquid portion of the blood that remains after blood cells have been removed.

serum sickness Hypersensitivity reaction following administration of an antiserum. Characterized by fever, hives, swollen lymph glands, joint pain and enlarged spleen.

service area The area where a health plan accepts members. For HMOs, it is also the area where services are provided. A health plan may terminate coverage for persons who move out of the plan's service area.

service guideline A type of practice guideline that presents the appropriate and inappropriate indications for the use of particular diagnostic and therapeutic procedures.

service substitution Use of lower cost, but still effective, service in place of a higher cost service.

sesamoid bone A bone embedded within a tendon. Sesamoid bones are typically found in locations where a tendon passes over a joint, such as the hand, knee, and foot. Functionally, they act to protect the tendon and to increase its mechanical effect.

sesamoidectomy Surgical removal of a sesamoid bone.

seton Material such as thread, wire, or gauze that is passed through subcutaneous tissues or through a cyst in order to form a sinus or fistula.

seton procedure A procedure in which a cord is run through a fistula tract. The procedure allows the fistula to continue to drain while it is healing.

severe acute respiratory syndrome A respiratory disease in humans which is caused by the SARS coronavirus.

severity modifier An adjustment that reflects the effect of patient factors, such as severity of illness, comorbidity, or risk of complications, on the relative work required to deliver a service.

sexual and gender disorders Mental disorders related to sexual dysfunction, paraphilias, and gender identity disorders.

sexual precocity Attainment of sexual maturity before the 6th birthday in girls and the 8th birthday in boys. This is an abnormal condition. Sexual development follows the usual pattern of normal puberty except the child's psychological sexuality is not mature. Cause is usually unknown. Sometimes caused by tumors of the hypothalamus or pineal gland. Other causes include Albright syndrome and untreated juvenile hypothyroidism.

SGGT Serum gamma-glutamyl-transferase.

SGOT Serum glutamic-pyruvic transaminase.

SGOT, SGPT Liver enzymes. Elevated for a variety of reasons. Checked for suspected liver disease, also for suspected mononucleosis, or to monitor the effect of long term drug therapy on the liver.

SGPT A test of serum glutamic pyruvic transaminase, an enzyme that is normally present in liver and heart cells. Elevated sgpt indicate heart or liver damage.

shared risk An arrangement in which financial liabilities are apportioned among two or more entities. For example, an HMO and the medical group may each agree to share the risk of excessive hospital cost over budgeted amounts on a 50/50 basis.

shared savings A provision of most prepaid health care plans where at least part of the providers' income is directly linked to the financial performance of the plan. If costs are lower than projections, a percentage of these savings are referred to the providers.

SHI Supplemental health insurance.

shigella A genus of bacteria that causes shigellosis.

shigellosis A food borne illness caused by infection by bacteria of the genus shigella. *Synonym:* bacillary dysentery.

Shilling test For vitamin B12 in the diagnosis of pernicious anemia. In injury cases, pernicious anemia is a variable that may be a non-proximate cause of degeneration of the brain and spinal cord.

Shirodkar's operation An operation for incompetent cervix in which the cervical os is closed with a surrounding purse-string suture. *Synonym:* cervical cerclage, cervical stitch.

short-term disability An injury or illness that keeps a person from working for a short time. The definition of short-term disability (and the time period over which coverage extends) differs among insurance companies and employers. Short-term disability insurance coverage is designed to protect an individual's full or partial wages during a time of injury or illness (that is not work-related) that would prohibit the individual from working.

short-term medical insurance Temporary major medical coverage designed to fill gaps in traditional medical coverage. Short-term plans typically last no longer than one year and cannot be renewed.

shoulder The part of the body between the neck and the upper arm.

shunt A hole or passage which moves, or allows movement of fluid from one part of the body to another.

shuntogram A radiographic method to evaluate the function and patency of a ventriculoperitoneal or ventriculoatrial shunt.

Shy-Dager syndrome Chronic idiopathic orthostatic hypotension.

sial(o)- Saliva, salivary gland.

sialoadenitis An infection of the salivary gland or the salivary duct.

sialodochoplasty Plastic repair of a salivary duct.

sialogram An x-ray of the salivary ducts and glands.

sialography The radiographic examination of the salivary glands. *Synonym:* radiosialography.

sialolithiasis The formation of stones in the salivary glands.

sialolithotomy Removal of calculus from a salivary gland or duct.

sickle cell anemia *See* Anemia, sickle cell.

sickle cell disease A disease in which the affected person makes an abnormal hemoglobin. Sickle cell disease is inherited.

sickle cell trait Anemia and other signs of sickle cell anemia do not occur in the person with sickle cell trait. People who have the trait are informed and counseled regarding the possibility of having an infant with sickle cell disease if both parents carry the trait. *See* Anemia, sickle cell.

sickling test One for demonstration of abnormal hemoglobin and the sickling phenomenon in erythrocytes.

SICU Surgical intensive-care unit.

side effect A problem caused by treatment. For example, medicine taken for high blood pressure may cause drowsiness. Most treatments have side effects.

SIDS Sudden infant death syndrome.

sigmoid colon Portion of the large intestine located in the left side of the abdomen. It connects to the descending colon above and the rectum below.

sigmoid torsion Twisting of the sigmoid portion of the large intestine.

sigmoid(o)- Sigmoid, sigmoid colon.

sigmoidoscopy Minimally invasive procedure for examining the large intestine from the rectum through the last part of the colon.

Simmons fusion Use of keystone-shaped graft in anterior fusion.

Simmons procedure Posterior osteotomy.

simple and unspecified goiter A simple enlargement of the thyroid gland, causing a swelling in the front part of the neck.

simple fractures Are fractures that occur along one line, splitting the bone into two pieces.

sin Without (sine).

single payer A proposed Federally sponsored universal health insurance coverage to all Americans. Employers would not be required to offer health insurance to their employees. Health insurance companies would not exist in the same capacity as they do today. The Government would establish payment rates for physicians, hospitals and other medical services.

single-vessel disease Disease involving only one of the coronary artery vessels. *See* Coronary artery disease.

sinistr(o)- Left, left side.

sinoatrial node The normal pacemaker for the heart is an area of specialized cells in the atrium called the sinoatrial or SA node. These cells automatically send out an electrical impulse to the rest of the heart telling it to contract.

sinogram A special x-ray procedure that is done with contrast media to visualize any abnormal opening (sinus) in the body.

sinus 1. A pouch or cavity in any organ or tissue, especially the paranasal sinus. 2. An abnormal cavity or passage such as a fistula, caused by the destruction of tissue.

sinus- of or pertaining to the sinus.

sinus of valsalva One of the anatomic dilations of the ascending aorta, which occurs just above the aortic valve.

sinus rhythm The normal rhythm of the heart originates in the sinoatrial node. It is called sinus rhythm.

sinusectomy Surgical removal of a sinus.

sinusitis Inflammation or infection of the sinuses. Usually refers to the eight sinuses adjacent to the nose.

sinusoid Any of the venous cavities through which blood passes in various glands and organs, such as the adrenal gland and the liver.

sinusoscopy Nasal or sinus endoscopy that includes puncture or cannulation to access the maxillary or sphenoid sinus cavities.

sinusotomy Incision into a sinus.

SIRS Systemic inflammatory response syndrome.

-sis Condition of.

SISI Short (small)-increment sensitivity index.

SISI test A hearing test used to determine differential sensitivity to changes in loudness.

site appropriateness listings A resource for the review of surgery and certain nonsurgical interventions that indicates the most appropriate settings for common procedures.

site-of-service differential The difference in the amount paid when the same service is performed in different practice settings, for example, an outpatient visit in a physician's office or a hospital clinic.

sito- Food, grain.

six-year Molar The first permanent tooth to erupt, usually between the ages of five and six.

Sjogren's syndrome Benign, chronic inflammation that results in diminished production of tears and saliva. Cause is unknown, but it is usually associated with rheumatoid arthritis or collagen vascular disease.

skeletal of or relating to or forming or attached to a skeleton.

skeletal fixation Stabilization of fractures using an external frame connected by rods, wires, nuts and bolts.

skeleton The hard structure (bones and cartilages) that provides a frame for the body.

Skene's glands Glands located on the anterior wall of the vagina, around the lower end of the urethra.

skilled care That level of care which requires the training and skills of a Registered Nurse; and is prescribed by a doctor for the medical care of the patient; and may not be provided by less skilled or less intensive care, such as custodial care or intermediate care.

Skilled Nursing Facility (SNF) A facility (which meets specific regulatory certification requiremints) which primarily provides inpatient skilled nursing care and related services to patients who require medical, nursing, or rehabilitative services but does not provide the level of care or treatment available in a hospital.

skin flap A mass of tissue for grafting, usually including skin, only partially removed from one part of the body so that it retains its own blood supply during transfer to another site.

skin graft A patch of skin that is surgically removed from one area of the body and transplanted to another one.

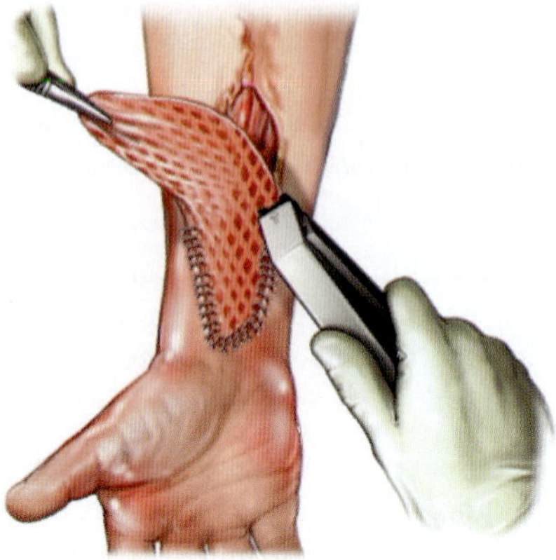

Skin graft.

skin lesion A superficial growth or patch of the skin that does not resemble the area surrounding it. They may take the form of bumps, blisters, or general sores. While many are benign (such as moles or freckles) some are the result of toxins (such as mosquito bites) or diseases (such as chicken pox or psoriasis).

skin tags A small benign tumor that forms primarily in areas where the skin forms creases, such as the neck, armpit, and groin. They may also occur on the face, usually on the eyelids.

skin test Any test in which an antigen is applied to the skin in order to observe the patient's reaction; used to determine exposure or immunity to infectious diseases, to identify allergens producing allergic reactions, and to assess ability to mount a cellular immunization program.

sleep apnea A cessation of airflow for at least 10 seconds. These cessations of breathing may be due to either an occlusion of the airway (obstructive sleep apnea), absence of respiratory effort (central sleep apnea), or a combination of these factors.

sleep study *See* polysomnography.

slit lamp A microscope using various magnifications combined with a strong light that can be focused into a slit for examining the eye.

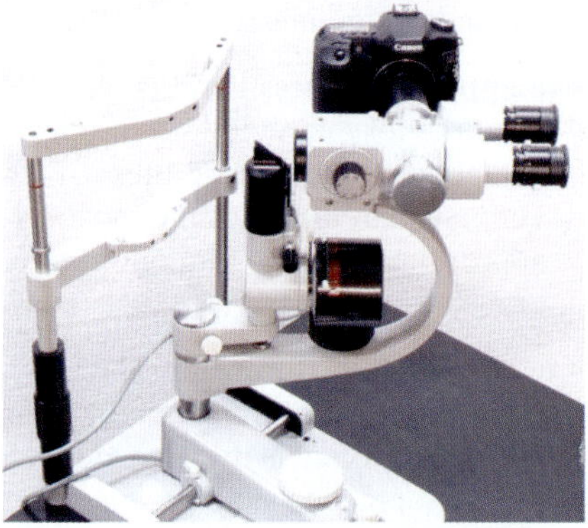

slit lamp

small cell lung cancer A disease in which malignant (cancer) cells form in the tissues of the lung. Small cell lung cancer is not commonly treated with surgery; radiation and chemotherapy are used instead.

Small Employer Health Insurance Availability Act In 1994 the General Assembly enacted modifications to the act expanding its scope to firms with 1-50 employees (previously 2-25 employees).

smallpox A highly contagious and frequently fatal viral disease characterized by a biphasic fever and a distinctive skin rash that left pock marks in its wake. The disease is caused by the variola virus. *Synonym:* variola.

SMD Senile macular degeneration.

SMI Supplementary Medical Insurance. Medicare Part B which helps pay for services other than hospital (Part A) services.

SMI premium Monthly premium paid by those individuals who have enrolled in the voluntary SMI program.

Smith fracture A fracture of the distal radius caused by falling onto flexed wrists. *Synonym:* reverse colles' fracture.

Smith Peterson procedure Lumbar spine osteotomy for correction of kyphotic deformity in ankylosing spondylitis.

Smith-Boyce operation Anatrophic nephrotomy.

Smith-Robinson operation Interbody spinal fusion through an anterior cervical approach.

Snellen chart One of several charts used to test vision. Letters, numbers or symbols are arranged on the chart in decreasing size from top to bottom.

SNF Skilled nursing facility.

SNF coinsurance For the 21st through 100th day of extended care services in a benefit period, a daily amount for which the beneficiary is responsible, equal to one-eighth of the inpatient hospital deductible.

SNOMED Standardized Nomenclature of Pathology.

snout reflex Similar to the Glabella, the patient is tapped lightly on the nose. Excessive grimace of the face is a positive sign and may be due to a brainstem lesion.

SOAP Subjective, Objective, Assessment, Plan (problem-oriented record).

SOB Shortness of breath.

SOC Standard of care.

social health maintenance organization A special type of health plan that provides the full range of Medicare benefits offered by standard Medicare HMOs, plus other services that include the following prescription drug and chronic care benefits, respite care, and short-term nursing home care; homemaker, personal care services, and medical transportation; eyeglasses, hearing aids, and dental benefits.

Social Security Act Public Law 74-271, enacted on August 14, 1935, with subsequent amendments. The Social Security Act consists of 20 titles, four of which have been repealed. The HI and SMI programs are authorized by Title XVIII of the Social Security Act.

Social Security Administration The Federal agency that, among other things, determines initial entitlement to and eligibility for Medicare benefits.

social worker Performs duties directly related to the health of the individual and the family in psychiatric and medical social work.

socioeconomic monitoring system A system of annual and supplemental surveys of physicians directed by the American Medical Association Center for Health Policy Research. The SMS provides information on a range of characteristics including physician's earnings, expense, work patterns, and fees.

sodium A body salt, also termed electrolyte. Kidney disease and some diseases of the adrenal gland and dehydration can cause abnormal results.

sodium, serum Sodium is an electrolyte and plays an important role in maintaining the normal amount of water and the acid-base balance in body fluids. Within the cells, sodium is involved in nerve stimulation. Serum sodium levels higher or lower than normal may be caused by various conditions, including diseases of the gastrointestinal tract, kidney and adrenal gland.

soft palate The movable fold suspended from the rear of the hard palate that closes off the nasal cavity from the oral cavity during swallowing or sucking.

solar plexus A complex network of nerves (a plexus) located in the abdomen. *Synonym:* celiac plexus.

Sole Community Hospital (SCH) A hospital which (1) is more than 50 miles from any similar hospital, (2) or is the exclusive provider of services to at least 75 percent of its service area populations or (3) has been designated as an SCH under previous rules. The Medicare DRG program makes special optional payment provisions for SCHs, most of which are rural, including providing that their rates are set permanently so that 75 percent of their payment is hospital-specific and only 25 percent is based on regional DRG rates.

solid tumors Growth of tissue of hard, unyielding substance. Differs from a tumor filled with fluid, such as a cystic tumor.

somat(o)-, somatico- Body, bodily.

somatoform disorders Disorders having the presence of physical symptoms that suggest a general medical condition but that are not fully explained by a general medical condition, by the direct effects of a substance, or by another mental disorder.

somatotropin A hormone produced by the anterior pituitary gland; promotes growth in humans.

somnolence A very sleepy state.

sonography *See* ultrasonography.

sonohysterography Imaging of the uterine cavity using an infusion of sterile saline through a soft plastic catheter placed in the cervix in conjunction with transvaginal ultrasound.

SOP Standard operating procedure.

space maintainer A dental appliance that fills the space of a lost tooth (or teeth) and prevents the other teeth from moving into the space; used especially in orthodontic and pediatric treatment.

spasm A painful and involuntary muscular contraction.

spasmo- Spasm.

spasmolytic A drug used to relieve or prevent spasms (especially of the smooth muscles).

spastic Relating to or characterized by spasm.

special benefit networks Provider networks for particular services, such as mental health, substance abuse, or prescription drugs.

special report An unlisted service or one that is unusual, variable, or new may require a special report demonstrating the medical appropriateness of the service.

specialist A physician who has special experience and expertise in a portion of the medical field. In most instances specific credentials, including residency placement and board certification must be acquired in order to qualify as a specialist.

specialty contractor A Medicare contractor that performs a limited Medicare function, such as coordination of benefits, and statistical analysis.

specialty differential The difference in the relative value or amount paid for the same service when performed by physicians in different specialties.

specialty health maintenance organization An organization that uses an HMO model to provide health care services in a subset or single specialty of medical care.

specialty plan A type of Medicare Advantage Plan that provides more focused health care for some people. These plans give you all your Medicare health care as well as more focused care to manage a disease or condition such as congestive heart failure, diabetes, or End-Stage Renal Disease.

specialty services Health care services that are generally considered outside standard medical-surgical services because of the specialized knowledge required for service delivery and management.

specificity Refers to the requirement to code to the highest number of digits possible when selecting ICD-9-CM codes.

specified disease insurance Insurance providing benefits, subject to a maximum amount, for expenses incurred in connection with the treatment of specified diseases, such as cancer.

specified low income medicare beneficiaries Medicare premiums (but not cost sharing) paid by Medicaid on behalf of certain low income eligibles.

specimen handling Procedures for collecting, preserving, and transporting of specimens sufficiently stable to provide accurate and precise results suitable for clinical interpretation.

SPECT An acronym for Single Photon Emission Computed Tomography, a nuclear medicine procedure in which a gamma camera rotates around the patient and takes pictures from many angles, which a computer then uses to form a tomographic (cross-sectional) image.

spectrin The major cytoskeleton protein, along with certain integral proteins, responsible for maintaining the biconcave shape of erythrocytes.

spectrophotometry A method of chemical analysis based on the absorption or attenuation by matter of electromagnetic radiation of a specified wavelength or frequency.

spectroscopy A noninvasive technique that uses the differential absorption properties of hemoglobin and myoglobin to evaluate tissue oxygenation and indirectly can measure regional hemodynamics and blood flow.

speech therapy Treatment of speech defects and disorders, especially through use of exercises and audio-visual aids that develop new speech habits.

speech-language therapy Treatment to regain and strengthen speech skills.

Speech Therapist (ST) Speech therapist are trained to evaluate and improve speech and community functioning.

Speed procedure (Kellogg Spinal fusion and anterior interbody fusion by Speed) using tibial cortical grafts.

spell of illness A period of consecutive days, beginning with the first day on which a beneficiary is furnished inpatient hospital or extended care services, and ending with the close of the first period of 60 consecutive days thereafter in which the beneficiary is in neither a hospital nor a skilled nursing facility.

spend down Procedure whereby Medicaid applicants use a portion of savings and other resources on medical expenses in order to meet Medicaid resource eligibility requirements.

sperm The male reproductive cell.

sperm agglutination test Any of various tests for the presence of antisperm antibodies as a cause of infertility, based on the ability of large multivalent isotypes such as igm or secretory iga to cross-link and agglutinate spermatozoa with such antibodies.

sperma-, spermo-, spermato- Semen, spermatozoa.

spermatic Consisting of or resembling sperm.

spermatic cord The cord-like structure in males formed by the vas deferens and surrounding tissue that run from the abdomen down to each testicle.

spermatocele A cyst-like mass within the epididymis usually filled with fluid and dead sperm cells.

spermatocystectomy Surgical excision of a seminal vesicle.

Spetzler fusion Approach to anterior C-1 to C-3 by using a transoral approach for fusion following excision of tumor.

sphenoid bone a single, irregular, wedge-shaped bone at the base of the skull, which forms a part of the floor of the anterior, middle, and posterior cranial fossae. This bone is referred to as the keystonc of the cranial floor because it articulates with all the other cranial bones.

sphenoid sinus Two large sinuses in the sphenoid bone. They are bordered with cells which secretes the mucus which keeps the nose from drying.

sphenoidectomy Surgical removal of the sphenoid sinus.

sphenoidotomy Surgical creation of an opening in the anterior wall of the sphenoidal sinus.

sphenopalatine ganglion A small parasympathetic ganglion in the upper part of the pterygopalatine fossa whose postsynaptic fibers supply the lacrimal, nasal, palatine and pharyngeal glands.

spherocytes Abnormally shaped red blood cells. Cells are sphere shape, in contrast to the doughnut shape of normal red blood cells.

spherocytosis Presence of spherocytes in the blood. Caused by some anemias. *See* Anemia.

sphincter A structure, usually a circular muscle, that normally maintains constriction of a natural body passage or orifice and which relaxes as required by normal physiological functioning.

sphincter of oddi Sphincter muscle of the bile duct.

sphincteroplasty Plastic repair of a sphincter.

sphincterotomy Incision into a sphincter muscle.

spica cast A cast which includes the trunk of the body and one or more limbs. *Synonym:* body cast.

spider vein A widened vein that can be seen through the surface of the skin.

spigelian hernia Abdominal hernia through the semilunar line.

spina bifida Inherited defective closure of the body encasement of the spinal cord through which the cord and meninges may protrude.

spinal of or relating to the spine or spinal cord; spinal cord.

spinal cord The longitudinal cord of nerve tissue that is enclosed in the spinal canal. It serves not only as a pathway for nervous impulses to and from the brain, but as a center for carrying out and coordinating many reflex actions independently of the brain.

spinal fusion A surgical technique used to combine two or more vertebrae. *Synonym:* spondylodesis.

spinal manipulation A therapeutic intervention performed on synovial joints in the spinal column. Spinal manipulation is most commonly performed by chiropractors, osteopathic physicians, and physical therapists.

spinal puncture A diagnostic and at times therapeutic procedure performed to collect a sample of cerebrospinal fluid (CSF) for analysis, or very rarely as a treatment to relieve increased intracranial pressure. *Synonym:* lumbar puncture.

spinal stenosis Reduction in the diameter of the spinal canal due to new bone formation which may result in pressure on the spinal cord or nerve roots.

spinal tap A diagnostic procedure performed to collect a sample of cerebrospinal fluid. *Synonym:* lumbar puncture.

spine The flexible bone column extending from the base of the skull to the tailbone. It is made up of 33 bones, known as vertebrae. The first 24 vertebrae are separated by discs known as intervertebral discs, and bound together by ligaments and muscles. Five vertebrae are fused together to form the sacrum and 4 vertebrae are fused together to form the coccyx. The spine is also referred to as the vertebral column, spinal column, or backbone..

spinocerebellar disease A disease involving both the spinal cord and the cerebellum.

spinous Shaped like a spine or thorn.

spirometry A test using a device called a spirometer to measure how much air the lungs can hold and how well the respiratory system is able to move air into and out of the lungs.

splanchn(i)-, splanchn(o)- Viscera.

splanchnicectomy Surgical resection of the splanchnic nerves and usually of the celiac ganglion for treatment of hypertension or pain.

spleen An organ located just below the liver that screens the blood for foreign particles and old blood cells.

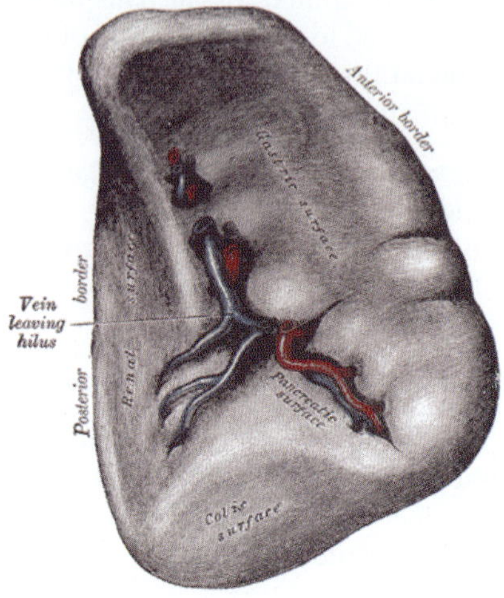

spleen

splen(o)- Spleen.

splenectomy Surgical removal of the spleen.

splenic of or relating to the spleen.

splenomegaly An enlargement of the spleen.

splenoplasty Surgical repair of spleen.

splenoportography X-ray visualization of the portal circulation that uses radiopaque material introduced into the spleen.

splenorrhaphy Suture of a ruptured spleen.

splint 1) An orthopedic mechanical device used to immobilize and protect a part of the body (as a broken leg). 2) The connection of two or more teeth so that they function as a stronger single structure.

spondyl(o)- of or pertaining to the spine, the vertebra.

spondylitis Inflammation of a spinal joint; characterized by pain and stiffness.

spondylolisthesis A defect in the construct of bone between the superior and inferior facets with varying degrees of displacement so the vertebra with the defect and the spine above that vertebra are displaced forward in relationship to the vertebrae below. It is usually due to a developmental defect or the result of a fracture.

spondylolysis Displacement of one vertebra over another with fracture of a posterior portion of the vertebra. A defect in the neural arch between the superior and inferior facets of vertebrae without separation at the defect and therefore no displacement of the vertebrae. It may be unilateral or bilateral and is usually due to a developmental defect but may be secondary to a fracture.

spondylopathy Any disease of the vertebrae.

spondylosis Degenerative arthritis (osteoarthritis) of the spinal vertebra and related tissue.

spontaneous abortion The spontaneous end of a pregnancy at a stage where the embryo or fetus is incapable of surviving, generally defined in humans at prior to 20 weeks of gestation. Miscarriage is the most common complication of early pregnancy. *Synonym:* miscarriage.

spontaneous dvt A clot that forms when there are no identified risk factors. of those who develop a spontaneous DVT, 20-40% have an inherited or acquired predisposition to thrombosis or thrombophilia.

SPP Suprapubic prostatectomy.

sprain Damage or tearing of ligaments or a joint capsule.

Sprengel's deformity A condition where the scapula (shoulder blade) on one or both sides are under-developed (hypoplastic) and abnormally high.

sprue Chronic disorder resulting from malabsorption of nutrients from the small intestine. It occurs in tropical and nontropical forms. *See* Tropical sprue; celiac disease.

squamos(o)- Denoting something as 'full of scales' or 'scaly'.

squamous cell carcinoma Cancer that begins in squamous cells, which are thin, flat cells that look like fish scales. *Synonym:* epidermoid carcinoma.

SSEP Somato-sensory evoked potential.

SSI Supplemental security income.

SSRI Selective serotonin re-uptake inhibitor.

SSS Sick sinus syndrome.

stabilization outcome (HHA) An outcome measure that assesses whether a specific health status attribute does not worsen between two time periods, as measured on the specified OASIS scale.

stabilizer Used to steady only the portion of the heart where the surgeon is sewing the bypass graft into place.

staff assisted dialysis Dialysis performed by the staff of the renal dialysis center or facility.

staff model Staff model is a type of HMO in which care is provided by physicians who are employees of the HMO. This contrasts with the independent practice association (IPA) HMO, in which independent physicians contract with the HMO.

Staff Model HMO An HMO that delivers health services through a group in which physicians are salaried employees who treat HMO members exclusively.

stages A comparative measure to determine how far a patient's cancer has spread.

stainless steel crown A pre-made metal crown, shaped like a tooth that is used to temporarily cover a seriously decayed or broken tooth; used most often on childrens teeth.

Stamey procedure A procedure for the treatment of stress incontinence.

standard benefits package Also referred to in some plans as minimum benefits or uniform benefits, this would include the basic package of preventive and acute care benefits to be offered by all health plans. The standard benefits package may be defined in terms of specific services or in terms of services to be included and excluded, allowing health plans to determine which services are rendered on the basis of appropriateness and medical necessity. The generosity of the standard benefit package will be a key political decision and will have wide ranging implications in terms of program costs, public support, and services available to previously uninsured populations.

standard claims processing system Certain computer systems currently used by carriers and Fiscal Intermediaries to process Medicare claims. For physician and lab claims, the system is Electronic Data Systems (EDS); for facility and other Part A provider claims the system is the Fiscal Intermediary Standard System (FISS), formerly known as the Florida Shared System (FSS); and for supplier claims the system is the Viable Information Processing System (VIPS).

standard community rating A type of community rating in which an MCO considers only community-wide data and establishes the same financial performance goals for all risk classes. *Synonym:* community rating.

standard of care A diagnostic and treatment process that a clinician should follow for a certain type of patient, illness, or clinical circumstance.

standard transaction Under HIPAA, this is a transaction that complies with the applicable HIPAA standard.

standards Authoritative statements of (a) minimum levels of acceptable performance or results, (b) excellent levels of performance or results, or (c) the range of acceptable performance or results, according to the Institute of Medicine.

standing committees Long-term advisory bodies on ongoing issues such as finance management, compliance, quality management, utilization management, strategic planning, and compensation.

standing referral A referral to a specialist provider that covers routine visits to that provider. It is a common practice to permit the gatekeeper to make referrals for only a limited number of visits (often 3 or fewer). In cases where the circumstances requires regular visits to a specialist, this type of referral eliminates the need to return to the gatekeeper each time the initial referral expires.

Stanford-Binet test A standardized test that assesses IQ and cognitive abilities in children and adults aged two to 23.

stapedectomy A procedure performed on the middle ear, in which the stapes is removed and (usually) replaced with an artificial part, in order to restore hearing.

stapedotomy A surgical procedure to improve hearing in otosclerosis in which a small opening is created in the stapes to secure a prosthetic device.

stapes One of the three bones in the middle ear. It transmits sound from the incus to the inner ear.

staph Staphylococcus, staphylococcal.

staphylococcal of or relating to the Staphylococcus bacteria.

staphylococcemia Infection caused by staphylococcus bacteria in the blood. May result in endocarditis, meningitis or osteomyelitis. *See* Meningitis; osteomyelitis.

staphylococcus aureus A bacteria, frequently part of the skin flora found in the nose and on skin. Staphylococcus aureus can cause a range of illnesses from minor skin infections, such as pimples, impetigo, boils (furuncles), cellulitis folliculitis, carbuncles, scalded skin syndrome and abscesses, to life-threatening diseases such as pneumonia, meningitis, osteomyelitis, endocarditis, toxic shock syndrome (tss), and septicemia.

staphyloma An abnormal protrusion of the uveal tissue through a weak point in the eyeball.

stapling The process of using special staples instead of sutures to close skin wounds and/or to connect or remove parts of the bowels or lungs.

Stark II The commonly used name for Federal laws and regulations that ban physician referral to entities with which the physician has a financial relationship.

Stark laws Ethics in Patient Referrals Act.

start of care (HHA) The time point when the home health agency initiates care and conducts a comprehensive assessment.

-stasis Stop, stand.

stat Immediately.

state certification Inspections of Medicare provider facilities to ensure compliance with Federal health, safety, and program standards.

state insurance department An administrative agency that implements state insurance laws and supervises (within the scope of these laws) the activities of insurance companies operating within the state.

state or local public health clinic A facility maintained by either state or local health departments that provides ambulatory primary medical care under the general direction of a physician.

state/private insurer long-term care partnerships Arrangements between some states and certain private insurance companies to provide long-term care insurance. Subject to the specific legal requirements for each state, these partnerships help protect the assets of enrollees who typically must become nearly impoverished before qualifying for Medicaid assistance for long-term care costs.

state survey Under 11864 of the Act, CMS has entered into agreemints with agencies of state governments, typically the agency that licenses health facilities within the state Health Departments, to conduct surveys of Medicare participating providers and suppliers for purposes of determining compliance with Medicare requirements for participation in the Medicare program.

state-mandated benefits Benefits for a variety of medical conditions that a given state requires of health insurance policies sold in that state.

statin therapy Treatment with statins, a class of drugs that lower cholesterol levels in people with or at risk of cardiovascular disease.

status epilepticus An epileptic seizure that lasts more than 30 minutes; a constant or near-constant state of having seizures. Status epilepticus is a health crisis, and requires immediate treatment.

Status location An indicator on a claim record describing the queue where the claim is currently situated and the action that needs to be performed on the claim.

-staxis Dripping, trickling.

STD Sexually transmitted disease.

steatorrhea Fatty stools.

Steffee plate Plate and screw device for posterolateral fusion fixation.

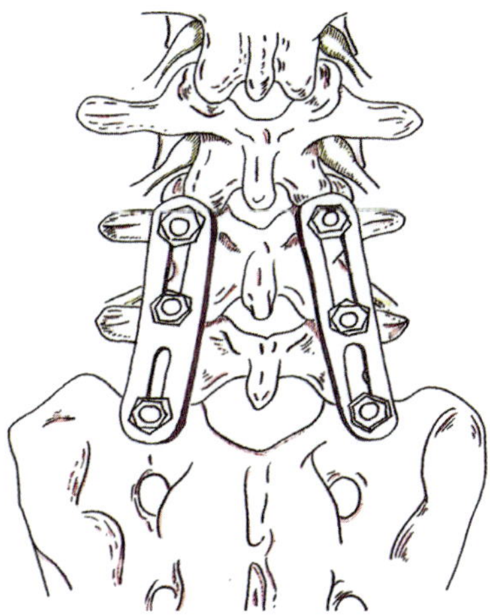

Steffee plate

Steindler advancement Plastic repair of the common flexor to restore elbow flexion.

Steindler stripping Surgical division of plantar fascia and muscle for plantar fasciitis.

Stein-Leventhal syndrome *See* Polycystic ovaries.

stem cell An embryonic or progenitor cell that can reproduce itself endlessly. Stem cells can develop into any cell type found in the body.

sten(o)- Denoting something as 'narrow in shape' or pertaining to narrowness.

stenger test A test to reveal feigned unilateral hardness of hearing.

stenosis Narrowing or stricture of any hollow structure, such as a blood vessel or bile duct.

Stensen duct The route that saliva takes from the parotid gland into the mouth. *Synonym:* parotid duct.

stent A small device that can be placed in the artery after angioplasty to ensure that the artery remains open.

step-down unit A ward or section of a ward in a hospital that is devoted to delivering sub-acute care to patients following a period of acute care.

stereognosis tests To examine for parietal lobe lesions, objects are placed in the patients hands and they are asked to identify them. Inability to identify shapes or discriminate between objects may indicate a (contralateral) parietal lobe lesion.

stereotactic surgery A minimally-invasive form of surgical intervention which makes use of a three-dimensional coordinates system to locate small targets inside the body and to perform on them some action such as ablation (removal), biopsy, lesion, injection, stimulation, implantation, radiosurgery (SRS) etc.

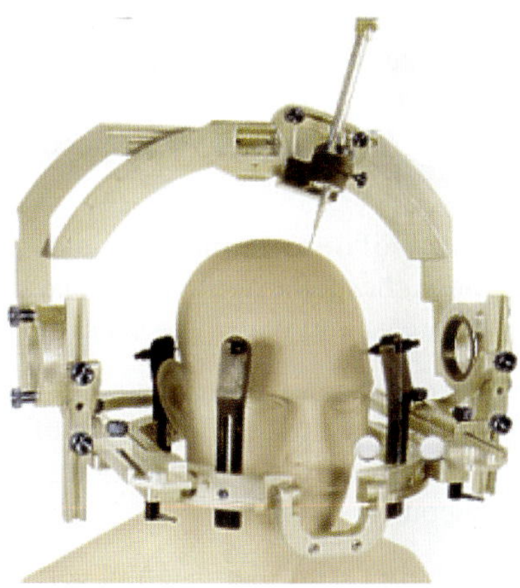

stereotactic surgery apparatus

stereotaxic techniques Techniques during brain surgery that use a system of three-dimensional coordinates to locate the site to be operated on.

sterilization A procedure which results in the inability to procreate.

sternal of or relating to or near the sternum.

sternoclavicular joint The joint connecting the sternum to the clavicle.

sternocleidomastoid muscle A paired muscle in the superficial layers of the anterior portion of the neck. It acts to flex and rotate the head.

sternotomy An incision into or through the sternum.

sternum The flat bone that articulates with the clavicles and the first seven pairs of ribs.

steroids A major class of lipids which have structures totally different from the other classes of lipids. Natural steroids include cholesterol and sex hormones. Steroid compounds are used in birth control pills, cortisone and anabolic steroids.

steth(o)- of or pertaining to the upper chest, chest, the area above the breast and under the neck.

Stevens-Johnson syndrome Severe, sometimes fatal, bullous form of erythema multiforme involving the mucous membranes.

Stoffel operation Division of certain motor nerves for the relief of spastic paralysis.

Stokes-Adams syndrome Condition caused by heart block with sudden attacks of unconsciousness and seizures.

stom(a) Mouth.

stoma An opening, either natural or surgically created, which connects a portion of the body cavity to the outside environment.

stomach The digestive organ located in the upper abdomen, under the ribs. The upper part of the stomach connects to the esophagus, and the lower part leads into the small intestine.

stomat(o)- of or pertaining to the mouth.

stomatitis An inflammation of the mucous lining of any of the structures in the mouth.

stomatoplasty Plastic repair of the mouth.

-stomy Creation of an opening.

stones Hard, unyielding substances. Stones may be made in the liver, gallbladder, blood vessels or urinary tract.

Stookey-Scarff procedure A ventriculostomy from the third ventricle to the prechiasmal and interpeduncular cisterns.

stool Fecal matter solid excretory product evacuated from the bowels.

stop loss insurance Describes two aspects in insurance. The policy-holder may be protected by a ceiling on the amount that must be paid out-of-pocket for deductibles and co-insurance for covered services and allowable charges in a policy year. A health plan may purchase insurance to protect the plan against costs that exceed specified levels.

stop-loss provisions A limit in a health insurance policy that provides for 100% payment of expenses after total patient out-of-pocket expenses exceed a certain contractual dollar amount.

storage-pool disease Metabolic disorder in which some substance accumulates in unusually large amounts.

strabismus More commonly known as crossed-eyes, is a vision condition in which a person cannot align both eyes simultaneously under normal conditions. One or both of the eyes may turn in, out, up or down.

strabismus surgery Procedure(s) performed to correct muscle imbalances surrounding the eye that cause problems with binocular vision.

strain Injury to a muscle (often caused by overuse); results in swelling and pain.

Strassman procedure Plastic repair on the uterus for the treatment of bicornuate uterus, a congenital uterine malformation where the uterus is heart-shaped with two joined cavities.

strategic planning committee The MCO committee responsible for directing the MCO's strategic direction and goals.

stratum corneum The outer most layer of the epidermis.

strayer procedure A surgical procedure for the treatment of gastrocnemius equinus contracture. *Synonym:* gastrocnemius recession.

strep Streptococcus.

streptococcal sore throat An infection of the oral pharynx and tonsils by streptococcus. Scarlet fever an infection caused by a bacterium called streptococcus.

streptococcus A group of bacteria, familiarly known as strep, that cause a multitude of diseases. In addition to strep throat, certain Streptococcus species are responsible for many cases of meningitis, bacterial pneumonia, endocarditis, erysipelas and necrotizing fasciitis.

streptococcus pneumoniae Pneumonia from streptococcal infection.

streptokinase treatment Treatment with streptokinase to dissolve blood clots in hollow blood vessels.

stress disorders, traumatic Anxiety disorders manifested by the development of characteristic symptoms following a psychologically traumatic event that is outside the normal range of usual human experience.

stress fracture A small crack in a bone usually resulting from repeated trauma or overuse.

stress incontinence Involuntary loss of urine in women that accompanies any action that suddenly increases pressure within the abdomen, such as lifting, sneezing, singing or laughing. Treatment may include exercises to strengthen the muscles of the pelvic floor or, if severe, surgery may be required.

stress test A variety of tests usually fall under the general term of stress test. These include stress or persantine thallium tests, dobutamine or stress echocardio-graphy, and traditional electrocardiographic stress tests.

stress tests Any of various tests that assess cardiovascular health and function after application of a stress, usually exercise, to the heart.

stricture An abnormal narrowing of a duct or lumen such as the bile duct, urethra or intestines.

stricturoplasty Surgical procedure for widening a structured segment of intestine that involves incision and closure in opposing directions.

stridor An abnormal, high-pitched, musical breathing sound caused by a blockage in the throat or larynx. Stridor can be indicative of serious airway obstruction from severe conditions such as epiglottitis, a foreign body lodged in the airway, or a laryngeal tumor.

strip-chart recorder Device that prints changes in electrical activity for measurement, such as EKG or tonometry.

stroboscopy A technique to gather information on the vibratory nature of the vocal cords. The technique involves the use of a strobe light which is linked to the frequency of the patient's voice.

stroke Sudden decrease in the blood supply to part of the brain, damaging the area so it cannot function normally. Decreased blood flow can be caused by a narrowed or closed-off artery, a blood clot or other embolus blocking the blood vessel, bleeding into the brain due to a ruptured blood vessel or rupture of an aneurysm in the brain. Symptoms may include inability to speak, inability to move part of the body, uncoordination of certain muscles, headache, vision disturbance, loss of consciousness, confusion, loss of bowel and bladder control. *Synonym:* cerebrovascular accident.

stroma Thickest and central layer of cells in the cornea.

Strümpell-Marie disease Ankylosing or rheumatoid spondylitis; arthritis of the spine resembling rheumatoid arthritis usually affecting young males.

STS Serologic test for syphilis.

Stuart-Prower factor A disorder caused by too little of a protein called factor X in the blood. *Synonym:* Factor X deficiency.

styloid process Refers to the slender, pointed process (protrusion) that serves as a point of muscle attachment for the temporal bone of the skull, the radius and ulna, and the 5th metatarsal of the foot.

styloidectomy Surgical removal of the radial styloid process.

Stypven time test A test measuring the clotting time of plasma after addition of Russell's viper venom, useful in evaluating patients with deficiencies in factor X.

sub- Beneath.

sub term Refers to listings appearing in the alphabetic index of ICD-9-CM under main terms and always indented two spaces to the right.

subacute bacterial endocarditis Chronic bacterial infection of the heart valves often caused by streptococcus or staphylococcus bacteria. Characterized by a slow, quiet onset, with fever, heart murmur, enlarged spleen and development of clumps of abnormal tissue (vegetations) on the flaps of a valve. Infected vegetations can break off and become an embolus. *See* Embolus.

subacute care Care given to patients who require less than a 30-day length of stay in a hospital and who have a more stable condition than those receiving acute care.

subacute hereditary tyrosinemia Metabolic disorder characterized by an excess of tyrosine in the blood.

subacute thyroiditis Inflammation of the thyroid gland usually following mumps, influenza or other viral illness. *See* Mumps; influenza. Symptoms include an enlarged thyroid gland (usually 2 to 3 days after the onset of fever), body aches and malaise. Thyroid may be painful, and you may have difficulty swallowing. Treatment may include medication to relieve pain and decrease inflammation. Thyroid hormone replacement may be needed if the condition lasts more than a few days.

subarachnoid hemorrhage Bleeding in the area between the brain and the thin tissues that cover the brain.

subauthorization The authorization of one health care service concurrently with the authorization of another service. For example, an authorization for hospitalization may cover surgery, anesthesia, pathology, and radiology.

subcapsular Below a capsule, especially the capsule of the cerebrum.

subcategories Refers to groupings of four-digit ICD-9-CM codes listed under three-digit categories.

subclavian Under the clavicle.

Subscriber The person responsible for payment of premiums or whose employment is the basis for eligibility for members in an HMO or other health plan.

Subscriber Contract A written agreement, which may also be called a subscriber certificate or a member certificate, describing an individual's health care policy.

subcutaneous Relating to or located below the epidermis.

subcutaneous tissue The bottom layer of the skin and is composed of fat cells, connective tissue, blood vessels and nerves.

subdural Below the dura mater but above the arachnoid membrane of the meninges.

subdural hematoma A form of traumatic brain injury in which blood gathers within the inner meningeal layer of the dura (the outer protective covering of the brain).

subdural hemorrhage A rapidly clotting collection of blood below the inner layer of the dura but external to the brain and arachnoid membrane. *Synonym:* subdural hematoma.

subdural puncture Perforation of the space between the dura mater and arachnoid membrane by a needle for injection of medication or aspiration of blood or other fluid.

subglottis The lower part of the larynx; the area from just below the vocal cords down to the top of the trachea.

sublingual Under the tongue.

subluxation Incomplete or partial dislocation of a bone in a joint.

submandibular gland A pair of salivary glands located beneath the floor of the mouth.

submaxillary gland A salivary gland inside the lower jaws.

subscriber *See* insured.

substance abuse detection Detection of drugs that have been abused, overused, or misused, including legal and illegal drugs. Urine screening is the usual method of detection.

substantial financial risk An incentive arrangement that places the physician or physician group at risk for amounts beyond the risk threshold, if the risk is based on the use or costs of referral services. The risk threshold is 25%. However, if the patient panel is greater than 25,000 patients, then the physician group is not considered to be at substantial financial risk because the risk is spread over the large number of patients. Stop loss and beneficiary surveys would not be required.

substernal Below the sternum.

subterms Are always indented two spaces to the right under main terms.

subungual Beneath a nail.

suckling reflex The patient's lip is stroked. If this produces a pout or sucking movements, the reflex is positive and is an indication of diffuse frontal lobe injury. Although this reflex is normal in the infant until weaning, the adult should have no suckling response. A Positive Suckling Reflex frequently accompanies dementia (the loss of acquired intelligence from disease, trauma or anoxia).

sulcus A groove.

sun protection factor Commonly seen on suntan ingredients as SPF, the sun protection factor is the amount of the protection a suntan product provides. The higher the SPF, the greater the protection.

super- In excess, above, superior.

superbill A multi-part form which provides sufficient information so that patients may file their own health insurance claim forms.

superficial thrombophlebitis Also called superficial vein thrombosis, this is when a blood clot or clots form in veins nearer to the surface.

superior above or near the head.

superior vena cava The large vein which returns blood to the heart from the head, neck and both upper limbs.

supernumerary tooth An extra tooth.

supination The opposite of pronation, the rotation of the forearm so that the palm faces anteriorly, or palm facing up. The hand is supine (facing anteriorly) in the anatomical position.

supplemental edit software A system, outside the Standard Claims Processing System, which allows further automation of claim reviews. It may be designed using the logic, or expertise of a medical professional.

supplemental health services Benefits offered by an HMO that exceed their basic health service requirements.

supplemental medical benefits Health care reform plans normally allow the acceptance of supplemental benefits, which are normally not covered by a standard benefit package. These include services not usually medically necessary such as organ transplant, or enhanced psychiatric services. Consumers would have to pay an additional premium for these benefits.

Supplemental Medical Insurance (SMI) Private health insurance, also called medigap, designed to supplement Medicare benefits by covering certain health care costs that are not paid for by the Medicare program.

supplemental services Optional services that a health plan may cover or provide in addition to its basic health services.

supplier Providers, other than practitioners, of health care services. Under Medicare, these include independent labs, durable medical equipment suppliers, ambulance services, orthotists, prosthetists, and portable X-ray providers.

supplies and materials Refers to items such as surgical trays, bandages, catheter sets, injectables, and other materials provided as part of a medical service or procedure.

supporting documentation Refers to the requirement that documentation in the patient's medical report must clearly support the procedures, services and supplies coded on the health insurance claim form.

suppositories Medicated dosage forms that are designed to be inserted into the rectal, vaginal, or urethral orifice of the body for absorption.

suppuration A bacterial contamination of tissue exudate.

suppurative Relating to or characterized by suppuration (formation of pus).

supra- Above, excessive.

supracondylar Above the condyle.

suprapubic Above, or anterior to, the pubic bone.

supratentorial Literally refers to an area of the brain but is used in medical records to indicate that the plaintiff's symptoms and complaints are functional and not organic.

surgical care only Refers to a situation where one physician performs a surgical procedure but preoperative and/or postoperative services are provided by another physician. This is reported by adding CPT modifier -54 to the procedure code.

surgical destruction the process of destroying tissue via surgical means.

surgical stapling A technique of closing incisions and wounds, or of joining and connecting tissues, in which staples are used as sutures.

surgical team Refers to the concomitant participation of several physicians, often of different specialties, in highly complex surgical procedures. This is reported by adding modifier -66 to the basic procedure code.

Surgicenter A separate, freestanding medical facility specializing in outpatient or same-day surgical procedures. Surgicenters drastically reduce the costs associated with hospitalizations for routine surgical procedures because extended inpatient care is not required for the specific disorders treated by them.

surplus The amount that remains when an insurer subtracts its liabilities and capital from its assets.

surrogate UPIN A temporary UPIN that a provider may use until one is assigned.

survey and certification process The activity conducted by state survey agencies or other CMS agents under the direction of CMS and within the scope of applicable regulations and operating instructions and under the provisions of 11864 of the Act whereby surveyors determine compliance or noncompliance of Medicare providers and suppliers with applicable Medicare requirements for participation. The survey and certification process for each provider and supplier is outlined in detail in the state Operations and Regional Office Manuals published by CMS.

suspension of payments The withholding of payment by an FI or carrier from a provider or supplier of an approved Medicare payment amount before a determination of the amount of the overpayment exists.

sustainable growth rate A system for establishing goals for the rate of growth in expenditures for physicians' services.

suture 1) The line formed by the junction of two bones or an immovable joint between two bones, especially of the skull.

2) Stitches used to hold tissue together or to close a wound.

SVPB Supraventricular premature beat.

SVT Supraventricular tachycardia.

Swan-Ganz catheter Flexible, flow-directed cardiac catheter featuring a balloon tip to measure pressure in the pulmonary artery.

Swanson procedure Total joint implant of the first metatarsal phalangeal joint.

sweat glands Are numerous small, tubular glands that are found nearly everywhere in the skin of humans and that secrete perspiration externally through pores to help regulate body temperature.

Swenson procedure A surgical procedure for the management of Hirschsprung's disease.

swinging flashlight test with the eyes fixed at a distance and a strong light shining before the intact eye, a crisp bilateral contraction of the pupil is noted; on moving the light to the affected eye, both pupils dilate for a short period, and on moving it back to the intact eye, both pupils contract promptly and remain contracted; indicative of minimal damage to the optic nerve or retina.

sx Signs or symptoms.

sy(l)-, sym-, syn-, sys- Indicates similarity, likeness, or being together.

Sydenham's chorea A disease characterized by rapid, uncoordinated jerking movements affecting primarily the face, feet and hands. *Synonym:* rheumatic chorea.

Syme's amputation An amputation at the ankle with removal of the malleoli and formation of a heel flap.

sympathectomy A surgical procedure that destroys nerves in the sympathetic nervous system. The procedure is done to increase blood flow and decrease long-term pain in certain diseases that cause narrowed blood vessels. It can also be used to decrease excessive sweating.

sympathetic of or relating to the sympathetic nervous system;.

sympathetic nerve Any nerve of the sympathetic system; especially, the axial chain of ganglions and nerves belonging to the sympathetic system.

sympathomimetics Drugs that mimic the effects of the sympathetic nervous system, such as adrenalin and phenylephrine.

symphysiotomy Division of the symphysis pubis to facilitate delivery.

symphysis the line or junction formed by a cartilaginous articulation between two bones without an intervening synovial membrane, this articulation often fuses as in the two bones and the two halves of the mandibles.

symphysis pubis The area in the front of the pelvis where the pubic bones meet.

symptom Any sensation or change in bodily function that is experienced by a patient and is associated with a particular disease.

syncope A spontaneous loss of consciousness caused by insufficient blood to the brain.

syndactylism A congenital anomaly in humans characterized by two or more fused fingers or toes.

syndactyly Birth defect in which there is partial or total webbing connecting two or more fingers or toes.

syndesmotomy Surgical division of a ligament.

syndrome A pattern of symptoms indicative of some disease.

synovectomy Surgical removal of the joint lining.

synovial fluid A clear fluid which serves as a lubricant in a joint, tendon sheath, or bursa.

synovitis Inflammation or infection of the synovium. *See* Synovium.

synovium A tissue that surrounds and protects the joints. It produces synovial fluid that nourishes and lubricates the joints.

syphilis A common venereal disease caused by the Treponema pallidum spirochete; symptoms change through progressive stages; can be congenital (transmitted through the placenta).

syphilis, late Final, destructive stage of the disease. Symptoms can occur anywhere from 1 to 35 years after initial infection.

syphilis, primary First stage of sexually transmitted infectious syphilis. Develops approximately 3 weeks after initial contact. Characterized by the eruption of one or more chancres (small, painless, fluid-filled lesions), usually on the genitals.

syphilis, secondary Develops 1 to 8 weeks after the initial chancre appears. It is characterized by a body rash. Symptoms often include headache, malaise, loss of appetite, sore throat and slight fever.

syphilitic of or relating to or infected with syphilis.

syringomyelia Condition characterized by abnormal cavities filled with liquid in the spinal cord.

system review An inventory of body systems obtained by asking a patient questions about physical signs or symptoms they may be experiencing.

Systematized Nomenclature of Medicine (SNOMED) - clinical terms A systematically organized computer processable collection of medical terminology covering most areas of clinical information such as diseases, findings, procedures, microorganisms, pharmaceuticals etc. It allows a consistent way to index, store, retrieve, and aggregate clinical data across specialties and sites of care. It also helps organizing the content of medical records, reducing the variability in the way data is captured, encoded and used for clinical care of patients and research.

Systemic Inflammatory Response Syndrome (SIRS) A serious condition in which there is inflammation throughout the whole body. It may be caused by a severe bacterial infection (sepsis), trauma, or pancreatitis. It is marked by fast heart rate, low blood pressure, low or high body temperature, and low or high white blood cell count. The condition may lead to multiple organ failure and shock.

systemic lupus erythematosus *See* Lupus erythematosus, systemic.

systole The part of the cycle during which the muscle contracts to empty the heart is called systole. The filling portion is diastole.

systolic The blood pressure when the heart is contracting.

T

T & A Tonsillectomy and adenoidectomy.

T cell leukemia virus A type of virus that infects T cells (a type of white blood cell) and can cause leukemia and lymphoma. Human T-cell leukemia virus type 1 is spread by sharing syringes or needles, through blood transfusions or sexual contact, and from mother to child during birth or breast-feeding. *Synonym:* HTLV-1.

Taarnhoj procedure Decompression of the trigeminal nerve root.

TAB Therapeutic abortion.

table of allowances *See* Schedule of allowances.

table of drugs and chemicals This table contains a classification of drugs and other chemical substances to identify poisoning states and external causes of adverse effects.

tabular list The portion of ICD-9-CM that lists codes and definitions in numeric order. Also known as Volume 1.

tabular list of **procedures** Refers to the list of codes and descriptions from Volume 3 of the ICD-9-CM. *Synonym:* Volume 3.

tachy- Denoting something as fast, irregularly fast.

tachycardia A rapid heart rate, exceeding the normal range for a resting heart rate.

TAH Total abdominal hysterectomy.

takeuchi procedure A procedure to establish a two coronary artery system a child with anomalous origin of the left coronary artery from the pulmonary artery.

talectomy Removal of the talus bone in the foot.

talus A bone in the tarsus of the foot that forms the lower part of the ankle joint through its articulations with the lateral and medial malleoli of the two bones of the lower leg, the tibia and fibula. *Synonym:* astragalus.

tamponade Blockage or closure (as of a wound or body cavity) by (or as if by) a tampon (especially to stop bleeding).

tarsal of or relating to or near the tarsus of the foot.

tarsal bone One of seven bones in each foot which forms part of the tarsus. The tarsal bones are the medial cuneiform, intermediate cuneiform, lateral cuneiform, navicular, cuboid, talus, and calcaneus bones.

tarsoconjunctival Pertaining to the tarsus of an eyelid and the conjunctiva.

tarsometatarsal joint Any of the three joints between the tarsal and metatarsal bones.

tarsorrhaphy A surgical procedure in which the eyelids are partially sewn together to narrow the opening (i.e. Palpebral fissure).

tarsus The part of the foot of a vertebrate between the metatarsus and the leg; in human beings the bones of the ankle and heel collectively.

tartar A common term for dental calculus, a hard deposit that adheres to teeth and produces a rough surface that attracts plaque.

TAT Thematic Apperception Test.

Tax Equity and Fiscal Responsibility Act (TEFRA) A Federal law that authorizes health plans to enter into arrangements with HCFA for cost and risk contracts.

Tax Incentives Tax deductions, credits, and rebates affecting insurance benefit decisions.

Tay-Sachs disease Inherited, rare disorder of the central nervous system in infants and young children. It causes progressive impairment and early death.

TB Tuberculosis.

tb skin test The standard method of determining whether a person is infected with Mycobacterium tuberculosis.

TC Technical component.

TDA Therapeutic drug assay.

teaching hospital A hospital that has an accredited medical residency training program and is typically affiliated with a medical school.

team surgery A single surgical procedure which requires the skills of more than two surgeons of different specialties, working together to carry out various portions of a complicated surgical procedure.

tear duct The which carries tears from the lacrimal sac into the nasal cavity. *Synonym:* nasolacrimal duct.

technical component The part of the relative value or fee for a procedure that represents the costs of doing the procedure excluding physician work.

technology assessment The term used to describe the evaluation process of new or existing diagnostic and therapeutic devices and procedures. Technology assessment evaluates the effect of a medical procedure, diagnostic tool, medical device, or pharmaceutical product. In the past, technology assessment meant primarily evaluating new equipment, focus-ing on the clinical safety and efficacy of an intervention, in today's health care world, it includes a broader view of clinical outcomes, such as the effect on a patient's quality of life, and the effect on society.

TEFRA Tax Equity and Fiscal Responsibility Act.

TEG Thrombelastography.

telangiectasia Small dilated blood vessels near the surface of the skin or mucous membranes.

telemedicine Professional services given to a patient through an interactive telecommunications system by a practitioner at a distant site.

telemetry Automatic transmission and measurement of data from remote sources by wire or radio or other means.

telephone services Non-face-to-face assessment and management services provided by a qualified health care professional to a patient via telephone.

telephonic analysis The analysis of ECG and pacemaker signals transmitted by telephone.

telephonic transmission The transmission of ECG and pacemaker signals by telephone for remote analysis.

teletherapy A form of radiotherapy in which penetrating radiation is directed at a patient from a distance.

temp Temporary.

temporal of or relating to the temples (the sides of the skull behind the orbit).

temporal arteries The arteries on each side of the head; the superficial temporal artery, the middle temporal artery, and the deep temporal artery.

temporal bone one of the two irregular bones on either side of the skull forming part of the lateral surfaces and base of the skull, and containing the organs of hearing. The temporal bones form the inferior sides of the cranium and part of the cranial floor.

temporal lobe The lobe of the cerebral hemisphere located down on the side just forward of the occipital lobe. The temporal lobe contains the auditory cortex which is responsible for hearing.

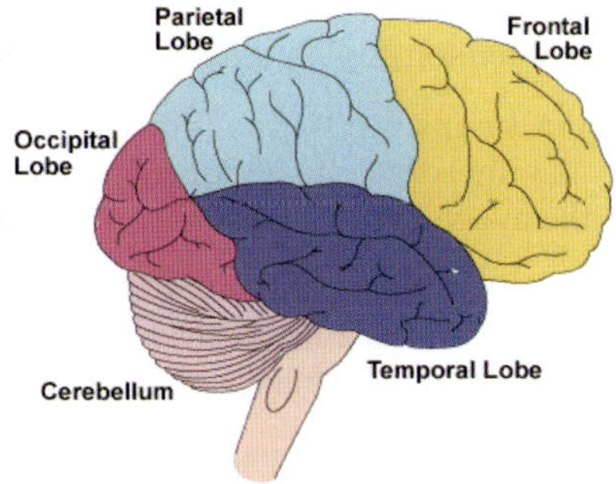

diagram of brain showing temporal lobe

temporal lobe epilepsy *See* Epilepsy, temporal lobe.

temporomandibular joint A small joint located in front of the ear where the skull and lower jaw meet. It permits the lower jaw (mandible) to move and function.

tendon A cord or band of inelastic tissue connecting a muscle with its bony attachment.

tendon reflex Contraction of the muscle caused by percussion of its tendon.

tenectomy Excision of a lesion of a tendon or of a tendon sheath.

tennis elbow A condition where the outer part of the elbow becomes sore and tender. It is a condition that is commonly associated with playing tennis and other racquet sports. *Synonym:* lateral epicondylitis.

tenodesis Suture of the end of a tendon to a bone.

tenolysis A surgical procedure to free a tendon from surrounding adhesions.

tenomyotomy Excision of a portion of a tendon and muscle.

tenon's capsule The fibrous tissue that lines the orbit and surrounds the eyeball.

tenonitis Inflammation of Tenon's capsule or the connective tissue within Tenon's space.

tenoplasty Plastic repair of a tendon.

tenorrhaphy Suture of a tendon.

tenosuspension The use of a tendon as a suspensory ligament.

tenosuture Suture of the divided ends of a tendon.

tenosynovectomy Excision or resection of a tendon sheath.

tenosynovitis The inflammation of the fluid-filled sheath (called the synovium) that surrounds a tendon. Symptoms include pain, swelling and difficulty moving the particular joint where the inflammation occurs.

tenotomy Surgical cutting or division of a tendon.

TENS Transcutaneous electrical nerve stimulator.

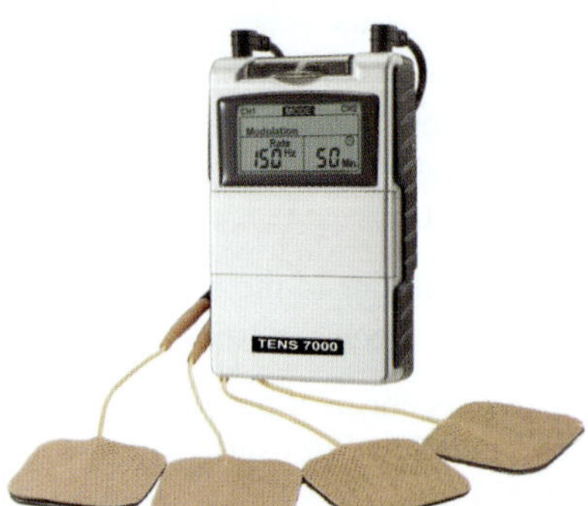

TENS unit

tensilon test An injection of edrophonium chloride (Tensilon) used to diagnosis myasthenia gravis.

-tension, -tensive blood pressure.

teratoma Tumor made up of several types of different tissue, none of which is native to the area in which it occurs. Most often found in ovaries and testes.

Terman-Merrill test A revision of the Stanford-Binet scale used to measure the intelligence of children.

termination provision A provider contract clause that describes how and under what circumstances the parties may end the contract.

termination with cause A contract provision, included in all standard provider contracts, that allows either the MCO or the provider to terminate the contract when the other party does not live up to its contractual obligations.

termination without cause A contract provision that allows either the MCO or the provider to terminate the contract without providing a reason or offering an appeals process.

tertiary care Highly specialized care given to patients who are in danger of disability or death often requiring sophisticated technologies (e.g., neurosurgeons or intensive care units).

testes Pair of male sex organs that lie within the scrotum and produce sperm and the male sex hormone, testosterone.

testicular of or referring to the testes.

testicular dysfunction Improper functioning of the testicles.

testosterone The sex hormone that stimulates development of male sex characteristics and bone and muscle growth;.

tetanus An acute and serious infection of the central nervous system caused by bacterial infection of open wounds; spasms of the jaw and laryngeal muscles may occur during the late stages.

tetanus toxoid A vaccine to prevent tetanus or to help boost the immune response to other vaccines.

tetralogy of Fallot A combination of four heart defects that are present together at birth. The four defects that constitute the tetralogy of Fallot are ventricular septal defect, pulmonary stenosis, right ventricular hypertrophy, and overriding aorta.

TFT Thyroid function test.

TGV Thoracic gas volume.

thalamus A large ovoid mass of gray matter situated in the posterior part of the forebrain that relays sensory impulses to the cerebral cortex.

thalassemia Inherited form of anemia in which red blood cells contain less hemoglobin than normal. *Synonym:* Mediterranean anemia, hereditary leptocytosis.

Thal-Nissen procedure Surgical treatment of reflux esophagitis.

thel(e)-, thel(o)- of or pertaining to a woman's teat, nipple [uncommon as a prefix].

theleplasty A plastic operation on the nipple.

thely- Denoting something as 'relating to a woman, feminine'.

thematic apperception test a projective test in which the subject tells a story based on each of a series of standard ambiguous pictures, so that the responses reflect a projection of some aspect of the subject's personality and current psychological preoccupations and conflicts.

therapeutic Tending to cure or restore to health.

therapeutic alternatives, equivalents, or substitution A drug that is believed to be therapeutically equivalent (i.e., will achieve the same outcome) to the exact drug prescribed by a physician is substituted by the dispensing pharmacist without the need to obtain the physician's permission.

therapeutic apheresis Enables hospitals to separate certain blood components from a patient and either replace or treat them before reinfusion.

therapeutic devices May include hospital beds, crutches, wheelchairs, ramps, intravenous pumps and respirators. Also see durable medical equipment and assistive technology.

therapeutic drug assays A test to measure the level of a therapeutic drug in human serum.

therapeutic exercise The prescription of bodily movement to correct an impairment, improve musculoskeletal function, or maintain a state of well-being.

therapeutic substitution The dispensing of a different chemical entity within the same drug class of a drug listed on a pharmacy benefit management plan's formulary. Therapeutic substitution always requires physician approval.

therm(o)- Heat.

thermal Relating to or associated with heat.

thermoablation A procedure using heat to remove tissue or a part of the body, or destroy its function.

thermocauterization Cautery by the application heat.

thermocoagulation The use of heat produced by high-frequency electric current for localized destruction of tissues.

thermography Measurement of the regional temperature of the body or an organ by infrared sensing devices, based on self-emanating infrared radiation.

thermotherapy The use of heat to treat a disease or disorder; heating pads or hot compresses or hot-water bottles are used to promote circulation in peripheral vascular disease or to relax tense muscles.

Thiersch's operation The application of a partial thickness skin graft.

third degree burn Occur when the epidermis is lost with damage to the subcutaneous tissue. Burn victims will exhibit charring and extreme damage of the epidermis.

Third-Party Administrator (TPA) Claims administration service conducted by entities specializing in the management of self-insured benefit programs. The TPA may collect premiums, determine employee eligibility, determine covered services, pay claims, prepare management information reports and provide other administrative services. The TPA is often able to provide reinsurance brokering, cost containment programs, and a full range of employee communication programs. Insurers may sell administrative services to self-insured employers, but this is described as "administrative services only.".

third-party payer Any payer of health care services other than the insured person. This can be an insurance company, HMO, PPO, or the federal government.

Thomas shunt A femoro-femoral shunt to provide vascular access for hemodialysis.

Thompson procedure An indirect lymphatic reconstruction incorporating a dermal flap.

Thompson test A test to determine the integrity of the Achilles' tendon.

thorac(i)-, thorac(o)-, thoracico- of or pertaining to the upper chest, chest; the area above the breast and under the neck.

thoracectomy An incision into the pleural space of the chest.

thoracentesis An invasive procedure to remove fluid or air from the pleural space for diagnostic or therapeutic purposes. A cannula, or hollow needle, is carefully introduced into the thorax, generally after administration of local anesthesia.

thoracic Of, relating to, or situated in or near the thorax.

thoracic surgery The specialty of treating problems in the chest cavity, except the heart, with surgery.

thoracic surgical procedures Surgery performed on the thoracic organs, most commonly the lungs and the heart.

thoracoabdominal Of, relating to, involving, or affecting the thorax and the abdomen.

thoracocentesis A procedure to remove excess fluid in the space between the lungs and the chest wall.

thoracolumbar Of, relating to, involving, or affecting the thoracic and lumbar sections of the spinal column.

thoracoplasty Surgical removal of part of the ribs to cause the collapse of a diseased lung.

thoracoscopy Examination of the inside of the chest, using a thoracoscope.

thoracostomy Surgical creation of an opening (stoma) into the chest cavity for drainage; used in the treatment of pleural effusion, pneumothorax, hemothorax and empyema.

thoracotomy An incision into the pleural space of the chest.

thorax The part of the human body between the neck and the diaphragm or the corresponding part in other vertebrates.

thromb(o)- of or relating to a blood clot, clotting of blood.

thrombectomy Surgical removal of an obstructing clot or foreign material from a blood vessel at the point of its formation.

thrombin The clotting factor that converts fibrinogen to fibrin.

thromboangiitis obliterans A rare disease in which blood vessels of the hands and feet become obstructed.

thrombocythemia An increase in the number of circulating blood platelets. *Synonym:* thrombocytosis.

thrombocytopenia Reduction of platelets in the blood, which reduces blood clotting and increases the risk of bleeding.

thrombocytosis Abnormal increase in the number of platelets. Often causes no symptoms. Usually occurs following removal of the spleen or with hemolytic anemias, hemorrhage or iron deficiency. May also occur in advanced cancer, Hodgkin's disease or other lymphomas. *Synonym:* thrombocythemia.

thromboembolism The blocking of a blood vessel by a blood clot dislodged from its site of origin.

thromboendarterectomy An operation to remove a thrombus from an occluded artery.

thrombolysis The breakdown (lysis) of blood clots by pharmacological means.

thrombolytic An agent that dissolves or splits up a thrombus.

thrombophilia A hereditary or acquired predisposition to develop blood clots. It is also referred to as hypercoagulable state or hypercoagulability.

thrombophlebitis Inflammation of a vein that occurs when a blood clot forms.

thromboplastin A plasma protein present in tissues, platelets, and white blood cells necessary for the coagulation of blood.

thrombosed Affected with or obstructed by a clot of coagulated blood.

thrombosis blood clot in a blood vessel.

thrombosis, venous (deep-vein thrombosis) blood clot that forms in a vein, usually in the lower leg or lower abdomen. It may partially or completely block blood flow or break off and travel to the lung. This is different from clots in superficial veins, which rarely break off. Symptoms include swelling and pain in the area and swelling of any part below the clot. Requires hospitalization for bed rest, observation and anticoagulation therapy.

thrombotic Relating to, caused by, or characterized by thrombosis.

thrombotic thrombocytopenic purpura A disease state in which red blood cells and platelets are destroyed and the body produces excessive blood clots which may damage the kidneys and nervous system.

thrombus A blood clot.

thrush Infection by yeast cells of the mouth, usually in infants.

thymectomy Surgical removal of the thymus gland.

thymus gland A gland located behind the breastbone that functions in the development of the immune system. The thymus is large in infancy and early childhood but begins to atrophy between ages eight and ten.

thyr(o)- Thyroid.

thyroglossal duct cyst A neck mass or lump that develops from cells and tissues remaining after the formation of the thyroid gland during embryonic development.

thyroid gland A two-lobed endocrine gland located in front of and on either side of the trachea. The thyroid gland produces producing various hormones, such as triiodothyronine and calcitonin.

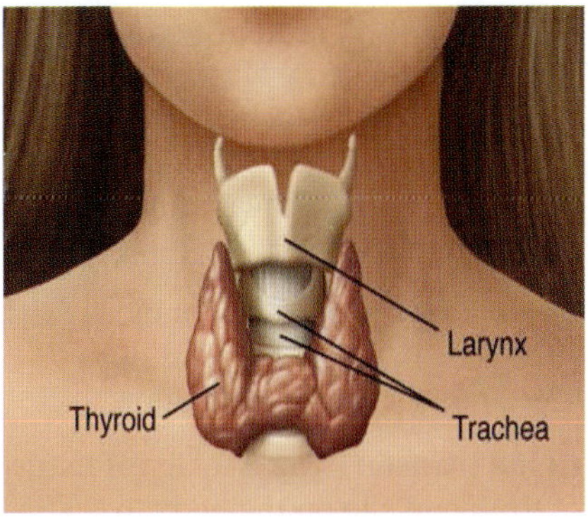

thyroid gland

thyroid profile Laboratory test of thyroid function including T3 uptake and T4 uptake.

thyroid stimulating hormone A hormone secreted by the front part of the pituitary gland. Thyroid stimulating hormone stimulates the production of thyroid hormone from the thyroid gland. It is sometimes taken in drug form to boost metabolism and reduce body weight.

thyroid suppression test After administration of liothyronine for several days, radioactive iodine uptake is decreased in normal persons but not in those with hyperthyroidism.

thyroidectomy Surgical removal of the thyroid gland.

thyroiditis Inflammation of the thyroid gland. Acute thyroiditis is caused by a bacterial infection and often results in formation of abscesses. Subacute thyroiditis usually follows a viral infection and is characterized by sore throat, fever, weakness and a painful, enlarged thyroid gland. Autoimmune thyroiditis is a chronic inflammation that can lead to Grave's disease (hyperthyroidism) or hypothyroidism if the thyroid gland diminishes in size.

thyrotomy An incision of the larynx through the thyroid cartilage.

thyrotoxic Refers to the state that is produced by excessive quantities of thyroid hormone.

thyrotoxicosis A condition resulting from excessive concentrations of thyroid hormones in the body, as in hyperthyroidism.

thyrotropin A hormone secreted by the anterior lobe of the pituitary gland that stimulates and regulates the activity of the thyroid gland. *Synonym:* thyroid stimulating hormone.

thyroxine An iodine-containing hormone produced by the thyroid gland, that increases the rate of cell metabolism and regulates growth.

thyroxine-binding globulin abnormalities Condition in which abnormal globulins circulating in the blood attach to thyroxin, one hormone made by the thyroid gland.

TIA Transient ischemic attack.

TIBC Total iron-building capacity.

tibia The inner and thicker of the two bones of the human leg between the knee and ankle.

tibial of or relating to the tibia.

tibio-fibular disease Disorders of the two big bones of the leg between the knee and ankle.

-tic Pertaining to.

tick-borne viral encephalitis An inflammation of the brain, caused by a tick-borne virus.

tilt-table test Tilt tables are used to maintain a head-down body posture during testing of cardiac response to identify patients with a vasodepressive or cardioinhibitory response as a cause of syncope.

tine test A multiple puncture tuberculin skin test used to aid in the medical diagnosis of tuberculosis.

tinea Refers to any of several diseases that can affect the scalp (tinea capitis), body (tinea corporis), nails (tinea unguium), feet (tinea pedis), groin (tinea cruris), and bearded skin (tinea harbae). *Synonym:* dermatophytosis.

Tinel's sign Procedure done to assess for a lesion or beginning regeneration of a nerve. Percussion is madc ovcr the site of a divided nerve and tingling is felt in the distal end of the limb.

tinnitus Noise or ringing in the ears.

tissue culture The growth of tissues and/or cells separate from the organism. This is typically facilitated via use of a liquid, semisolid, or solid growth medium, such as broth or agar. T.

tissue expansion Process whereby tissue adjacent to a soft tissue defect is expanded by means of a subcutaneously implanted reservoir. The procedure is used in reconstructive surgery for injuries caused by trauma, burns, or ablative surgery.

tissue factor A protein exposed to the blood when a blood vessel is injured. The tissue factor sets off a chain reaction – the coagulation cascade – that activates a series of clotting factors.

tissue harvesting The removal of organs or tissue for reuse, for example, for transplantation.

tissue transfer The transfer of tissue from one site on the body to another.

tissue transplantation Transference of tissue within an individual, between individuals of the same species, or between individuals of different species.

tissue typing A procedure in which the tissues of a prospective donor and recipient are tested for compatibility prior to transplantation.

Title XIX Medicaid.

Title XVII Medicare.

TKA Total knee arthroplasty.

TLSO Thoracolumbosacral orthosis.

TLV Total lung volume.

TMJ Temporomandibular joint (syndrome).

TMR Transmyocardial revascularization.

toco- Childbirth.

tocolysis Any drug treatment modality designed to inhibit uterine contractions in pregnant women at risk for preterm labor.

tocolytic agents Drugs that prevent preterm labor and immature birth by suppressing uterine contractions.

-tome Cutting instrument.

Tommaselli syndrome (disease) Fever and hematuria due to quinine overdose.

tomography Imaging methods that result in sharp images of objects located on a chosen plane and blurred images located above or below the plane.

Tompkins metroplasty A procedure used to treat infertility through excision of a septum dividing a uterus or to correct some other abnormality in uterine shape.

-tomy Cutting operation.

tono- Tone, tension, pressure.

tonography Recording of changes in intraocular pressure due to sustained pressure on the eyeball.

tonometry A procedure for the measurement of the fluid pressure inside the eye (intraocular pressure). One of the tests for glaucoma.

tonsil Either of two masses of lymphatic tissue one on each side of the oral pharynx.

tonsillar of or relating to the tonsils.

tonsillectomy Surgical removal of a tonsil or tonsils.

tonsillitis An infection and swelling of the tonsils.

tonsils Clumps of lymphoid tissue at the back of the throat.

-tony Tension.

tooth bud The early embryonic structure that becomes a tooth.

tooth extraction The surgical removal of a tooth.

tooth preparation Procedures carried out with regard to the teeth or tooth structures preparatory to specified dental therapeutic and surgical measures.

tooth remineralization Therapeutic technique for replacement of minerals in partially decalcified teeth.

tooth replantation Reinsertion of a tooth into the alveolus from which it was removed or otherwise lost.

top(o)- Place, topical.

topical Pertaining to the surface of a body part.

Tornwaldt's abscess Abscess of the adenoids.

tort A negligent or intentional civil wrong not arising out of a contract or statute that injures someone in some way and for which the injured person may sue the wrongdoer for damages.

tort reform Efforts to change the procedural or substantive rules for malpractice claims in the judicial system. Examples include reductions in statutes of limitations, mandatory offsets for collateral sources of payment, caps on non-economic damages, periodic payments of large awards, and limits on attorneys' contingency fees.

torticollis A condition in which the head is tilted toward one side (cervical rotation), and the chin is elevated and turned toward the opposite side (cervical extension).

torus Common bony protuberance on the palate or lower jaw.

TOS Type of Service.

total abdominal hysterectomy Surgical removal of the uterus and cervix.

total bilirubin The level of pigment in the blood. Elevations can be associated with liver disease or breakdown or red blood cells. Slight increases are sometimes seen without significance.

total cholesterol or hdl ratio The ratio of total cholesterol to HDL cholesterol is the most useful measure of cardiovascular risk. Most health professionals consider a ratio of 4 (or under) to be very low risk. For example, a person with a total cholesterol of 200 and HDL of 50 is at lower risk for heart disease than someone with a total level of 180 and HDL of 30.

total obstetrical care Complete obstetrical care which includes the antepartum care, delivery and postpartum care. Providers are reimbursed a global payment for the total physician services related to the pregnancy from the initial diagnosis of the pregnancy until the end of the postpartum period. The provider is reimbursed one fee for all physician services regardless of the number of visits or possible complications with the pregnancy.

total protein This is a combination of albumin and globulin, which are proteins. Abnormal values occur in liver disease and poor nutrition.

Tourette's syndrome A tic disorder characterized by repeated involuntary movements and uncontrollable vocal sounds. This disorder usually begins during childhood or early adolescence.

Touroff operation Ligation of subclavian artery.

tox(i)-, tox(o)-, toxico- Toxin, poison.

toxemia Presence of toxins in the bloodstream. Also called blood poisoning. *See* Eclampsia; pre-eclampsia.

toxic of or relating to or caused by a toxin or poison.

toxic adenoma Small, benign nodule in the thyroid gland that secretes thyroid hormone. Cause is unknown. Second most common cause of hyperthyroidism. Symptoms are the same as those in Grave's disease except there is no protrusion of the eyes. *See* Grave's disease.

toxic nodular goiter Tumor of the thyroid gland with nodules. Causes overactivity of the thyroid gland.

toxicology The study of the toxic or harmful effects of substances on the body.

toxicosis Any disease condition due to poisoning.

toxic-shock syndrome Disease characterized by sudden onset of fever, diarrhea, vomiting, sore throat, aching muscles, falling blood pressure and skin rash on palms and soles of the feet. Has been reported most often as occurring in women who use super-absorbent tampons during menstrual periods. The germ that causes the disease is normally found in the nose, mouth and vagina.

toxins Poisons, usually produced by or occurring in a microorganism.

toxoplasmosis An infection caused by the parasite named toxoplasma gondii that can invade tissues and damage the brain, especially in a fetus and in a newborn baby. Symptoms include fever, fatigue, headache, swollen lymph glands, and muscle aches and pains.

TPA Third party administrator.

TPN Total parenteral nutrition.

trabeculectomy A surgical procedure used in the treatment of glaucoma to relieve intraocular pressure by removing part of the eye's trabecular meshwork and adjacent structures.

trabeculoplasty Photocoagulation of the trabecular meshwork of the eye by means of a laser. It is used in the treatment of glaucoma.

trabeculotomy Surgical opening of the canal of Schlemm to treat glaucoma.

trach Tracheostomy.

trache(o)- Trachea.

trachea The airway that leads from the larynx to the lungs. *Synonym:* windpipe.

tracheal Relating to or resembling or functioning like a trachea.

tracheitis Inflammation of the trachea.

trachel(o)- of or pertaining to the neck.

trachelectomy Surgical removal of the cervix.

tracheloplasty Plastic repair of the uterine cervix.

trachelorrhaphy Suture of the uterine cervix.

tracheobronchoscopy Inspection of the interior of the trachea and bronchi.

tracheoesophageal fistula An abnormal connection (fistula) between the esophagus and the trachea.

tracheomalacia Degeneration of the elastic and connective tissue of the trachea.

tracheopharyngeal fistula Fistulas intentionally created for prosthetic or surgical voice restoration after laryngectomy or that develop after radiotherapy or surgical interventions.

tracheoplasty Plastic repair of the trachea.

tracheoscopy Examination of the interior of the trachea.

tracheostoma An opening through the neck and into the trachea.

tracheostomy Surgical formation of an opening into the trachea through the neck, or the opening so created.

tracheotomy Surgical incision of the trachea.

trachoma A severe, chronic and contagious conjunctival eyelid and corneal infection caused by a virus that leads to corneal blood vessel formation, corneal clouding, conjunctival and eyelid scarring, and dry eyes.

tracing (only) Refers to the output of an electrocardiogram, without interpretation or report.

traction The act of pulling on a bone or limb (as in a fracture) to relieve pressure or align parts in a special way during healing;.

tractotomy Surgical severing or incising of a nerve tract.

trading partner [HIPAA] External entity with whom business is conducted, i.e. Customer. This relationship can be formalized via a trading partner agreement. (Note a trading partner of an entity for some purposes, may be a business associate of that same entity for other purposes.).

trans- Denoting something as moving or situated 'across' or 'through'.

transabdominal Across the abdominal wall or through the abdominal cavity.

transaction Under HIPAA, this is the exchange of information between two parties to carry out financial or administrative activities related to health care.

transaction change request system A system established under HIPAA for accepting and tracking change requests for any of the adopted HIPAA transaction standards via a single web site. *See* www.hipaa-dsmo.org.

transcatheter Performed through the lumen of a catheter. Includes the delivery of intravascular devices such as balloon, coils and stents to dilate or close cardio-vascular defects.

transcervical Performed through the cervical opening of the uterus.

transcondylar fracture A fracture that occurs transversely and distally to the epicondyles of any one of the long bones.

transcutaneous Through the unbroken skin; refers to medications applied directly to the skin (creams or ointments) or in time-release forms (skin patches).

transducers Any device or element which converts an input signal into an output signal of a different form.

transection To divide by cutting transversely.

transferase deficiency Deficiency of any group of enzymes called transferase. Transferase enzymes catalyze the transfer from one molecule to another of a chemical group that does not exist in a free state during the transfer.

transferrin Substance present in the blood. It is essential for transportation of iron from the intestine into the blood. It makes iron available to the bone marrow, where red blood cells are produced.

transforaminal injection An injection of long acting steroid into the opening at the side of the spine where a nerve roots exits.

transfusion The introduction of blood or blood plasma into a vein or artery.

transfusion medicine The branch of medicine that is concerned with the transfusion of blood and blood components.

transient cerebral ischemia The reduction or loss of oxygen to the cerebrum; prolonged ischemia may lead to cerebral infarction.

transient ischemic attacks Temporary decrease in blood supply to part of the brain. The affected part of the brain is temporarily unable to function normally.

transient patients Patients who receive treatments on an episodic basis and are not part of a facilities regular caseload (i.e. Patients who have not been permanently transferred to a facility for ongoing treatments).

transillumination Passage of light through body tissues or cavities for examination of internal structures.

translocation Removal to another place. In genetics, the shifting of a segment or fragment of one chromosome into another part.

transplant The surgical procedure that involves removing a functional organ from either a deceased or living donor and implanting it in a patient needing a functional organ to replace their nonfunctional organ.

transplant surgery The specialty of replacing failing organs with donated organs with surgery.

transplantation Transference of a tissue or organ, alive or dead, within an individual, between individuals of the same species, or between individuals of different species.

transplantation, autologous Transplantation from another site in or on the body of the individual receiving it.

transplantation, heterologous Transplantation between animals of different species.

transplantation, heterotopic Transplantation of tissue typical of one area to a different recipient site. The tissue may be autologous, heterologous, or homologous.

transplantation, homologous Transplantation between individuals of the same species. Usually refers to genetically disparate individuals in contradistinction to isogeneic transplantation for genetically identical individuals.

transplants Organs, tissues, or cells taken from the body for grafting into another area of the same body or into another individual.

transportability [HIPAA] A signed document that can be transported (over an insecure network) to another system, while maintaining the integrity of the document.

transposition Any abnormal position of the organs of the body.

transureteroureterostomy Suture of the transected end of one ureter into the intact opposite.

transurethral resection of prostate (TURP) Surgical removal of a portion of the prostate through the urethra.

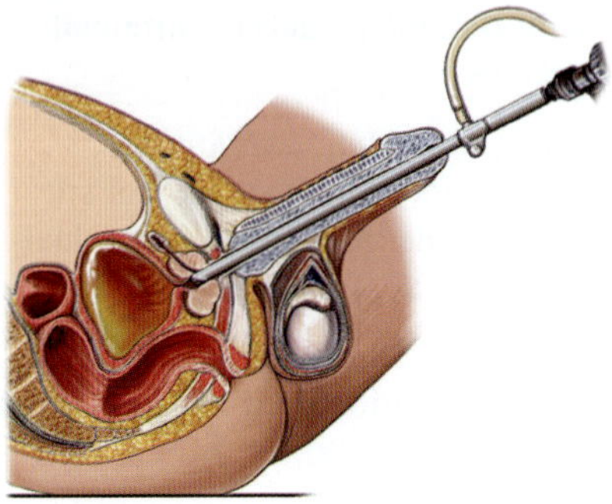

tranurethral resection of the prostate

transverse Extending or lying across; in a crosswise direction; at right angles to the long axis.

transverse plane divides the body into a superior (or upper) and an inferior (or lower) section. *Synonym:* horizontal plane.

trapezium The wrist bone on the thumb side of the hand that articulates with the 1st and 2nd metacarpals.

trapezoid The wrist bone between the trapezium and the capitate bones.

trauma Any injury , whether physically or emotionally inflicted. Trauma has both a medical and a psychiatric definition. Medically, trauma refers to a serious or critical bodily injury, wound, or shock.

Trauma Center An emergency room that is equipped and staffed to care for serious traumatic injuries. Emergency rooms are classified as Level 1, 2 and 3 trauma centers, with Level 1 being the highest care level. Generally, a Level 1 trauma center will be a large emergency room that has most medical specialties (especially trauma, surgery, orthopedics, and neurosurgery) available on-site or on short notice, has good access to CT Scanning and other technology such as MRI, and is able to care for multiple traumatic injuries of both blunt and penetrating nature.

trauma code development An MSP investigation process triggered by receipt of a Medicare claim with a diagnosis indicating traumatic injury.

trauma surgery The specialty of treating injuries from car crashes, gunshot wounds, stabbings and other traumatic injuries with surgery.

Treacher Collins syndrome Mandibulofacial dystosis limited to the orbit and malar regions.

Treatment Facility A residential or non-residential facility or program licensed, certified or otherwise authorized to provide treatment of substance abuse or mental illness pursuant to the law or jurisdiction in which treatment is received.

treatment options The choices you have when there is more than one way to treat your health problem.

trematode infection The infection of the digestive tract by adult parasitic flatworms called cestodes or tapeworms.

trench mouth Gum disease characterized by severe mouth sores and loss of tissue.

Trendelenburg operation 1) Surgical removal of a pulmonary embolus. 2) Ligation of the great saphenous vein for the treatment of varicose veins in the leg.

trephination The removal of a circular disk of the cranium. It is performed with a trephine, a small circular saw with a center pin mounted on a hollow metal shaft to which is attached a transverse handle.

treponema pallidum The bacteria that causes syphilis.

treponemal antigen test Any of various tests detecting specific anti-treponemal antibodies in serum in the diagnosis of the Treponema pallidum infection of syphilis.

tretinoin A prescription drug related to vitamin A used to treat acne and other skin disorders.

trh Thyrotropin-releasing hormone. Chemical substance secreted by the hypothalamus. Regulates secretion of thyroid-stimulating hormone (TSH) by the pituitary gland.

TRICARE Formerly known as the Civilian Health and Medical Program of the Uniformed Services (CHAMPUS), is a health care program of the United States Department of Defense Military Health System. TRICARE provides civilian health benefits for military personnel, military retirees, and their dependents, including some members of the Reserve Component. The TRICARE program is managed by TRICARE Management Activity (TMA) under the authority of the Assistant Secretary of Defense (Health Affairs). TRICARE is the civilian care component of the Military Health System, although historically it also included health care delivered in the military medical treatment facilities.

triage The process by which patients are sorted or classified according to the type and urgency of their conditions.

triceps reflex Testing for lesions at the C6-C7 level, the patient flexes his arms or places them on his hips. The short tendon above the elbow is tapped for a reflex response in the triceps muscle.

trich(i)-, trichia, trich(o)- of or pertaining to hair, hair-like structure.

trichiasis A medical term for abnormally positioned eyelashes that grow back toward the eye, touching the cornea or conjunctiva.

trichinosis A parasitic disease caused by eating raw or under-cooked pork and wild game infected with the larvae of a species of roundworm trichinella spiralis commonly called the trichina worm. *Synonym:* trich-inellosis, trichiniasis.

trichogram The result of examining plucked hairs under a microscope.

trichomonas vaginalis A parasitic protozoan that causes trichomoniasis.

trichomoniasis A common sexually transmitted disease caused by the parasite trichomonas vaginal is and infecting the urinary tract or vagina.

tricuspid Having three flaps or cusps.

tricuspid aortic valve The normal aortic valve has three cusps or leaflets, and is therefore called tricuspid (as opposed to a bicuspid aortic valve).

tricuspid regurgitation Abnormal flow of blood backward through the tricuspid valves.

tricuspid stenosis Closure of the tricuspid valves.

tricuspid valve A valve between the atrium and the ventricle that prevents the back flow of blood pumped from the atrium to the ventricle.

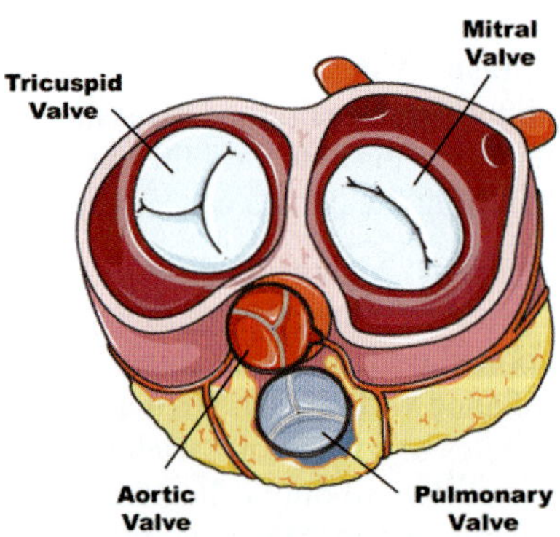

illustration of heart values

trigeminal The main sensory nerve of the face and motor nerve for the muscles of mastication.

trigeminal nerve The main sensory nerve of the face and motor nerve for the muscles of chewing.

triglycerides A blood fat related to calories and starch (sweets) in the diet. High levels can impair circulation and lead to hardening of the arteries. Alcohol also will increase the value. Fast overnight test for accurate test results.

trigonitis Inflammation of the urinary bladder, localised in the trigone.

trigonocephaly A malformation characterized by a triangular configuration of the skull, due in part to premature synostosis of the cranial bones with accompanying compression of the cerebral hemispheres.

tri-iodothyronine (t3-3) toxicosis Crisis in uncontrolled hyperthyroidism caused by the release of too much thyroid hormone. Thyroid storm may be preceded by infection or stress, or it may occur spontaneously. Also may occur after surgical removal of the thyroid gland (thyroidectomy). Characterized by high fever, rapid pulse, severe difficulty breathing, fear, restlessness, irritability and exhaustion. The person may become delirious, lapse into a coma and die of heart failure. *Synonym:* thyroid storm.

triploidy Presence in humans of 69 chromosomes (3 full sets). Frequently causes miscarriages.

-tripsy Crushing.

trisegmentectomy The removal of the true right lobe of the liver in continuity with most or all of the medial segment of the left lobe.

trisomy Addition of a third chromosome to an otherwise normal cell.

trochanter One of the bony prominences developed near the upper extremity of the femur to which muscles are attached.

trochar Instrument with a blunt component inside a sharp tube. Used to pierce the wall of a body cavity, such as the chest or abdomen.

trochlear nerve Either of the two cranial nerves on either side that control the superior oblique muscles of the eyes.

-trophy Nourishment, development, tissue.

tropical sprue Chronic form of malabsorption accompanied by diarrhea; occurs in the tropics and subtropics.

truncus arteriosus A rare type of congenital heart disease characterized by a single blood vessel arising from the right and left ventricles, instead of the normal two (pulmonary artery and aorta).

trypanosomiasis An infection caused by a type of protozoan parasite of the genus trypanosoma that causes sleeping sickness and other diseases in man and animals (usually transmitted by insects).

TSH Thyroid Stimulating Hormone. It is produced by the pituitary gland at the base of the brain. TSH promotes the growth of the thyroid gland and stimulates it to produce more thyroid hormones. If there is an excessive amount of thyroid hormones, the pituitary gland stops producing TSH, reducing thyroid hormone production. This process helps maintain a relatively constant level of thyroid hormones circulating in the blood.

TSS Toxic shock syndrome.

Tsuli procedure Expansive, multiple laminectomy for severe cervical spondylosis.

Tsutsugamushi disease A mite-borne infectious disease characterized by fever, headache, a raised rash, swollen glands and a dark crusted ulcer at the site of the chigger (mite larva) bite.

TT Tetanus toxoid.

tt-4 Total (serum) thyroxine.

TTN Transient tachypnea of the newborn.

tubal ligation A form of female sterilization, in which the fallopian tubes are severed and sealed or pinched shut, in order to prevent fertilization.

tubal pregnancy An abnormal pregnancy that occurs outside the womb (uterus).

tubectomy Surgical removal of the Fallopian tubes. *Synonym:* salpingectomy.

tuberculin test One of several skin tests to determine past or present tuberculosis infection. A purified protein derivative of the tubercle bacilli, called tuberculin, is introduced into the skin by scratch, puncture, or intradermal injection.

tuberculoma A non-neoplastic mass, usually in the lungs or brain, caused by a localized tuberculous infection.

tuberculosis A common and often deadly infectious disease caused by mycobacteria, in humans mainly mycobacterium tuberculosis. Tuberculosis usually attacks the lungs but can also affect the central nervous system, the lymphatic system, the circulatory system, the genitourinary system, the gastro-intestinal system, bones, joints, and even the skin.

tuberculous Constituting or afflicted with or caused by tuberculosis or the tubercle bacillus.

tuberosity A projection or protuberance, especially one at the end of a bone for the attachment of a muscle or tendon.

tuboplasty A surgical operation to correct a fallopian tube obstruction or adhesion, to achieve a pregnancy in women with tubal infertility.

tubular epithelial damage Damage to the lining cells of kidney tubules.

tubular function Normal function of kidney tubules.

tularemia Infectious bacterial disease of rodents that is transmissible to man by infected insects or direct contact. Symptoms include fever, headache, pneumonia, ulcerations in the digestive tract or ulcers on the skin, depending on the site of entry into the body. *Synonym:* rabbit fever, deer fly fever, O'Hara's fever.

tumor New growth of tissue in which multiplication of cells is uncontrolled and progressive.

tumor registrar Identifies, registers and maintains records of all cancer patients by utilizing the tumor registry data system. Analyzes registry data and disseminates information in accordance with professional ethics.

tunica vaginalis The serous covering of the testis.

TUR Transurethral resection.

Turner's sign Discoloration of the groin following acute pancreatitis.

Turner's syndrome Chromosome abnormality seen in about 1 in 3,000 live female births. It is marked by the absence of one sex chromosome. Characterized by short stature, primary amenorrhea and lack of development of secondary sex characteristics. Other features, which may or may not occur, include webbed neck, low set ears, broad shield-like chest, hypertension, heart abnormalities and learning disorders. Treatment includes hormone therapy. *See* Amenorrhea; hypertension.

TURP transurethral resection of the prostrate.

TVC Timed vital capacity.

TVH Total vaginal hysterectomy.

TW Total work.

TX Treatment.

tylectomy Surgical removal of a tumor from the breast. *Synonym:* lumpectomy.

tympan(o)- Eardrum.

tympanic membrane A thin membrane that separates the external ear from the middle ear.

tympanic nerve A branch of the glossopharyngeal nerve found near the ear.

tympanomastoidectomy A mastoidectomy with excision of the tympanic membrane.

tympanometry An examination used to test the condition of the middle ear and mobility of the eardrum (tympanic membrane) and the conduction bones by creating variations of air pressure in the ear canal.

tympanoplasty Reconstructive surgery for the tympanic membrane.

tympanosclerosis A condition characterized by the presence of masses of hard, dense connective tissue around the auditory ossicles in the middle ear.

tympanostomy Surgical puncture of the tympanic membrane, as for the removal of fluid or the drainage of pus.

tympanotomy Surgical puncture of the tympanic membrane. *Synonym:* myringotomy.

typhoid Serious infection marked by intestinal inflammation and ulceration; caused by Salmonella typhosa ingested with food or water.

typhoid fever An illness caused by the bacterium salmonella enterica serovar typhi. *Synonym:* enteric fever.

typhus Rickettsial disease transmitted by body lice and characterized by skin rash and high fever.

U

U & C Usual and customary.

UA Urinalysis.

UB-04 The health insurance claim form and instruction set used by hospitals and other institutional providers to file Medicare Part A insurance claims with Medicare Fiscal Intermediaries. The paper version of the UB-04 is also known as the CMS1540. The UB-04 incorporates the National Provider Idenifier (NPI), taxonomy, and additional codes.

UB-92 Claim form used prior to introduction of the UB-04 form.

UCC Urgent care center.

UCG Urinary chorionic gonadotropin.

Uchida procedure A sterilization procedure that involves suturing the fallopian tubes in back of the uterus.

UCR Usual, customary and reasonable.

UGI Upper gastrointestinal.

-ula, -ule Small.

ulcer Round, crater-like lesion of the skin or mucous membrane resulting from tissue death.

ulceration 1. A circumscribed inflammatory and often suppurating lesion on the skin or an internal mucous surface resulting in necrosis of tissue 2. The process of ulcer formation; the process of becoming ulcerated.

ulcerative of or relating to or characterized by ulceration.

ulcerative colitis Serious, chronic inflammatory disease of the large intestine (colon). Characterized by ulceration and episodes of bloody diarrhea.

ulna The inner and longer of the two bones of the human forearm.

ulnar Relating to or near the ulna.

ULQ Upper left quadrant.

ultra- Beyond, excessive.

ultrafiltration The separation of particles from a suspension by passage through a filter with very fine pores.

ultrasonic guidance The use of ultrasound to guide the insertion of needles, catheters or other medical procedures.

ultrasonography The visualization of deep structures of the body by recording the reflections of echoes of pulses of ultrasonic waves directed into the tissues.

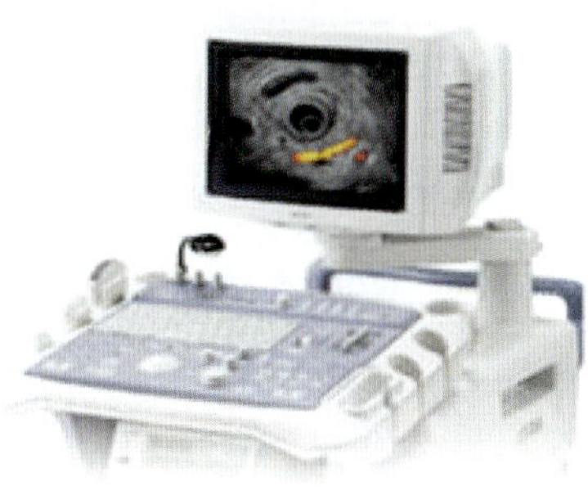

ultrasound equipment

ultraviolet light therapy The use of ultraviolet light to treat psoriasis or eczema.

umbilectomy Surgical excision of the naval. *Synonym:* omphalectomy.

umbilic- of or pertaining to the navel, the umbilicus.

umbilical of or referring to the umbilicus.

umbilical artery Either of a pair of arteries passing through the umbilical cord to carry impure blood from the mammalian fetus to the placenta.

umbilical cord Cord that transports blood, oxygen and nutrients to the baby from the placenta.

umbilical hernia A usually self-correcting hernia of the intestines in which protrusion occurs through the abdominal wall in the region of the navel.

umbilical vein A vein passing through the umbilical cord and conveying purified, nutrient-rich blood from placenta to fetus.

umbilicus Scar where the umbilical cord was attached.

un(i)- One.

unassigned claim A claim submitted for a service or supply by a provider who does not accept assignment.

unbundling Separating a service into its individual components and billing for each component separately. Also refers to a trend in insurance benefits contracting where the purchaser unbundles or contracts separately for specific services.

uncompensated Care The charges for services rendered by providers which are not paid for by the recipient and for which there is usually no third-party coverage. Uncompensated care is usually either charity care or bad debt.

unconjugated bilirubin Fat-soluble form of bilirubin that circulates in loose association with plasma proteins. Also called indirect bilirubin.

ungui- of or pertaining to the nail, a claw.

unicondylar knee arthroplasty Surgical repair of the knee using an implant on one side of the knee, instead of over the entire surface of the knee joint.

uniform claim form All insurers and self-insurers would be required to use a single claims form and standardized format for electronic claims.

Uniform Health Data Act Amendment of this act ensures that discharge data currently required of hospitals resides with the state and can be publicly released without prior permission of the hospitals. In addition, the act calls upon the Delaware Health Care Commission to study the feasibility of broadening its scope to apply to other health care facilities, such as nursing homes and ambulatory surgical centers.

Uniform Hospital Discharge Data Set A defined set of data that gives a minimum description of a hospital discharge. It includes data on age, sex, race, residence of patient, length of stay, diagnosis, physicians, procedures, disposition of the patient and sources of payment.

unilateral Involving only one part or side.

Unique Provider Identification Number (UPIN) A six character identifier (one alpha, five numeric) assigned to physicians by the Centers for Medicare & Medicaid Services.

uninsured People who lack health insurance.

universal access Access to health insurance coverage for everyone.

unlisted code A CPT code with a description including the term unlisted. Unlisted codes are used only when a cpt code which specifically describes the service or procedure is unavailable. A report is usually required by third party payers.

unna boot A special gauze bandage, which can be used for the treatment of venous stasis ulcers and other venous insufficiencies of the leg. It can also be used as a supportive bandage for sprains and strains of the foot, ankle and lower leg.

Unschuld's sign Cramping in the calves of the legs, as seen in early diabetes mellitus.

unusual anesthesia Occasionally, a procedure, which usually requires either no anesthesia or local anesthesia, because of unusual circumstances must be done under general anesthesia. This circumstance may be reported by adding the modifier -23 to the procedure code of the base procedure.

UOQ Upper outer quadrant.

UOS Unit of service.

upcoding The process of selecting a code for a service that is more intense, extensive, or has a higher charge, than the service actually provided.

UPIN Unique Physician Identification Number.

upper respiratory infection An inflammation of the nose, sinuses, ears or throat, caused by a viral infection.

upper respiratory tract The nose and throat and trachea.

UR Utilization review.

ur(o)- of or pertaining to urine, the urinary system; (specifically) pertaining to the physiological chemistry of urine.

URC Utilization review committee.

urea The chief solid component of urine.

urea breath test Rapid diagnostic procedure used to identify infections by Helicobacter pylori.

Urgent Care Center A medical facility where ambulatory patients can be treated without an appointment, and receive immediate, non-emergency care. The urgent care center may be opened 24 hours a day; patients calling an HMO after hours with urgent, but not emergent, clinical problems, are often referred to these facilities.

uremia Presence in blood of excessive amounts of protein metabolism byproducts, such as urea. Results in a toxic condition (as occurs in kidney failure) characterized by nausea, vomiting, dizziness, convulsions and coma.

ureter Tube that carries urine from the kidney to the bladder.

ureteral Refers to the ureter.

ureteral stent A surgical device implanted in patients with damaged ureters that holds the ureter open so that urine can flow freely from the kidneys to the bladder.

ureterectomy Surgical removal of the ureter.

ureterocalycostomy A procedure used to join healthy ureter proximal to the lower calyceal system.

ureterocele Prolapse of the end of the ureter where it joins the bladder. The condition may lead to obstruction of urine flow and result in hydronephrosis and loss of kidney function. Surgery is required to prevent permanent kidney damage.

ureteroenterostomy Anastomosis of one or both ureters to the wall of the intestine.

ureterography Radiography of the ureter after injection of a contrast medium.

ureterolithotomy The open surgical removal of a stone from the ureter.

ureterolysis The operation of freeing the ureter from adhesions.

ureteroneocystomy The removal of the lower part of the ureter, and sometimes a small part of the bladder.

ureteroneocystostomy Surgical transplantation of a ureter to a different site in the bladder.

ureteropelvic junction Site of origin of the ureter from the renal pelvis.

ureteroplasty Plastic repair of a ureter.

ureteropyelography Radiography of the ureter and renal pelvis.

ureteropyelostomy Surgical formation of a junction of the ureter and the renal pelvis.

ureterorrhaphy Suture of a ureter.

ureteroscopy An examination of the upper urinary tract, usually performed with an endoscope that is passed through the urethra, bladder, and then directly into the ureter. The procedure is useful in the diagnosis and the treatment of disorders such as kidney stones.

ureterosigmoidostomy A surgical procedure where the ureters are diverted into the sigmoid colon.

ureterostomy Surgical formation of an opening in the ureter for external drainage of the urine; cutaneous route utilizes a ureteral orifice emerging through the skin.

ureterotomy Incision of a ureter.

ureteroureterostomy End-to-end anastomosis of the two portions of a transected ureter.

ureterovesical Pertaining to a ureter and the bladder.

ureters Muscular ducts that propel urine from the kidneys to the urinary bladder.

urethra Hollow anatomical structure that leads from the bladder to outside the body.

urethral of or relating to the urethra.

urethral stricture A narrowing of the urethra caused by injury or disease such as urinary tract infections or other forms of urethritis.

urethrectomy Surgical removal of the urethra.

urethritis Inflammation or infection of the urethra.

urethrocele Prolapse of the urethra into the vagina.

urethrocutaneous fistula A fistula between the ureter and the skin.

urethrocystography Radiography of the urethra and bladder that utilizes a radiopaque substance.

urethrocystopexy Fixation of urethra and bladder for stress incontinence.

urethrocystoscopy *See* cystourethroscopy.

urethrolysis An anti-incontinence operation that involves the cutting of obstructive adhesions (fibrous tissue bands) that fix the urethra to the pubic bone.

urethromeatoplasty Plastic repair of the urethral canal.

urethropexy Surgical suspension of the urethra from the posterior surface of the pubic symphysis in order to correct urinary stress incontinence.

urethroplasty Open surgical procedure for urethral reconstruction to treat urethral stricture.

urethrorrhaphy Suture of the urethra.

urethroscopy Examination of the urethra by means of the urethroscope.

urethrostomy Surgical formation of a permanent opening of the urethra at the perineal surface.

urethrotomy Surgical incision of a stricture of the urethra.

urethrovaginal of or relating to the urethra and the vagina.

urgent care Health care provided in situations of medical duress that have not reached the level of emergency. Claim costs for urgent care services are typically much less than for services delivered in emergency rooms.

Urgent Care Facility Location, distinct from a hospital emergency room, an office, or a clinic, whose purpose is to diagnose and treat illness or injury for unscheduled, ambulatory patients seeking immediate medical attention.

URI Upper respiratory infection.

uri(c)-, urico- Uric acid.

uric acid A material, which, if in excess, can deposit stones in the kidney or in the joints and cause gout.

uric acid test Test measures the amount of uric acid in a blood sample. High levels of uric acid in the blood can cause solid crystals to form within joints. This causes a painful condition called gout.

urin- of or pertaining to urine, the urinary system.

urinalysis Examination of urine by chemical, physical, or microscopic means.

urinary bladder The organ that collects urine excreted by the kidneys prior to disposal by urination.

urinary calculus A stone in the urinary tract.

urinary diversion Temporary or permanent diversion of the flow of urine through the ureter away from the bladder in the presence of a bladder disease or after cystectomy.

urinary frequency Urinating too often, at too frequent intervals, not due to an unusually large volume of urine, but rather to a decrease in the capacity of the bladder to hold urine.

urinary incontinence The loss of bladder control causing leakage of urine.

urinary sphincter A collective name for the muscles used to control the flow of urine from the urinary bladder.

urinary system The organ system that produces, stores, and eliminates urine. In humans it includes two kidneys, two ureters, the bladder, the urethra, and the penis in males.

unique user identification The combination name/number assigned and maintained in security procedures for identifying and tracking individual user identity.

urodynamics The investigation of functional disorders of the lower urinary tract, i.e. The bladder and the urethra.

uroflowmetry A test that measures the volume of urine released (excreted) from the body, the speed with which it is excreted, and how long the excretion takes.

urogenital of or relating to the urinary and reproductive systems.

urogenital surgical procedures Surgery performed on the urinary tract or its organs and on the male or female genitalia.

urography Radiography of any part of the urinary tract.

urokinase treatment Treatment with the enzyme urokinase found in urine. Enzyme activates the system that dissolves blood clots in the body.

urostomy A stoma (artificial opening) for the urinary system. A urostomy is made in cases where long-term drainage of urine through the bladder and urethra is not possible.

URQ Upper right quadrant.

urticaria The transient appearance of slightly raised patches of skin which are redder or paler than the surrounding skin and often attended by severe itching. *Synonym:* hives.

URVG Uniform relative value guide.

US ultrasound.

user authentication The provision of assurance of the claimed identity of an entity.

user-based access A security mechanism used to grant users of a system access based upon the identity of the user.

USN Ultrasonic nebulization.

USP United states pharmacopeia.

USPHS United states public health service.

Usual, Customary and Reasonable Charges (UCR) Charges for health care services in a geographical area that are consistent with the charges of identical or similar providers in the same geographic area.

uter(o)- of or pertaining to the uterus or womb.

uterine of or involving the uterus.

uterine adnexa The uterine appendages the ovaries, uterine tubes, and ligaments of the uterus.

uterine leiomyoma One or more smooth, firm, painful, often waxy nodules arising from cutaneous or subcutaneous of the uterus.

uterine monitoring Measurement or recording of contraction activity of the uterine muscle. It is used to determine progress of labor, obstetric and assess status of pregnancy.

uterine prolapse Bulging of the uterus into the vagina.

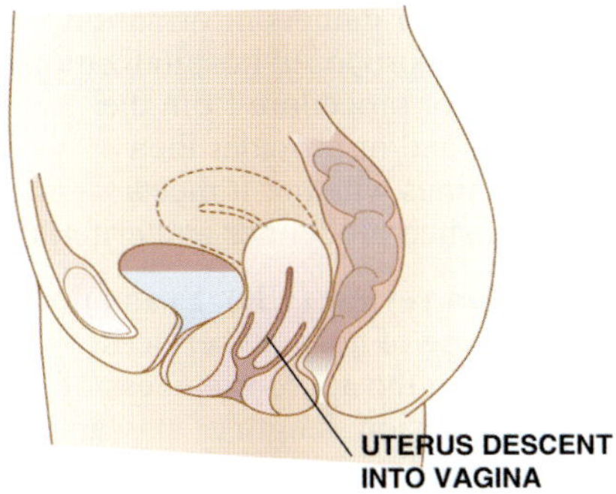

uterine prolapse

uterus A hollow muscular organ in the pelvic cavity of females; contains the developing fetus.

UTI Urinary tract infection.

Utilization The patterns of use of a service or type of service within a specified time, usually expressed in a rate per unit of population-at-risk for a given period (e.g., the number of hospital admissions per year per 1,000 persons in a geographic area).

utilization guidelines A utilization review resource that indicates accepted approaches to care for common, uncomplicated health care services.

Utilization Review Committee (URC) Committee that reviews utilization issues brought to it by the medical director, often approving or reviewing policy regarding coverage, reviewing utilization patterns of providers, and approving or reviewing the sanctioning process against providers.

utilization management The process of evaluating the necessity, appropriateness and efficiency of health care services. A review coordinator gathers information about the proposed hospitalization service or procedure from the patient and/or provider then determines whether it meets established guidelines and criteria.

utilization review (UR) Evaluation of the use of hospital services, including the appropriateness of the admission, length of stay and ancillary services. Review may be conducted concurrently, retrospectively, or in combination. The process uses objective clinical criteria to ensure that the services are medically necessary and provided at the appropriate level of care. UR is conducted by the hospital for its own quality assurance and risk management system, using norms, criteria and standards adopted by its medical staff. Reports summarizing the findings and action taken as a result of the process are regularly provided to the hospital board.

Hospitals conduct their own internally accountability system and comply with multiple delegated and non-delegated UR systems simultaneously. This occurs because of the hospital's legal responsibilities as well as each payer requiring its covered population to comply with its unique system as a condition of claims payment.

Utilization Review Accreditation Commission (URAC) A Washington-based, not-for-profit corporation formed in 1990 and dedicated to improving the quality of utilization review in the health care industry by providing a method of evaluation and accreditation of utilization review programs.

utilization review organization An external organization that conducts reviews to assess the medical appropriateness of suggested courses of treatment for patients, thereby providing the patient and the purchaser increased assurance of the value and quality of health care services.

UV Ultraviolet.

UVA Long-wavelength ultraviolet light.

UVB Medium-wavelength ultraviolet light.

uvea The middle coat of the eyeball, consisting of the choroid in the back of the eye and the ciliary body and iris in the front of the eye.

uveitis Inflammation of the uvea of the eye.

UVL Ultraviolet light.

UVR Ultraviolet radiation.

uvula A small pendant fleshy lobe at the back of the soft palate.

uvulectomy Surgical removal of the uvula.

uvulopalatopharyngoplasty A surgical procedure used to remove tissue in the throat.

uvulopharyngoplasty A procedure to treat snoring that involves trimming the uvula and the palate.

V

V codes Specific ICD-9-CM codes used to identify encounters for reasons other than illness or injury, for example, immunization.

V flutter Ventricular flutter.

VA Veterans administration.

vaccination Administering a vaccine as a precaution against contracting a disease.

vaccine Immunogen consisting of a suspension of weakened or dead pathogenic cells injected in order to stimulate the production of antibodies.

VAD Ventricular assist device.

vagin- of or pertaining to the vagina.

vagina The lower part of the female reproductive tract; a moist canal in female mammals extending from the labia minora to the uterus.

vaginal of or relating to the vagina.

vaginal douching The washing of the vagina cavity or surface with a solution. Agents or drugs can be added to the irrigation solution.

vaginal hysterectomy A procedure in which the uterus is surgically removed through the vagina. One or both ovaries and fallopian tubes may be removed during the procedure as well.

vaginal prolapse A condition in which structures such as the uterus, rectum, bladder, urethra, small bowel, or the vagina itself may begin to prolapse, or fall, out of their normal positions.

vaginal smears Collection of pooled secretions of the posterior vaginal fornix for cytologic examination.

vaginectomy Surgical removal of the vagina.

vaginismus An involuntary spasm of the muscles surrounding the vagina. The spasms close the vagina.

vaginogram Radiographic study of the vagina using a contrast medium.

vaginoplasty A surgical procedure designed to rejuvenate and tighten a woman's vagina.

vaginorrhaphy Suture of the vagina.

vaginoscopy Examination of the vagina, usually by means of an endoscope.

vaginotomy Incision of the vagina.

vagotomy The surgical cutting of the vagus nerve to reduce acid secretion in the stomach.

vagus nerve A mixed nerve that supplies the pharynx and larynx and lungs and heart and esophagus and stomach and most of the abdominal viscera.

valgus Turned outward; especially of a deformity in which part of a limb is twisted away from the center of the body.

vallecula epiglottica A depression just behind the root of the tongue between the folds in the throat.

value-added network A vendor of EDI data communications and translation services.

valvectomy Surgical excision of a valve, especially a heart valve.

valvotomy Incision into a stenosed cardiac valve to relieve the obstruction.

valvular heart disease Complication of diseases that distort or destroy heart valves. Valvular heart disease can be narrowed valves (stenosis) that obstruct blood flow or widened or scarred valves that allow blood to leak backward into the heart (insufficiency or regurgitation). Disorder may be inherited or caused by another disease, such as rheumatic fever, hypertension, atherosclerosis, endocarditis or syphilis (rarely). Disease outcome depends on the underlying condition. Many complications and symptoms can be controlled with medication or cured with surgery.

valvuloplasty A surgical procedure to open a stenotic (stiff) heart valve.

Van Den Bergh test A test to determine whether jaundice in a patient is due to haemolysis or to disease of the liver or bile duct.

Van Hook's operation End-to-end anastomosis of the two portions of a transected ureter. *Synonym:* ureteroureterostomy.

varic(o)- Swollen or twisted vein.

varicella An acute contagious disease caused by herpes varicella zoster virus; causes a rash of vesicles on the face and body.

varices Enlarged veins, arteries or lymph vessels.

varicocele Dilatation of the veins associated with the spermatic cord in the testes.

varicose vein Enlarged, twisted veins found near the surface of the skin.

variola A highly contagious and frequently fatal viral disease characterized by a biphasic fever and a distinctive skin rash that left pock marks in its wake. The disease is caused by the variola virus. *Synonym:* smallpox.

vas deferens The tube connecting the testes with the urethra.

vas(o)- Duct, blood vessel.

vasc Vascular.

vascular of or relating to the blood vessels of the body.

vascular insufficiency Inadequate peripheral blood flow.

vascular shunt A surgical procedure used in surgical by-pass operations to divert blood flow during an operation from the aorta into a plurality of arteries serving different organs of the body.

vascular surgery Operative procedures for the treatment of vascular disorders.

vascularization The development of blood vessels (usually capillaries) within a tissue.

vasculitis Inflammation of a blood vessel.

vasculo- blood vessel.

vasectomy Surgical procedure that removes all or part of the vas deferens (usually as a means of sterilization); is sometimes reversible.

vasoactive Causing constriction or dilation of blood vessels.

vasoconstriction State in which blood vessels are tightened or narrowed. Can be caused by the nervous system sending messages to the blood vessels to constrict. Can also be induced by medications.

vasoconstrictor agents Drugs used to cause constriction of the blood vessels.

vasodilator agents Drugs used to cause dilation of the blood vessels.

vasogram An X-ray study of the vas deferens.

vasography A specialized x-ray sometimes used in the diagnosis or treatment of male infertility. It involves injecting a radiographic dye into the vas deferens and ejaculatory ducts. An x-ray is taken once the dye is injected.

vasomotor Relating to the nerves and muscles that cause the blood vessels to constrict or dilate.

vasoplasty Plastic repair to reverse sterility procedures.

vasopneumatic device Pressure application by special equipment to reduce swelling.

vasopressin Hormone made by the hypothalamus and stored in the pituitary gland. Effects include contraction of the muscular layer of small blood vessels, contraction of the smooth muscles of the intestinal tract and stimulation of contraction of the uterus. Also called anti-diuretic hormone. Has specific effect on kidney tubules stimulating resorption of water, causing a concentration of the urine.

vasospasm Refers to a condition in which blood vessels spasm, leading to vasoconstriction. This can lead to tissue ischemia and death.

vasotomy Surgical incision into or division of the vas deferens.

vasovasostomy Surgical anastomosis or fistulization of the spermatic ducts to restore fertility in a previously vasectomized male.

VBAC Vaginal birth after cesarean.

VBG Venoaortocoronary artery bypass graft.

VCG Vectorcardiogram.

VCU Voiding cystourethrogram.

VD Venereal disease.

VDRL test A flocculation test for syphilis using VDRL antigen, which contains cardiolipin, cholesterol, and lecithin, to test heat-inactivated serum.

vein A blood vessel that carries blood from the capillaries toward the heart; all veins except the pulmonary carry unaerated blood.

vein stripping A surgical procedure to remove varicose veins.

velocimetry The measurement of the velocity of fluids.

ven- of or pertaining to the (blood) veins, a vein [used in terms pertaining to the vascular system].

vena cava A very large vein that returns blood from organs and extremities to the right side of the heart.

vena caval filter A device inserted to prevent PE in patients with DVT and/or PE when anticoagulants fail or cannot be used.

veneer A plastic or porcelain facing bonded directly to a tooth to improve its appearance. *Synonym:* laminate.

venereal of or relating to the external sex organs.

venereal disease A disease that is contracted and transmitted by sexual contact, caused by microorganisms that survive on the skin or mucus membranes.

venesection Phlebotomy.

venipuncture Puncture of a vein through the skin in order to withdraw blood for analysis or to start an intravenous drip or to inject medication or a radiopaque dye.

venogram An x-ray of a vein injected with a radiopaque contrast medium.

venography An X-ray that takes pictures of blood flow through the veins in a certain area of the body. During the test, a special dye (contrast material) is put into the veins so they can be seen clearly on an X-ray picture.

venorrhaphy Suture of a vein.

venotomy The surgical opening of a vein.

venous of or contained in or performing the function of the veins.

venous cutdown Creation of a small incised opening in a vein to permit the passage of a needle or cannula for withdrawal of blood, administration of medication, or in diagnostic or therapeutic catheterization.

venous embolism and thrombosis A mass of clotted blood or other material moved by the blood from one vein and forced into a smaller one.

venous hypertension Pressure in veins that is higher than normal.

venous thromboembolism The collective term for deep vein thrombosis and pulmonary embolism.

venous thrombosis blood clot in a vein.

venovenostomy The surgical formation of an anastomosis between two veins. *Synonym:* phlebophlebostomy.

ventilation The bodily process of inhalation and exhalation; the process of taking in oxygen from inhaled air and releasing carbon dioxide by exhalation.

ventilation-perfusion scan A test used to evaluate both air flow (Ventilation or V) and blood flow (Perfusion or Q) in the lungs to determine whether a person has experienced a pulmonary embolism.

ventilator A mechanical device that assists or replaces that natural mechanism for breathing.

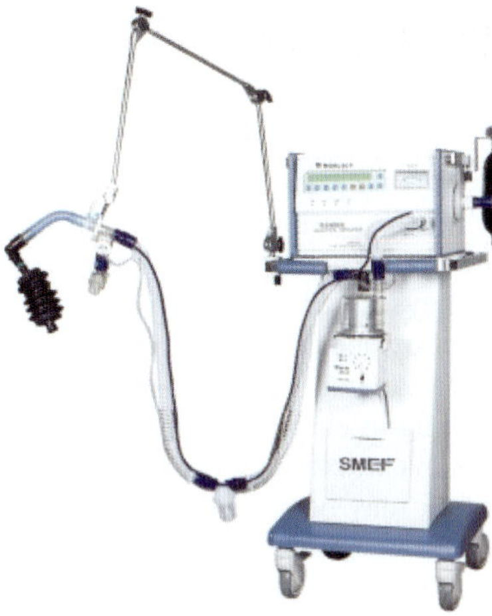

ventilator equipment

Ventilator Dependent A person who must rely on a ventilator for survival, whether for a short time, or intermittent time but frequently, or constantly.

ventr(o)- of or pertaining to the belly; the stomach cavities.

ventral front side of the body. *Synonym:* anterior.

ventricle A chamber of an organ.

ventricles 1. One of four connected cavities in the brain; is continuous with the central canal of the spinal cord and contains cerebrospinal fluid 2. A chamber of the heart that receives blood from an atrium and pumps it to the arteries.

ventricular of or relating to a ventricle (of the heart or brain).

ventricular function The performance or strength of the main pumping chamber of the heart is called ventricular function.

ventriculocisternostomy The surgical formation of an opening between the ventricles of the brain and the cerebello-medullary cistern.

ventriculography X-ray examination of the ventricles of the brain after the introduction of a contrast medium.

ventriculomyotomy Resection of myocardial tissue for idiopathic hypertrophic subaortic stenosis. *Synonym:* ventriculomyomectomy.

VEP Visual evoked potential.

VER Visual evoked response.

vermiform appendix A wormlike diverticulum of the cecum.

vermilionectomy Excision of the vermilion border of the lip.

vermont (krag) procedure Posteriorly placed internal fixation device.

vermont (krag)instrumentation Posteriorly placed internal fixation device.

verruca plana A flat wart.

vertebra One of the 33 bones of the spinal column. A cervical, thoracic, or lumbar vertebra has a cylinder-shaped body anteriorly and a neural arch posteriorly (composed primarily of the laminae and pedicles as well as the other structures in the posterior aspect of the vertebra) that protects the spinal cord.

vertebral of or relating to or constituting vertebrae.

vertebral column Consists of a series of 33 irregularly shaped bones, called vertebrae. These 33 bones are divided into five categories depending on where they are located in the backbone. *Synonym:* backbone, spine, spinal column.

vertebral-artery disease Disease (usually hardening of the artery) in the vertebral artery, a large artery that supplies blood to the neck, vertebrae, cerebellum and other parts of the brain and spinal cord.

vertebroplasty A procedure that involves injecting bone cement into the vertebrae to stabilize fractures, resulting in significant pain relief and restoration of mobility in many patients.

vertical dimension The arbitrary space between the upper and lower jaws upon closure that may decrease over time due to wear, shifting or damage to the teeth.

vertiginous syndromes Disorders that cause vertigo (dizziness).

vesic(o)- of or pertaining to the bladder.

vesical of or relating to a bladder (especially the urinary bladder).

vesication Formation of a blister.

vesicle A small anatomically normal sac or bladder like structure (especially one containing fluid).

vesicocentesis Transabdominal aspiration of fetal urine.

vesicostomy Surgical creation of a stoma between the anterior bladder wall and the skin of the lower abdomen, for temporary or permanent lower urinary tract diversion.

vesicoureteral reflux Condition in which urine flows backward from the bladder into the ureters and kidneys. Because the bladder empties poorly, a urinary tract infection may result, possibly leading to chronic pyelonephritis and even to kidney damage. The reflux may be caused by a congenital defect, a bladder infection or a neurogenic bladder. Sometimes cause is unknown. Treatment includes administration of antibiotics. Rarely, surgery may be required.

vesicourethropexy A term used to describe a wide variety of surgical procedures performed to relieve stress urinary incontinence (SUI). The procedures all ultimately result in repositioning of the urethra and bladder neck.

vesicouterine closure Surgical closure of a vesicouterine fistula.

vesicovaginal fistula A fistula between bladder and uterus.

vesiculectomy Excision of a vesicle, especially the seminal vesicles.

vesiculitis Inflammation of a vesicle, and particularly of the seminal vesicles behind the male bladder.

vesiculogram A radiograph of the seminal vesicles.

vesiculography The use of special X-ray equipment and a dye to examine the seminal vesicles and related structures. Vesiculography is most often used when prostate disease or cancer is suspected.

vesiculotomy Incision into a vesicle, especially the seminal vesicles.

vestibular Pertaining to an oral cavity in the middle of the inner ear.

vestibular function test Test to evaluate the function and structure of the inner ear and/or brain.

vestibular neuronitis Acute, sustained dysfunction of the peripheral vestibular system with secondary nausea, vomiting, and vertigo.

vestibule Any of various bodily cavities leading to another cavity (as of the ear or vagina).

vestibulitis A condition which causes redness and pain of the vestibule. Vestibulitis is an inflammation of this skin and the mucous secreting glands found in the skin.

vestibuloplasty Surgical modification of gingival-mucous membrane relationships in the vestibule of the mouth.

Veterans Administration (VA) A Federal agency responsible for veterans including VA hospitals and Veterans' benefits. Also see domiciliary care.

VF Ventricular fibrillation.

VFT Vestibular function tests.

viable Capable of life. For example, a viable premature baby is one who is able to survive outside the womb.

videoradiography An x-ray system in which the image obtained by intensification fluoroscopy is displayed on a television screen or recorded on videotape.

villusectomy Excision of a synovial villus.

Vincent disease (gingivitis) Necrotizing ulcerative gingivitis; trench mouth; characterized by gingival erythema and pain, fetid odor, and necrosis and sloughing giving rise to a gray pseudomembrane.

VIQ Verbal intelligence quotient.

viral encephalitis An inflammation of the brain.

viral exanthemata Other skin eruptions occurring as a symptom of an acute viral or coccal disease.

viral hepatitis A liver inflammation due to a viral infection. It may present in acute or chronic forms. The most common causes of viral hepatitis are the five unrelated hepatotropic viruses hepatitis A, hepatitis B, hepatitis C, hepatitis D, and hepatitis E.

viral pneumonia An inflammation of the lungs caused by infection with a virus.

Virchow's triad The 3 factors identified with the development of blood clots; blood vessel injury, interruption of blood flow and thrombophilia (the increased tendency toward blood clotting).

viremia The presence of a virus in the blood.

virilization Process in which secondary male sexual characteristics are acquired by a female, usually the result of dysfunction of the adrenal gland(s) or hormone medication. Also called masculinization.

virtual private network A technical strategy for creating secure connections, or tunnels, over the Internet.

virus Ultramicroscopic infectious agent that replicates itself only within cells of living hosts; many are pathogenic.

viscer(o)- of or pertaining to the internal organs, the viscera.

viscera Internal organs collectively (especially those in the abdominal cavity).

visceral Relating to or affecting the viscera.

viscosity The resistance of a fluid which is being deformed by either shear stress or extensional stress.

visual acuity Clearness of vision. The ability to distinguish details and shapes of objects. *Synonym:* central vision.

visual cortex The region of the cerebral cortex occupying the entire surface of the occipital lobe and receiving the visual data from the lateral geniculate body of the thalamus.

visual field Field of vision measured by special tests.

visual field examination An examination to determine the total area in which objects can be seen in the peripheral vision while the eye is focused on a central point.

vital capacity The maximum volume of air that a person can exhale after maximum inhalation.

vital signs Pulse, respiration and temperature.

vitamin Any of a group of organic substances essential in small quantities to normal metabolism.

vitamin a deficiency May result in abnormal visual adaptation to darkness (night blindness), dry skin, dry hair, broken fingernails, and decreased resistance to infections.

vitamin d deficiency A deficiency of vitamin D2 or D3, required for normal growth of teeth and bones, and produced in general by ultraviolet irradiation of sterols found in milk, fish, and eggs.

vitiligo An acquired skin disease characterized by patches of unpigmented skin (often surrounded by a heavily pigmented border).

vitrectomy Removal of the whole or part of the vitreous body in treating endophthalmitis, diabetic retinopathy, retinal detachment, intraocular foreign bodies, and some types of glaucoma.

vitreoretinopathy Retinopathy with vitreous complications.

vitreous of or relating to or constituting the vitreous humor of the eye.

VLBW Very low birth weight.

VLDL cholesterol calc Very-low-density lipoprotein (VLDL) cholesterol is one of the three major types of blood cholesterol combined with protein. VLDL cholesterol contains the highest amount of triglyceride. VLDL cholesterol is considered bad cholesterol because elevated levels may be associated with an increased risk of coronary artery disease.

VNA Visiting Nursing Association.

vocal cord Either of two pairs of bands or folds of mucous membrane in the throat that project into the larynx.

vocational rehabilitation The process of facilitating an individual in the choice of or return to a suitable vocation. When necessary, assisting the patient to obtain training for such a vocation.

voiding pressure studies Simultaneous measurement of bladder contraction, urinary flow, and sphincter electromyogram.

volar plate A very thick ligament that prevents hyperextension injuries. If the force is sufficient enough, the joint may be dislocated.

Volhard's test A test for kidney function.

Volkman contracture A permanent flexion contracture of the hand at the wrist, resulting in a claw-like deformity of the hand and fingers.

volume (behavioral) offset The change in the volume of services that occurs in reaction to a change in fees. A 50 percent volume offset means that half of the savings from fee reductions will be offset by increase volume of services.

Volume 1 Refers to the tabular list of diagnosis codes of ICD-9-CM.

Volume 2 Refers to the alphabetic index of diagnosis codes of ICD-9-CM.

Volume 3 Procedure codes used only for hospital coding. Volume 3 contains both a numeric listing and an alphabetic index.

Volume Performance Standard (VPS) A mechanism to adjust Medicare physician fee updates based on how annual increases in actual Part B expenditures compare to previously predicted rates of increase.

voluntary agreement Agreements between CMS and various insurers and employers to exchange Medicare information and group health plan eligibility information for the purpose of coordinating health benefit payments.

voluntary enrollee Certain individuals aged 65 or older or disabled, who are not otherwise entitled to Medicare and who opt to obtain coverage under Part A by paying a monthly premium.

volvulus Abnormal twisting of the intestine which can impair the blood flow to the intestine. Volvulus can lead to gangrene and death of that segment of the gastrointestinal tract, intestinal obstruction, perforation of the intestine, and peritonitis.

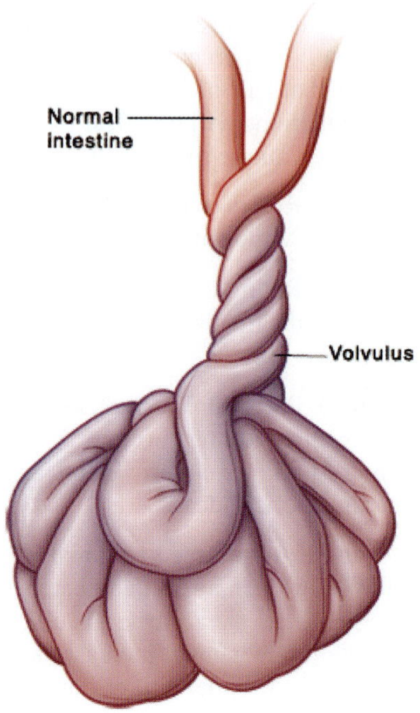

volvulus

vomer A roughly triangular bone that forms the inferior and posterior of the nasal septum.

Von Hippel-Lindau disease A rare, autosomal dominant genetic condition in which hemangioblastomas are found in the cerebellum, spinal cord and retina. These are associated with several pathologies including renal angioma, renal cell carcinoma and phaeochromocytoma.

Von Recklinghausen disease Neurofibromatosis characterized by café au lait spots, intertriginous freckling, iris hamartomas and other neurofibromas.

Von Willebrand's disease Inherited disorder characterized by abnormally slow clotting of the blood, causing spontaneous nosebleeds or bleeding of the gums. Due to a deficiency of blood factor VIII. Excessive bleeding can also occur following surgery or during menstruation. *Synonym:* angiohemophilia, vascular hemophilia.

VSD Ventricular septal defect.

vulva The external genital organs of the female.

vulvar of or relating to the vulva.

vulvectomy Surgical removal of the vulva.

vulvodynia Pain in the vulva characterized by itching, burning, stinging or stabbing in the area around the opening of the vagina.

vulvovaginitis Inflammation or infection of the vulva and vagina.

V-Y plasty A surgical method for lengthening tissues in one direction by cutting in the lines of a V, sliding the two segments apart, and closing in the lines of a Y.

W

w/o Without.

Wada activation test A test performed in selected cases before embolization or occlusion of intracranial vessels that provides subjective evidence whether selected blood vessels can be permanently occluded without loss of neurologic or cranial nerve function.

WAIS Wechsler adult intelligence scale.

waiting periods A period of time an individual must wait to become eligible for benefits for a specific condition(s) after overall coverage has commenced.

waiver of liability provision A provision which states that if the provider informed the beneficiary in writing before the item or service was furnished that Medicare is likely to deny payment for the item or service rendered as not reasonable and necessary, and obtained his or her agreement to pay, the provider's liability is waived and payment is made to the provider by the beneficiary.

Waldenstrom's macroglobulinemia Rare, progressive disorder associated with abnormal proteins in the blood, swollen lymph glands, enlarged liver and spleen, anemia and bone marrow changes. *See* Anemia.

Waldius procedure Total knee arthroplasty using a hinged metal knee replacement.

Walsh prostatectomy Radical retropubic prostatectomy.

warfarin effect Refers to the effect of thinning of the blood by a medication known as warfarin or coumadin.

warfarin therapy Therapy with warfarin, the oral anticoagulant most frequently used to control and prevent thromboembolic disorders.

Warren shunt A surgical procedure in which the distal splenic vein (a part of the portal venous system) is attached to the left renal vein (a part of the systemic venous system). It is used to treat portal hypertension and its main complication (esophageal varices)..

Wasserman test An antibody test for syphilis.

Wassmund osteotomy Surgical treatment of anterior alveolar protrusion.

Waterston procedure An anastomosis between the ascending aorta and the right or main pulmonary artery.

Watson-Jones procedure A surgical procedure for ankle stabilization.

WBC White blood cell.

Weber's test A vibrating tuning fork is placed in the center of the patient's forehead. If the patient reports that the sound originates in the midline of the forehead, there is no impairment in air conduction. When the sound is referred to the involved or damaged side, the Weber test is positive. When there is disease of the cochlea or nerve deafness, the sound is lateralized to the opposite side, the test is said to be negative.

wedge excision A surgical procedure to remove a triangle-shaped slice of tissue.

wedge resection A surgical procedure to remove a triangle-shaped slice of tissue followed by repair. It may be used to remove a tumor and a small amount of normal tissue around it.

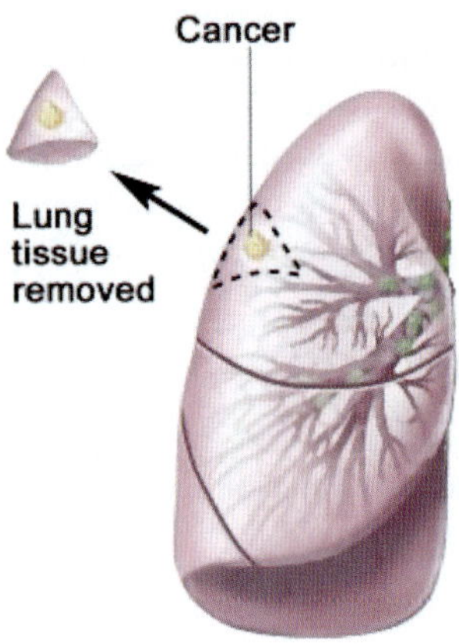

wedge resection of lung

wedging Crowding, forcing or pushing into a limited space.

WEDI Workgroup for Electronic Data Interchange.

Wegener's granulomatosis Progressive disease characterized by lesions in the bronchi and lungs, scarring of small arteries and widespread inflammation of all organs of the body.

well-baby care Preventative health services, including immunizations, for young children within an age range specified by the health plan.

wellness programs Health promotion programs.

Wenckebach phenomenon Cardiac arrhythmia where the P-R interval grows progressively longer until a beat is dropped.

Wernicke-Posadas disease A systemic mycosis caused by of dust particles containing arthroconidia of Coccidioides immitis.

Wertheim Bohlman fusion Use of iliac crest graft and wire fixation from occiput to C-2 for occipital cervical fusion.

Wertheim operation A radical hysterectomy for treatment of uterine cancer, in which as much as possible of the vagina is excised, and lymph nodes are excised throughout a broad area.

West Nile virus An infectious disease caused by a virus spread to humans by the bite of an infected mosquito.

Westergren test A blood test that detects and monitors inflammation in the body.

Western blot A technique in molecular biology, used to separate and identify proteins.

wet mount Sometimes called a vaginal smear, is a test to find the cause of vaginitis, or inflammation of the vagina and the area around the vagina.

wheelchair management Direct one-on-one assessment, fitting and/or training in the use of manual or power driven wheelchairs.

Wheeler knife procedure A stab incision technique.

wheezing Relating to breathing with a whistling sound.

Whipple procedure A procedure is performed to address chronic pancreatitis and cancer of the pancreas, ampulla of Vater, duodenum, and the distal bile duct. *Synonym:* pancreatico-duodenectomy.

Whipple's disease A rare, systemic infectious disease caused by the bacterium Tropheryma whipplei. Whipple's disease primarily causes malabsorption but may affect any part of the body including the heart, lungs, brain, joints, and eyes. *Synonym:* intestinal lipodystrophy.

whirlpool therapy Involves the use of agitated water in order to relieve pain, improve circulation, and/or to promote wound healing (e.g., ulcers, exfoliative skin conditions). The use of whirlpool therapy requires supervision and should be reported for each 15 minute time period.

white blood cells Refers to any of various blood cells that help protect the body from infection and disease. White blood cells include neutrophils, eosinophils, basophils, lymphocytes, and monocytes. *Synonym:* leucocyte.

Whitecloud and Larocca fusion Anterior technique for cervical spine fusion using fibular graft.

Whitman astragalectomy A surgical operation for removal of the talus bone (astragalus) for stabilization of the ankle.

Whitman procedure Surgical procedure for the treatment of adolescent coxa vara.

Whitmore disease An infectious disease caused by a gram-negative bacterium, burkholderia pseudomallei, found in soil and water.

WHO World Health Organization.

whole blood A general description for a sample of blood taken from the venous or arterial circulation. It is composed of blood cells, platelets, and plasma.

whooping cough A highly contagious disease caused by bacteria. The most prominent symptom of whooping cough is a distinctive, uncontrollable cough, followed by a sharp, high-pitched intake of air. *Synonym:* pertussis.

Wick catheter technique A procedure for measurement of intramuscular pressure.

Widal serum test An agglutination test for the detection of agglutinins.

Wilks syndrome Myasthenia gravis.

Wilm's tumor Rapidly developing malignant tumor of the kidneys in children under 5 years of age.

Wilson's syndrome Degeneration of the liver and the nucleus of the lens in the eye.

Wiltse plate Screw plate device for posterior spinal stabilization.

Wiltse procedure Bilateral lateral spine fusion for spondylolisthesis.

windpipe Common term for the trachea.

Winiwarter operation Osteotomy for hallux valgus.

Winter procedure A surgical procedure for prolonged low-flow priapism.

Wintrobe test A test for erythrocyte sedimentation rate.

Wirsung duct The pancreatic duct.

WISC Wechsler Intelligence Scale for Children.

Wisconsin (Drummond) interspinous instrumentation Series of wires, rods, and buttons for multisegmental spine stabilization.

wisdom teeth The third (last) molars that usually erupt between the age of 18-25.

Wiskott-Aldrich syndrome Inherited immunodeficiency disorder only affecting males. Characterized by severe bleeding, eczema, recurrent infections and an increased risk of developing malignancy. Causes early death with an average life span of 4 years.

withhold A percentage of payment or set dollar amounts that are deducted from the payment to the physician group or physician that may or may not be returned depending on specific predetermined factors.

Witzel operation Temporary gastrostomy used to treat vicious circle vomiting.

wnl Within normal limits.

Wolff-Parkinson-White syndrome Intermittent rapid heartbeat or atrial fibrillation with characteristic changes in an electrocardiogram.

womb Common term for the uterus.

work capacity evaluation Assessment of physiological capacities in relation to job requirements.

Work-Up The total patient evaluation, which may include laboratory assessments, radiologic series, medical history, and diagnostic procedures.

workers' compensation Programs established by state law to provide medical benefits and compensation for injuries and diseases that occur in the course of employment. The workers compensation program is financed by covered employers insured or self-insured under property and casualty lines and is mandatory for employers in almost all states.

workers' compensation indemnity benefits Benefits that replace an employee's wages while the employee is unable to work because of a work-related injury or illness.

World Health Organization (WHO) A specialized agency of the United Nations that acts as a coordinating authority on international public health. As well as coordinating international efforts to monitor outbreaks of infectious diseases, such as SARS, malaria, swine flu, and AIDS the WHO also sponsors programs to prevent and treat such diseases. The WHO supports the development and distribution of safe and effective vaccines, pharmaceutical diagnostics, and drugs. The WHO organization maintains the International Classification of Diseases (ICD) medical code set.

wound repair Refers to the process of repairing or closing a wound. Wound repair is defined as simple, intermediate or complex.

Simple wound repair Refers to superficial wounds involving mostly the dermis, epidermis, or subcutaneous tissues.

Intermediate wound repair Refers to wounds that require closure or one or more layers of deeper subcut-aneous tissue and fascia.

Complex wound repair Refers to scar revision, debridement, and the use of stents or retention sutures.

W-plasty A procedure to prevent the contracture of a straight-line scar in which the edges of a wound are trimmed in the shape of a W and closed.

WPW Wolf-Parkinson-White (syndrome).

XYZ

X12 An ANSI-accredited group that defines EDI standards for many American industries, including health care insurance. Most of the electronic transaction standards mandated or proposed under HIPAA are X12 standards.

xanth(o)- Denoting a yellow color, an abnormally yellow color.

xanthines Class of drugs that stimulate the brain and smooth muscles, such as bronchial tubes and the heart. This family of drugs includes caffeine, theophylline, aminophylline and others.

xenograft Tissue from an animal of one species used as a temporary graft (as in cases of severe burns) on an individual of another species.

xenograft valves Artificial valves made from animal tissue are called xenografts. Most often the valves are made from pig aortic valves. More recently, some valves have been made from cow tissues.

xenografts The cells of one species transplanted to another species.

xenotransplantation The transplantation of living cells, tissues or organs from one species to another, such as from pigs to humans.

xeroderma A mild form of ichthyosis characterized by abnormal dryness and roughness of the skin.

xerophthalmia Abnormal dryness and thickening of the mucous membrane lining of the eyelids and white part of the eye and cornea. Caused by vitamin-A deficiency or certain eye diseases.

xeroradiography The process of making a type of dry x-ray in which a picture of the body is recorded on paper rather than on film.

xerosis An abnormal dryness of the skin or mucus membranes.

xerostomia Dry mouth or decrease in the production of saliva.

x-match Crossmatch.

x-ray A diagnostic test that uses invisible electromagnetic energy beams to produce images of tissues, bones and organs onto film.

xx Normal female sex chromosome type.

xy Normal male sex chromosome type.

-y Condition or process of.

yag Yttrium-aluminum-garnet (laser).

yatapoxvirus A virus that causes tumors in primates.

yaws A contagious tropical disease caused by the spirochete treponema pertenue, character-ized by yellowish or reddish tumors, which often resemble currants, straw-berries, or raspberries.

yellow fever An acute systemic (body wide) illness caused by a virus called a flavivirus. In severe cases, the viral infection causes a high fever, bleeding into the skin, and necrosis (death) of cells in the kidney and liver.

yellow vision Objects appear yellow. One symptom of digitalis toxicity.

YOB Year of birth.

YTD Year-to-date.

Zenker's diverticulum Pharyngo-esophageal diverticulum; the most common diverticulum at the junction of the esophagus and the pharynx.

ZES Zollinger-Ellison syndrome.

Ziegler's operation V-shaped iridectomy for forming an artificial pupil.

zo(o)- Animal, animal life.

Zollinger-Ellison syndrome Syndrome with three features; severe ulcers of the stomach or small intestine, extreme hyper-secretion of stomach acid and tumors of the pancreas. Treatment includes anti-ulcer medication, but complete surgical removal of the stomach may be required.

zoonotic Other diseases that can be passed from animals, whether wild or domesticated, to humans.

z-plasty A plastic repair technique that is used to improve the funct-ional and cosmetic appearance of scars.

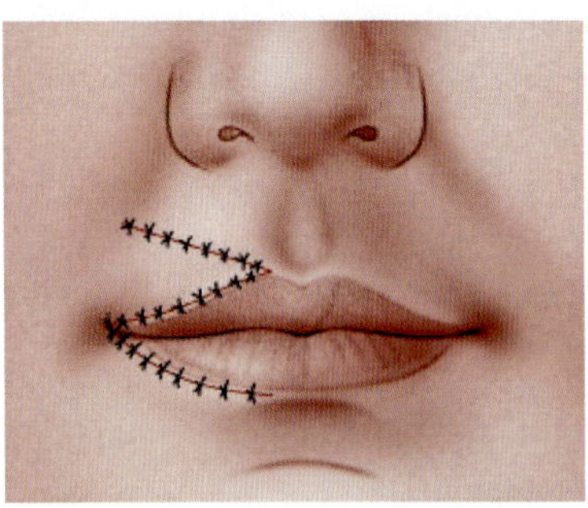

zygoma Generally refers to the zygomatic bone, a bone of the human skull commonly referred to as the cheekbone or malar bone.

zygomatic of or relating to the cheek region of the face.

zygomatic arch The part of the temporal bone of the skull that forms the prominence of the cheek. *Synonym:* zygomatic bone, zygoma, malar bone, cheek bone, yoke bone.

zygomatic bone the triangular bones on either side of the face below the eyes, commonly referred to as the cheekbones, they form the prominences of the cheeks and part of the outer wall and floor of the orbits.

METRIC CONVERSION

Length

1 centimeter (cm) = 10 millimeters (mm)
1 inch = 2.54 centimeters (cm)
1 foot = 0.3048 meters (m)
1 foot = 12 inches
1 yard = 3 feet
1 meter (m) = 100 centimeters (cm)

Volume

1 US tablespoon = 3 US teaspoons
1 US fluid ounce = 29.57353 milliliters (ml)
1 US cup = 16 US tablespoons
1 US cup = 8 US fluid ounces
1 US pint = 2 US cups
1 US pint = 16 US fluid ounces
1 liter (l) = 33.8140227 fluid ounces
1 liter (l) = 1000 milliliters (ml)
1 US quart = 2 US pints
1 US gallon = 4 US quarts
1 US gallon = 3.78541178 liters

Weight

1 milligram (mg) = 0.001 grams (g)
1 gram (g) = 0.001 kilograms (kg)
1 gram (g) = 0.035273962 ounces
1 ounce = 28.34952312 grams (g)
1 ounce = 0.0625 pounds
1 pound (lb) = 16 ounces
1 pound (lb) = 0.45359237 kilograms (kg)
1 kilogram (kg) = 1000 grams
1 kilogram (kg) = 35.273962 ounces
1 kilogram (kg) = 2.20462262 pounds (lb)

Temperature

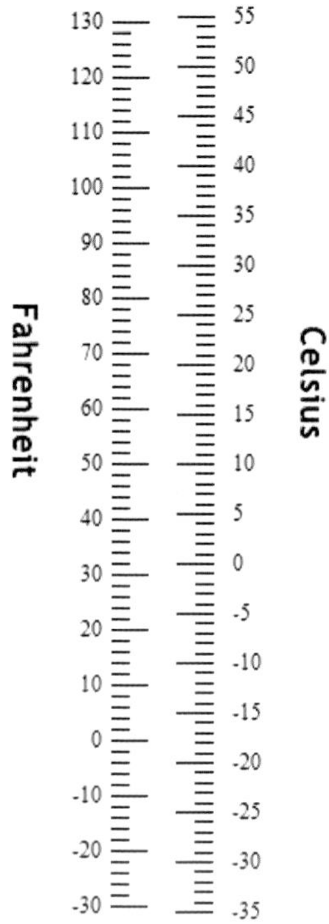